Cannabinoids and Pain

Samer N. Narouze
Editor

Cannabinoids and Pain

Springer

Editor
Samer N. Narouze
Western Reserve Hospital
Center For Pain Medicine
Cuyahoga Falls, OH
USA

ISBN 978-3-030-69185-1 ISBN 978-3-030-69186-8 (eBook)
https://doi.org/10.1007/978-3-030-69186-8

This Springer imprint is published by the registered company Springer Nature Switzerland AG
The registered company address is: Gewerbestrasse 11, 6330 Cham, Switzerland

To my wife, Mira, and my children, John, Michael, and Emma—the true love and joy of my life. Without their continued understanding and support, I could have not completed this book.

This book is also dedicated to the memory of my father, who always had faith in me, and to my mother for her ongoing love and guidance.

Preface

Cannabis has been used throughout history for an array of medical indications ranging from pain to curing cancer, in addition to recreational, religious, and spiritual purposes. Since 1970, marijuana has been classified at the federal level as a Schedule I substance under the controlled substance act and defined as a drug with no currently accepted medical use and a high potential for abuse.

To date, medical cannabis is legalized in two-thirds of US states. In the November 2020 elections, four more states voted to legalize marijuana for recreational purposes. More recently, in December 2020, The House of Representatives passed a legislation legalizing marijuana at the federal level. Regardless whether the Senate will take up the legislation or not, this reflects a whooping change in the public attitude towards cannabis.

Policy makers have outpaced clinical research, creating a critical mismatch between the state legalization of medical cannabis and the lack of knowledge and education among pain physicians. We conducted a national survey among pain physicians in 2019 to measure participants' attitudes, beliefs, preparedness, and knowledge regarding medical cannabis. The survey revealed a mismatch between pain physicians' favorable attitude regarding the legitimacy of using medical cannabis and their lack of preparedness and education.

This reflects the current enthusiastic climate surrounding medicinal cannabis and cannabinoids. Physicians and patients are hoping for novel pain treatments amid the current opioids crisis. However, there is ongoing uncertainty due to conflicting laws between federal and state governments. This conflict coupled with lack of education creates a "gray area" surrounding the use of medical cannabis, which can lead to confusion, apprehension, and frustration among pain physicians and patients alike.

There is a great necessity for a comprehensive yet easy-to-follow book on cannabinoids and pain. I was fortunate to gather some of the national and international experts to contribute to the book, each one writing about their area of expertise, and for this reason, I am very proud of this book. The main objective of the book is to provide physicians managing pain with a comprehensive resource on "all that you need to know" about cannabinoids and pain. Among the target groups are pain physicians, primary care physicians, internists, physiatrists, rheumatologists, neurologists, orthopedists, and spine specialists.

The book comprises 40 chapters organized into 9 parts, covering the basic science and clinical applications of cannabinoids in pain management.

The first part reviews cannabis history, regulations, and terminology. The second and third parts cover cannabinoids pharmacology from the endocannabinoids system and cannabinoid receptors to phytocannabinoids (THC and CBD) and the synthetic ones.

The fourth part focuses on medical cannabis strains and the model of a specialized cannabis clinic. It elaborates on practical recommendations for the use of medical cannabis, dosing and monitoring, as well as patient safety considerations.

The fifth part addresses the mechanisms of action and clinical evidence of cannabinoid-based medicine in pain disorders. While Part VI reviews the exciting concept of cannabinoids as a substitute for opioids.

Part VII is devoted to the various challenges with medical cannabis, product safety and quality control, and mental health risks. It highlights the cannabis negative impact on brain development and use during pregnancy and in adolescents. More challenges are discussed in Part VIII regarding cannabis impairment and adverse events, vaping hazards, and cannabis use disorder. The final part discusses future directions of cannabinoids.

A couple of notes about the book: the text has been augmented with several instructive tables, illustrations, and images, and the information described are based on the current review of the available literature as well as the authors' experience.

The advancement in our knowledge about cannabinoid-based medications, as the federal government will ease up barriers to clinical research, will lead to better understanding of the potential role of cannabis in the treatment of various pain disorders and how to incorporate it in clinical practice. It is my hope that this book will encourage and stimulate all physicians and healthcare providers interested in cannabinoid-based medications and pain management.

Cuyahoga Falls, OH, USA Samer N. Narouze
18 December 2020

Acknowledgments

In preparing *Cannabinoids and Pain* textbook, I had the privilege of gathering highly respected national and international experts in the field. My sincere thanks to Dr. Caroline MacCallum, MD (Department of Medicine and Faculty Pharmaceutical Sciences, University of British Columbia, Canada), for her valuable contributions and agreeing to serve as the assistant editor of the book.

This book would not have been complete without the essential practical chapters by Dr. Maria Fernanda Arboleda, MD (Research Department, Santé Cannabis, Montreal, Canada).

I cannot thank enough Dr. Christina Le-Short, MD, and her colleagues at the Department of Pain Medicine, The University of Texas MD Anderson Cancer Center, and the Department of Neurology, The University of Texas McGovern Medical School.

Special thanks to Michael Boivin, BSc Phm, consultant pharmacist (Ontario, Canada), and Glenn Rech, RPH senior clinical pharmacist (Akron, OH), for their help with the pharmacology part.

I would also like to acknowledge my esteemed colleagues Drs. Nathan Harrison, MD, and Yashar Eshraghi, MD, at the University of Queensland and Ochsner Health System for agreeing to contribute essential chapters.

I do appreciate the help and support from Dr. Qian Chen, MD (NYU Langone Health), Dr. Ignacio Badolia, MD (University of Pennsylvania), and Dr. Amita Kundra MD (NYU Long Island School of Medicine).

I am very blessed that these experts agreed to contribute to my book, and I am very grateful to everyone.

Conflict of Interest

Caroline A. MacCallum is the Medical Director of Greenleaf Medical Clinic and Chief Medical Officer for Translational Life Sciences. She is on the Board of Directors for the Green Organic Dutchman. She is an advisor to Andira, Active Patch Technologies and Dosist. She previously advised Emerald Health Therapeutics, Vitality Biopharma, and Strainprint. She has attended advisory board meetings for Syqe Medical, Shoppers Drug Mart, and Scientus Pharma. Additionally, she has provided medical consultation and/or received support for industry sponsored continuing medical education from: Aleafia, Spectrum, Tilray, Numinus, Aurora & MD Briefcase.

Contents

Part I Introduction to Cannabis

1 **History of Cannabis** 3
Alexander Shustorovich and Samer N. Narouze

2 **Cannabis Regulations** 9
Yashar Eshraghi and Dustin Duracher

3 **The Demand for Medical Cannabis Education** 15
Christina Le-Short and Samer N. Narouze

4 **Pain Physicians and Medical Cannabis: Attitudes, Believes, Preparedness and Knowledge** 19
Samer N. Narouze, Sameh M. Hakim, Lynn Kohan, and Dmitri Souza

5 **Cannabis Terminology** 31
Maria Fernanda Arboleda and Erin Prosk

Part II Cannabinoids Pharmacology

6 **The Endocannabinoid System** 39
Glenn R. Rech and Samer N. Narouze

7 **Cannabinoid Receptor 1 (CB1)** 47
Glenn R. Rech and Samer N. Narouze

8 **Cannabinoid Receptor 2 (CB2)** 55
Glenn R. Rech and Samer N. Narouze

9 **Endocannabinoids: Anandamide and 2-Arachidonoylglycerol (2-AG)** 63
Danielle Despina Pete and Samer N. Narouze

10 **Phytocannabinoids: Tetrahydrocannabinol (THC)** 71
Priodarshi Roychoudhury, Ning Nan Wang, and Samer N. Narouze

11 Phytocannabinoids: Cannabidiol (CBD) 79
Priodarshi Roychoudhury, Ning Nan Wang, and Samer N. Narouze

12 Other Phytocannabinoids................................ 87
Hance Clarke, Priodarshi Roychoudhury, and Samer N. Narouze

13 Cannabis Drug Interactions............................. 93
George Polson, Matthew Chung, Salman Hirani, and Christina Le-Short

Part III Pharmaceutical Cannabinoids

14 Dronabinol (Marinol®) 105
Juliet Gaisey and Samer N. Narouze

15 Nabilone (Cesamet).................................... 109
Nathan J. Harrison and Hunter Simpson

16 Cannabidiol (Epidiolex) 113
Nathan J. Harrison

17 Nabiximols (Sativex®) 119
Michael Boivin

Part IV Medical Cannabis

18 Cannabis Strains to Chemovars 129
Michael Boivin

19 The Model of a Medical Cannabis Clinic 135
Maria Fernanda Arboleda and Erin Prosk

20 Barriers for the Prescription of Cannabinoid-Based Medicines.. 145
Maria Fernanda Arboleda and Erin Prosk

21 Practical Recommendations for the Use of Medical Cannabis 153
Maria Fernanda Arboleda and Erin Prosk

22 Cannabinoid-Based Medicines: Dosing, Titration & Monitoring 167
Caroline A. MacCallum, Lauren de Freitas, Lindsay A. Lo, and Michael Boivin

23 Cannabinoid-Based Medicines: Patient Safety Considerations... 179
Caroline A. MacCallum, Lindsay A. Lo, and Michael Boivin

Part V Cannabinoids and Pain

24 Cannabinoids and Pain: Mechanisms of Action 191
Samer N. Narouze

25 Cannabinoids and Pain: Clinical Evidence 205
Caroline A. MacCallum, Lauren Eadie, and Samer N. Narouze

26 Cannabinoids and Cancer Pain 211
Matthew Chung, Barlas Benkli, Salman Hirani, and Christina Le-Short

Part VI Cannabinoids as a Substitute for Opioids

27 Cannabinoids as a Substitute for Opioids: Basic Science and Clinical Evidence 223
Caroline A. MacCallum, Lauren de Freitas, Lauren Eadie, and Samer N. Narouze

28 Cannabinoids as a Substitute for Opioids: Suggested Algorithm 231
Tolulope Oso, Salman Hirani, Matthew Chung, Barlas Benkli, and Christina Le-Short

29 Perioperative Management of Patients on Cannabis/Cannabinoids 237
Amita Kundra

Part VII The Challenges with Medical Cannabis

30 The Colorado Experience 243
Alexander Shustorovich

31 Product Safety and Quality Control 249
Caroline A. MacCallum, Lindsay A. Lo, Fonda Betts, and Michael Koehn

32 Cannabinoids and Brain Development 259
Samer N. Narouze

33 Cannabinoids and Mental Health Risks 271
Caroline A. MacCallum, Lauren de Freitas, and Shaohua Lu

34 Cannabinoids and Adolescence 281
Caroline A. MacCallum and Lauren de Freitas

35 Cannabinoids and Child Development: During and After Pregnancy 287
Qian Cece Chen and Samer N. Narouze

Part VIII Cannabis Impairment and Use Disorder

36 Cannabinoid-Related Adverse Events and Impairment 293
Caroline A. MacCallum, Lauren de Freitas, Lindsay A. Lo, Lauren Eadie, and Jeffrey R. Brubacher

37 Cannabis Vaping Hazards 307
Qian Cece Chen and Samer N. Narouze

38 Cannabis Use Disorder 313
Samer N. Narouze, Caroline A. MacCallum, and Lauren de Freitas

39 Cannabis Withdrawal 317
Yinan Chen and Christina Le-Short

Part IX Cannabinoids Future Directions

40 Cannabinoids Future Research 325
Ignacio Badolia

Index 333

Contributors

Maria Fernanda Arboleda, MD Research Department, Santé Cannabis Clinic, Montreal, QC, Canada

Ignacio Badolia Anesthesiology and Critical Care, University of Pennsylvania, Philadelphia, PA, USA

Barlas Benkli Department of Neurology, The University of Texas McGovern Medical School, Houston, TX, USA

Fonda Betts Greenleaf Medical Clinic, Langley, BC, Canada

Michael Boivin, BSc Phm CommPharm Consulting, Barrie, ON, Canada

Jeffrey R. Brubacher Department of Emergency Medicine, Faculty of Medicine, UBC, Vancouver, BC, Canada

Qian Cece Chen Department of Anesthesiology, Perioperative Care, and Pain Medicine, NYU Langone Health, New York, NY, USA

Yinan Chen Department of Pain Medicine, Division of Anesthesiology and Critical Care, The University of Texas MD Anderson Cancer Center, Houston, TX, USA

Matthew Chung Department of Pain Medicine, Division of Anesthesiology, Critical Care and Pain Medicine, The University of Texas MD Anderson Cancer Center, Houston, TX, USA

Hance Clarke Department of Anesthesia and Pain Management, Toronto General Hospital, Centre for Cannabinoid Therapeutics, University Health, Network, University of Toronto, Toronto, ON, Canada

Lauren de Freitas, MSc Centre for Addiction and Mental Health, Toronto, ON, Canada

Dustin Duracher Department of Anesthesiology & Critical Care Medicine, University Ochsner Health System University of Queensland Ochsner Medical School, New Orleans, LA, USA

Lauren Eadie, MD Department of Medicine, Faculty of Medicine, University of British Columbia, Vancouver, BC, Canada

Yashar Eshraghi Department of Anesthesiology & Critical Care Medicine, Ochsner Health System University of Queensland Ochsner Medical School, New Orleans, LA, USA

Louisiana State University School of Medicine, New Orleans, LA, USA

Juliet Gaisey Department of Physical Medicine and Rehabilitation, Johns Hopkins Hospital, Baltimore, MD, USA

Sameh M. Hakim Faculty of Medicine, Ain Shams University, Cairo, Egypt

Nathan J. Harrison Ochsner Health Systems, Department of Anesthesiology and Critical Care Medicine, New Orleans, LA, USA

Salman Hirani Department of Pain Medicine, Division of Anesthesiology, Critical Care and Pain Medicine, The University of Texas MD Anderson Cancer Center, Houston, TX, USA

Department of Anesthesiology and Perioperative Medicine, Oregon Health and Science University, Portland, OR, USA

Michael Koehn CannSolve Medical Clinic, Mental Health Agency and Cannabis Education Centre, Kamloops, BC, Canada

Lynn Kohan Department of Anesthesiology and Pain Medicine, University of Virginia, Charlottesville, VA, USA

Amita Kundra South Shore Hospital Department of Anesthesiology, Northwell Health, Bay Shore, NY, USA

Christina Le-Short Department of Pain Medicine, Division of Anesthesiology, Critical Care and Pain Medicine, The University of Texas MD Anderson Cancer Center, Houston, TX, USA

Lindsay A. Lo, BSc H Department of Psychology, Queen's University, Kingston, ON, Canada

Shaohua Lu Department of Psychiatry, Faculty of Medicine, University of British Columbia, Vancouver, BC, Canada

Caroline A. MacCallum, MD Department of Medicine, Faculty of Medicine, University of British Columbia, Vancouver, BC, Canada

Samer N. Narouze, MD Western Reserve Hospital, Center For Pain Medicine, Cuyahoga Falls, OH, USA

Tolulope Oso Department of Anesthesia, The University of Texas McGovern Medical School, Houston, TX, USA

Danielle Despina Pete Ohio Northern University, Ada, OH, USA

George Polson Department of Pain Medicine, Division of Anesthesiology, Critical Care and Pain Medicine, The University of Texas MD Anderson Cancer Center, Houston, TX, USA

Department of Physical Medicine and Rehabilitation, Baylor College of Medicine, Houston, TX, USA

Erin Prosk, MSc Research Department, Santé Cannabis Clinic, Montreal, QC, Canada

Glenn R. Rech Western Reserve Hospital, Cuyahoga Falls, OH, USA

Priodarshi Roychoudhury Department of Anesthesia and Pain Management, Toronto General Hospital, University of Toronto, Toronto, ON, Canada

Alexander Shustorovich Department of Physical Medicine & Rehabilitation, Johns Hopkins University School of Medicine, Baltimore, MD, USA

Hunter Simpson Ochsner Health Systems, Department of Anesthesiology and Critical Care Medicine, New Orleans, LA, USA

Dmitri Souza Western Reserve Hospital, Cuyahoga Falls, OH, USA

Ning Nan Wang Department of Anesthesia and Pain Management, Toronto Western Hospital, University of Toronto, Toronto, ON, Canada

Part I

Introduction to Cannabis

History of Cannabis

1

Alexander Shustorovich and Samer N. Narouze

In modern day, "cannabis is the most widely cultivated, trafficked and abused illicit drug. About 147 million people, 2.5% of the world population, consume cannabis compared with [only] 0.2% consuming cocaine and 0.2% consuming opiates" [1]. Its widespread use is not a recent phenomenon or trend. It is one of the oldest domestic plants in the history of mankind, and its utilization can be traced back to more than 10,000 years ago in ancient China [2]. Humanity has used cannabis for its medicinal, spiritual, and textile properties for thousands of years across many cultures and civilizations. However, despite its prevalence throughout history, it is currently recognized as a Schedule I controlled substance under the Controlled Substances Act of 1970, defined as having a high potential for abuse, with no currently accepted medicinal use in the United States [3].

The earliest account of medicinal cannabis use is believed to be around 2800 BC, by the Father of Chinese medicine, Shen Nung. In the medical compendium *Pen Ts'ao*, Shen Nung determined the female plant had a very high source of yin, contained a potent medicine, and prescribed *chu-ma* (female hemp) for treatment of various ailments, including rheumatoid arthritis, nausea, constipation, and anxiety [4]. Shen Nung deemed the herb as "one of the Superior Elixirs of Immortality" because of its routine use and multiple beneficial effects [4]. Over the centuries, Chinese physicians continued to prescribe cannabis and further developed their understanding of its medicinal properties. The famous Chinese surgeon, Hua T'o, used cannabis as an anesthetic during complex surgeries such as colon resection, laparotomies, and thoracotomies [5]. In 2006, Jiang et al. identified rare, well-preserved archeological specimens of cannabis in the 2500-year-old Yanghai Tombs of China [2], demonstrating physical evidence of cannabis use in ancient spiritual practices.

Although cannabis origins are rooted in Asia, it has propagated westward through both trade and human migration. Accounts of cannabis utility are found in various scriptures from India, the Middle East, Egypt, and Europe [4]. In Romania, archeologists have found evidence of cannabis used as a sacrament in the form of incense residue at a gravesite of Proto-Indo-Europeans who occupied the area 5000 years ago. The root word, *canna*, is identified in the Indo-European language, which is regarded as the primordial dialect of English, German, Latin, Greek, Persian, and Sanskrit languages [4]. It has similarities with the early reference of cannabis as *qunabu* in ancient Mesopotamia (considered the advent of civilized human culture) [4]. Use of the word

A. Shustorovich (✉)
Department of Physical Medicine & Rehabilitation, Johns Hopkins University School of Medicine, Baltimore, MD, USA

S. N. Narouze
Western Reserve Hospital, Center For Pain Medicine, Cuyahoga Falls, OH, USA
e-mail: narouzs@hotmail.com

S. N. Narouze (ed.), *Cannabinoids and Pain*, https://doi.org/10.1007/978-3-030-69186-8_1

qunabu begins to increase around 250 BC to describe the source of oil, fiber, and medicine [6]. Meissner described medicinal application of oils and incense prepared from the plant as its "aroma was pleasing to the Gods" [7]. In Dr. Russo's seminal paper on clinical cannabis in ancient Mesopotamia, he recounts use of cannabis anointment to treat the "Hand of Ghost," now believed to be early descriptions of epilepsy disorder. Other ancient Mesopotamian uses include treatment of the cardiovascular, pulmonary, musculoskeletal, and skin disorders [8].

Similar preparations, tinctures, and anointments were used for both healing and spiritual purposes in ancient Egypt. Known by the name *sm-sm-t*, the herb was considered a creation of the sun god, Ra, and was used in ceremonies honoring the dead [4]. Remnants of the plant have been found in pharaoh burial grounds, such as Ramses II, dating back to 1200 BC. Common ailments were treated with mixtures of honey and cannabis as identified in various Egyptian medical texts [4]. Recently, residues of cannabinoids such as Δ9-teterahydrocannabinol (THC), cannabidiol (CBD), and cannabinol (CBN) were detected at the Judahite Shrine of Arad dated from the ninth to the early sixth centuries BCE (Iron IIA–IIC) [9].

Further progression to the Western world was inevitable with expansion of commerce and culture to the West. William O'Shaughnessy, an Irish physician during the mid-nineteenth century, introduced cannabis into Western medicine as a treatment for tetanus and other convulsive diseases. Around the same time, French physician Jean-Jacques Moreau de Tours experimented with cannabinoid preparations for mental health disorders [10].

North American cultivation and use of cannabis/hemp blossomed in the seventeenth century, but quickly wilted during the 1900s. In 1851, cannabis was included in the third edition of the *United States Pharmacopoeia* (USP) [10]. Subsequent amendments and revisions provided detailed recipes for tincture and extract formulations for use as an analgesic, hypnotic, and anticonvulsant [8]. After the Mexican Revolution of 1910, a large influx of Mexican immigrants into the United States introduced recreational use of cannabis. Regarded as the "Marijuana Menace," the plant became strongly associated with new coming immigrants, giving root to the fear and prejudice exploited by anti-drug campaigners during the Great Depression [11, 12]. During this period, Harry J. Anslinger became the first Commissioner of the Federal Bureau of Narcotics (FBN) in 1930. Anslinger denounced the herb, using propaganda such as "Reefer Madness," to escalate public and government concerns. Due to quickly increasing use (among immigrants and citizens) and concerns about safety, states were encouraged by the federal government to begin outlawing the plant in the early 1930s [10, 11]. However, national prohibition did not take shape until the signing of the Marijuana Tax Act of 1937, which regulated the production, distribution, and use of cannabis within the United States [10]. With growing national hatred toward the marijuana plant, the American Medical Association reluctantly removed cannabis from the USP with the publication of the twelfth edition in 1942 [10].

Due to Anslinger's persistence, the United States continued to regard marijuana as an "evil weed" until the publication of the La Guardia Report in 1944 shed some doubt on popular belief [12]. Contrary to prior research, the report showed that cannabis use did not induce "violence, insanity, or sex crimes, or lead to addiction or other drug use" [11]. Despite these profound findings, the La Guardia Report was not well regarded, and sentencing laws became more strict during the civil rights movements of the 1960s. Ironically, due to a changing political and cultural climate during the civil rights movement, marijuana use increased in the counterculture of the 1960s and 1970s [11]. The prevalence of cannabis use peaked in the late 1970s, "when more than one-third of high school seniors (37 percent in 1976) and one in eight Americans over 12 years old (12.8 percent in 1979) reported past-month use" [10]. Concerned parents nationwide formed a conservative parental movement that lobbied for more strict marijuana regulation. With the creation of the US Drug Enforcement Agency

(DEA) and persistent parental groups, turmoil persisted into the 1980s. A series of significant legislature was passed during the 1970s and 1980s, which severely restricted cultivation, research, and access of marijuana. Cannabis was rescheduled as a Schedule I controlled substance under the Controlled Substances Act of 1970 [3], the Anti-Drug Abuse Act of 1986 issued mandatory sentences based on the amount of the drug involved, and a "new War on Drugs" was declared by President George Bush Senior in 1989 echoing the fears of the early nineteenth century [11].

Yet there remained hope for this persistent weed. The National Organization for the Reform of Marijuana Laws (NORML) was founded in the early 1970s and resisted state and federal restrictions. Activists fought for reform as the laws were viewed as crude and ineffective in reducing marijuana abuse. States and localities slowly began to look for alternatives in policy to reduce a growing economic burden, prioritizing decriminalization rather than pursuing possession offenses [11]. The Shafer Commission, appointed by President Nixon, considered law reform to decriminalize personal use of marijuana, but President Nixon rejected the recommendation [11]. Nonetheless, decriminalization efforts spanned the United States over the next few decades throughout individual states [13]. A 12-year study from 1990 to 2002, analyzing drug offenses, demonstrated that 82% of the increase in drug arrests nationally (450,000) was primarily for minor marijuana possession charges, which translated roughly to $4 billion per year of resources being dedicated to marijuana alone [14]. The United States was spending billions of dollars jailing people for non-violent crimes and restricting cannabis research and medicinal applications through enforcement of outdated prohibition laws.

The passage of Proposition 215 in 1996 legalized medicinal use of cannabis in California and is considered a monumental change in marijuana legislature because it catalyzed marijuana law reformation over the next 20 years [11]. In 2012, Colorado and Washington became the first two states to legalize the recreational use of cannabis, with Amendment 64 and Initiative 502, respectively [15]. By January 2016, 21 states had various levels of decriminalization of marijuana possession offenses, 26 states had legalized medical marijuana use, and another 16 states had adopted cannabidiol (CBD)-only laws [13]. A 2016 survey showed that the primary use of cannabis in the United States remained recreational (89.5% of adult cannabis users), with about 10.5% use for solely medical purposes,and 36.1% reporting a mixed medical/recreational use [16]. Initiatives and referenda have continued to be drafted and proposed within state and federal governments. In fact, marijuana legislature was a major topic of discussion in the 2020 presidential election, and most candidates challenged the President of the United States, taking positions on cannabis reform [17]. As noted in Fig. 1.1, states have various combinations of marijuana reform, and continued changes are expected. For example, in 2020, Vermont began to tax and regulate recreational cannabis sales [18].

Recent preclinical studies in animals have increased our understanding of the mechanisms of cannabinoid-induced analgesia and have facilitated strategies for treating pain in humans. Multiple mechanisms have been proposed including inhibition of the release of neurotransmitters from presynaptic junctions, modulation of postsynaptic activity, activation of descending inhibitory pain pathways, and reduction of neural inflammation [19]. The active compounds are various cannabinoids, such as cannabidiol (CBD) and tetrahydrocannabinol (THC), that bind to endocannabinoid receptors to produce anxiolytic, analgesic, and psychoactive effects [20]. THC is the psychoactive component that causes euphoria and "high" via the CB1 receptors, while other cannabinoids, such as cannabidiol (CBD), lack this affinity. Therefore, it was theorized that the non-psychoactive compounds were responsible for the plant's therapeutic effects [20]. Recent meta-analyses of clinical trials that examined the use of medicinal cannabis for chronic pain demonstrated a moderate amount of evidence supporting analgesic activity of cannabinoids, especially for neuropathic pain. However, the

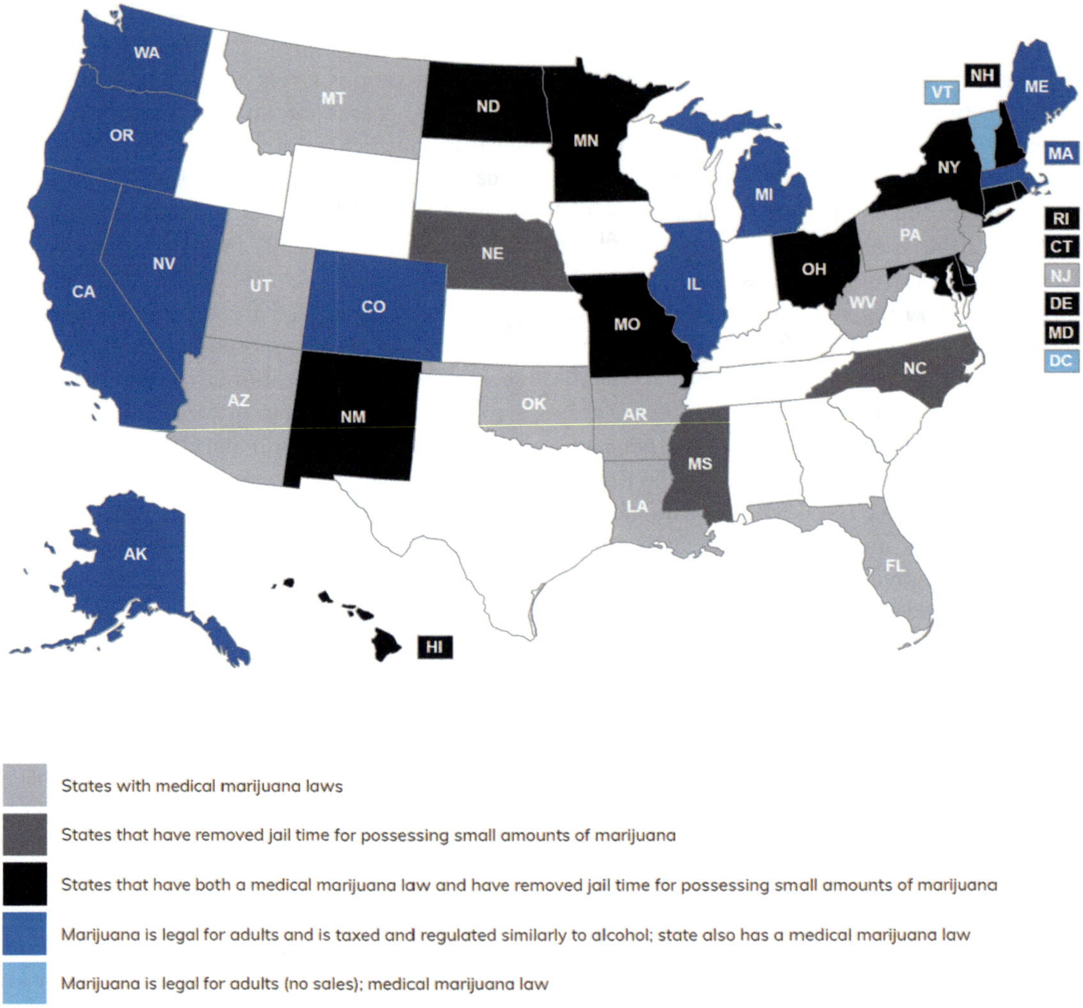

Fig. 1.1 Map of US state cannabis policies. (Source: mpp.org with permission (2019))

heterogeneity and small sample sizes of the studies are a major limitation. Nonetheless, the therapeutic properties and relatively benign side effect profile of cannabis have made it a favorable alternative remedy for chronic pain [20].

In 2018, the federal government passed the 2018 farm bill which legalized low-THC hemp (hemp defined as any cannabis plant that has 0.3 percent or less of THC) nationwide and effectively removed it from the restrictions of the Controlled Substances Act [21]. In near synchrony, the hemp industry boomed throughout the country, capitalizing on mass production of CBD oils, balms, lotions, and tinctures without FDA regulation. Currently, the only FDA-approved CBD extract is Epidiolex, indicated for severe epileptic conditions (Lennox-Gastaut syndrome and Dravet syndrome) [22]. In anticipation of Canadian legalization of marijuana, cannabis stocks surged in 2018, but due to relatively high taxation and surprising deficits in supply, the cannabis bubble quickly burst in the beginning of 2019. Legalization of cannabis in Canada has only shown increased use in one age group (45–64), without any significant changes in the other age groups. Traffic fatalities have shown a minimal increase after legalization, but this data has been extrapolated from US states with legal recreational use [23]. It is important to note that the overall risk equilibrates to states without legal recreational use after the first year [23]. Nonetheless, cannabis acceptance is here to stay, and legislative reform (medicinal and recreational) continues to evolve. At the time of publication, 15 US states and the District of Columbia have legalized marijuana for adults over the age of 21, and marijuana is legal for medical use in 36 US states. The end of marijuana prohibition is near and, at this rate, may be fully legalized within our lifetimes.

References

1. World Health Organization. Management of substance abuse: cannabis https://www.who.int/substance_abuse/facts/cannabis/en/.
2. Jiang H, Li X, Zhao Y, et al. A new insight into Cannabis sativa (Cannabaceae) utilization from 2500-year-old Yanghai Tombs, Xinjiang, China. J Ethnopharmacol. 2006;108(3):414–22. https://doi.org/10.1016/j.jep.2006.05.034.
3. Drug Enforcement Administration Office of Diversion Control. Schedules of controlled substances. (b) Placement on schedules; findings required. (1) Schedule I. Springfield, Virginia: U.S. Department of Justice; 1970. [Accessed 5 Aug 2016]. Title 21 United States Code (USC) Controlled Substances Act. Subchapter I–Control and enforcement Part B–Authority to control; standards of controlled substances §812. [also known as Controlled Substances Act, 21 United States Code § 812(b) (1), 1970]. Available at: www.deadiversion.usdoj.gov/21cfr/21usc/812.htm.
4. Bennett C. Early/ancient history. In: Holland J, editor. The pot book: a complete guide to cannabis. Rochester: Park Street Press; 2010.
5. Abel EL. Marihuana, the first twelve thousand years. New York: Plenum Press; 1980.
6. Barber EW. Pre-historic textiles: Princeton University Press; 1989.
7. Meissner B. Babylonian und assyrian. 1925.
8. Russo EB. History of cannabis and its preparations in saga, science, and sobriquet. Chem Biodivers. 2007;4(8):1614–48. https://doi.org/10.1002/cbdv.200790144.
9. Arie E, Rosen B, Namdar D. Cannabis and frankincense at the Judahite shrine of Arad. Tel Aviv. 2020;47(1):5–28. https://doi.org/10.1080/03344355.2020.1732046.
10. National Academies of Sciences, Engineering, and Medicine; Health and Medicine Division; Board on Population Health and Public Health Practice; Committee on the Health Effects of Marijuana: An Evidence Review and Research Agenda. The Health Effects of Cannabis and Cannabinoids: The Current State of Evidence and Recommendations for Research. Washington, DC: National Academies Press; 2017, 2, Cannabis. Available from: https://www.ncbi.nlm.nih.gov/books/NBK425762/.
11. PBS Frontline Marijuana Timeline. https://www.pbs.org/wgbh/pages/frontline/shows/dope/etc/cron.html.
12. Leal-Galicia P, Betancourt D, Gonzalez-Gonzalez A, Romo-Parra H. A brief history of marijuana in the western world. Rev Neurol. 2018;67(4):133–40.
13. Pacula RL, Smart R. Medical Marijuana and Marijuana Legalization. Annu Rev Clin Psychol. 2017;13:397–419. https://doi.org/10.1146/annurev-clinpsy-032816-045128.
14. King RS, Mauer M. The war on marijuana: the transformation of the war on drugs in the 1990s. Harm Reduct J. 2006;3:6. https://doi.org/10.1186/1477-7517-3-6.
15. Coffman, Keith; Neroulias, Nicole (November 6, 2012). Colorado, Washington first states to legalize recreational pot. Reuters. Retrieved 9 Feb 2018.
16. Schauer GL, King BA, Bunnell RE, Promoff G, McAfee TA. Toking, vaping, and eating for health or fun: marijuana use patterns. Am J Prev Med. 2016;50(1):1–8.
17. Levenson MS. Here's where the 2020 presidential candidates stand on cannabis. Leafly. https://www.leafly.com/news/politics/2020-presidential-candidates-marijuana-positions. Published February 10, 2020. Accessed 2 Apr 2020.
18. Marijuana Policy Project. https://www.mpp.org. Accessed 5 Apr 2020.
19. Vučković S, Srebro D, Vujović KS, Vučetić Č, Prostran M. Cannabinoids and pain: new insights from old molecules. Front Pharmacol. 2018;9:1259. https://doi.org/10.3389/fphar.2018.01259.
20. VanDolah HJ, Bauer BA, Mauck KF. Clinicians. 2019; guide to cannabidiol and hemp oils. Mayo Clin Proc. 2019;94(9):1840–51. https://doi.org/10.1016/j.mayocp.2019.01.003.
21. 115th congress (2017–2018): agriculture improvement act of 2018, Congress.gov (2018), https://www.congress.gov/bill/115th-congress/house-bill/2/text (last visited Dec 26, 2018).
22. FDA approves first drug comprised of an active ingredient derived from marijuana to treat rare, severe forms of epilepsy. U.S. food and drug administration. https://www.fda.gov/news-events/press-announcements/fda-approves-first-drug-comprised-active-ingredient-derived-marijuana-treat-rare-severe-forms. Published June 25, 2018. Accessed 2 Apr 2020.
23. Leyton M. Cannabis legalization: did we make a mistake? Update 2019. J Psychiatry Neurosci. 2019;44(5):291–3. https://doi.org/10.1503/jpn.190136.

Cannabis Regulations

2

Yashar Eshraghi and Dustin Duracher

Introduction

Currently, the climate surrounding medicinal cannabis and its derived products is filled with both enthusiasm from patients and physicians searching for novel treatments and uncertainty due to conflicting laws between federal and state governments. This confliction creates a "gray area" surrounding the use of medical cannabis, which can lead to confusion and apprehension from physicians and patients alike. At the core of this conflict is the Controlled Substances Act (CSA) enacted by Congress in 1970. Under this act, cannabis and cannabis-derived products are classified as Schedule I drugs, which indicates a lack of accepted medical use for the drug and enacts strict regulations on possession, manufacturing, dispensing, and clinical research involving these substances [1–4]. Despite federal regulations, the use of cannabis for medical purposes has moved mainstream with nearly all US states decriminalizing either cannabis or cannabis-derived products (cannabinoids) for specific medicinal purposes [3]. The medical community has also reevaluated cannabis as a potential medical intervention. This chapter aims to provide physicians and other healthcare providers with an up-to-date understanding of the current legal framework surrounding medical cannabis.

Y. Eshraghi (✉)
Department of Anesthesiology & Critical Care Medicine, Ochsner Health System University of Queensland Ochsner Medical School, New Orleans, LA, USA

Louisiana State University School of Medicine, New Orleans, LA, USA
e-mail: yashar.eshraghi@ochsner.org

D. Duracher
Department of Anesthesiology & Critical Care Medicine, University Ochsner Health System University of Queensland Ochsner Medical School, New Orleans, LA, USA

Federal Regulations

In 1970, Congress enacted the Controlled Substances Act (CSA), which consolidated all prior federal laws related to the handling of substances that possess the potential for abuse [3, 4]. Under the CSA, substances are categorized into five schedules based on their medical efficacy and potential for abuse. Schedule I is the most restrictive. Criteria for substances under Schedule I include no accepted medical use, lack of accepted safety for the substance under medical supervision, and the high potential for abuse [1, 4]. Substances under Schedule I include marijuana and its cannabinoid derivatives, THC, mescaline, psilocybin, peyote, heroin, MDMA, and LSD [4]. The CSA specifically defines marijuana as:

> The term 'marihuana' means all parts of the plant *Cannabis sativa L.*, whether growing or not; the seeds thereof; the resin extracted from any part of

S. N. Narouze (ed.), *Cannabinoids and Pain*, https://doi.org/10.1007/978-3-030-69186-8_2

> such plant; and every compound, manufacture, salt, derivative, mixture, or preparation of such plant, its seeds or resin. Such term does not include mature stalks, oil or cake made from the seeds of such plant, any other compound, manufacture, salt, derivative, mixture or preparation of such mature stalks (except the resin extracted there from), fiber, oil, or cake, or the sterilized seed of such plant which is incapable of germination. 21 USC 802(16) [3].

From this definition, cannabis and all cannabinoids derived from the plant are classified as Schedule I, and those who possess, dispense, or prescribe said substances are in violation of the DEA and can theoretically face criminal charges.

Placing cannabis and cannabinoids under Schedule I hinders the ability to perform clinical trials with cannabis; it restricts access to patients and limits the ability of physicians to "prescribe" these substances to their patients. Under the CSA, Schedule I substances can only be legally possessed and/or dispensed as part of a federally approved research program. In order to be approved for such research, investigators, and all involved manufactures and distributors, must secure a Schedule I substance-specific registration (license) [4]. In addition, cannabis used for research must be obtained through a facility contracted with the National Institute on Drug Abuse (NIDA). Currently, the only facility contracted with NIDA to grow marijuana for research purposes is the University of Mississippi.

Given that cannabis and its derivatives are Schedule I drugs and can only be dispensed through a federally approved research program, physicians can only "recommend" their patients use medical cannabis but cannot formally write a prescription [1, 3]. According to a 2002 federal appeals court decision *Conant v. Walters*, the First Amendment prohibits the federal government from prosecuting physicians "on the basis of the content of doctor-patient communications" [2]. The court also ruled that physicians should not be held liable for a patient's actions after said communications. However, physicians violate the federal law if they prescribe or dispense marijuana and may be charged with an "aiding and abetting" violation of the federal law if they advise patients on how to obtain it [1]. Though various states' laws allow the distribution of cannabis through dispensaries to patients who have recommendations from their physicians, this remains in conflict with the CSA.

Substances categorized under Schedule II are, however, less restrictive and familiar to physicians and patients alike. Criteria for Schedule II includes high potential for abuse, and abuse of the substance may lead to severe psychological of physical dependence, but there is currently an accepted medical use in the United States. Common drug classes listed under Schedule II are opioids and stimulants. Similar to Schedule II, drugs in Schedules III–V have an accepted medical use in the United States and a sequential de-escalating abuse potential. Schedules II–V impose fewer restrictions on drugs within these categories and allow for a more liberal investigation of these substances by physicians. For instance, any physician who holds a Schedule II, III, IV, or V prescriber registration can perform research on these substances without special approval from the DEA, and FDA-approved drugs within Schedules II–V can be prescribed legally in clinical practice [3, 4]. Proponents of medical cannabis often urge rescheduling of cannabis from Schedule I to Schedule II to allow for more robust, high-quality research in hopes of forming universal, evidence-based recommendations on the use of cannabis or cannabis-derived products in treating varying illnesses.

Having an "accepted medical use," or lack thereof, is the defining difference between Schedule I and Schedule II. Interestingly enough, the CSA does not define the concept of accepted medical use. However, the DEA has developed criteria that a substance must meet before it can be accepted for medical use. These include the following: the drug's chemistry must be known and reproducible, there must be adequate safety studies, there must adequate and well-controlled studies proving efficacy, the drug must be accepted by qualified experts, and the scientific evidence must be widely available [3]. The only exception to these criteria for proving accepted medical use is the FDA approval of a substance as a prescription medication.

FDA approval does allow for "differential scheduling" of products that are derived from a parent compound (e.g., cannabinoids from cannabis) in a more restrictive schedule. For example, the FDA has not approved a marketing application for cannabis as a whole, but it has approved one cannabis-derived (Epidiolex) and three cannabis-related pharmaceutical medications (Marinol, Syndros, Cesamet) for patient use when prescribed by a healthcare provider. Marinol and Syndros, approved for the treatment of anorexia associated with weight loss in AIDS patients, contain the active ingredient dronabinol, a synthetic delta-9-tetrahydrocannabinol (THC) [8]. Marinol was moved to Schedule II following FDA approval in 1985 and was eventually moved to Schedule III upon petition by the manufacturer [4]. Cesamet contains the active ingredient nabilone (synthetically derived THC) and was placed in Schedule II after its approval in 1985 for nausea and vomiting associated with chemotherapy. Finally, Epidiolex, which contains a purified form of cannabidiol (CBD), was approved for the treatment of seizures associated with Lennox-Gastaut syndrome or Dravet syndrome in patients 2 years of age and older [8]. Contrarily, recent (2016) rescheduling petitions have been denied based on the conclusions by the DEA and FDA that marijuana still has no currently accepted medical use, lacks accepted safety for use under medical supervision, and has a high potential for abuse [5]. Until more high-quality, reproducible data on the efficacy and safety of standardized cannabis preparations exist, it is likely that cannabis will remain in Schedule I.

State Cannabis Laws

In 1996, California became the first state to decriminalize marijuana for medicinal use. The Compassionate Use Act of 1996 allowed qualifying patients and caregivers to cultivate and possess cannabis for medicinal purposes [3]. Since then, a total of 33 states, and the District of Columbia, have approved the use of cannabis for medical use. In addition, 13 states allow the use of low-THC, high-cannabidiol (CBD) products for medical use. Limited interference by the federal government has been a catalyst for the expansion of state-regulated medical cannabis programs (Fig. 2.1).

In 2009, the Department of Justice issued a memorandum to US Attorneys stating federal funds should not be used to prosecute persons acting within their own state medical laws [1]. Most recently, an amendment to the Consolidated Appropriations Act of 2018 restricts the DOJ from using federal funds to interfere with a state's implementation of medical marijuana laws [4].

While most states share similar laws regarding medical cannabis use, facets of those laws can vary on a state by state basis. In most states, patients must obtain a recommendation from a physician based on a predetermined qualifying medical condition. All states involved allow such patients to use and possess small amounts of cannabis or CBD products for medical purposes without being criminalized; however, amounts permissible vary from state to state. Definitions of qualifying medication conditions also vary by state but typically include chronic debilitating diseases such cancer, cachexia related to chronic disease, chronic pain, HIV-AIDS, and seizure disorders [1]. In states that have collected data on patient-reported qualifying medical conditions, chronic pain is, by far, the most common reported condition for medical cannabis use (67.5% in 2016) [6]. Of most concern to physicians and other permissible healthcare providers is the lack of uniform quality control standards for the production of cannabis products intended for medical use. For instance, California requires laboratory testing of cannabis and derived products to ensure they meet quality standards mandated by the state, while Arizona does not have state-mandated testing [7]. As there are no uniform methods of quality control testing, it is up to recommending physicians or healthcare providers to familiarize themselves with state policies regarding production quality standards to ensure the safety of the products they are recommending to patients.

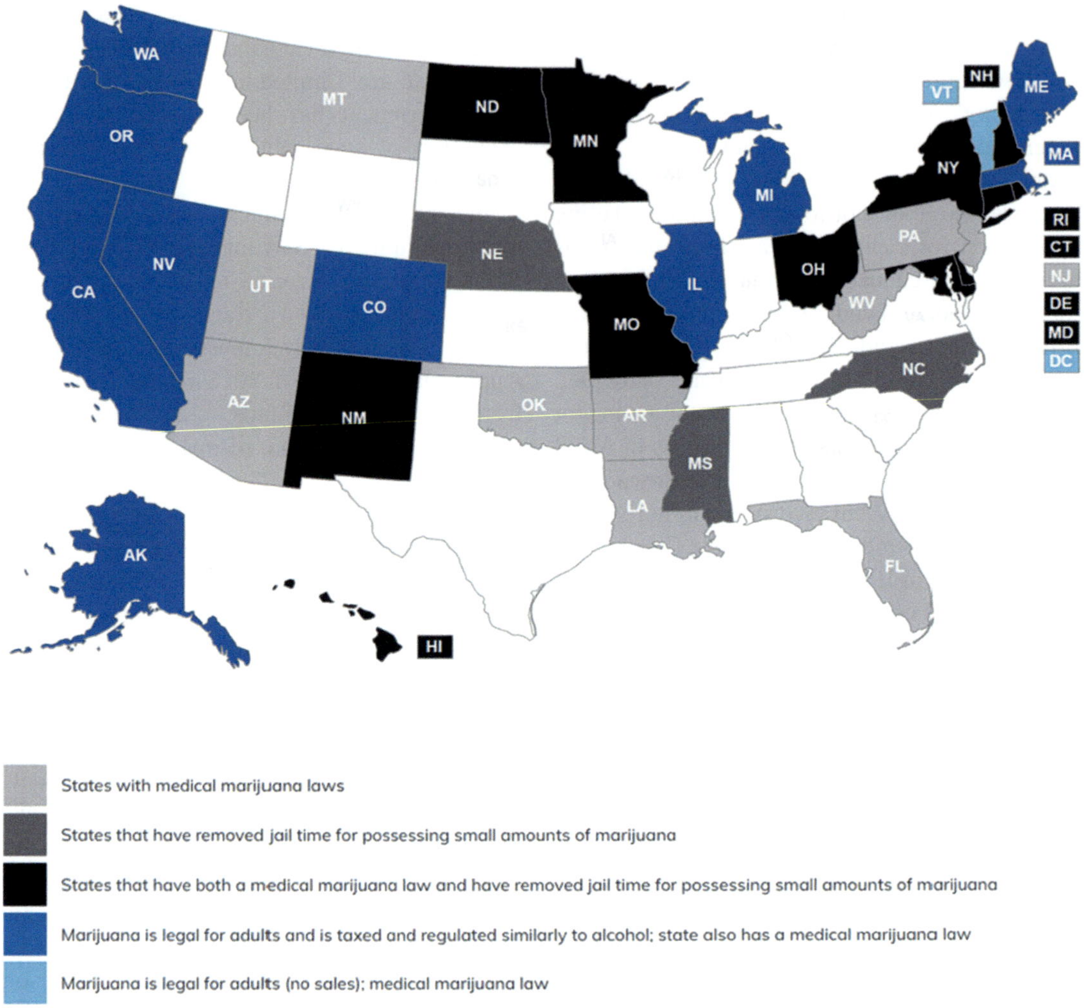

Fig. 2.1 Map of state cannabis policies. (Source: mpp.org with permission (2019))

Research Expansion

Despite failures in rescheduling marijuana from Schedule I to Schedule II, recent attempts have been made by Congress to deregulate and expand research and manufacturing of marijuana for medicinal purposes. The American Society of Anesthesiologists (ASA) has recently endorsed two bipartisan bills that aim to expand and expedite the ability to perform rigorous studies on marijuana. H.R. 601, the Medical Cannabis Research Act of 2019, was introduced into the House of Representatives in 2019 and is currently under review by the Subcommittee on Crime, Terrorism, and Homeland Security. The aim of this bill is to expand cannabis research by increasing the number of federally registered manufactures of cannabis for legitimate research purposes. It would also authorize healthcare providers of the Department of Veterans Affairs to provide recommendations to veterans regarding participation in federally approved cannabis clinical trials. If this bill were enacted, in its first year it would require the Attorney General to increase the number of cannabis manufactures for legitimate research purposes from its current number of one (University of Mississippi) to at least three. In addition, the Attorney General would be required to conduct annual assessments on whether there is an adequate and uninterrupted supply of cannabis for legitimate research purposes, and it would allow the Attorney General to increase the number of manufactures on a yearly basis to maintain an adequate supply of cannabis for medical research [9].

The second bill endorsed by the ASA, the Cannabidiol and Marijuana Research Expansion Act, aims to deregulate and expedite both the research and manufacturing application pathway. For both research and manufacturing applications, the bill would require an action by the Attorney General within 60 days of receiving a completed application. The AG can accept/deny the application or request supplemental information from the applicant. If supplemental information is requested, the AG will be required to either accept or deny the application no later than 30 days upon receipt of supplemental material. In addition, once an application is granted for research purposes, the registrant may amend or supplement their research protocol without reapplying if the registrant does not change the quantity/type/source of drug or the conditions under which the drug is stored, tracked, or administered. In an effort to expand access to marijuana for research purposes, the bill would allow appropriately registered research groups to grow and possess their own marijuana for the purpose of medical research for drug development. Finally, the bill would require the Department of Health and Human Services, National Institutes of Health, and other responsible federal agencies to submit a report on several topics: the potential therapeutic effects of CBD and marijuana on major medical conditions, the side effects of increasing THC levels on the human body, the developing adolescent brain, cognitive abilities, the barriers to researching marijuana and recommendations on how such barriers might be overcome, and recommendations for safeguarding the potency and purity of marijuana-derived products in the United States [10].

Conclusion

With an increasing number of states legalizing cannabis for medical use and with chronic pain being the most commonly cited qualifying condition by patients, current and future pain physicians will undoubtedly face a growing number of inquiries about cannabis use from their patient populations. Given the current legal climate surrounding cannabis, physicians are placed in a difficult situation as they are operating under conflicting laws at both the federal and state levels. Also, varying standards of quality control measures among states and a lack of FDA-approved cannabis-derived medications for chronic pain, pain physicians may potentially risk harming a patient by "recommending" a product whose content, safety profile, and dosage cannot be precisely quantified. There is a huge demand for higher-quality research on the safety profile and efficacy of standardized reproducible cannabis preparations.

References

1. Hoffmann DE, Weber E. Medical marijuana and the law. N Engl J Med. 2010;362(16):1453–7. https://doi.org/10.1056/nejmp1000695.
2. Annas GJ. Medical marijuana, physicians, and state law. N Engl J Med. 2014;371(11):983–5. https://doi.org/10.1056/nejmp1408965.
3. Mead A. Legal and regulatory issues governing cannabis and cannabis-derived products in the united states. Front Plant Sci. 2019;10:697. https://doi.org/10.3389/fpls.2019.00697.
4. Mead A. The legal status of cannabis (marijuana) and cannabidiol (CBD) under U.S. law. Epilepsy Behav. 2017;70:288–91. https://doi.org/10.1016/j.yebeh.2016.11.021.
5. Drug Enforcement Administration. Denial of petition to initiate proceedings to reschedule marijuana. Administration DE, editor. 81 Fed. Reg; 2016. p. 53699.
6. Boehnke KF, Gangopadhyay S, Clauw DJ, Haffajee RL. Qualifying conditions of medical cannabis license holders in the United States. Health Aff. 2019;38(2):295–302. https://doi.org/10.1377/hlthaff.2018.05266.
7. Milley J. Which states do not require medical marijuana testing and why not, 2018? 2018. Available at: https://droseaz.com/which-states-do-not-require-medical-marijuana-testing-and-why-not/. Accessed 5 Jan 2020.

8. FDA regulation of cannabis and cannabis-derived products, including cannabidiol (CBD). (8/3/2020). https://www.fda.gov/news-events/public-health-focus/fda-regulation-cannabis-and-cannabis-derived-products-including-cannabidiol-cbd#approved. Accessed 31 Aug 2020.
9. Rep. Gaetz, Matt. H.R.601 – 116th congress (2019-2020): Medical Cannabis Research Act of 2019. https://www.congress.gov/bill/116th-congress/house-bill/601?q={"search":["medical+cannabis+research+act"]}. Accessed 31 Aug 2020.
10. Senator Feinstein, Dianne S. 2032 – 116th congress (2019–2020): Cannabidiol and Marihuana Research Expansion Act, 2019. https://www.congress.gov/bill/116th-congress/senate-bill/2032/text?r=11. Accessed 31 Aug 2020.

The Demand for Medical Cannabis Education

3

Christina Le-Short and Samer N. Narouze

Medical marijuana is legalized in two-thirds of US states and used for various conditions including epilepsy, multiple sclerosis, post-traumatic stress disorder, chronic pain, cancer-related adverse effects, and Crohn's disease [1, 2]. However, policy-makers have outpaced clinical research and have thus created a critical mismatch between state legalization and the lack of knowledge and education among physicians. As more states loosen their legislation surrounding marijuana use, health-care providers are increasingly expected to advise patients regarding its health benefits and safe use. Despite the growing public interest, medical teaching and training at the medical school and post-graduate levels are widely lacking.

At all levels, from student to attending physician, health providers feel unprepared to address medical marijuana concerns. A recent primary care physicians' survey showed that half of physicians were not ready to answer patient's questions on medical cannabis or they did not want to [3]. Two-thirds of medical school deans reported their graduates were "not at all prepared" to prescribe medical marijuana, and a quarter reported their graduates were not even ready to answer questions about the drug [4]. In a survey of post-graduate medical trainees, the majority (89.5%) of residents and fellows felt "not at all prepared" to prescribe medical marijuana, while 35.3% felt "not at all prepared" to answer questions. The vast majority (84.9%) reported receiving no education in medical school nor residency on medical marijuana. In fact across the nation, only nine percent of medical school curricula, documented in the Association of American Medical Colleges (AAMC) Curriculum Inventory database, contain educational content on medical marijuana [4].

Despite the lack of preparedness and training, the majority of medical students have a desire to learn more about medical cannabis. In a 2020 survey of medical students at the George Washington University School of Medicine, 60% of students reported receiving no cannabis education in medical school, while 77.2% believed there should be more formal education on the subject. The majority of students felt "not at all prepared" to counsel patients on the hazards or benefits of cannabis [5]. Beyond physicians in training, a survey of pharmacy students found that nearly 80% of students felt the topic of medical cannabis should be added to existing curricula [6]. This widespread lack of preparedness reflects a failure on the part of medical schools to adapt to changing laws and a changing culture around marijuana.

C. Le-Short (✉)
Department of Pain Medicine, Division of Anesthesiology, Critical Care and Pain Medicine, The University of Texas MD Anderson Cancer Center, Houston, TX, USA
e-mail: cle2@mdanderson.org

S. N. Narouze
Western Reserve Hospital, Center For Pain Medicine, Cuyahoga Falls, OH, USA
e-mail: narouzs@hotmail.com

S. N. Narouze (ed.), *Cannabinoids and Pain*, https://doi.org/10.1007/978-3-030-69186-8_3

When medical knowledge is insufficient, it is unsurprising that public knowledge is even more so. Kruger et al. compared cannabis users' knowledge about cannabis risks and effectiveness in treating medical conditions against existing empirical evidence. They reported considerable discrepancies. In a survey of 472 adults who frequently used cannabis (85% for health or medical purposes), only 18% had received drug information from their primary care provider. Others derived their knowledge from personal experience or hearsay. The majority of participants' beliefs correlated with the National Academies of Sciences, Engineering, and Medicine (NASEM)'s conclusions for effectiveness and risk. However more than half of participants believed cannabis was effective in treating cancer, depressive symptoms, and epilepsy, all conditions contrary to NASEM's conclusions. Unsurprisingly, cannabis users who had received information from their health-care provider had better knowledge of medical effectiveness compared to others [7].

The Veterans Health Administration (VHA) conducted a survey on clinician knowledge surrounding cannabis use with 249 responses from primary care providers across 39 US states and the District of Columbia. They found significant knowledge gaps in policy, terminology, and current evidence base. Overall, the VHA providers felt uncomfortable discussing key aspects of cannabis use with their patients, evidencing the need for more widespread clinician education [8].

It is a physician's duty and responsibility to educate themselves on the health concerns of their patients, and thus it should be the medical educator's responsibility to assure the next generation of physicians is better prepared. However, there are several challenges that prevent the implementation of medical marijuana education in our medical schools, clinics, and hospitals. Firstly, there is an overall dearth of high-quality evidence regarding its use. And thus, there is a disconnect between prescribers, patients, and evidence. For instance, chronic pain remains the most common indication for medical cannabis use; however the evidence regarding its use is inconclusive [9–11]. Without high-quality studies and requisite knowledge syntheses, developing evidence-based education becomes nearly impossible.

Second, stigma surrounding marijuana makes it difficult to make unbiased judgments. In the aforementioned surveys, several providers, educators, and students did not feel the study of cannabis was important or should be included in medical school education. This in part is due to the medical community as a whole behaving dismissive of the issue. Many patients may find themselves wishing to learn more about the medical uses of marijuana but feel embarrassed to bring this up with their provider. Other patients are already using medical marijuana, but don't know how to tell their doctors for fear of being scolded. This inconsideration of the use of cannabis and possible underlying bias needs to be further explored.

Third, many state's policies are in conflict with federal policy, where cannabis remains a Drug Enforcement Agency (DEA) Schedule I substance with no defined medical use. In states where marijuana is not legal for medical or recreational use, educators may feel uncomfortable speaking about any benefits of an illicit drug.

Across specialties, there are concerns there is a knowledge gap among medical practitioners, students, and the general public. There is a significant need to implement comprehensive evidence-based cannabis education plans in the USA to educate patients, health professionals, and the general public. Medical educators may be wary about teaching such a controversial and politically charged topic. But they do not need to make moral statements on medical marijuana in order to communicate the evidence that is already known. Medical cannabis is already a therapeutic option in the majority of US states and frequently requested by patients. Physicians must do more to address and get ahead of their patients' knowledge on cannabis and approach patient concerns with an open mind.

References

1. Federation of state medical boards. Model guidelines for the recommendation of marijuana in patient care. 2016. https://www.ncbi.nlm.nih.gov/pmc/articles/PMC6041497/pdf/ajpe6296.pdf. Accessed 22 Mar 2020.
2. National Academies of Sciences, Engineering, and Medicine. The health effects of cannabis and cannabinoids: current state of evidence and recommendations for research. Washington, DC: National Academies Press; 2017.
3. Philpot LM, Ebbert JO, Hurt RT. A survey of the attitudes, beliefs and knowledge about medical cannabis among primary care providers. BMC Fam Pract. 2019;22(1):17.
4. Evanoff AB, Quan T, Dufault C, Awad M, Bierut LJ. Physicians-in-training are not prepared to prescribe medical marijuana. Drug Alcohol Depend. 2017;180:151–5.
5. Benadides A, Gregorio N, Gupta P, Kogan M. Medical students are unprepared to counsel patients about medical cannabis and want to learn more. Complement Ther Med. 2020;48:102237.
6. Caligiuri F, Ulrich E, Welter K. Pharmacy student knowledge, confidence and attitudes toward medical cannabis and curricular coverage. Am J Pharm Edu. 2018;82(5):6296.
7. Kruger DJ, Kruger JS, Collins RL. Cannabis enthusiasts' knowledge of medical treatment effectiveness and increased risks from cannabis use. Am J Health Promot. 2020;34(4):436–9. https://doi.org/10.1177/0890117119899218.
8. Kansagara D, Morasco B, Iacocca M, Bair M, Hooker E, Becker W. Clinician knowledge, attitudes, and practice regarding cannabis: results from a National Veterans Health Administration Survey. Pain Med. 2020;21(11):3180–6. https://doi.org/10.1093/pm/pnz322.
9. Bonn-Miller MO, Boden MT, Bucossi MM, Babson KA. Self reported cannabis use characteristics, patterns and helpfulness among medical cannabis users. Am J Drug Alcohol Abuse. 2014;40(1): 23–30.
10. Nugent SM, Morasco BJ, O'Neil ME, et al. The effects of cannabis among adults with chronic pain and an overview of general harms: a systematic review. Ann Intern Med. 2017;167(5):319–31.
11. Compton WM, Han B, Hughes A, Jones CM, Blanco C. Use of marijuana for medical purposes among adults in the United States. JAMA. 2017;317(2):209–10.

Pain Physicians and Medical Cannabis: Attitudes, Believes, Preparedness and Knowledge

4

Samer N. Narouze, Sameh M. Hakim, Lynn Kohan, and Dmitri Souza

Introduction

Cannabis has been used throughout history for an array of medical indications from pain to curing cancer, in addition to recreational, religious, and spiritual purposes [1].

Marijuana is the most commonly used illicit drug in the United States. An estimated 26.0 million Americans aged 12 or older in 2017 were current users of marijuana. This number of past month marijuana users corresponds to 9.6 percent of the population aged 12 or older [2].

Since 1970 marijuana has been classified at the federal level as a Schedule I substance under the Controlled Substance Act and defined as a drug with no currently accepted medical use and a high potential for abuse [3, 4]. To date, 47 out of the 50 states allow some form of medical marijuana. Thirty-three states and the District of Columbia currently have passed legislation for a "comprehensive medical marijuana program," according to the National Conference of State Legislatures [5]. In addition, 13 states allow only the use of low tetrahydrocannabinol (THC)/high cannabidiol (CBD) ratio products. Moreover, a number of states have also decriminalized the possession of small amounts of marijuana.

While medical marijuana is legalized in two-thirds of the US states, policy-makers have outpaced clinical research and medical education, creating a critical mismatch between the state legalization of medical marijuana and the lack of knowledge, education, and preparedness among physicians.

A recent primary care physicians' survey showed that one-half of physicians either were not ready to or did not want to answer patient's questions on medical cannabis [6].

Two-thirds and one-quarter of medical school curriculum deans reported that their graduates were not at all prepared to prescribe and answer questions about medical marijuana, respectively [7]. Almost all residents and fellows (89.5%) felt not at all prepared to prescribe medical marijuana, while 35.3% felt not at all prepared to answer questions. The vast majority of residents and fellows (84.9%) reported receiving no education in medical school or residency on medical marijuana. Only 9% of medical school curricula document in the Association of American Medical Colleges (AAMC) Curriculum Inventory database content on medical marijuana [7].

Recently, there have been two bipartisan bills that aim to expand and expedite the ability to perform rigorous studies on marijuana. H.R. 601,

S. N. Narouze (✉)
Western Reserve Hospital, Center For Pain Medicine, Cuyahoga Falls, OH, USA
e-mail: narouzs@hotmail.com
Twitter: @NarouzeMD

S. M. Hakim
Faculty of Medicine, Ain Shams University, Cairo, Egypt

L. Kohan
Department of Anesthesiology and Pain Medicine, University of Virginia, Charlottesville, VA, USA

D. Souza
Western Reserve Hospital, Cuyahoga Falls, OH, USA

S. N. Narouze (ed.), *Cannabinoids and Pain*, https://doi.org/10.1007/978-3-030-69186-8_4

the Medical Cannabis Research Act of 2019, was introduced into the House of Representatives in 2019 and is currently under review by the Subcommittee on Crime, Terrorism, and Homeland Security. The aim of this bill is to expand cannabis research by increasing the number of federally registered manufactures of cannabis for legitimate research purposes [8]. The second bill, the Cannabidiol and Marijuana Research Expansion Act, aims to deregulate and expedite both the research and manufacturing application pathway [9].

This reflects the current enthusiastic climate surrounding medicinal cannabis and cannabinoids. Physicians and patients are hoping for novel pain treatments amid the current opioid crisis. However, there is ongoing uncertainty due to conflicting laws between federal and state governments. This conflict coupled with lack of education creates a "gray area" surrounding the use of medical cannabis, which can lead to confusion, apprehension, and frustration among pain physicians.

We conducted a national survey for pain physicians with the aim to advance our understanding of the attitudes, beliefs, preparedness, and knowledge of pain physicians regarding medical cannabis and cannabinoids [10]. This will help the pain medicine community identify the current barriers and knowledge gaps.

Development and Description of the Applied Questionnaire

The questionnaire employed for the present survey was adapted from that used previously by Philpot and colleagues for surveying attitudes, beliefs, and knowledge of primary care providers regarding medical cannabis [7]. The original questionnaire was adapted by the present authors to fit the purpose of surveying pain physicians. The adapted questionnaire was presented to a small group of experts in pain medicine to gather their suggestions and proposals for making it more fitting to pain physicians. The survey was modified accordingly and was structured into five principal domains:

- Domain A (legitimacy): Attitude regarding the legitimacy or appropriateness of using cannabis for medical purposes
- Domain B (symptoms): Knowledge regarding pain-related symptoms for which medical cannabis could be helpful
- Domain C (quality of life): Beliefs regarding functional aspects related to the quality of life in chronic pain patients that medical cannabis could improve
- Domain D (worries): Worries and concerns regarding the recommendation of medical cannabis to chronic pain patients
- Domain E (preparedness): Practitioners' beliefs that they have gained enough knowledge and education regarding medical cannabis during their training

In addition to the five principal domains that measured participants' attitudes, beliefs, preparedness, and knowledge regarding medical cannabis, we added two blocks of questions for relevant demographic and professional information:

- Block A (experience with medical cannabis): Information regarding registration in a medical cannabis program, ever recommending medical cannabis to patients, and caring for patients on medical cannabis
- Block B (personal): Personal information including age, gender identity, and years since graduation from medical school

The modified questionnaire was tested on a training sample of 30 participants to examine internal consistency of each domain. For domains A through E, which measured attitudes, knowledge, beliefs, and preparedness regarding medical cannabis, participants were asked to score their responses on a scale graded from 0 to 100 by moving a pointer on a graded scale. For blocks A and B (experience with medical cannabis and personal data, respectively), participants chose a single response out of three possible choices. A reliability analysis was carried out on the training sample for domains A through E separately. For domains B (symptoms), C (quality of life), and D (worries), the reliability index (Cronbach's α) was 0.900, 0.902, and 0.886, respectively, denoting high internal validity. When we removed any item from these domains, the corresponding reliability index decreased. Therefore, we retained all items in these domains. For domains A (legitimacy) and E (preparedness), the reliability index was low (Cronbach's α = 0.413 and 0.561, respectively) denoting low internal consistency. One item in domain A (my patients frequently request medical cannabis) was inconsistent with poor correlation with the other two items (r = −0.268 and −0.038, respectively). When we removed that item, the reliability index increased to 0.834. So we removed that item and retained the other two. For domain E (preparedness), one item (I attended medical conferences specifically to learn about medical cannabis) was inconsistent and correlated poorly with the other three items (r = 0.124, −0.017, and −0.150, respectively). When we removed that item, the reliability index increased to 0.765. Subsequently we removed that item, too.

The ultimate questionnaire, which has been applied for the main sample, is shown in Appendix 1. The questionnaire was entered into the Qualtrics^{XM} survey software website and was accessed and scored by participants in the same way as that used for the training sample. The American Society of Regional Anesthesia and Pain Medicine (ASRA) distributed the survey to their active members (acute and chronic pain physicians) by email with the web link.

Statistical Analysis

Data were analyzed using IBM© SPSS© Statistics version 22 (IBM© Corp., Armonk, NY) and JMP® version 14.3.0 (SAS Institute Inc., Cary, NC). Categorical variables were presented as number and percentage, and numerical variables as mean, standard deviation, and quartiles.

For all domains measuring attitudes, knowledge, or beliefs (domains A through E), the questions were formulated such that higher scores denoted higher trend for the dimension measured by the domain. Except for domain D which measured worry or concern regarding recommending medical cannabis to a patient, a higher score on all other domains denoted a more favorable attitude toward use of medical cannabis. So, in order to make a higher score on any domain denote more favorable attitude toward use of cannabis, we subtracted the scores for domain D from 100 and used the calculated score to denote comfort or ease with recommending medical cannabis to chronic pain patients. For data analysis and presentation, we referred to domain D as "Ease with recommending medical cannabis to chronic pain patients."

For each participant, we calculated a mean score for each domain by averaging the scores of all items (questions) within the same domain. In addition, we calculated an overall score for the questionnaire by averaging the scores of all five domains. Thus, for any participant, the score on any domain, as well as the overall score, could range from a minimum of 0 (least favorable) to 100 (most favorable) regarding use of cannabis.

Associations between continuous variables and nominal variables on two levels were examined using point biserial correlation (r_{pb}). Kendall's tau-b rank correlation (τ_b) was used to test associations between continuous and ordinal variables. Correlations between continuous variables were examined using the Spearman rank correlation (Superman's ρ). The Bonferroni method was used to adjust the critical P value for the number of comparisons in order to maintain the alpha error at <0.05. Hence, a two-tailed $P < 0.001$ was considered statistically significant.

Results

All active members of the ASRA were invited via electronically sent mails to take part in the survey. Out of 1536 members who received the email, 334 (21.7%) logged into the survey website during the period from January 29, 2020, to March 15, 2020. Of those who logged into the website, only 325 entered valid responses to one or more items of the questionnaire with an effective response rate of 21.2%. All survey participants and responses were anonymous, and they were asked to take the survey only once. There were no financial or other material incentives provided for survey participants.

Table 4.1 shows the demographic and professional characteristics of participants. The majority (*n* = 178, 59%) were 30 to 50 years of age, 114 (38.3%) were over 50 years of age, and only 6 (2%) were below 30 years of age. About two-thirds of participants (*n* = 199, 66.8%) were males, about one-third (*n* = 98, 32.0%) belonged to the female gender, and only 1 (0.3%) participant was non-binary.

Most of participants (*n* = 187, 65.8%) had been graduated from medical school for more than 10 years. About one-fifth of participants (*n* = 57, 20.1%) had been graduated for 5 to 10 years, and only 40 (14.1%) participants had been graduated for less than 5 years.

Table 4.1 Demographic and professional characteristics of participants

Variable		Valid responses Number	Percentage
Age	*<30 years*	6	2.0
	30–50 years	178	59.7
	>50 years	114	38.3
	Total	298	100.0
Gender	*Male*	199	66.8
	Female	98	32.9
	Non-binary	1	0.3
	Total	298	100.0
Time since graduated from medical school	*<5 years*	40	14.1
	5–10 years	57	20.1
	>10 years	187	65.8
	Total	284	100.0
Registered to recommend medical cannabis in one's state	*Yes*	39	13.0
	No	262	87.0
	Total	301	100.0
Ever recommended medical cannabis for patients	*Yes*	93	30.9
	No	208	69.1
	Total	301	100.0
Taking care of patients on medical cannabis	*Yes*	228	75.7
	No	73	24.3
	Total	301	100.0

Data are presented as valid number and percentage

Regarding experience with medical cannabis, only 39 (13.0%) participants were currently registered in a medical cannabis program in their states, 93 (30.9%) recommended medical cannabis for their patients at least once, and 228 (75.7%) were taking care of patients on medical cannabis (Fig. 4.1).

Table 4.2 shows the scores of participants on each domain items, while Table 4.3 shows the averaged score for each of the five principal questionnaire domains.

In order of decreasing magnitude, the participants' scores were most favorable regarding the legitimacy of medical cannabis where 75% of participants scored 50 or higher, 50% scored 76 or higher, and 25% scored 91 or higher on the 100-point scale for this domain (mean ± SD score, 67 ± 29).

The participants' scores were less favorable regarding the symptoms cannabis could help (75% scored 37 or more, 50% scored 56 or more, and 25% scored 67 or more; mean ± SD score, 53 ± 22) and regarding the ease with recommending cannabis for patients (75% scored 23 or more, 50% scored 50 or more, and 25% scored 79 or more; mean ± SD score, 50 ± 32).

The participants' scores were least favorable regarding the quality of life aspects helped by cannabis (75% scored 23 or more, 50% scored 50 or more, and 25% scored 79 or more; mean ± SD score, 40 ± 23) and regarding the preparedness to recommend medical cannabis for patients (75% scored 16 or more, 50% scored 31 or more, and 25% scored 42 or more; mean ± SD score, 32 ± 21).

The overall trend of participants for recommending medical cannabis to their patients was moderately favorable with 75% of participants scoring 38 or higher, 50% scoring 49 or higher, and only 25% scoring 61 or higher on the 100-point overall scale (mean ± SD overall score, 50 ± 17) (Fig. 4.2).

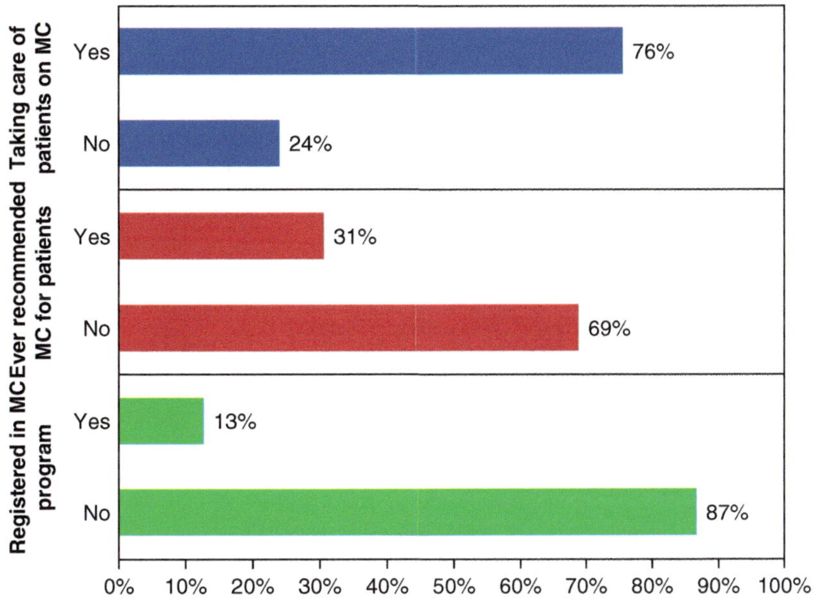

Fig. 4.1 Percentage of participants registered in medical cannabis program, those who had ever recommended medical cannabis for patients, and those who were actually taking care of patients on medical cannabis. *MC*, medical cannabis

Table 4.2 Scoring of participants' attitudes, knowledge and beliefs regarding use of medical cannabis

Domain	Valid responses	Score		Score percentiles		
		Mean	SD	25th	50th	75th
A. Legitimacy of medical cannabis						
Physicians should be able to offer cannabis for certain medical conditions	325	72	30	50	81	100
Medical cannabis is a legitimate medical therapy	324	63	31	40	69	90
B. Symptoms cannabinoids may help						
Pain	311	55	28	32	52	76
Seizures	301	59	29	38	65	80
Muscle spasms	304	46	27	25	50	68
Anxiety	303	57	30	35	61	80
Insomnia	302	52	31	27	51	79
Depression	297	36	28	10	31	54
Nausea/Vomiting	305	64	28	50	70	85
C. Quality of life aspects cannabinoids may benefit in patients with CPS						
Energy level	293	30	24	10	25	50
Mood	295	45	27	21	50	61
Social engagement	293	38	27	13	34	55
Sense of hope	294	42	27	20	42	58
D. Ease with prescription of medical cannabis to patients with CPS						
I'm not worried of getting sued because of discrepancy between state and federal regulations	296	50	37	11	50	90
I'm not worried of getting in trouble 'later' like what has happened with the opioid crisis	297	49	35	18	50	81
Preparedness to prescribe medical cannabis to patients with CPS						
I'm prepared enough to answer patients' questions about medical cannabis	297	48	31	21	50	73
I had enough education regarding medical cannabis during my training	292	22	25	4	11	30

CPS chronic pain syndromes, *SD* standard deviation

Table 4.3 Participants' scores on the five principal domains of the questionnaire and their overall scores on the questionnaire

Domain and dimension	Valid N	Score		Score percentiles		
		Mean	SD	25th	50th	75th
A. Legitimacy of MC	325	67	29	50	76	91
B. Symptoms helped by MC	312	53	22	37	56	67
C. Quality of life aspects improved by MC	191	40	23	23	42	54
D. Ease with recommending MC	301	50	32	23	50	79
E. Preparedness to recommend MC	298	32	21	16	31	42
Overall score	326	50	17	38	49	61

MC medical cannabis, *N* number, *SD* standard deviation

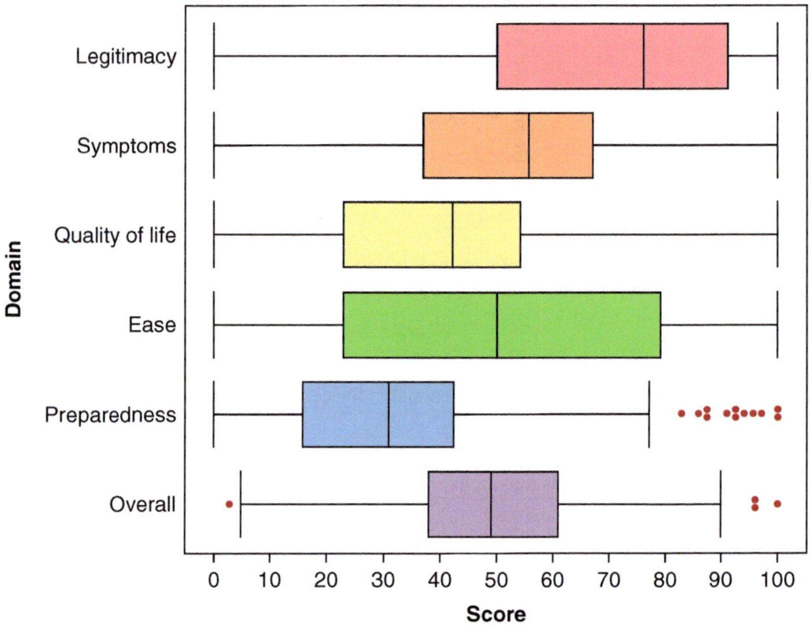

Fig. 4.2 Box plot illustrating the participants' scores on each of the five principal domains of the questionnaire and the averaged score of all five domains (overall score). Box represents the interquartile range. Line inside the box represents the median. Whiskers represent minimum and maximum values excluding outliers (red markers)

Table 4.4 summarizes the associations between demographic and professional characteristics of participants and their scores on the five principal domains of the questionnaire.

There was very weak positive association between registration in a medical cannabis program and the participants' overall score (r_{pb}, 0.199; *P* value, 0.0005) (Fig. 4.3). Besides, there was weak positive association between the participants' ever recommending cannabis to patients and their scores for the legitimacy (r_{pb}, 0.286; *P* value, <0.0001), symptoms (r_{pb}, 0.260; *P* value <0.0001), and preparedness (r_{pb}, 0.323; *P* value, <0.0001) domains. There was similarly weak positive association between the participants' ever recommending cannabis to patients and their overall score as well (r_{pb}, 0.335; *P* value, <0.0001) (Fig. 4.4).

Otherwise, no statistically significant association was observed between the participants' scores for any of the domains and their age, gender identity, time since graduation from medical school, or taking care for patients on medical cannabis (all *P* values > critical *P* of 0.001).

Table 4.5 presents a correlation matrix summarizing the associations among the participants'

Table 4.4 Association between demographic and professional characteristics of participants and their scores on the five principal domains of the questionnaire

		Domain					
Variable	Measure of association	Legitimacy	Symptoms	Quality of life	Ease	Preparedness	Overall
Age	Kendall τ_b	−0.086	−0.106	−0.068	0.096	−0.025	−0.058
	P-value	0.074	0.025	0.250	0.043	0.607	0.222
	N	297	298	189	296	293	298
Male gender	Kendall τ_b	0.091	0.000	−0.064	−0.077	0.100	0.040
	P-value	0.061	0.993	0.285	0.108	0.038	0.400
	N	297	298	189	296	293	298
Time since graduated from medical school	Kendall τ_b	−0.074	−0.127	−0.124	0.044	0.023	−0.059
	P-value	0.124	0.007	0.039	0.357	0.631	0.213
	N	283	284	177	282	282	284
Registration in a medical cannabis program	r_{pb}	0.134	0.085	0.098	0.160	0.158	0.199
	P-value	0.020	0.143	0.178	0.006	0.006	**0.0005**
	N	300	301	190	298	296	301
Ever recommending medical cannabis for patients	r_{pb}	0.286	0.260	0.177	0.085	0.323	0.335
	P-value	**<0.0001**	**<0.0001**	0.015	0.145	**<0.0001**	**<0.0001**
	N	300	301	190	298	296	301
Taking care of patients on medical cannabis	r_{pb}	0.107	0.035	0.049	−0.024	0.181	0.084
	P-value	0.065	0.547	0.498	0.679	0.002	0.148
	N	300	301	190	298	296	301

N valid number, r_{pb} point biserial correlation coefficient, τ_b Kandall's tau-b correlation coefficient

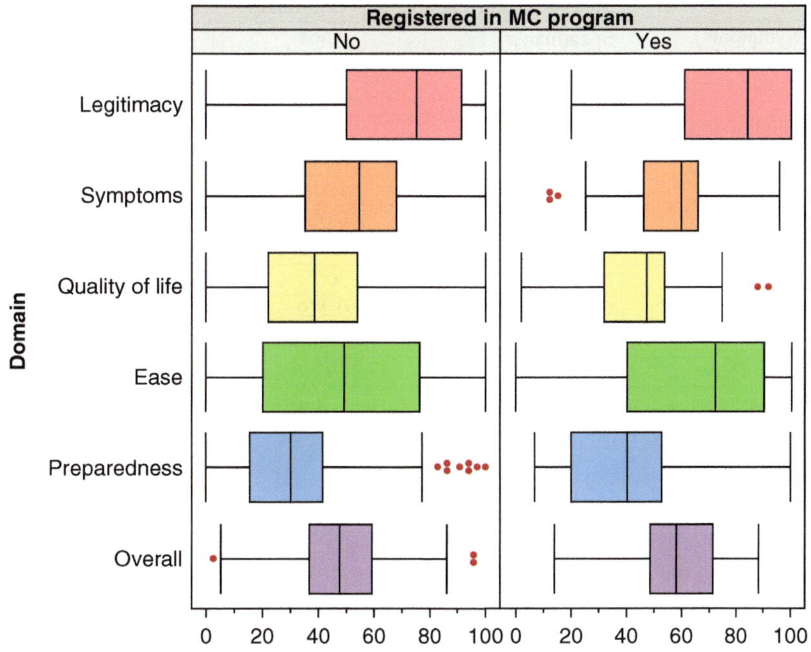

Fig. 4.3 Box plot illustrating the relation between registration of participants in a medical cannabis program and their scores on the five principal Domains of the questionnaire. Box represents the interquartile range. Line inside the box represents the median. Whiskers represent minimum and maximum values excluding outliers (red markers). *MC*, medical cannabis

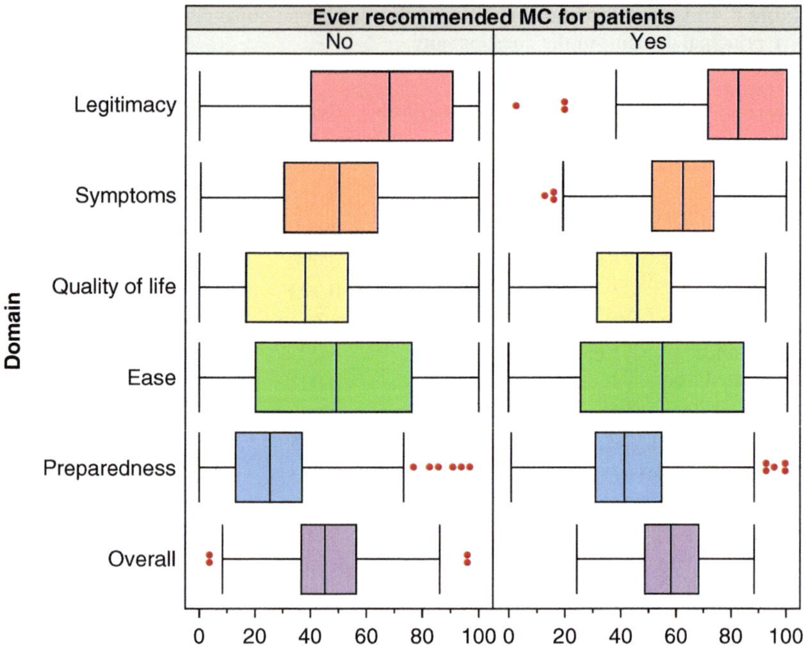

Fig. 4.4 Box plot illustrating the relation between ever recommending medical cannabis to patients by participants and their scores on the five principal domains of the questionnaire. Box represents the interquartile range. Line inside the box represents the median. Whiskers represent minimum and maximum values excluding outliers (red markers). *MC*, medical cannabis

Table 4.5 Correlation matrix illustrating the correlations among the participants' scores on the principal domains of the questionnaire

	Measure of correlation	Legitimacy	Symptoms	Quality of life	Ease
Symptoms	Spearman ρ	0.661			
	P-value	**<0.0001**			
	N	311			
Quality of life	Coefficient	0.486	0.691		
	P-value	**<0.0001**	**<0.0001**		
	N	190	191		
Ease	Coefficient	0.024	0.005	0.045	
	P-value	0.679	0.926	0.538	
	N	300	301	190	
Preparedness	Coefficient	0.279	0.259	0.168	−0.074
	P-value	**<0.0001**	**0.0001**	0.021	0.205
	N	297	298	188	296

N valid number, ρ Spearman correlation coefficient (rho)

scores on the principal domains of the questionnaire.

There was a strong positive correlation between the participants' scores on the symptoms domain and their scores on the legitimacy (Spearman ρ, 0.661; P value, <0.0001) and quality of life (Spearman ρ, 0.691; P value, <0.0001) domains. On the other hand, there was moderate positive correlation between the participants' scores on the legitimacy and quality of life domains (Spearman ρ, 0.486; P value, <0.0001).

There was only weak positive correlation between participants' score on the preparedness domain and their scores on the legitimacy (Spearman ρ, 0.279; P value, <0.0001) and symptoms (Spearman ρ, 0.259; P value, <0.0001) domains (Fig. 4.5).

Discussion

The present survey helped to elucidate the attitudes, beliefs, knowledge, and preparedness of pain practitioners regarding the use of medical cannabis for patients with chronic pain disorders. Previous studies tried to explore the attitudes or practices of primary care providers [7] or palliative care providers [11] regarding medical cannabis.

The findings of the present survey were very interesting. The participants' trend was most favorable regarding the legitimacy of medical cannabis. Their trend was less favorable for the symptoms cannabis could help and for the ease with recommending cannabis to patients. The participants' trend was least favorable for the quality of life aspects helped by cannabis and for

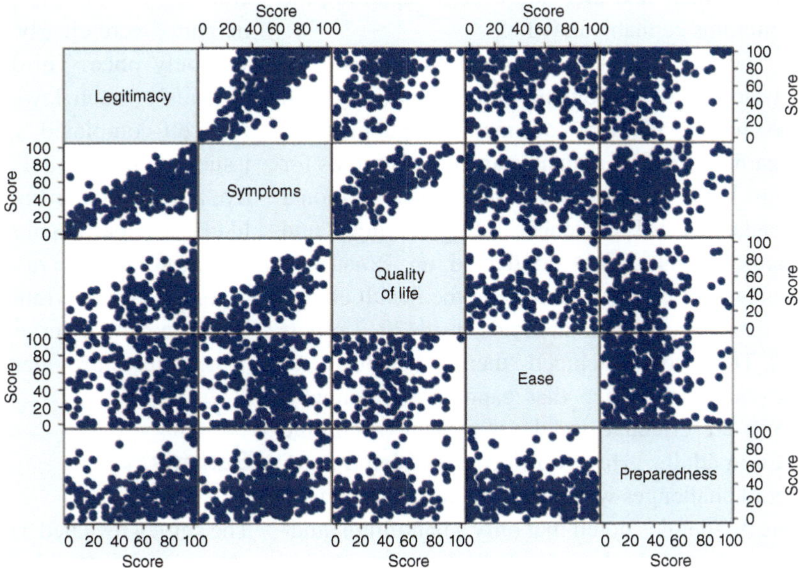

Fig. 4.5 Scatter plot matrix illustrating correlations among the participants' scores on the principal domains of the questionnaire. Markers represent individual observations. *QoL*, Quality of life

the preparedness to recommend medical cannabis to patients. Overall, the participants' trend for recommending medical cannabis to their patients was moderately favorable with 75% of participants scoring 38 or higher, 50% scoring 49 or higher, and only 25% scoring 61 or higher on the 100-point overall scale.

There was a strong correlation between the participants' knowledge regarding the symptoms cannabis may help and their beliefs regarding the legitimacy of medical cannabis and the potential quality of life improvements. In addition, there was also a significant, though weaker, correlation between the participants' beliefs regarding the legitimacy of medical cannabis and the quality of life aspects that may be improved by medical cannabis. Notably, the least strong correlations were between the participants' sense of preparedness to recommend medical cannabis to patients and their beliefs regarding the legitimacy of medical cannabis and their knowledge regarding the symptoms cannabis may help.

The survey response highlights the need for physicians' education and training specially with the recent plethora of medical publications regarding medical cannabis and cannabinoids for pain with inconsistent results. The National Academies of Sciences, Engineering, and Medicine (NASEM) conducted an exhaustive review of medical literature on the health effects of cannabis and cannabinoids in its 2017 report [1]. The report concluded "there is conclusive or substantial evidence that cannabis or cannabinoids are effective for the treatment of chronic pain in adults." However, they identified a number of challenges with research gaps and barriers. The Academies noted that only a handful of studies evaluated the benefit of dispensary cannabis in the United States and that little is known about dosing or side effects. On the other hand, the Cochrane Database of Systematic Reviews in 2018 concluded that "the potential benefits of cannabis-based medicine (herbal cannabis, plant-derived or synthetic THC, THC/CBD oromucosal spray) in chronic neuropathic pain might be outweighed by their potential harms" [12]. The College of Family Physicians of Canada released a simplified guideline for prescribing medical cannabinoids in primary care. The College recommended strongly against the use of medical cannabinoids for acute pain, headache, fibromyalgia, osteoarthritis, and back pain while suggesting that they should be considered only for intractable neuropathic pain after failure of multiple analgesics [13].

The present study has a few limitations. First, the sampling process was rather selective, in that we invited only ASRA members to participate in our survey. Despite ASRA being one of the largest pain societies, the trends of its members may not be plainly extrapolated to all pain practitioners as they may share uncharacteristic academic, clinical, or cultural attitudes. We also postulate that a larger, more representative pain physician's sample will likely yield a larger education gap. Secondly, all participants made their entries online so that, owing to privacy issues, we could not preclude multiple or duplicate entries by the same participant. However, participants were clearly instructed to take the survey only once. Thirdly, the response rate was obviously much lower than that recommended for self-completed questionnaires [14]. This issue may be relevant if subjects with more negative attitudes regarding medical cannabis are less likely to participate [15]. Nonetheless, the observed response rate is practically close to that reported by previous investigators who conducted a similar survey on a different population of healthcare providers [7].

Summary

The survey revealed a mismatch between the pain physicians' favorable attitude regarding the legitimacy of using medical cannabis and their lack of preparedness. While the participants' trend was most favorable regarding the legitimacy of medical cannabis, it was least favorable for the preparedness to recommend medical cannabis to pain patients. The survey results will help the pain medicine community identify the current barriers and knowledge gaps.

Conflict of Interest None.

Medical Cannabis Questionnaire

A. Place a mark on the line below each item indicating your level of agreement with the following statements:

Physicians should be able to offer cannabis for certain medical conditions

Don't agree at all ●————● Extremely agree

Medical cannabis is a legitimate medical therapy

Don't agree at all ●————● Extremely agree

B. Place a mark on the line below each item indicating how helpful you think cannabinoids are for the following symptoms:

Pain

Not at all ●————● Extremely helpful

Seizures

Not at all ●————● Extremely helpful

Muscle spasms

Not at all ●————● Extremely helpful

Anxiety

Not at all ●————● Extremely helpful

Insomnia

Not at all ●————● Extremely helpful

Depression

Not at all ●————● Extremely helpful

Nausea/Vomiting

Not at all ●————● Extremely helpful

C. Place a mark on the line below each item indicating how beneficial you think cannabinoids are for the following aspects in patients with chronic pain syndromes:

Energy level

Not at all ●————● Extremely beneficial

Mood

Not at all ●————● Extremely beneficial

Social engagement

Not at all ●————● Extremely beneficial

Sense of hope

Not at all ●————● Extremely beneficial

D. Place a mark on the line below each item indicating how worried you may be regarding prescribing medical cannabis to your patients:

I'm worried of getting sued because of discrepancy between state and federal regulations

Not at all ●————● Extremely worried

I'm worried of getting in trouble 'later' like what has happened with the opioid crisis

Not at all ●————● Extremely worried

I feel worried or uncomfortable recommending medical cannabis for my patients

Not at all ●————● Extremely worried

E. Place a mark on the line opposite each item indicating how prepared you are for prescribing medical cannabis to your patients:

I'm prepared enough to answer patients' questions about medical cannabis

Not at all ●————● Extremely agree

I had enough education regarding medical cannabis during my training

Not at all ●————● Extremely agree

I think I don't need to see more research before offering medical cannabis for my patients

Not at all ●————● Extremely agree

F. Check a response to the following questions:

Are you registered to recommend medical cannabis in your state?

Yes

No

Have you ever recommended medical cannabis for your patients?
Yes
No
Do you take care of patients on medical cannabis?
Yes
No
G. Please check a response to the following questions:
How long have been graduated from medical school?
<5 years
5–10 years
>10 years
What is your age?
<30 years
30–50 years
>50 years
What is your gender?
Male
Female
Non-binary

References

1. National Academies of Sciences, Engineering, and Medicine. The health effects of cannabis and cannabinoids: Current state of evidence and recommendations for research. Washington, DC: National Academies Press; 2017.
2. Substance Abuse and Mental Health Services Administration. Key substance use and mental health indicators in the United States: results from the 2017 National Survey on Drug Use and Health (HHS Publication No. SMA 18-5068, NSDUH Series H-53). Rockville: Center for Behavioral Health Statistics and Quality, Substance Abuse and Mental Health Services Administration; 2018. Retrieved from. https://www.samhsa.gov/data/sites/default/files/cbhsq-reports/NSDUHFFR2017/NSDUHFFR2017.pdf. Accessed 25 Apr 2020.
3. FDA regulation of cannabis and cannabis-derived products: questions and answers. https://www.fda.gov/news-events/public-health-focus/fda-regulation-cannabis-and-cannabis-derived-products-questions-and-answers. Accessed 29 Apr 2020.
4. United states drug enforcement administration (DEA) drug scheduling. https://www.dea.gov/drug-scheduling Accessed 29 Apr 2019.
5. State medical marijuana laws. National conference of state legislatures (NCSL). http://www.ncsl.org/research/health/state-medical-marijuana-laws.aspx#3. Accessed 25 Apr 2020.
6. Philpot LM, Ebbert JO, Hurt RT. A survey of the attitudes, beliefs and knowledge about medical cannabis among primary care providers. BMC Fam Pract. 2019;20(1):17. https://doi.org/10.1186/s12875-019-0906-y. PMID: 30669979; PMCID: PMC6341534.
7. Evanoff AB, Quan T, Dufault C, Awad M, Bierut LJ. Physicians-in-training are not prepared to prescribe medical marijuana. Drug Alcohol Depend. 2017;180:151–5.
8. Rep. Gaetz, Matt. H.R.601 – 116th congress (2019–2020): Medical Cannabis Research Act of 2019. 2019. https://www.congress.gov/bill/116th-congress/house-bill/601?q={"search":["medical+cannabis+research+act"]}. Accessed 25 Apr 2020.
9. Senator Feinstein, Dianne. S.2032 – 116th congress (2019–2020): cannabidiol and marihuana research expansion act. 2019. https://www.congress.gov/bill/116th-congress/senate-bill/2032/text?r=11. Accessed 25 Apr 2020.
10. Narouze S, Hakim SM, Kohan L, Adams D, Souza D. Medical cannabis attitudes and beliefs among pain physicians. Reg Anesth Pain Med. 2020; https://doi.org/10.1136/rapm-2020-101658. Online ahead of print. PMID: 32759172
11. Luba R, Earleywine M, Farmer S, Slavin M. Cannabis in end-of-life care: examining attitudes and practices of palliative care providers. J Psychoactive Drugs. 2018;50(4):348–54. https://doi.org/10.1080/02791072.2018.1462543. PMID: 29714640.
12. Mücke M, Phillips T, Radbruch L, Petzke F, Häuser W. Cannabis-based medicines for chronic neuropathic pain in adults. Cochrane Database Syst Rev. 2018;(3):CD012182. https://doi.org/10.1002/14651858.CD012182.pub2.
13. Allan GM, Ramji J, Perry D, et al. Simplified guideline for prescribing medical cannabinoids in primary care. Canad Fam Phys. 2018;64(2):111–1204.
14. Sitzia J, Wood N. Response rate in patient satisfaction research: an analysis of 210 published studies. Int J Qual Health Care. 1998;10(4):311–7. https://doi.org/10.1093/intqhc/10.4.311. PMID: 9835247.
15. French K. Methodological considerations in hospital patient opinion surveys. Int J Nurs Stud. 1981;18(1):7–32. https://doi.org/10.1016/0020-7489(81)90004-3. PMID: 6906348.

Cannabis Terminology

5

Maria Fernanda Arboleda and Erin Prosk

Introduction

Cannabis has been used therapeutically for thousands of years to relieve various symptoms. However almost 100 years of cannabis prohibition during the twentieth century caused a gap in clinical use and research. There are still significant gaps in the understanding of cannabis and its components and their pharmacological and potential therapeutic benefits. The use of cannabis for medical purposes has increased dramatically in the last 10 years, and chronic pain is one of the main reasons reported for its use [1]. There is a wide variability of preferences for different cannabinoid-based medicines reported among patients living with chronic pain. The majority prefer oral administration and low delta-9-tetrahydrocannabinol (THC) concentrations. However, less than 3% of patients receiving advice from medical professionals, therefore, many patients rely on their own research or support from cannabis retailers for product selection [2].

To build a foundation of medical cannabis knowledge, it is important to start by learning about the cannabis plant and its main components and therapeutic characteristics and familiarize one's self with the common terminology, both scientific and colloquial to be able to discuss with patients and their families. Informed and accessible discussion with patients supports improved patient communication and trust and may contribute to improved outcomes. Such understanding of basic cannabis properties and common terminology also allows for a better communication among clinicians interested in the cannabis field.

The aim of this chapter is to review the fundamentals of cannabis plants and provide simple definitions of the terminology related to cannabinoid-based treatments.

General Aspects of the Cannabis Plant

The cannabis plant is one of the oldest documented plants to be used not only for well-known therapeutic and spiritual reasons but also as a source of food and textile fiber. Originated from central Asia, the cannabis plant belongs to the family Cannabaceae that contains only two genera, *Humulus*, commonly known as hops, and *Cannabis*. Some debate is ongoing related to the taxonomy of cannabis classification and whether the *Cannabis* genus is composed of only one or more species that may vary according to geographical origin, morphological characteristics, chemotype differences, and genetic sequencing [3, 4]. Some authors have suggested that three different species exist, *C. sativa, C. indica*, and C. *ruderalis*. Other researchers have proposed

M. F. Arboleda (✉) · E. Prosk
Research Department, Santé Cannabis Clinic, Montreal, QC, Canada
e-mail: mfarboleda@santecannabis.ca

S. N. Narouze (ed.), *Cannabinoids and Pain*, https://doi.org/10.1007/978-3-030-69186-8_5

that *Cannabis* genus is monotypic and that these previously mentioned subpopulations represent subspecies of *C. sativa L.* [5, 6].

Cannabis sativa is a dioecious species; this means that male and female flowers develop on separate plants. New genetics, termed *cultivars* but more commonly "varieties" or "strains," are developed via pollination of female plants by pollen from male plants. Rarely, it develops as a hermaphrodite with male and female flowers on the same plant. Moreover, the plant can reach a height of 16 ft (5 m), and it grows in a variety of habitats and altitudes. The active molecules, known as cannabinoids, as well as abundant terpenes and flavonoids are primarily produced by the female flowers. Generally, cannabis developed for medical purposes is cultivated as female plants that are propagated by cloning, cuttings from "mother" plants in hopes of uniform, stable production of specific chemotypes. Cultivars are grown indoors or in closed greenhouses as a way to control environmental conditions such as light, temperature, humidity, and chemical profile [4]. More recently, the combination of popularity of cannabis extracts, improvements in commercial manufacturing equipment, and methodology and evolution of cannabis production regulations has allowed for the emergence of significant commercial outdoor cultivation.

Differences Between C. *sativa* and C. *indica*

Cannabis taxonomy has been subject of a long debate. Whether separate species or subspecies, *Cannabis sativa*, subspecie *sativa* differs from *Cannabis indica*, subspecie *indica* mainly on its phenotypic characteristics and geographical origins. *Sativa* cultivars were originally cultivated for industrial use for fiber and for culinary utility in equatorial regions and are phenotypically characterized as tall plants with widely spaced branches and long thin leaves. Contrarily, *indica* cultivars are characteristically short plants with broader leaves, originating from mountainous regions in Southern Asia.

Interestingly, as anecdotal data primarily from non-medical use, consumers report *sativa*-predominant varieties to elicit uplifting, cerebral effects versus *indica*-predominant varieties that are associated with relaxation and analgesic effects. However, such anecdotal reporting has not been validated by any placebo-controlled studies or randomized controlled trials. It is also widely accepted that all commercial cultivars in North America are hybrids of *sativa* and *indica.* Traditionally, the phenotype and origin of the plant are unlikely to determine its therapeutic effects. This will depend only on the chemovar classification and main cannabinoid component, such as THC-predominant (chemotype I), THC-cannabidiol (CBD) balanced (chemotype II), and CBD-predominant (chemotype III) chemotypes [7, 8].

Terpenes, which are produced in the glandular trichomes of female flowers (small, hair-like glands), are responsible for cannabis odor and flavor and may also produce specific pharmacological effects [9]. A hypothesized, but widely referenced, theory,describes a potential *entourage effect* whereby cannabinoids and terpenes act synergistically to produce specific pharmacological effects and may contribute to the tolerability of certain cannabis cultivars [10].

Cannabinoids are synthetized in the glandular trichomes of female flowers [11] and include tetrahydrocannabinolic acid (THCA) and cannabidiolic acid (CBDA). Both compounds are progressively decarboxylated during maturation, especially during drying of cannabis flowers, and accelerated upon heating to convert into THC and CBD [12].

Cannabis Versus Hemp

Widely misunderstood, cannabis or "marijuana" and hemp are actually from the same cannabis plant species. *Hemp* is a term to describe a collection of cannabis cultivars with specific properties, namely, high production of fiber and seeds with minimal production of THC. The main differences between cannabis and hemp [6] are summarized in Table 5.1.

Table 5.1 Differences between cannabis (or "marijuana") and hemp

Characteristics	Cannabis (marijuana)	Hemp
Phenotype	Short plant and large flower production	Tall plant and small flower
Cannabinoid concentration	Traditionally, high-THC concentrations in flowers and, more recently, some high-CBD *cultivars* have been developed	THC must measure less than 0.3% w/w
Uses	Medical and non-medical or *recreational* use	Variety of commercial and industrial products such as fiber, textile, seeds, source of dietary fiber, omega-3 and omega-6, building material, and paper.
Legal status	Legalized in Canada since October 2018, cultivation controlled by a specific division of Health Canada. Still a Schedule 1 substance in the USA, legalized by many states both for medical and non-medical use	Legalized in Canada since 1998, cultivation requires a specific license from Health Canada. Recently legalized in the USA via the 2018 Farm Bill

The Endocannabinoid System (ECS)

The ECS is an interesting biological system composed of cannabinoid receptor proteins, such as CB1 and CB2, as well as endogenous lipid-based neurotransmitters known as endocannabinoids, such as *anandamide* (AEA) and *2-arachidonoylglycerol* (2-AG). THC acts as a partial agonist of the G protein-coupled cannabinoid receptors, CB1 and CB2, producing the majority of psychoactive and specific therapeutic effects of cannabis [13]. Conversely, CBD is a non-intoxicating phytocannabinoid that exerts other therapeutic properties and is still under study to better understand its pharmacological activity [14].

Key Terminology

A glossary of the most common and relevant terms for medical cannabis and related uses are presented in more detail below.

Cannabis
All plant materials, components, and derivative products of the cannabis plant, including flowers, leaves, seeds, stalks, and other materials and cannabis resins, extractions, and other derivative products.

Cannabis is listed in Schedule 1 of the Controlled Substances Act in the USA, reserved for substances with no currently accepted medical use and a high potential for abuse. The removal of cannabis from Schedule 1 has been proposed several times dating back to 1972.

Cannabinoid-based medicines or treatments
A general term used to describe therapeutic cannabis or cannabinoid-based products where cannabinoids are the primary active pharmaceutical ingredient. This term is applied regardless of origin as plant-derived or synthetic cannabinoids.

Cannabinoid-based medicines may be approved or unapproved medical treatments, but generally are regulated and legally accessible though availability of products is varied in different countries and jurisdictions.

Pharmaceutical or prescription cannabinoids
Cannabinoid-based treatments have been approved as medical treatments for specific indications. They must be prescribed by a licensed healthcare practitioner according to applicable local regulations and are available through pharmacies. In Canada, there are two products authorized as cannabinoid-based pharmacological treatments, nabilone (Cesamet®) and nabiximols (Sativex®), whereas in the USA, nabilone,

dronabinol (Marinol®), and Epidiolex® are available.

Medical cannabis
Cannabis-based treatments that have not been approved as medical treatments but have been legalized and regulated for patient access. Medical cannabis is differentiated from non-medical cannabis by a unique access program and a required medical authorization. Medical cannabis products may be available in many forms such as dried cannabis, cannabis extracts, oil, capsules, edibles, or topical products.

Cultivars (varieties, strains)
Distinct cultivars of the cannabis plant, having unique genetic signature and expressing distinct chemical composition. Colloquially referred to as strains.

Phytocannabinoids
Cannabinoids that are produced by the cannabis plant, primarily in the female flowers. More than 100 unique cannabinoids have been identified [15, 16].

Delta-9-tetrahydrocannabinol (THC)
THC is the primary cannabinoid in almost all strains of cannabis, and almost all therapeutic effects of cannabis can be attributed to THC. THC is the primary psychoactive and intoxicating agent and is responsible for most adverse effects related to cannabis use.

Cannabidiol (CBD)
CBD is usually the secondary cannabinoid found in cannabis; however recent research into its analgesic, anti-epileptic, anxiolytic, and anti-inflammatory properties has encouraged the selective breeding of cannabis strains with high concentration of CBD and minimal THC concentration.

Cannabinol (CBN)
The degradation molecule of both THC and CBD, CBN is often found in significant concentration in cannabis products that have been stored for several months. The effects of CBN have not been well-studied; however preclinical evidence suggests that it may produce sedating, mild psychoactive, and mild analgesic effects.

Cannabigerol (CBG)
The pre-cursor compound, CBG is a non-psychoactive cannabinoid found in higher concentration in immature cannabis plants. In addition, CBG is often found in higher concentrations in hemp plants and other low-THC cultivars. The effects have not been well-studied.

THC-A, CBD-A, etc.
Acidic forms of cannabinoids, existing in the natural plant or in "fresh" or "raw" unprocessed prior to decarboxylation via drying or manufacturing such as for oral administration products.

Terpenes
Aromatic compounds that exist in unique profiles in different strains. May provide some therapeutic benefit and may contribute to the varying effects of different strains of cannabis.

Some of the most common terpenes found in cannabis are D-limonene (commonly found in citrus essential oils), beta-myrcene, linalool (common to lavender), alpha-pinene, and beta-caryophyllene (common to black pepper) [9, 17].

Entourage effect
A proposed theory that cannabinoids and terpenes act synergistically to produce specific pharmacological effects and may contribute to the tolerability of certain cannabis cultivars [10].

Endocannabinoid system (ECS)
The body system made up of cannabinoid receptors, endogenous cannabinoids or *endocannabinoids*, and the enzymes that synthesize or degrade them. The ECS has been widely studied and has been identified as an important modulatory system to support homeostasis of many body functions including appetite, sleep, mood, memory, and pain sensation, among others [12, 13, 18].

Cannabinoid receptors
The group of receptor proteins that bind with endocannabinoids and phytocannabinoids. The most well-described are the G protein-coupled receptors CB1 and CB2, located in the central and peripheral nervous systems. Additionally, other receptors are known to bind endocannabinoids, often termed *orphan cannabinoid receptors.*

Endocannabinoids
The endogenous cannabinoids produced by the body and active at cannabinoid receptors. The most well-known endocannabinoids are anandamide (AEA) and 2-arachidonolyglycerol (2-AG) though several hundreds have been identified.

Cannabis Products and Accessories

Marijuana, Marihuana
The historical slang term *marihuana* or *marijuana* usually refers to dried cannabis of high-THC concentration. The term has recently been dropped from legal and regulatory legislation in Canada in favor of the term *cannabis*; however the use of the term continues globally and within social discussion.

Cannabis extracts
Highly concentrated preparations of cannabis which are produced via a variety of manufacturing techniques, such as cannabinoid and terpenoid supercritical CO2 extraction, and highly flammable solvents such as ethanol, isopropyl alcohol, butane, or hexane.

Concentrates (Hashish, Shatter, Dab, Wax) Slang terms for highly concentrated preparations of cannabis utilizing various methodologies. The potency of concentrates can be up to 90% THC by weight. Various methods of administration are used to inhale these products, but electronic pen-style vaporizers and glass bongs are common. Concentrates have gained popularity among recreational cannabis consumers [19] and should not be recommended for medical purposes [20].

Pipe or Bong
A pipe is a glass or metal device designed to combust or inhale cannabis smoke. Similarly, a bong is a glass smoking device which combines water with the cannabis smoke and may increase the cannabinoid potency.

Vaporizer
An electronic device designed to heat dried cannabis or cannabis extracts to specific temperature allowing for vaporization and required decarboxylation of active ingredients. Importantly, vaporizer temperatures stay well below the temperature of combustion limiting. Some vaporizers for dried cannabis have been recognized as medical devices [21, 22] and may be eligible for insurance coverage.

Recently, the use of unregulated, illicit cannabis extract vaporizers (also known as electronic cigarettes or vape pens) has produced serious adverse events including lung toxicity and even death [23, 24].

Conclusion

Understanding the general information about the cannabis plant and the basic terminology that describes medical cannabis and related uses is key for effective communication with patients and medical professionals. Once the main concepts are familiarized, clinicians are ready to move forward to explore other important areas of understanding such as the pharmacology of cannabinoid-based treatments and practical considerations for its safe use.

The cannabis plant has a fascinating history and unique, still understudied pharmacology. There is much discovery to be made in order to understand its therapeutic potential and relationship with the human body.

References

1. Pergam SA, Woodfield MC, Lee CM, Cheng G-S, Baker KK, Marquis SR, et al. Cannabis use among patients at a comprehensive cancer center in a state with legalized medicinal and recreational use. Cancer. 2017;123(22):4488–97.
2. Boehnke KF, Scott JR, Litinas E, Sisley S, Clauw DJ, Goesling J, et al. Cannabis use preferences and decision-making among a cross-sectional cohort of medical Cannabis patients with chronic pain. J Pain. 2019;20(11):1362–72.
3. Grof CPL. Cannabis, from plant to pill. Br J Clin Pharmacol. 2018;84(11):2463–7.
4. Klumpers LE, Thacker DLA. Brief background on Cannabis: from plant to medical indications. J AOAC Int. 2019;102(2):412–20.
5. Sawler J, Stout JM, Gardner KM, Hudson D, Vidmar J, Butler L, et al. The genetic structure of Marijuana and Hemp. PLoS One. 2015;10(8):e0133292.
6. ElSohly MA, Radwan MM, Gul W, Chandra S, Galal A. Phytochemistry of Cannabis sativa L. Prog Chem Org Nat Prod. 2017;103:1–36.
7. Lewis MA, Russo EB, Smith KM. Pharmacological Foundations of Cannabis Chemovars. Planta Med. 2018;84(4):225–33.
8. Russo EB. Current therapeutic Cannabis controversies and clinical trial design issues. Front Pharmacol. 2016;7:309.
9. Russo EB. Taming THC: potential cannabis synergy and phytocannabinoid-terpenoid entourage effects. Br J Pharmacol. 2011;163(7):1344–64.
10. Worth T. Unpicking the entourage effect. Nature. 2019;572:S12–3.
11. Livingston SJ, Quilichini TD, Booth JK, Wong DCJ, Rensing KH, Laflamme-Yonkman J, et al. Cannabis glandular trichomes alter morphology and metabolite content during flower maturation. Plant J. 2020;101(1):37–56.
12. Russo EB. Beyond Cannabis: plants and the endocannabinoid system. Trends Pharmacol Sci. 2016;37(7):594–605.
13. Di Marzo V, Piscitelli F. The endocannabinoid system and its modulation by phytocannabinoids. Neurotherapeutics. 2015;12(4):692–8.
14. Russo EB. Cannabidiol claims and misconceptions. Trends Pharmacol Sci. 2017;38(3):198–201.
15. Bridgeman MB, Abazia DT. Medicinal cannabis: history, pharmacology, and implications for the acute care setting. Pharm Therap. 2017;42(3):180.
16. Ahmed SA, Ross SA, Slade D, Radwan MM, Khan IA, ElSohly MA. Minor oxygenated cannabinoids from high potency Cannabis sativa L. Phytochemistry. 2015;117:194–9.
17. Booth JK, Bohlmann J. Terpenes in Cannabis sativa - from plant genome to humans. Plant Sci. 2019;284:67–72.
18. Mechoulam R, Parker LA. The endocannabinoid system and the brain. Annu Rev Psychol. 2013;64:21–47.
19. Sagar KA, Lambros AM, Dahlgren MK, Smith RT, Gruber SA. Made from concentrate? A national web survey assessing dab use in the United States. Drug Alcohol Depend. 2018;190:133–42.
20. Cavazos-Rehg PA, Krauss MJ, Sowles SJ, Floyd GM, Cahn ES, Chaitan VL, et al. Leveraging user perspectives for insight into cannabis concentrates. Am J Drug Alcohol Abuse. 2018;44(6):628–41.
21. Abrams DI, Vizoso HP, Shade SB, Jay C, Kelly ME, Benowitz NL. Vaporization as a smokeless cannabis delivery system: a pilot study. Clin Pharmacol Ther. 2007;82(5):572–8.
22. Hazekamp A, Ruhaak R, Zuurman L, van Gerven J, Verpoorte R. Evaluation of a vaporizing device (volcano) for the pulmonary administration of tetrahydrocannabinol. J Pharm Sci. 2006;95(6):1308–17.
23. Perrine CG, Pickens CM, Boehmer TK, King BA, Jones CM, DeSisto CL, et al. Characteristics of a multistate outbreak of lung injury associated with E-cigarette use, or vaping - United States, 2019. MMWR Morb Mortal Wkly Rep. 2019;68(39):860–4.
24. Dicpinigaitis PV, Trachuk P, Fakier F, Teka M, Suhrland MJ. Vaping-associated acute respiratory failure due to acute lipoid pneumonia. Lung. 2020;198(1):31–3.

Part II

Cannabinoids Pharmacology

The Endocannabinoid System

6

Glenn R. Rech and Samer N. Narouze

Introduction

The endocannabinoid system (ECS) present in all animals, including vertebrates (mammals, birds, reptiles, and fish) and invertebrates (sea urchins, leeches, mussels, nematodes, and others), arose in the phylogeny concurrently with the development of the nervous system [1]. The hydra (*H. vulgaris*), a cnidarian in the class Hydrozoa, is one of the first animals with a neural network. The major function of the ECS in this primitive organism was determined by De Petrocellis in 1999, to control its feeding response [2]. The ECS was discovered secondary to the discovery of the structure of the psychotropic phytocannabinoid, Δ-9-tetrahydrocannabinol (THC). Cannabinoid receptor 1 was found during the search for the biological target(s) for THC [3].

There are at least two types of cannabinoid receptors, CB1 and CB2; both are protein coupled. CB1 receptors are expressed predominantly at nerve terminals and mediate inhibition of transmitter release, whereas CB2 receptors are found mainly on immune cells. The ECS system also includes endogenous agonists for cannabinoid receptors. These endogenous agonists are synthesized on demand and removed from their sites of action by cellular uptake and intracellular enzymatic hydrolysis [4].

G. R. Rech (✉)
Western Reserve Hospital, Cuyahoga Falls, OH, USA

S. N. Narouze
Western Reserve Hospital, Center For Pain Medicine, Cuyahoga Falls, OH, USA
e-mail: narouzs@hotmail.com

Brief History of Cannabis and Hemp

The utilization of cannabis for pain can be traced back to ancient Chinese texts, dating to 2900 B.C. The *Shennong Ben Cao Jing*, a Chinese encyclopedia on agriculture and medicine, contains the oldest written record of cannabis as a medicine, recommending cannabis for constipation, rheumatic pain, female reproductive tract disorders, and malaria [5].

In terms of American history, it was reported that in 1492 Christopher Columbus brought cannabis as rope of hemp into the New World. Without hemp, Columbus would never have been able to discover the New World. The sails and ropes of his three ships were made of hemp. The cracks between the planks were filled with hemp to make the ships watertight. No other natural fiber can withstand the forces of the open ocean and the stresses of salt water. Moreover, the hold of his flagship, the Santa Maria, was filled with hemp seeds. These served not only as a protein-rich source of nutrition for the crew; they were being shipped so that hemp could be planted in any newly discovered regions. Furthermore, the ships' lamps were fueled using hemp oil, and these lamps allowed Columbus to read the Bible, the pages of which were made of hemp, in the

S. N. Narouze (ed.), *Cannabinoids and Pain*, https://doi.org/10.1007/978-3-030-69186-8_6

evening in his nightshirt, which was also made of hemp. In short, hemp was an essential part of Columbus's 7-month long sea voyage [6].

In 1619, Jamestown colony law declared that all settlers were required to grow cannabis. George Washington grew cannabis for fiber production at Mount Vernon as his primary crop.

Components of the Endocannabinoid System (ECS)

The ECS system is composed of receptors, transporters, and enzymes that support and control the various actions of endogenous cannabinoids (eCBs), both in the central nervous system and at the periphery. It is striking that at least 12 receptors are activated by eCBs in the same cell. both on the plasma membrane (where they can have an extracellular or an intracellular binding site) and in the nucleus [7].

The discovery of cannabinoid receptors, followed by endogenous cannabinoids and their regulatory metabolic and catabolic enzymes, led to the identification of the endocannabinoid system [8] (Table 6.1).

1. Cannabinoid receptors [CB1, CB2, and, the ionotropic cannabinoid receptor, transient receptor potential vanilloid 1 (TRPV1)]
2. Endogenous cannabinoids [or endocannabinoids, anandamide (AEA), and 2-arachidonoylglycerol (2-AG)]
3. The regulatory metabolic and catabolic enzymes [fatty acid amide hydrolase (FAAH), monoacylglycerol lipase (MAGL), and others]

Another recent article expresses the opinion of the composition of the ECS to include receptors with an extracellular binding site such as CB1 and CB2, as well as G protein-coupled orphan receptors (GCPRs) 55 and 119; receptors with an intracellular binding site such as transient receptor potential vanilloid 1 (TRPV1), TRPV2, TRPV3, TRPV4, TRPA1, and TRPM8; and transcription factors such as nuclear peroxisome proliferator-activated receptors (PPARs). Three subtypes of PPARs are known: PPAR-alpha, PPAR-delta, and PPAR-gamma [7].

Table 6.1 The endocannabinoid system

Components of the endocannabinoid system	
Cannabinoid receptors	CB1 and CB2 Transient receptor potential vanilloid 1 (TRPV1), TRPV2, TRPV3, TRPV4, TRPA1, and TRPM8 G protein-coupled orphan receptors (GCPRs): GCPR55 and GCPR119 Nuclear peroxisome proliferator-activated receptors (PPARs): PPAR-alpha, PPAR-delta, and PPAR-gamma
Endogenous cannabinoids (endocannabinoids)	Anandamide (AEA) 2-Arachidonoylglycerol (2-AG) 2-Arachidonyl glyceryl ether (2-AGE, Noladin ether) Virodhamine Palmitoylethanolamide N-Arachidonoyl dopamine N-Arachidonylglycine Oleamide Oleoylethanolamine
Transporters	Anandamide membrane transporter (AMT) Endocannabinoid membrane transporter (EMT)
Metabolic enzymes	Fatty acid amide hydrolase (FAAH) Monoacylglycerol lipase (MAGL)

eCBs and Their Signal Transduction Pathways

Both CB1 and CB2 receptors are members of the GPCR family. AEA and 2-AG, the two well-documented endogenous cannabinoids, possess distinct properties. AEA is a high-affinity partial agonist of CB1 receptors and almost inactive at CB2 receptors. 2-AG acts as a full agonist at both CB receptors with moderate to low affinity [9]. The basal level of 2-AG is approximately 1000 times higher than AEA in the brain [10]. In most cases, 2-AG is expressed in the postsynaptic membrane. It is then released into and traverses the extracellular space, by an unknown mechanism, where it binds to the CB1 receptor. Activated CB1 receptors suppress the release of neurotransmitters by inhibiting voltage-gated Ca2+ channels, reducing Ca2+ influx and inhibiting adenylyl cyclase, which reduces cAMP production. Both CB1 and CB2 receptors activate mitogen-activated protein kinase (MAPK) enzymes which are involved in a wide variety of vital signaling cascades in many cellular responses, including cell proliferation, migration, transformation, and death [11]. CB2 receptors, commonly referred to as "peripheral" cannabinoid receptors, are expressed mainly on immune cells, such as macrophages, CD4+ T cells, CD8+ T cells, B cells, natural killer cells, monocytes, and polymorphonuclear neutrophils. The extent of their expression in healthy central nervous system tissue is quite controversial [12].

Complexity of the Endogenous Cannabinoid System

Receptor-mediated activation by eCBs depends on their cellular concentration, which in turn depends on a balance between synthesis and degradation operated by different biosynthetic and hydrolytic enzymes. ECBs have a short (approximately 15 minutes) period of activity [7]. Metabolic enzymes and transporters are responsible for their timely delivery at the right concentration and to the right target within the cell (Fig. 6.1). CB2 receptors have been found on microglia cells. Microglia are derived from macrophages and can be viewed as the resident immune cells of the brain where they monitor the brain for pathological damage. In response to specific signals within the brain, they transition between different states of activity. The expression of CB2 receptors depends on the activation state of the cell [12].

Interestingly, cannabidiol (CBD) does not activate CB1 or CB2 receptors, which likely accounts for its lack of psychotropic activity. However, CBD interacts with many other signaling systems, including the orphan GPCR and GPR55 receptors [13].

CB_1 and CB_2 Receptor

The discovery in 1990 that an orphan G protein-coupled receptor (SKR6) derived from a rat cerebral cortex mediates pharmacological effects of THC established the identity of the first cannabinoid receptor CB1 [14]. In 1993, a G protein-coupled receptor (CX5) expressed in the human promyelocytic leukemic cell line HL60 was as a second cannabinoid receptor and named CB2 [15]. Both CB1 and CB2 are G protein-coupled receptors (GPCR), also called seven-transmembrane receptor. Protein located in the cell membrane binds extracellular substances and transmits signals from these substances to an intracellular molecule called a G protein (guanine nucleotide-binding protein). CB_1 receptors are densely populated in the nervous system, substantia nigra, pars reticulata, and globus pallidus [16]. CB2 receptors have been located mainly on immune cells [12].

Other Receptors

If we include components that respond to endogenous endocannabinoids, the non-selective cationic channel type-1 vanilloid receptor (transient receptor potential vanilloid 1, TRPV1), usually activated by capsaicin, heat, and acid, should be included. TRPV1 is activated by AEA, but not 2-AG [17].

Peroxisome proliferator-activated receptors (PPARs) are import modulators of cellular metabolism in metabolically active tissues including liver and adipose tissue. PPARs are nuclear receptors which, when activated, transactivate target genes involved in metabolic regulation, energy homeostasis, and cell differentiation. The cannabinoid AEA can bind to PPARα [18].

GPR55 has been labeled as an orphan cannabinoid receptor. The status of GPR55 as a cannabinoid receptor is controversial. GPR55 is abundantly expressed in large-diameter dorsal root ganglion (DRG) neurons [19].

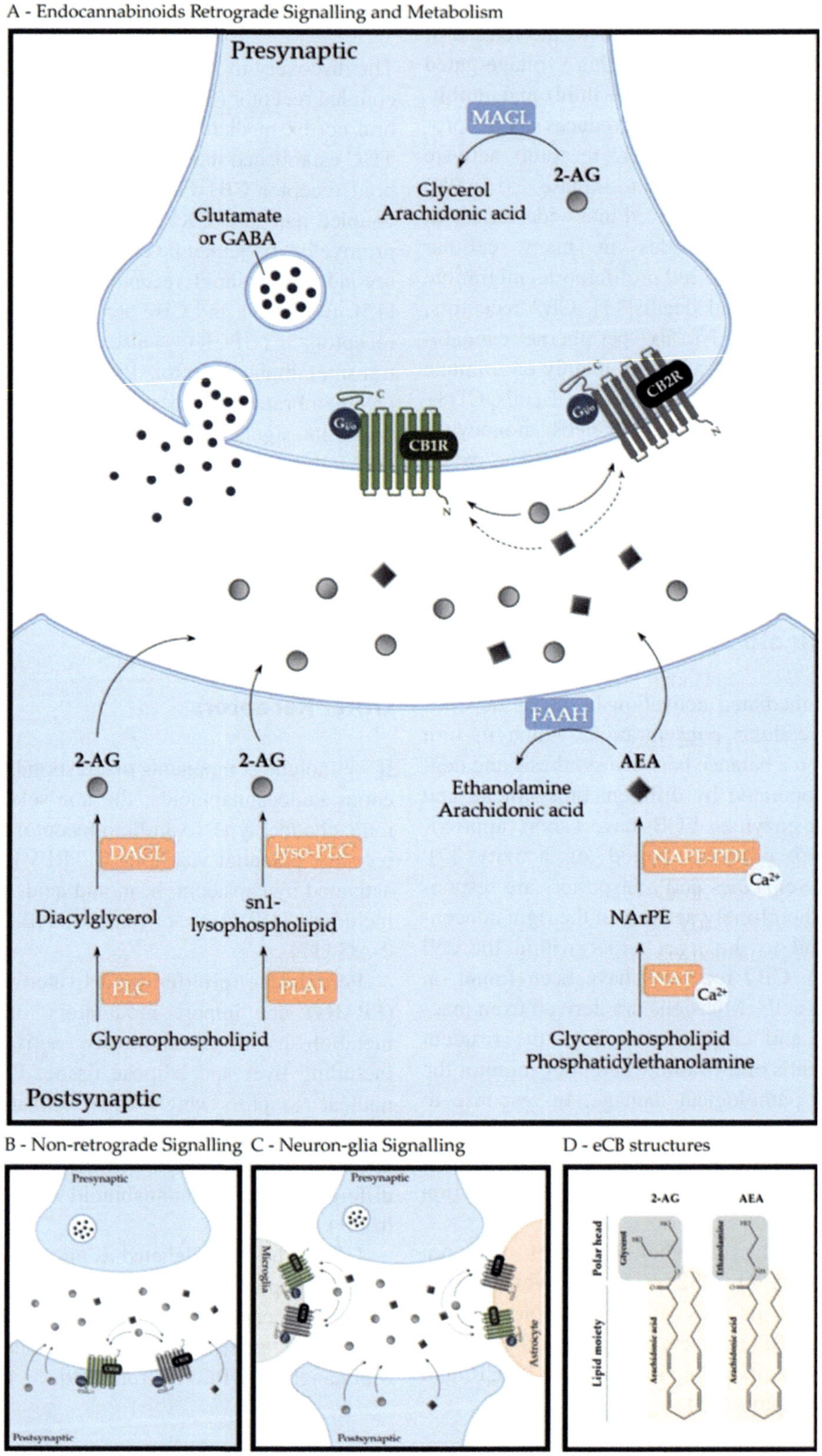
A - Endocannabinoids Retrograde Signalling and Metabolism
Presynaptic
MAGL
2-AG
Glycerol
Arachidonic acid
Glutamate
or GABA
CB1R
CB2R
FAAH
2-AG
2-AG
AEA
Ethanolamine
Arachidonic acid
DAGL
lyso-PLC
NAPE-PDL
Ca2+
Diacylglycerol
sn1-
lysophospholipid
NArPE
PLC
PLA1
NAT
Ca2+
Glycerophospholipid
Glycerophospholipid
Phosphatidylethanolamine
Postsynaptic
B - Non-retrograde Signalling
Presynaptic
Postsynaptic
C - Neuron-glia Signalling
Presynaptic
Microglia
Astrocyte
Postsynaptic
D - eCB structures
2-AG
AEA
Polar head
Lipid moiety
Glycerol
Ethanolamine
Arachidonic acid
Arachidonic acid

Fig. 6.1 The endocannabinoid signaling and metabolism. (**a**) 2-Arachidonoglycerol (2-AG) is synthesized by two different metabolic pathways: via the cleavage of diacylglycerol by diacylglycerol lipase (DAGL), where diacylglycerol is released from membrane phospholipids by phospholipase C (PLC), or via the action of phospholipase A1 (PLA1), releasing an sn-1 lysophospholipid from membrane phospholipids, which is cleaved by lyso-PLC in order to generate 2-AG. On the other hand, a calcium-dependent trans-acylase (NAT) acts on glycerophospholipids and phosphatidylethanolamine, resulting in N-arachidonoyl-phosphatidylethanolamine (NArPE), which is then cleaved by a calcium-dependent NAPE (N-acyl-phosphatidylethanolamine)-specific phospholipase D (NAPE-PLD), releasing N-arachidonoylethanolamine (anandamide, AEA) from membrane lipids. While hydrolysis of AEA occurs postsynaptically, via fatty acid amide hydrolase (FAAH) into arachidonic acid and ethanolamine, 2-AG is hydrolyzed by monoacylglycerol lipase (MAGL) into arachidonic acid and glycerol presynaptically. AEA and 2-AG are usually synthesized postsynaptically and are released "on demand" to the synaptic cleft, where they modulate presynaptic glutamatergic or GABAergic signaling by binding to CB1R or CB2R. (**b**) Non-retrograde signaling. AEA and 2-AG signal autocrinally and non-retrogradely the postsynaptic neuron, modulating synaptic transmission. (**c**) Neuron-glia signaling. Endocannabinoids produced by neurons can bind to the cannabinoid receptors expressed in astrocytes and microglia. This neuron-glia signaling is able to modulate several responses. (**d**) eCB structures. 2-AG and AEA have similar molecular structures. They are both polar ester lipids formed by the bond of the omega-6 fatty acid arachidonic acid with either glycerol (to form 2-AG) or ethanolamine (to form AEA). (Source: https://www.ncbi.nlm.nih.gov/corecgi/tileshop/tileshop.fcgi?p=PMC3&id=442443&s=87&r=4&c=3. Rodrigues RS, et al. Cannabinoid Actions on Neural Stem Cells: Implications for Pathophysiology. Molecules. 2019 Apr 5;24(7):1350. doi: https://doi.org/10.3390/molecules24071350. This article is an open-access article distributed under the terms and conditions of the Creative Commons Attribution (CC BY) license (http://creativecommons.org/licenses/by/4.0/))

Transporters

The eCBs, anandamide (AEA), and 2-arachidonoylglycerol (2-AG) activate cell-surface CB1 and CB2 receptors and additional intracellular CB receptors [20]. In the brain, Wilson and Nicoll identified eCBs as retrograde signaler, involving these retrograde messengers that locally initiate a signaling cascade in the presynaptic axon terminal [21]. How do these eCBs move to locations of activity? Early observations suggest that eCBs are accumulated via a transporter. These carriers have been labeled anandamide membrane transporter (AMT) or endocannabinoid membrane transporter (EMT) [22].

Enzymes

2-AG and AEA are enzymatically hydrolyzed by fatty acid amide hydrolase (FAAH) or monoacylglycerol lipase (MAGL). For AEA, the principal metabolic pathway is hydrolysis to arachidonic acid by an enzyme fatty acid amide hydrolase (FAAH). 2-AG can be metabolized by FAAH; however in the brain MAGL is the more important enzyme [23].

Physiological Actions of ECS

The presence of ECS in vertebrates, mammals, and humans implies a role in several physiological processes, including appetite, cancer, cardiovascular diseases, fertility, immune functions, memory, reward, coordination, temperature control, neuroprotection, and pain modulation [17] (Fig. 6.2).

The regulation of pain is one of the earliest medical requests of the cannabinoids. Numerous studies have documented the analgesic effects of cannabinoids in various types of pain, including chemical, mechanical, thermal, neuropathic, and inflammatory pain [24].

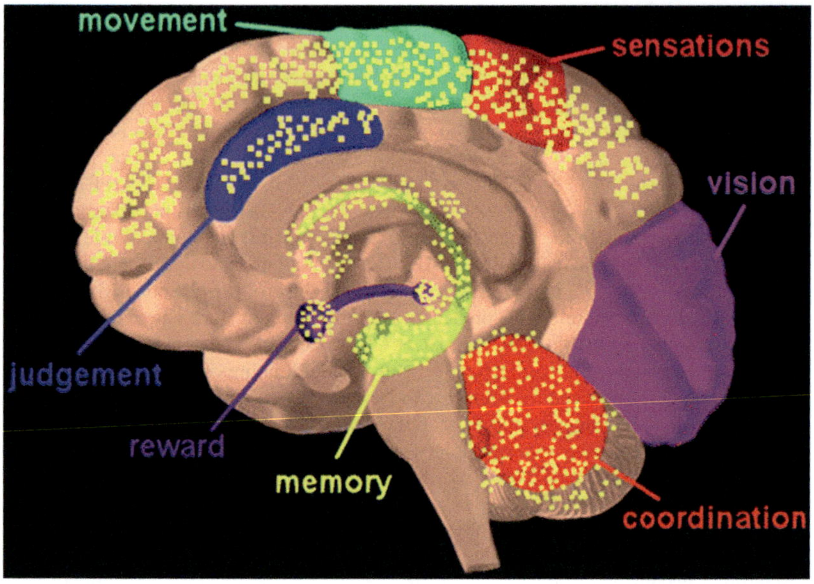

Fig. 6.2 Endocannabinoid system functions. https://www.drugabuse.gov/sites/default/files/thc_brain.gif

In approximately 30 years, the endogenous cannabinoid system has been discovered, components identified and isolated, and characterized physiologic properties. Antinociceptive properties have been allocated to the main cannabinoid receptors, CB1 and CB2. Further research is essential to characterize the integration of the ECS within the pain model.

References

1. Silver RJ. The endocannabinoid system of animals. Animals. 2019;9:686.
2. De Petrocellis L, Melck D, Bisogno T, Miline A, Marzo V. Finding of the endocannabinoid signaling system in Hydra, a very primitive organism: possible role in the feeding response. Neuroscience. 1999;92:377–87.
3. Gaoni Y, Mechoulam R. Isolation structure and partial synthesis of an active constituent of hashish. J Am Chem Soc. 1964;86:1646–7.
4. Pertwee R. The therapeutic potential of drugs that target cannabinoid receptors or modulate the tissue levels or actions of endocannabinoids. AAPS J. 2005;7:E625–54.
5. Touw M. The religious and medicinal uses for cannabis in China, India and Tibet. J Psychoactive Drugs. 1981;13:23–4.
6. Columbus and Cannabis. https://hashmuseum.com/en/collection/columbus-and-cannabis. Retrieved on July 11, 2020.
7. Maccarrone M. Missing pieces to the endocannabinoid puzzle. Trends Mol Med. 2019;26(3):263–72. https://doi.org/10.1016/j.molmed.2019.11.002.
8. Pacher P, Kunos G. Modulating the endocannabinoid system in human health and disease- successes and failures. FEBS J. 2013;280(9):1918–43. https://doi.org/10.1111/febs.12260.
9. Pertwee RG, Howlett AC, Abood ME, Alexander SPH, DiMarzo V, Elphick MR, Greasley PJ, et al. International Union of basic and clinical pharmacology. LXXIX. Cannabinoid receptors and their ligands: beyond CB1 and CB2. Pharmacol Rev. 2010;62:588–631.
10. Zou S, Kumar U. Cannabinoid receptors and the endocannabinoid system: signaling and function in the central nervous system. Int J Mol Sci. 2018;19(3):833. https://doi.org/10.3390/ijms19030833.
11. Dhopeshwarkar A, Mackie K. CB2 cannabinoid receptors as a therapeutic target. What does the future hold? Mol Pharmacol. 2014;86(4):430–7. https://doi.org/10.1124/mol.114.094649.
12. Atwood BK, Mackie K. CB2: a cannabinoid receptor with an identity crisis. Br J Pharmacol. 2010;160(3):467–79. https://doi.org/10.1111/j.1476-5381.2010.00729.x.
13. Devinsky O, Cilio MR, Cross H, Fernandez-Ruiz J, et al. Cannabidiol: pharmacology and potential therapeutic role in epilepsy and other neuropsychiatric disorders. Epilepsia. 2014;55(6):791–802. https://doi.org/10.1111/epi.12631.
14. Matsuda LA, Lolait SJ, Brownstein MJ, Young AC, Bonner TI. Structure of a cannabinoid receptor and functional expression of the cloned cDNA. Nature. 1990;346(6284):561–4. https://doi.org/10.1038/346561a0.

15. Munro S, Thomas KL, Abu-Shaar M. Molecular characterization of a peripheral receptor for cannabinoids. Nature. 1993;365(6441):61–5. https://doi.org/10.1038/365061a0.
16. Herkenham M, Lynn AB, Little MD, Johnson MR, Melvin LS, de Costa BR, Rice KC. Cannabinoid receptor localization in brain. Proc Natl Acad Sci U S A. 1990;87(5):1932–6. https://doi.org/10.1073/pnas.87.5.1932.
17. Battista N, Di Tommaso M, Bari M, Maccarrone M. The endocannabinoid system: an overview. Front Behav Neurosci. 2012;6:9. https://doi.org/10.3389/fnbeh.2012.00009. eCollection 2012
18. Dalton GD, Bass CE, Van Horn CG, Howlett AC. Signal transduction via cannabinoid receptors. CNS Neurol Disord Drug Targets. 2009;8(6):422–31.
19. Lauckner JE, Jensen JB, Chen HY, Lu CH, Hille B, Mackie K. GPR55 is a cannabinoid receptor that increases intracellular calcium and inhibits M current. Proc Natl Acad Sci U S A. 2008;105(7):2699–704. https://doi.org/10.1073/pnas.0711278105.
20. Fowler CJ. Transport of endocannabinoids across the plasma membrane and within the cell. FEBS J. 2013;280(9):1895–904. https://doi.org/10.1111/febs.12212.
21. Wilson RI, Nicoll RA. Endogenous cannabinoids mediate retrograde signalling at hippocampal synapses. Nature. 2001;410(6828):588–92. https://doi.org/10.1038/35069076.
22. Di Marzo V, Fontana A, Cadas H, Schinelli S, Cimino G, Schwartz J-C, Plomelli D. Formation and inactivation of endogenous cannabinoid anandamide in central neurons. Nature. 1994;372(6507):686–91. https://doi.org/10.1038/372686a0.
23. Ghafouri N, Tiger T, Razdan R, Mahadevan A, Pertwee R, Martin B, Fowler C. Inhibition of Monoacylglycerol Lipase and fatty acid amide hydrolase by analogues of 2-Arachidonoylglycerol. Br J Pharmacol. 2004;143(6):774–84. https://doi.org/10.1038/sj.bjp.0705948.
24. Donvito G, Nass ST, Wilkerson JI, Curry ZA, et al. The endogenous cannabinoid system: a budding source of targets for treating inflammatory and neuropathic pain. Neuropsychopharmacology. 2018;43(1):52–79. https://doi.org/10.1038/npp.2017.204.

Cannabinoid Receptor 1 (CB1)

7

Glenn R. Rech and Samer N. Narouze

CB1 Receptors

The CB1 receptor was discovered after the isolation of Δ-9-tetrahydrocannabinol (THC), the main psychoactive component of marijuana [1]. CB1 is encoded by the gene CNR1, located on chromosome 6, and consists of 472 amino acids in humans (Fig. 7.1). CB1 along with CB2 belongs to the superfamily of G protein-coupled receptors (GPCRs). These receptors are characterized by a conserved structure consisting of an extracellular N-terminal domain, seven transmembrane domains, and a C-terminal intracellular tail (Fig. 7.2). When CB1 receptors are activated, adenylyl cyclase is inhibited, mitogen-associated protein kinase is activated, and calcium and potassium ion channels are regulated by signaling through $G_{i/o}$ proteins [2]. CB1 was first discovered in the brain. Later, by using autoradiography, in situ hybridization, and immunohistochemistry, CB1 was proven to be the most widely expressed receptor protein from the GPCR family in the brain [3]. Ligand binding sites for CB1 are distributed widely in the brain at various levels depending on the regions and the neuron types within a given region. High levels are observed in the innermost layers of the olfactory bulb, hippocampus, lateral part of the striatum, target nuclei of the striatum (i.e., globus pallidus, entopeduncular nucleus, substantia nigra pars reticulata), and cerebellar molecular layer. The thalamus, other nuclei in the brain stem, and spinal ventral horn are low in ligand binding. Generally low levels of ligand binding in the lower brain stem areas that control cardiovascular and respiratory functions may explain why high doses of cannabinoids are not lethal [4].

The CB1 receptors are also expressed in the peripheral nervous system. In the peripheral nervous system, the CB1 receptors are mostly expressed in the sympathetic nerve terminals. Agonists binding to the CB1 receptors are associated with the cardiovascular system: promote pro-inflammatory effects [5]. Likewise agonist binding to the CB1 receptors expressed within the gastrointestinal tract may contribute to obesity. CB1 receptors are also found in the liver, muscles, bones, reproductive system, and skin [5].

CB1 Receptor Physiology, Pathology, and Pharmacology

Like many GPCRs, the CB1 receptors are primarily located in the cell membrane where they are activated by their ligands. However considerable observations have reported predominant intracellular localization of CB1 receptors in

G. R. Rech (✉)
Western Reserve Hospital, Cuyahoga Falls, OH, USA

S. N. Narouze
Western Reserve Hospital, Center For Pain Medicine, Cuyahoga Falls, OH, USA
e-mail: narouzs@hotmail.com

S. N. Narouze (ed.), *Cannabinoids and Pain*, https://doi.org/10.1007/978-3-030-69186-8_7

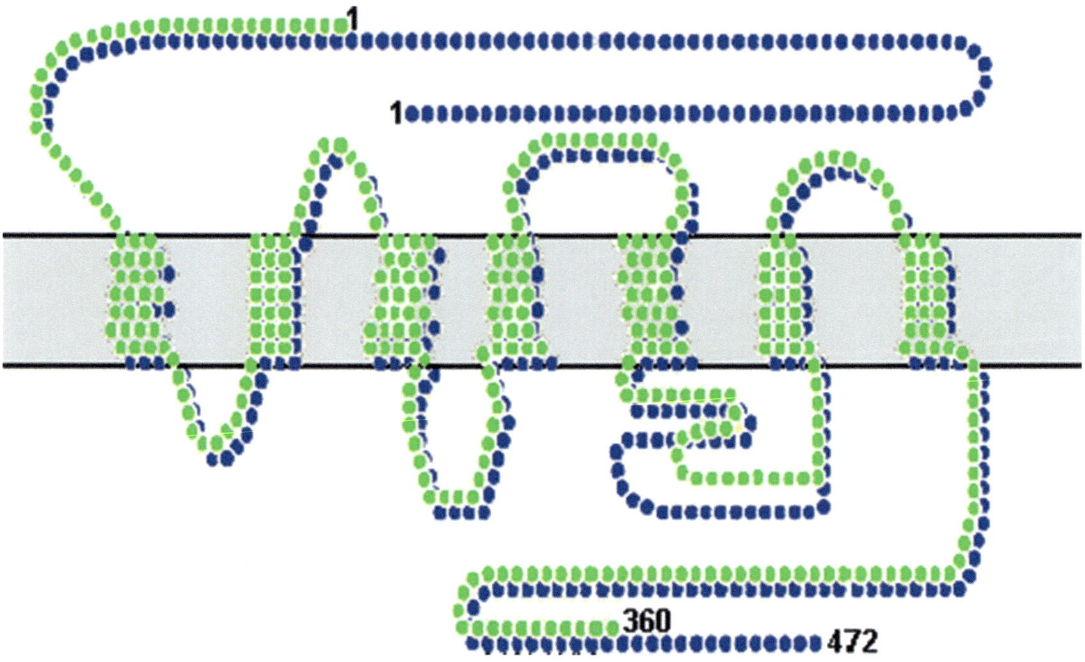

Fig. 7.1 CB1 receptor, blue, and CB2 receptor, green. https://commons.wikimedia.org/wiki/File:Cb1_cb2_structure.png

diverse cell types. Following agonist stimulation, the CB1 receptors are endocytosed and targeted for degradation [6]. Clathrin, a protein described as a triskelion with three kinked legs that radiate from a central vertex, provides a pit for invagination of the plasma receptor, placing them into the cellular cytoplasm [7]. Additionally, diverse intracellular localization of endogenously expressed CB1 receptors was reported in studies using antibodies that recognize an N-terminal epitope of the receptor [2].

The level and duration of CB1 signaling activity are regulated by the two distinct processes of desensitization and endocytosis. Desensitization begins within seconds of agonist exposure and involves phosphorylation of agonist-activated receptors by GPCR kinases. β-arrestin 1 and β-arrestin 2 immediately bind to the agonist-occupied, phosphorylated GPCR which prevents G protein-mediated signal transduction, while the GPCR-arrestin complex associates with clathrin to initiate GPCR endocytosis [2] (Fig. 7.3).

CB1 signaling involvement has also been discovered from within neuronal cells. Cannabinoid receptor-interacting protein 1a ($CRIP_{1a}$) binds to the CB1 receptor C-terminus and can attenuate constitutive CB1 receptor-mediated inhibition of Ca^{2+} channel activity. Thus, CRIP1a appears to act as a broad negative regulator of CB1 receptor function [8].

CB1 Signaling

CB1 receptors are located mainly on the presynaptic terminal. The presynaptic localization indicates that cannabinoids modulate neurotransmitter release from axon terminals. The effect of cannabinoids on synaptic function consists of inhibition of release of a variety of neurotransmitters as well as the electrical activity accompanying depolarization. The neurotransmitters whose release is inhibited by activation of cannabinoid receptors include L-glutamate, GABA, noradrenaline, dopamine,

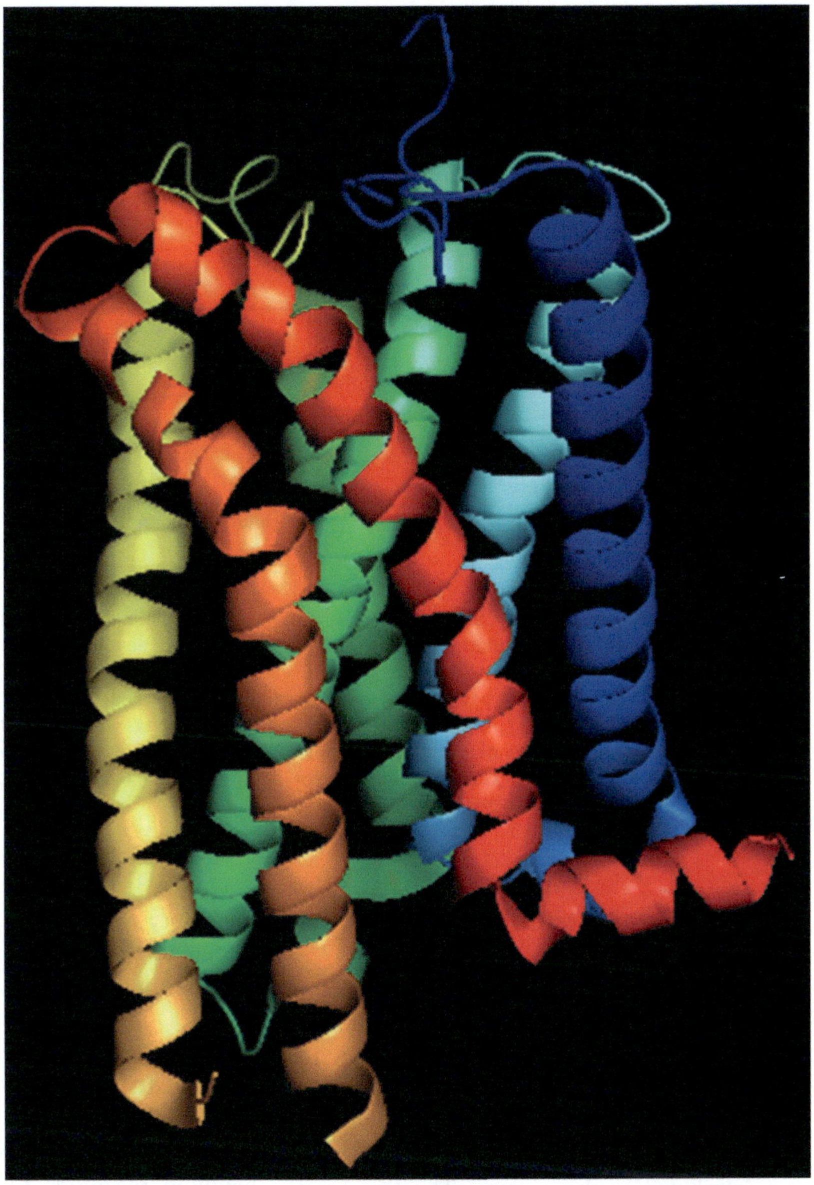

Fig. 7.2 CB1 receptor. https://commons.wikimedia.org/wiki/File:Cannabinoid_CB1_Receptor.png

serotonin, and acetylcholine [9]. Therefore, depending on the state of the presynaptic terminal, endocannabinoids induce either suppression of inhibition or suppression of excitation, namely, depolarization-induced suppression of inhibition (DSI) or depolarization-induced suppression of excitation (DSE). DSI is a form of fast retrograde signaling from postsynaptic neurons back to inhibitory cells that innervate them [10]. DSE, likewise, is a form of fast retrograde signaling from postsynaptic neurons back to excitatory cells that innervate them [11].

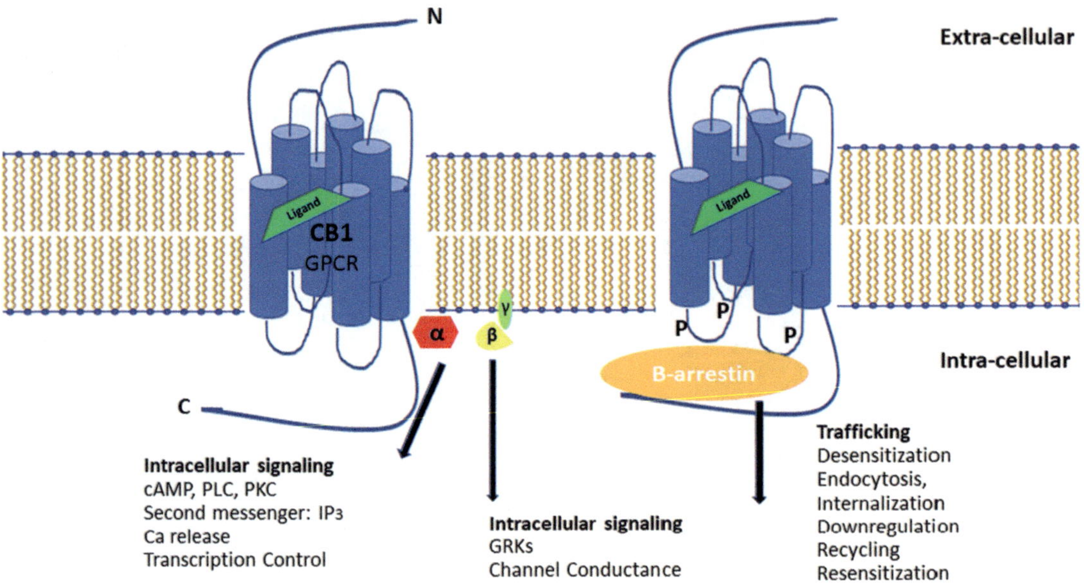

Fig. 7.3 CB1 receptor signaling and biased agonism. Upon agonist binding and stimulation of cannabinoid receptors, G proteins dissociate into α and βγ subunits activating intracellular signaling pathways. G protein-coupled receptor kinases (GRKs) phosphorylate the intracellular domains of agonist-activated G protein-coupled receptors. The phosphorylated (P) cannabinoid receptor-β-arrestin complex initiates endocytosis, internalization, and desensitization. Modified from Howlett and Abood [18]. cAMP, cyclic adenosine monophosphate; CB1, cannabinoid receptor type 1; DAG, diacylglycerol; GPCR, G protein-coupled receptor; GRKs, G protein- coupled receptor kinases; IP3, inositol triphosphate; PKC, protein kinase C; PLC, phospholipase C. Used with permission from Samer Narouze, MD, PhD

CB1 Receptor Distribution

Understanding the distribution of CB1 receptors has proved helpful to both predict and understand the effects of cannabinoids. For example, the high CB1 receptor levels found in the cortex, basal ganglia, and cerebellum coincide with the prominent effects cannabinoids have on functions attributed to these areas. The low levels present in the medullary nuclei responsible for regulating respiration are consistent with the limited effects cannabinoids have on the respiratory center [4].

Neocortex

In the neocortex, almost all neurons expressing CB1 at high or moderate levels are likely to be inhibitory due to the tight correlation between glutamate decarboxylase and CB1 mRNA expression [12].

Hippocampus

The hippocampus expresses high levels of cannabinoid receptors. One of the most common effects of cannabinoid intoxication in humans and animals is the impairment of spatial working memory due to activation of astroglial CB1 receptors. The proposed process is described by activation of the astroglial CB1 receptor to increase ambient glutamate, which in turn activates NR2B-containing N-methyl-D-aspartate receptors (NMDAR). Activation of NR2B-containing NMDAR triggers α-amino-3-hydroxy-5-methyl-isoxazole propionic acid receptor (AMPAR) internalization at CA3-CA1 synapses. These events ultimately induce long-term depression of synaptic CA3-CA1 firing and spatial working memory (SWM) [13, 14].

Hypothalamic

Hypothalamic pro-opiomelanocortin (POMC) neurons promote satiety. CB1 receptors are critical for central regulation of food intake. POMC neurons have been considered as key drivers of cessation of feeding. CB1 activation increases feeding, and notably, CB1 activation also promotes neuronal activity of POMC cells. This paradoxical increase in POMC activity was crucial for CB1-induced feeding because designer-receptors-exclusively-activated-by-designer-drugs (DREADD)-mediated inhibition of POMC neurons diminishes, whereas DREADD-mediated activation of POMC neurons enhances CB1-driven feeding. The POMC gene encodes both the anorexigenic peptide α-melanocyte-stimulating hormone and the opioid peptide β-endorphin. CB1 activation selectively increases β-endorphin but not α-melanocyte-stimulating hormone release in the hypothalamus. Noteworthy, naloxone, an opioid receptor antagonist, blocked acute CB1 receptor activation-induced feeding [15].

CB1 activation had a bimodal effect, in which lower doses of the CB1 agonist, ACEA, induced depolarization of POMC neurons (200 nM), while higher doses hyperpolarized these cells (1 μM) [15]. Using immunolabeling, CB1 receptors were detected in both GABAergic and glutamatergic presynaptic terminals of POMC neurons.

Midbrain Periaqueductal Gray; Brain Stem Rostral Ventromedial Medulla

The midbrain PAG is part of the descending inhibitory system responsible for inhibiting pain processing at the spinal cord level. The PAG sends mono-synaptic projections to the rostral ventromedial medulla (RVM) modulating ON- and OFF-cells. When activated these cells are responsible, respectively, for facilitating and inhibiting pain at the spinal cord level [16]. This PAG-RVM circuitry expresses several neurotransmitters systems; among them is the cannabinoid system [17].

CB1 receptors, the most abundant cannabinoid receptor, are present in nervous system areas involved in modulating nociception, and evidence supports a role of the endocannabinoids in pain modulation. However, widespread distribution accompanied by expression on various presynaptic neuron clouds research on antinociceptive agents.

Tolerance

Cannabinoid tolerance develops in the absence of pharmacokinetic changes. Therefore, biochemical and/or cellular changes are responsible for this adaptation [18]. One hypothesis for tolerance development is that receptors lose function during chronic agonist stimulation. The phenomenon of receptor downregulation has been observed with cannabinoid receptors. A comprehensive study examining the time course of changes in cannabinoid-stimulated [^{35}S]GTPγS binding and cannabinoid receptor binding in both rat brain sections and membranes, following daily Δ^9-THC treatments for 3, 7, 14, and 21 days, found time-dependent decreases in both [^{35}S]GTPγS binding and [^{3}H]WIN 55212-2 and [^{3}H]SR141716 binding in the cerebellum, hippocampus, caudate-putamen, and globus pallidus, with regional differences in the rate and magnitude of downregulation and desensitization [19]. β-arrestin 2 regulates CB1 receptor signaling and adaptation in a central nervous system region-dependent manner [20, 21].

CB1 receptor downregulation following chronic cannabis exposure in humans has also been reported using positron emission tomography [22]. Interestingly, regional specificity of downregulation was also observed in cannabis-dependent people, with reduction in cortical areas but not in non-cortical areas [23]. The receptor downregulation correlated with years of cannabis smoking and was reversible upon cessation. The authors concluded that cortical CB1 cannabinoid receptor downregulation is a neuro-adaptation that may promote cannabis dependence in human brain [22, 23].

CB1 Receptor Ligands

CB1 receptor ligands are summarized in Table 7.1.

Ligands affect CB1 differently than CB2 and point to principles that could inform rational and selective drug design. The yin-yang relationship of CB1 and CB2 will facilitate the design of selective drugs [24] (Fig. 7.4).

Table 7.1 Cannabinoid receptor 1 (CB1) ligands

Agonists	Full	Endocannabinoid	2-Arachidonoylglycerol (2-AG)
		Synthetic	AM-2201 CP 55,940 JWH-018 WIN 55,212-2
	Partial	Endocannabinoid	Anandamide (AEA) 2-Arachidonyl glyceryl ether (2-AGE, noladin ether)
		Phytogenic	Tetrahydrocannabinol (THC)
		Synthetic	JWH-073
	Selective	Endocannabinoid	Oleamide
		Phytogenic	Epigallocatechin (EGCG) Epicatechin Kavain Yangonin
	Unspecified efficacy	Endocannabinoid	N-Arachidonoyl dopamine (NADA)
		Phytogenic	Cannabinol 11-Hydroxy-THC (THC metabolite)
		Synthetic	Levonantradol HU-210 Minocycline
Allosteric modulators	NAM	Endocannabinoid	Pregnenolone Pepcan-12
		Phytogenic	Cannabidiol (CBD)
		Synthetic	Fenofibrate GAT100 GAT228 PSNCBAM-1 RVD-Hpα
	PAM	Endocannabinoid	Lipoxin A4
		Synthetic	ZCZ-011
Inverse agonists		Synthetic	Rimonabant Taranabant
Antagonists		Endocannabinoid	Virodhamine
		Phytogenic	Cannabigerol (CBG) Tetrahydrocannabivarin (THCV)
		Synthetic	Ibipinabant Otenabant

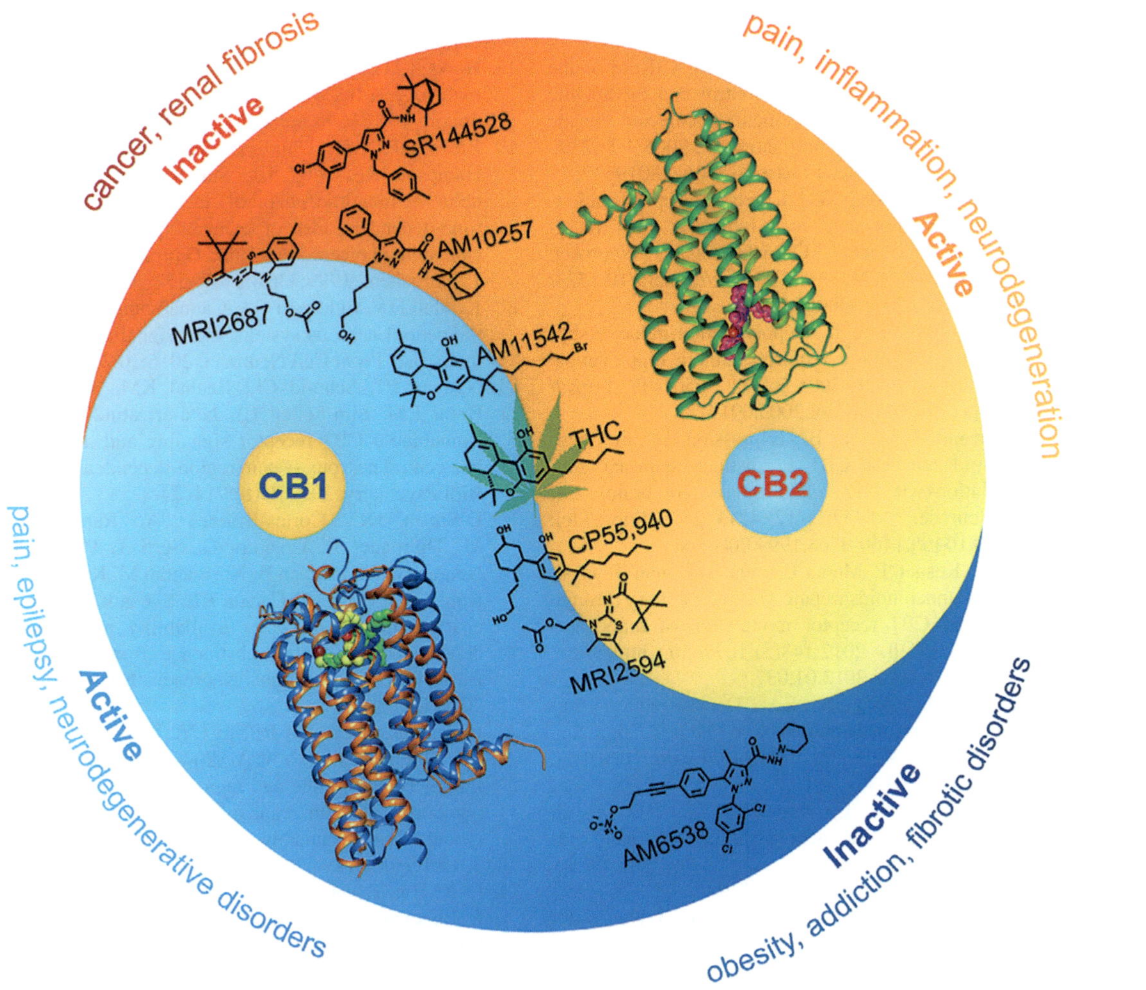

Fig. 7.4 The yin-yang relationship of CB2 and CB1 receptors. Ligands affect CB2 differently than CB1 receptors. (Adopted from Li X et al., Ref. [24], with permission)

References

1. Matsuda LA, Lolait SJ, Brownstein MJ, Young AC, Bonner TI. Structure of a cannabinoid receptor and functional expression of the cloned cDNA. Nature. 1990;346(6284):561–4. https://doi.org/10.1038/346561a0.
2. Howlett AC, Blume LC, Dalton GD. CB1 Cannabinoid receptors and their associated proteins. Curr Med Chem. 2010;17(14):1382–93. https://doi.org/10.2174/092986710790980023.
3. Kano M, Ohno-Shosaku T, Uchigashima Y, Watanabe M, Hashimotodani M. Endocannabinoid-mediated control of synaptic transmission. Physiol Rev. 2009;89(1):309–80. https://doi.org/10.1152/physrev.00019.2008.
4. Mackie K. Distribution of Cannabinoid receptors in the central and peripheral nervous system. Handb Exp Pharmacol. 2005;(168):299–325. https://doi.org/10.1007/3-540-26573-2_10.
5. Pacher P, Kunos G. Modulating the endocannabinoid system in human health and disease- successes and failures. FEBS J. 2013;280(9):1918–43. https://doi.org/10.1111/febs.12260.
6. Rozenfeld R. Type 1 Cannabinoid receptor trafficking: all roads lead to lysosome. Traffic. 2011;12(1):12–8. https://doi.org/10.1111/j.1600-0854.2010.01130.x.
7. Royle SJ. The cellular functions of clathrin. Cell Mol Life Sci. 2006;63(16):1823–32. https://doi.org/10.1007/s00018-005-5587-0.
8. Smith TH, Blume LC, Straiker A, Cox JO, et al. Cannabinoid receptor-interacting protein 1a modulates CB1 receptor signaling and regulation.

Mol Pharmacol. 2015;87(4):747–65. https://doi.org/10.1124/mol.114.096495.
9. Manzanares J, Julian M, Carrascosa A. Role of the cannabinoid system in pain control and therapeutic implications for the management of acute and chronic pain episodes. Curr Neuropharmacol. 2006;4(3):239–57. https://doi.org/10.2174/157015906778019527.
10. Kreitzer AC, Regehr WG. Cerebellar depolarization-induced suppression of inhibition is mediated by endogenous Cannabinoids. J Neurosci. 2001;21(20):RC174. https://doi.org/10.1523/JNEUROSCI.21-20-j0005.2001.
11. Straiker A, Mackie K. Depolarization-induced suppression of excitation in murine autaptic hippocampal neurons. J Physiol. 2005;569(Pt 2):501–17. https://doi.org/10.1113/jphysiol.2005.091918.
12. Marsicano G, Lutz B. Expression of the cannabinoid receptor CB1 in distinct neuronal subpopulations in the adult mouse forebrain. Eur J Neurosci. 1999;11(12):4213–25. https://doi.org/10.1046/j.1460-9568.1999.00847.x.
13. Han J, Kesner P, Metna-Laurent M, Duan T, et al. Acute Cannabinoids impair working memory through Astroglial CB1 receptor modulation of hippocampal LTD. Cell. 2012;148(5):1039–50. https://doi.org/10.1016/j.cell.2012.01.037.
14. Hassabis D, Maguire EA. Deconstruction episodic memory with construction. Trends Cogn Sci. 2007;11(7):299–306. https://doi.org/10.1016/j.tics.2007.05.001.
15. Koch M, Varela L, Kim JG, Kim JD, et al. Hypothalamic POMC neurons promote cannabinoid-induced feeding. Nature. 2015;519(7541):45–50. https://doi.org/10.1038/nature14260.
16. Mascarenhas DC, Gomes KS, Sorregotti T, Nunes-de-Souza RL. Blockade of cannabinoid CB1 receptors in the dorsal periaqueductal gray unmasks the antinociceptive effect of local injections of anandamide in mice. Front Pharmacol. 2017;8:695. https://doi.org/10.3389/fphar.2017.00695. eCollection 2017
17. Palazzo E, Rossi F, Maione S. Role of TRPV1 receptors in descending modulation of pain. Mol Cell Endocrinol. 2008;286(1–2 Suppl 1):S79–83. https://doi.org/10.1016/j.mce.2008.01.013.
18. Howlett AC, Abood ME. CB1 and CB2 receptor pharmacology. Adv Pharmacol. 2017;80:169–206. https://doi.org/10.1016/bs.apha.2017.03.007.
19. Breivogel CS, Childers SR, Deadwyler SA, Hampson RE, Vogt LJ, Sim-Selley LJ. Chronic delta9-tetrahydrocannabinol treatment produces a time-dependent loss of cannabinoid receptors and cannabinoid receptor-activated G proteins in rat brain. J Neurochem. 1999;73(6):2447–59.
20. Kendall DA, Yudowski GA. Cannabinoid receptors in the central nervous system: their signaling and roles in disease. Front Cell Neurosci. 2016;10:294.
21. Nguyen PT, Schmid CL, Raehal KM, Selley DE, Bohn LM, Sim-Selley LJ. beta-arrestin2 regulates cannabinoid CB1 receptor signaling and adaptation in a central nervous system region-dependent manner. Biol Psychiatry. 2012;71(8):714–24.
22. D'Souza DC, Cortes-Briones JA, Ranganathan M, Thurnauer H, Creatura G, Surti T, Planeta B, Neumeister A, Pittman B, Normandin M, Kapinos M, Ropchan J, Huang Y, Carson RE, Skosnik PD. Rapid changes in CB1 receptor availability in Cannabis dependent males after abstinence from Cannabis. Biol Psychiatry Cogn Neurosci Neuroimaging. 2016;1(1):60–7.
23. Hirvonen J, Goodwin RS, Li CT, Terry GE, Zoghbi SS, Morse C, Pike VW, Volkow ND, Huestis MA, Innis RB. Reversible and regionally selective down-regulation of brain cannabinoid CB1 receptors in chronic daily cannabis smokers. Mol Psychiatry. 2012;17(6):642–9.
24. Li X, Hua T, Vemuri K, Ho JH, Wu Y, Wu L, Popov P, Benchama O, Zvonok N, Locke K, Qu L, Han GW, Iyer MR, Cinar R, Coffey NJ, Wang J, Wu M, Katritch V, Zhao S, Kunos G, Bohn LM, Makriyannis A, Stevens RC, Liu ZJ. Crystal structure of the human cannabinoid receptor CB2. Cell. 2019;176(3):459–467.e13. https://doi.org/10.1016/j.cell.2018.12.011.

8 Cannabinoid Receptor 2 (CB2)

Glenn R. Rech and Samer N. Narouze

Cannabinoid 2 Receptor

The cannabinoid type 2 (CB2) receptor is a G protein-coupled receptor that was cloned in 1993 and consists of 360 amino acids in humans. This is somewhat shorter than the 472 amino acid long CB1 receptor. It is encoded by the gene CNR2, located on chromosome 1. As is common with G protein-coupled receptors, the CB2 receptor has seven transmembrane spanning domains, a glycosylated extracellular N-terminus, and an intracellular C-terminus (Fig. 8.1).

It shares only 44% sequence homology with CB1 receptor at the protein level in humans. Two isoforms of CB2 receptor have been identified [1]. Traditionally, CB2 receptors have been considered as the peripheral cannabinoid receptors. Later, these receptors have been located throughout the central nervous system exhibiting several unique features [2]. Compared with CB1 receptors, CB2 receptors located in the brain have lower expression levels than CB1 receptors. Brain CB2 receptors are highly inducible [3].

Unfortunately, CB2 receptors' modulation of neuronal functions, including ion channels, receptors, synaptic transmission, and plasticity, has not been well investigated. Reasons put forth include (1) lack of highly selective CB2 receptor antibodies, (2) lack of full knockout CB2 receptor mice, and (3), under some conditions, CB1 and CB2 receptors can form a heteromer, which makes the identification of CB2 receptors' function even more complex and difficult [2].

G. R. Rech (✉)
Western Reserve Hospital, Cuyahoga Falls, OH, USA

S. N. Narouze
Western Reserve Hospital, Center For Pain Medicine, Cuyahoga Falls, OH, USA
e-mail: narouzs@hotmail.com

CB2 Receptor Physiology and Pharmacology

CB2 receptors share the seven-transmembrane structure, although about 25% shorter than CB1 receptors. Receptor modulation triggers adenylyl cyclase inhibition and promotes MAPK activation. Initial experiments failed to detect functional coupling of CB2 receptors to G protein gated inwardly rectifying potassium channels and calcium channels. The failure to detect ion channel modulation can be attributed to the functional selectivity of the ligands used in the earliest studies [4].

CB2 receptor-mediated pertussis toxin-sensitive $G_{i/o}$ protein stimulation leads to inhibition of adenylyl cyclase and decreased cAMP levels. Pertussis toxin, which blocks the function of the heterotrimeric G_i and G_o proteins through ADO ribosylation, attenuates the ability of agonists to inhibit cAMP accumulation in both CB2 and CB1 cells [5].

CB2 receptors appear to poorly modulate calcium channels or inwardly rectify potassium channels. This is a key difference between CB1

S. N. Narouze (ed.), *Cannabinoids and Pain*, https://doi.org/10.1007/978-3-030-69186-8_8

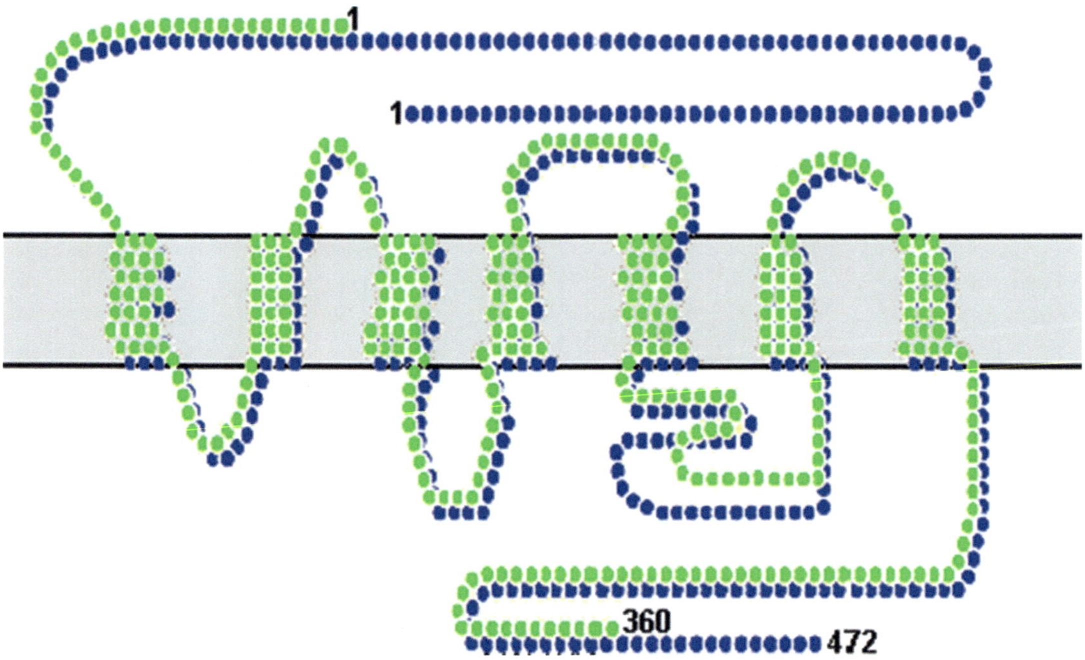

Fig. 8.1 CB1 receptor, blue, and CB2 receptor, green. https://commons.wikimedia.org/wiki/File:Cb1_cb2_structure.png

and CB2 receptors [5]. Of further interest, CB2 receptors from different species often have different pharmacological responses to identical drugs, complicating the drug discovery process [6].

Most G protein-coupled receptors undergo some degree of internalization following agonist binding. Like CB1 receptors, CB2 receptors internalize in response to an agonist, but in varying degrees [7].

CB2 receptors are highly inducible. CB2 receptor mRNA levels often increase by as much as 100-fold following nerve injury or during inflammation [7].

CB2 Receptor Distribution

Human CB2 receptors are expressed in two isoforms, labelled hCB2A and hCB2B. Human hCB2A promoter transcription is stronger in the testis and brain regions, whereas hCB2B promoter transcription is stronger in the spleen, leucocytes, and other peripheral tissues. hCB2A expression in brain regions was observed in the amygdala, caudate, putamen, nucleus accumbens, cortex, hippocampus, and cerebellum at low levels [8].

CB2 receptors have been labelled as "peripheral cannabinoid receptor." Munro and colleagues cloned a receptor for cannabinoids that is not expressed in the brain but rather in macrophages in the marginal zone of the spleen [9]. CB2 receptor mRNA has been identified in many immune tissues. Macrophages, CD4+ T cells, CD8+ T cells, B cells, natural killer cells, monocytes, and polymorphonuclear neutrophils have the highest levels of mRNA [10].

Microglia are derived from macrophages and can be viewed as the resident immune cells of the brain where they monitor the brain for pathological damage. In response to specific signals within the brain, they transition between different states of activity. The expression levels of CB2 receptors in microglia vary depending on the activation state of the cell [11]. CB2 receptors modulate microglial migration and infiltration into brain areas with active neuroinflammation and degeneration [10].

Stempel et al. have demonstrated CB2 receptors on postsynaptic pyramidal neuronal cells located in the hippocampus. The authors suggested, on a cellular level within the hippocampus, CB1 receptors expressed presynaptically and CB2 receptors expressed postsynaptically modulate neuro-chemical transmission [12].

CB2 Signaling

Around the time that CB1 and CB2 receptors were cloned, anandamide and 2-arachidonylglycerol (2-AG) were identified as endogenous cannabinoid agonists. 2-AG is a high-efficacy agonist at the CB2 receptor [13]. Both Δ-9-THC and anandamide display lower relative intrinsic activity for CB2 receptor than for CB1 [14].

Dhopeshwarkar et al. describe a phenomenon in which different agonists activate distinct (or overlapping) intracellular signaling pathways, termed *functional selectivity*. Functional selectivity, or biased agonism or stimulus trafficking, is noted as different agonists activating signaling pathways with different potencies. A balanced agonist activates all pathways similarly, whereas a biased agonist shows bias toward subset pathways [7].

CB2 ligands show functional selectivity. Shoemaker et al. found that endocannabinoids activated distinct signaling pathways with varied and order potencies in CHO cells transfected with CB2 receptors. 2-AG was most potent in activating the extracellular signal-regulated kinases 1/2 (ERK1/ERK 2), but higher concentrations were needed to inhibit adenylyl cyclase and induce calcium passing [13].

CB2 Chronic Pain Models

The regulation of pain is one of the earliest medical applications of cannabinoids. Numerous studies have documented the analgesic effects of cannabinoids in different types of pain, including chemical, mechanical, thermal, neuropathic, and inflammatory pain. CB2 receptors have been labelled the "peripheral cannabinoid receptor" resulting from initial isolation in the spleen of a rat.

Complete Freund's adjuvant (CFA) model, which induces nociception and rodent paw swelling, osteoarthritis (OA) produced by intra-articular injection of monosodium iodoacetate (MIA), and the collagen-induced arthritis (CIA) model are well-characterized long-term inflammatory pain models. CB2 receptor gene expression was significantly upregulated in dorsal root ganglion (DRGs) ipsilateral to injury under inflammatory and neuropathic pain conditions, suggesting that these receptors play an integral role in the modulation of chronic inflammatory pain [15, 16].

Burston et al. studied the arthritis-producing chemical into the knee joint of rats. They determined the expression and localization of CB2 receptors were significantly increased in the ipsilateral spinal cord of the MIA-treated rats . Systemic administration of a CB2 receptor agonist (JWH133) attenuated the knee pain associated with MIA-induced arthritis in the rat model. The authors concluded that acute activation and upregulation of spinal CB2 receptors selectively attenuate spinal neuronal processing of noxious inputs, and JWH133 attenuated the development and maintenance of pain behavior (weight bearing on the affected knee joint) [17].

Neuropathic pain is a severe chronic, debilitating condition associated with nerve injury. Assessing neuropathic pain behavior in rodents is crucial to validate pain models. Using complementary genetic and pharmacological approaches, distinct components of the cannabinoid system (i.e., genetic deletion, -/- CB1, -/- CB2 receptors) have emerged as promising targets to treat neuropathic pain. Presently, models show both CB1 and CB2 receptor agonists contribute to antinociceptive effects [15].

Microglia are one of the first spinal cord cell types to be activated with peripheral nerve injury, which continues for several months. Stimulation of CB2 receptors expressed on immune cells by either NESS400 or JWH-015, two known CB2 agonists, led to the attenuation of pain hypersensitivity in several animal models of neuropathy. There was a parallel decrease in microglial activation and an increase in anti-inflammatory cytokines [18].

Tolerance

The CB2 receptor is desensitized and internalized following agonist treatment in vitro [4]. The first studies were conducted in human CB2-transfected CHO cells and demonstrated that phosphorylation at S352 appears to play a key role in the loss of responsiveness of the CB2 receptor to CP-55,940. Furthermore, SR144528 could regenerate the desensitized CB2 receptors by activating a phosphatase that dephosphorylated the receptor [19]. Atwood et al. observed marked functional selectivity of cannabinoid receptor internalization, where WIN55,212-2 did not produce internalization, nor did most of the aminoalkylindoles tested. They reported that Δ-9-THC did not produce any internalization of HEK-293 cells expressing rat CB2, but compounds that are structurally similar to Δ-9-THC notably JWH133, THCV, and HU210 did [4].

Another study utilizing cultured rat microglia cells revealed chronic exposure to 2-AG increased CB2 receptor internalization [20]. Hence, the pharmacological properties and phosphorylation state of the CB2 receptor can be regulated by both agonists and antagonists, but this appears to be agonist selective. Whether this is also true in vivo remains to be defined [21].

Alternatively, Deng et al. demonstrated in a mouse model that chronic cannabinoid CB2 receptor activation reverses paclitaxel-induced allodynia without tolerance or cannabinoid receptor 1-dependent withdrawal. Tolerance was also not observed with the administration of a CB2 receptor analog AM1710 [22].

An overwhelming body of evidence indicates that cannabinoids produce antinociceptive effects in inflammatory and neuropathic rodent pain models. CB2 receptors are expressed in the central nervous system. The challenges going forward include distinction among cell types associated with CB2 receptor binding, agonists which are species specific, and identification of agonists exclusively binding to CB2 receptors.

CB2 Receptor Ligands

CB2 receptor ligands are summarized in Table 8.1.

Ligands affect CB2 differently than CB1 and point to principles that could inform rational and selective drug design. The yin-yang relationship of CB2 and CB1 will facilitate the design of selective drugs [23] (Fig. 8.2).

Pepcan-12 will be reviewed as one example. Pepcan-12 (RVD-hemopressin) is the major peptide of a family of endogenous peptide endocannabinoids (pepcans) shown to act as negative allosteric modulators (NAM) of CB1 receptors. On the other hand, it acts as a potent CB2 receptor positive allosteric modulator (PAM). It significantly potentiated the effects of CB2 receptor agonists, including the endocannabinoid 2-arachidonoyl glycerol (2-AG), for GTPγS binding and cAMP inhibition (5–10 fold). The wide occurrence of this endogenous hormone-like CB2 receptor PAM, with unforeseen opposite allosteric effects on cannabinoid receptors, suggests its potential role in peripheral pathophysiological processes [24] (Fig. 8.3).

Table 8.1 CB2 receptor ligands

Agonists	Full	Endocannabinoid	2-Arachidonoylglycerol (2-AG) 2-Arachidonyl glyceryl ether
		Phytogenic	β-Caryophyllene
		Synthetic	CP55940 HU-210 HU-243 HU-308 JWH-018 JWH-133 L-759633 L-759656 Olorinab UR-144 WIN 55,212-2
	Partial	Endocannabinoid	Anandamide (AEA) Virodhamine
		Phytogenic	Tetrahydrocannabinol (THC) Cannabinol (CBN) N-Alkylamide 3,3′-Diindolylmethane
	Selective	Synthetic	AM1241 (ab120934) Gp 1a (ab120344)
	Unspecified efficacy	Synthetic	AM-1221 AM-1235 AM-2232 JWH-007 JWH-015
Allosteric modulators	PAM	Endogenous peptide endocannabinoids (pepcans)	Pepcan-12 (RVD-hemopressin)
		Synthetic	Compound C2
Inverse agonists		Phytogenic	? Cannabidiol (CBD)
		Synthetic	6-Iodopravadoline (AM-630) BML-190 (indomethacin morpholinylamide, ab143353) JTE-907 SR-144528 (ab146185)
Antagonists			Iodopravadoline, AM-630 AM-10257 SR144528 TM-38837

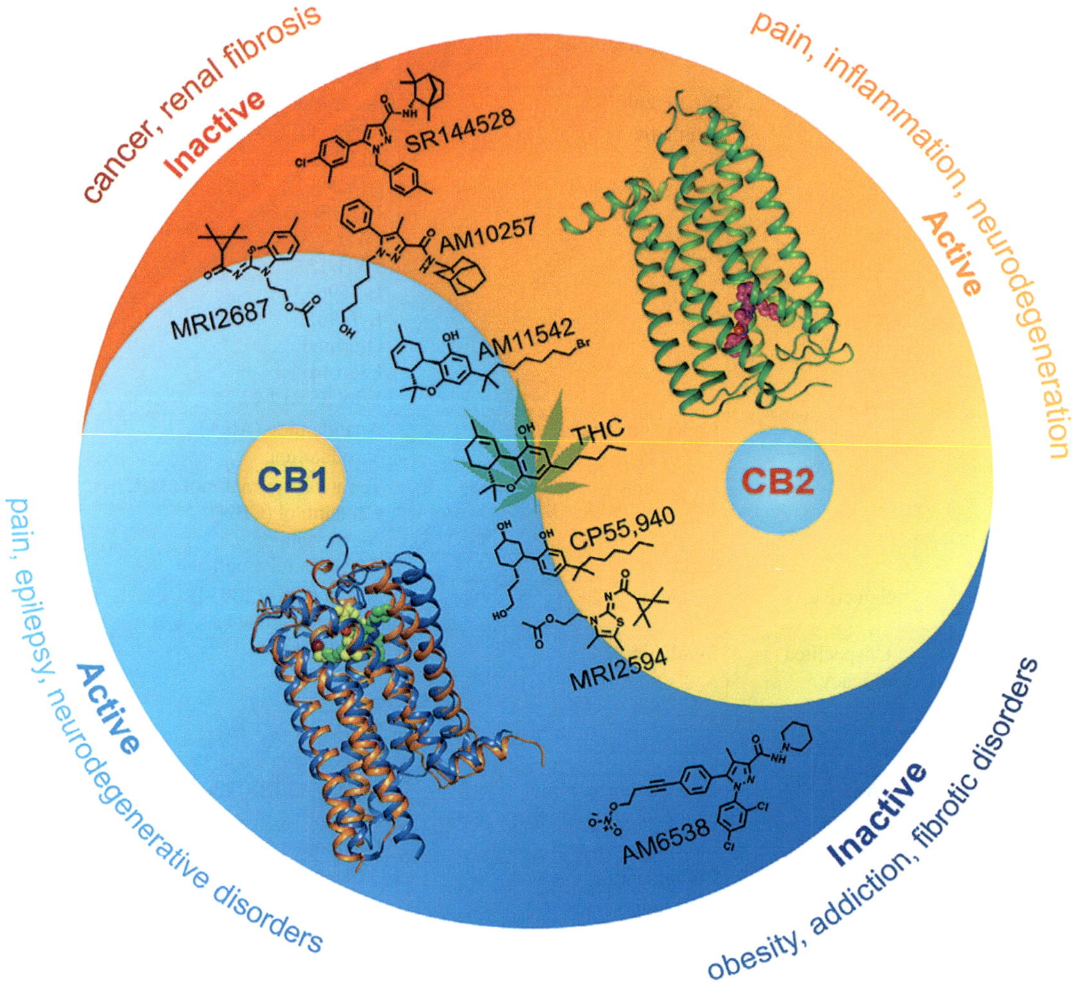

Fig. 8.2 The yin-yang relationship of CB2 and CB1 receptors. Ligands affect CB2 differently than CB1 receptors. (Adopted from Li X et al., Ref. [23], with permission)

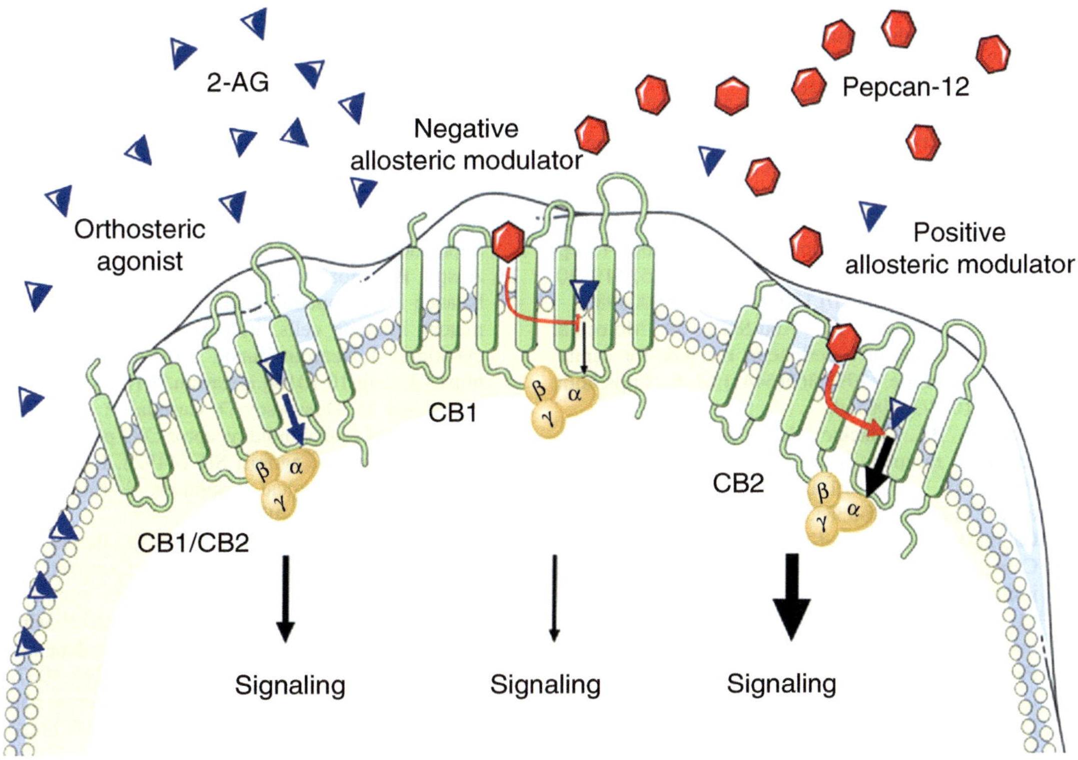

Fig. 8.3 Illustration showing the opposite effects of pepcan-12 on CB1 and CB2 receptor G protein signaling. In the presence of the endocannabinoid 2-AG, pepcan-12 acts as a negative allosteric modulator (NAM) of CB1 and as a positive allosteric modulator (PAM) of CB2. (Adopted from Petrucci V et al., Ref. [24], open access)

References

1. Zhang HY, Bi GH, Li X, Li J, Qu H, Zhang SJ, Li CY, Onaivi ES, Gardner EL, Xi ZX, Liu QR. Species differences in Cannabinoid receptor 2 and receptor responses to cocaine self-administration in mice and rats. Neuropsychopharmacology. 2015r;40(4):1037–51. https://doi.org/10.1038/npp.2014.297.
2. Chen DJ, Gao M, Gao FF, Su QX, Wu J. Brain cannabinoid receptor 2: expression, function and modulation. Acta Pharmacol Sin. 2017\;38(3):312–6. https://doi.org/10.1038/aps.2016.149.
3. Miller LK, Devi LA. The highs and lows of cannabinoid receptor expression in disease: mechanisms and their therapeutic implications. Pharmacol Rev. 2011;63(3):461–70. https://doi.org/10.1124/pr.110.003491.
4. Atwood BK, Wager-Miller J, Haskins C, Straiker A, Mackie K. Functional selectivity in CB(2) cannabinoid receptor signaling and regulation: implications for the therapeutic potential of CB(2) ligands. Mol Pharmacol. 2012;81(2):250–63. https://doi.org/10.1124/mol.111.074013.
5. Felder CC, Joyce KE, Briley EM, Mansouri J, Mackie K, Blond O, Lai Y, Ma AL, Mitchell RL. Comparison of the pharmacology and signal transduction of the human cannabinoid CB1 and CB2 receptors. Mol Pharmacol. 1995;48(3):443–50.
6. Mukherjee S, Adams M, Whiteaker K, Daza A, Kage K, Cassar S, Meyer M, Yao BB. Species comparison and pharmacological characterization of rat and human CB2 cannabinoid receptors. Eur J Pharmacol. 2004;505(1–3):1–9. https://doi.org/10.1016/j.ejphar.2004.09.058.

phospholipids into N-arachidonoyl-phosphatidylethanolamine (NAPE). NAPE is hydrolyzed by a phospholipase D-like enzyme to create anandamide, making this the major pathway for anandamide biosynthesis [6]. The breakdown of anandamide is mediated by fatty acid amide hydrolase (FAAH) [4]. Once reuptake occurs into the cell, FAAH breaks anandamide down into arachidonic acid and ethanolamine. Other breakdown pathways of anandamide include hydrolysis by N-acylethanolamine-hydrolyzing acid amidase (NAAA) and oxygenation by cyclooxygenase-2 (COX-2), lipoxygenase isoenzymes (LOX), and cytochrome P450 [7–10] (Fig. 9.3).

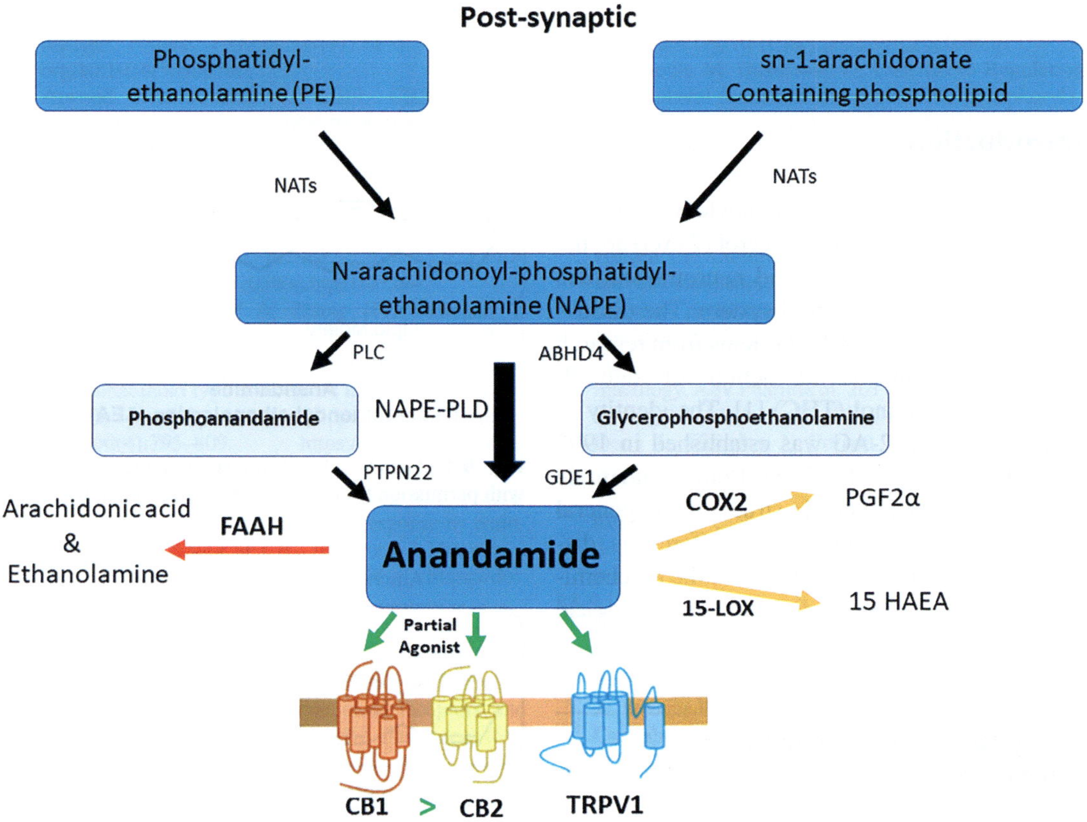

Fig. 9.3 Biosynthesis and metabolism of anandamide. Green arrows, binding and activation; red arrow, metabolism and breakdown; yellow arrows, oxidation. ABDH4 α/β-hydrolase domain type-4, CB1 cannabinoid receptor 1, CB2 cannabinoid receptor 2, COX2 cyclooxygenase 2, FAAH fatty acid amide hydrolase, GDE1 glycerophosphodiester phosphodiesterase 1, MAGL monoacylglycerol lipase, NAPE-PLD N-acylphosphatidylethanolamine-specific phospholipase D, NATs N-acyltransferases, PA phosphatidic acid, PLCβ phospholipase Cβ, PLD phospholipase D, 15-LOX 15-lipoxygenase, PTPN22 protein tyrosine phosphatase non-receptor type 22, PGF2α prostaglandin F2alpha-ethanolamide, 15 HAEA 15(S)-HETE ethanolamide, TRPV1 transient receptor potential vanilloid type-1 channel. (Reprinted with permission from ©Samer Narouze, MD, PhD)

2-AG

2-AG belongs to the monoacylglycerol class and is derived from the AA-containing phospholipids as anandamide. The corresponding on-demand synthesis driven by calcium-dependent biosynthesis pathways also yields 2-AG. Diacylglycerol (DAG) is the precursor to 2-AG.

This synthesis pathway is a two-step process activating phospholipase C (PLC) to generate diacylglycerol (DAG), which is then hydrolyzed by DAG lipase to form 2-AG, and is thought to occur on postsynaptic neurons in dendritic spines and somato-dendritic compartments [5].

Another minor pathway forms 2-AG from phosphatidic acid hydrolysis [10] (Fig. 9.4).

The breakdown of 2-AG is mediated by a membrane-associated enzyme, monoacylglycerol lipase (MAGL), which dissociates 2-AG into AA and glycerol [4].

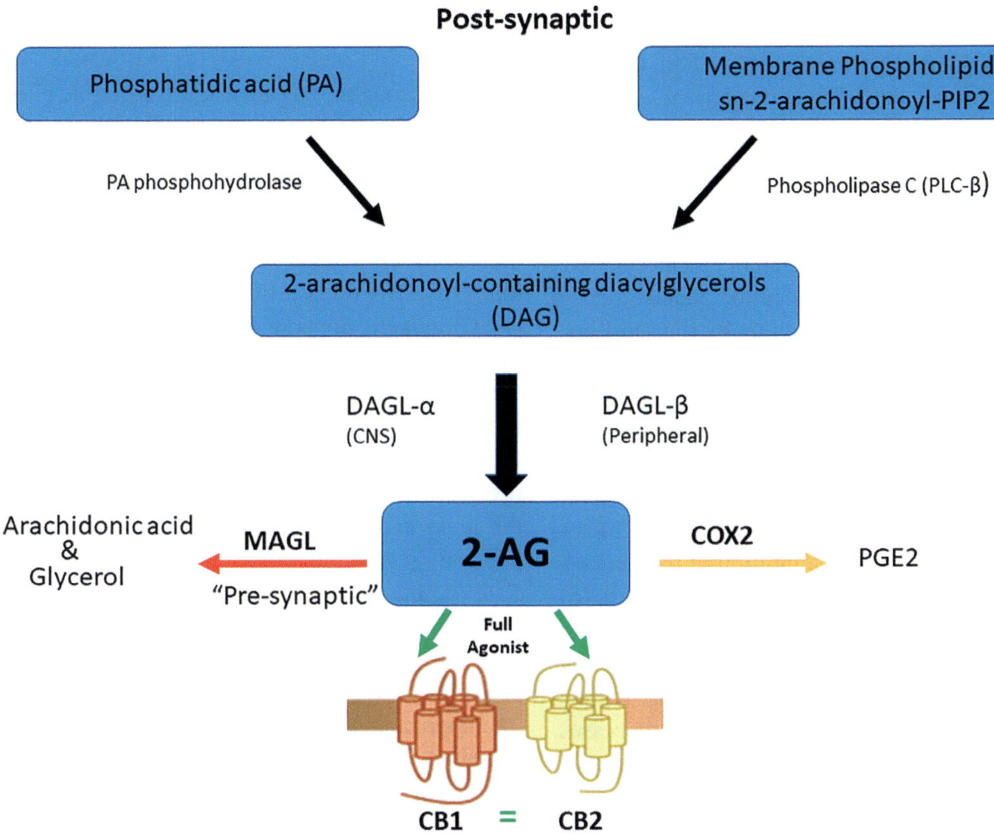

Fig. 9.4 Biosynthesis and metabolism of 2-AG. Green arrows, binding and activation; red arrow, metabolism and breakdown; yellow arrow, oxidation. 2-AG 2-arachidonoyl-glycerol, CB1 cannabinoid receptor 1, CB2 cannabinoid receptor 2, COX2 cyclooxygenase 2, DAG diacylglycerol, DAGL-α and DAGL -β diacylglycerol lipase-α and diacylglycerol lipase-β, MAGL monoacylglycerol lipase, PA phosphatidic acid, PLCβ phospholipase Cβ, PLD phospholipase D, 15-LOX 15-lipoxygenase, PGE2 prostaglandin E2-glycerol ester, PIP2 sn-2-arachidonoyl-phosphatidylinositol-4,5-bisphosphate, TRPV1 transient receptor potential vanilloid type-1 channel. (Reprinted with permission from ©Samer Narouze, MD, PhD)

Endocannabinoids' Mechanism of Action

As with the biochemical and breakdown pathways, the endocannabinoids display slight differences in their mechanism of action. The differences noted here are important to the overall action of the endocannabinoids in pain modulation.

Anandamide

Anandamide is a partial agonist at both CB1 and CB2 receptors, but a full agonist at the ion channel receptor transient receptor potential vanilloid type 1 (TRPV1) [11]. Anandamide shows a selectivity for the CB1 receptor [11]. Although anandamide is a partial agonist, it has a higher affinity to the CB1 receptor than 2-AG [1]. Once actions are carried out at the receptor, anandamide is thought to possibly be taken up by transport proteins on both neurons and glia that mediate endocannabinoid uptake [5]. Anandamide can play a dual role in nociception: antinociceptive at cannabinoid receptors and pronociceptive at the TRPV1 receptor [11]. Anandamide has a noted "tetrad effect" when injected into mice. The tetrad is a combination of inhibition of motor activity, catalepsy, hypothermia, and hypoalgesia [6]. Anandamide helps regulate pain, depression, appetite, memory, and fertility. High areas of anandamide synthesis take place in brain regions important to memory, higher thought processes, and movement control [12].

2-AG

2-AG is a full agonist at CB1 and CB2 receptors. 2-AG relays signals via a retrograde signaling cascade. When 2-AG is released, it controls the activity of the complementary presynaptic neuron by binding to the CB1 receptor [5]. Different mechanisms have been proposed as to how 2-AG is induced to leave the postsynaptic cell. It is thought 2-AG may be secreted by simple diffusion or the use of passive carrier proteins may be required to secrete 2-AG [5]. Once bound to CB1, activation leads to inhibition of neurotransmitter release in the presynaptic cell via inhibition of voltage-activated calcium channels and enhancement of inwardly rectifying K^+ channels in the cell [5]. With 2-AG being present at higher levels in nervous tissue than anandamide, 2-AG may have a greater role in analgesia and antinociception.

Plasticity of Endocannabinoid Signaling

The endocannabinoids are a highly synaptic plastic system. In regard to synaptic plasticity, endocannabinoids' synaptic plasticity is thought to be due to the depolarization-induced suppression of inhibition mechanism [4]. Endocannabinoids are mobilized as needed by postsynaptic cells to inhibit GABA release from presynaptic neurons [4]. Glutamate, dopamine, and muscarinic receptor stimulus leads to the synthesis of endocannabinoids. The endocannabinoids mediate long-term depression and heterosynaptic long-term potentiation [4]. When looking at the involvement of 2-AG and anandamide, 2-AG is the main endocannabinoid involved in synaptic plasticity regulation.

2-AG has a broad effect in neuronal plasticity and retrograde signaling. 2-AG mediates long-term depression at the hippocampus, cerebellum, prefrontal cortex, and ventral tegmental area. At the hippocampal neurons, a study using MAG-L inhibitors in mice demonstrated that 2-AG modulated both depolarization-induced suppression of inhibition and depolarization-induced suppression of excitation [4]. 2-AG also synapses at the Purkinje cells in the cerebellum. Various studies in rodents revealed 2-AG to be required in mGluR-dependent plasticity and long-term depression in Purkinje cells [4]. At the prefrontal cortex, 2-AG is responsible for short- and long-term forms of plasticity leading to modifications of cognitive and motivational functions [4]. 2-AG is found to play a role in enabling subthreshold doses of dopamine D1 and D2 receptor agonists to increase the firing activity at the nucleus accumbens neurons [4]. This evidence shows 2-AG to play a role in the ventral tegmental area modulating the reward pathway [4]. 2-AG is a key neuromodulator involved in various synaptic plasticities in key brain regions.

Anandamide regulates synaptic transmission with mechanisms different from classical retrograde action as seen with 2-AG. Anandamide mediates short- and long-term forms of synaptic plasticity through an anterograde mechanism. Postsynaptic NAPE-PLD localization in the cerebellum is congruent with the autocrine action of anandamide at TRPV1 receptors [4]. While 2-AG mediates short-term depression through CB1 receptor-dependent retrograde signaling, anandamide is released by a postsynaptic mGluR5-dependent mechanism and modulates long-term depression through postsynaptic TRPV1 activation. Both endocannabinoids cooperate by using different strategies to modulate synaptic plasticity in brain regions that govern highly dynamic processes [4].

Endocannabinoids in Pain

Endocannabinoids regulate various cerebral functions including nociception, mood, appetite, and memory. For the purpose of this chapter, nociception and pain modulation will be discussed in depth. There has been an interest in the role of exogenously administered cannabinoid compounds to induce analgesic effects. When noxious stimuli occur, there is an increase in endocannabinoid release, thus leading to pain modulation effects [12]. Animal studies show endocannabinoids to have analgesic actions in the periphery, spinal, and supraspinal pain pathways [12].

Peripheral Mechanisms

The cannabinoid receptors in the periphery play a vital role in analgesia. Antinociceptive effects are noticed when anandamide and 2-AG are administered locally and systemically. Models of inflammatory pain show elevated concentrations of anandamide and 2-AG in peripheral tissues [11]. CB2 receptors are also present in the periphery leading to 2-AG mainly regulating actions at these receptors. 2-AG has been studied to show multiple mechanisms leading to pain modulation which include inhibiting production and release of reactive oxygen species and cytokines, and in addition 2-AG will release peripheral endogenous opioids [11]. There is more research describing the anti-inflammatory and antinociceptive mediated actions of 2-AG compared to anandamide. There are also CB1 receptors in the periphery that localize on sensory afferent terminals where endocannabinoids act to gate the transduction of pain from noxious stimuli [11].

Spinal Mechanisms

A vital region for pain processing occurs at the dorsal horn in the spinal cord. Endocannabinoids are shown to have antinociceptive effects at this region and phase of the pain-signaling pathway due to high expression of CB1 receptors. At this level, 2-AG inhibits the release of pronociceptive neurotransmitters from primary afferent terminals mediated by CB1 receptors [11]. In contrast, anandamide was shown to have effects on acute and chronic pain via mediation of CB1 receptors expressed on inhibitory interneurons and glial cells [11]. To get a better picture for when each of the endocannabinoids takes effect, a surgical incision model was used to assess spinal levels of endocannabinoids. Hours after a peripheral surgical incision, there was a marked decrease in anandamide concentrations, whereas no changes in 2-AG concentration were observed [11]. Anandamide concentrations returned to baseline as nociceptive behavior subsides [11]. 2-AG concentrations increased at a later time point in conjunction with glial cell activation, CB2 receptor upregulation, and resolution of the pain state [11].

Anandamide exerts its actions at the onset of pain, whereas 2-AG plays a role in the resolution of pain. This research shows the difference in the timing of endocannabinoid actions of pain modulation.

Supraspinal Mechanisms

Endocannabinoids modulate ascending pain signals in the thalamus, descending signals in the brain stem, and pain sensation in the frontal-limbic circuits [11]. Anandamide has a biphasic effect on the supraspinal level of pain modulation. Anandamide is released due to stimulation of the periaqueductal gray (PAG) or peripheral inflammatory insult [5]. In acute pain, anandamide that is released causes antinociceptive actions. When high concentrations of anandamide occur due to prolonged stimulation, anandamide modulates pronociceptive responses via TRPV1 binding [5].

Anandamide and 2-AG have a synergistic yet differential role regarding pain signaling at the spinal and supraspinal levels. Stress-induced analgesia exhibits a synergistic effect of anandamide and 2-AG modulation. Signaling at the PAG can result in induction of descending inhibitory GABAergic signaling to the spinal cord, thus mediating stress-induced analgesia [5]. In a prolonged foot shock modulation study, both endocannabinoids were found to be released in the ipsilateral lumbar V dorsal root ganglion upon stimulation [4]. The CB1 receptors at the dorsal root ganglion and CB2 receptors at the periphery involve a synergistic interplay between anandamide and 2-AG [4]. The signaling mechanism is strengthened when the molecular pathway switches. Petrosino et al. uncovered that both endocannabinoid levels were enhanced after 3 and 7 days of chronic constriction injury at the sciatic nerve of a rat [4]. After the 3-day mark, endocannabinoid levels were increased only at the spinal cord and PAG. However, after 7 days, elevated concentrations were detected in the rostral ventral medulla as well [4]. This study provides evidence of endocannabinoid cooperation regarding synergistic involvement in the regulation of pain. This combined effort is present at both the spinal and supraspinal levels and can modulate chronic pain states.

Chronic pain enhances the endocannabinoid signaling effects of both anandamide and 2-AG. An upregulation of CB2 receptors found in such pain states would benefit from endocannabinoid agonism [5]. 2-AG signaling cascades from microglial cells mediate effects in persistent pain [5]. Although CB2 receptors are widely studied in the literature for chronic pain, CB1 receptors were also shown to provide antinociceptive benefit when agonists are present. The spinal level endocannabinoids have the greatest modulation of pain in chronic pain states displaying a synergistic benefit of the endocannabinoid agonists.

Anandamide has also been shown to interact with other neurotransmitter systems that may play a role in nociception. Cannabinoids might directly inhibit 5-HT_3 receptors, leading to analgesia and neuroprotection effects [6]. Anandamide exerts part of its CNS effects through the 5-HT_3 receptors [6]. Kimura et al. found micromolar concentrations of anandamide to bind to 5-HT_1 and 5-HT_2 receptors, thus further describing the role of anandamide in other neurotransmitter systems [6]. The combined efforts of anandamide binding at 5-HT and cannabinoid receptors will have a positive influence on therapeutic outcomes for pain.

Conclusion

Anandamide and 2-AG are key lipid mediators of the endocannabinoid system. Although similar in function, the endocannabinoids have a different biochemical synthesis and breakdown pathway. This system of neurotransmitters is highly plastic, with altered expression and function due to physiological state. Anandamide and 2-AG play a vital role in pain modulation at the peripheral, spinal, and supraspinal levels of the pain processing system. Throughout previous research, endocannabinoids are shown to have a differential but synergistic involvement in pain states. Acute and chronic nociception is modulated by these endocannabinoids. The site-specific actions of anandamide and 2-AG provide crucial pharmacological actions in the regulation of pain.

References

1. Hillard CJ. Biochemistry and pharmacology of the endocannabinoids arachidonylethanolamide and 2-arachidonylglycerol. Prostaglandins Other Lipid Mediat. 2000;61(1-2):3–18.
2. Devane WA, Hanus L, Breuer A, Pertwee RG, Stevenson LA, Griffin G, Gibson D, Mandelbaum A, Etinger A, Mechoulam R. Isolation and structure of a brain constituent that binds to the cannabinoid receptor. Science. 1992;258(5090):1946–9.
3. Mechoulam R, Ben-Shabat S, Hanus L, Ligumsky M, Kaminski NE, Schatz AR, Gopher A, ALmog S, Martin BR, Compton DR, Pertwee RG, Griffin G, Bayewitch M, Barg J, Vogel Z. Identification of an endogenous 2-monoglyceride, present in canine gut, that binds to cannabinoid receptors. Biochem Pharmacol. 1995;50(1):83–90.
4. Luchicch A, Pistis M. Anandamide and 2-arachidonoylglycerol: pharmacological properties, functional features, and emerging specificities of the two major endocannabinoids. Mol Neurobiol. 2012;46:374–92.
5. Reggio PH. Endocannabinoid binding to the cannabinoid receptors: what is known and what remains unknown. Curr Med Chem. 2010;17(14):1468–86.
6. Mechoulam R, Fride E, Marzo VD. Endocannabinoids. Eur J Pharmacol. 1998;359(1):1–18.
7. Ueda N, Tsuboi K, Uyama T. N-acylethanolamine metabolism with special reference to N-acylethanolamine-hydrolyzing acid amidase (NAAA). Prog Lipid Res. 2010;49(4):299–315.
8. Yu M, Ives D, Ramesha CS. Synthesis of prostaglandin E2 ethanolamide from anandamide by cyclooxygenase-2. J Biol Chem. 1997;272(34):21181–6.
9. Bornheim LM, Kim KY, Chen B, Correia MA. The effect of cannabidiol on mouse hepatic microsomal cytochrome P450-dependent anandamide metabolism. Biochem Biophys Res Com- mun. 1993;197(2):740–6.
10. Iannotti FA, Di Marzo V, Petrosino S. Endocannabinoids and endocannabinoid-related mediators: targets, metabolism and role in neurological disorders. Prog Lipid Res. 2016;62:107–28. https://doi.org/10.1016/j.plipres.2016.02.002.
11. Woodhams SG, Sagar DR, Burston JJ, Chapman V. The role of the endocannabinoid system in pain. Handb Exp Pharmacol. 2015;227:119–43. https://doi.org/10.1007/978-3-662-46450-2_7.
12. Manzanares J, Julian MD, Carrascosa A. Role of the cannabinoid system in pain control and therapeutic implications for the management of acute and chronic pain episodes. Curr Neuropharmacol. 2006;4(3):239–57.

Phytocannabinoids: Tetrahydrocannabinol (THC)

10

Priodarshi Roychoudhury, Ning Nan Wang, and Samer N. Narouze

Phytocannabinoids

Introduction

Phytocannabinoids are natural products derived from cannabis either interacting directly with cannabinoid receptors or sharing chemical similarity with endocannabinoids or both [1]. *Cannabis sativa* is a flowering plant belonging to the family Cannabaceae. Eighteen chemical families including 500 different chemical compounds have been identified in the flower and leaves of cannabis so far [2]. Among these chemical compounds,100 active phytocannabinoids have been identified within *cannabis sativa* alone [3]. Apart from Δ9-tetrahydrocannabinol (THC), cannabidiol (CBD), and cannabinol (CBN), which are the most popular phytocannabinoids, others identified include tetrahydrocannabivarin (THCV), cannabigerol (CBG), and cannabichromene (CBC) [4]. In contrast to THC and CBD, these phytocannabinoids have poor affinities for the cannabinoid receptors [5] and display a complex range of physiological interaction and mechanism of action which is still poorly understood [6].

The relative concentration of different cannabinoids and other chemical components varies greatly based on the strain, soil, climatic conditions, and the cultivation techniques [7]. Besides phytocannabinoids, *Cannabis sativa* contains additional pharmacologically active molecules, such as terpenoid and β-caryophyllene, that are members of other chemical families. They also interact and mediate potential therapeutic actions through cannabinoid receptors [8]. Several cannabis terpenoids, for instance, limonene, linalool, and β-myrcene, have been discovered in other plants as well [9].

Both active and inactive forms of phytocannabinoids coexist in the living plant. Inactive monocarboxylic acids (tetrahydrocannabinolic acid, THCA) and active decarboxylated forms (THC) coexist [10]. Smoking, or heating the herb, leads to the transformation of these chemicals by decarboxylation and pyrolysis (Fig. 10.1). For instance, combustion above 120 degree Celsius leads to decarboxylation of THCA to THC [11]. Pyrolysis, or thermal decomposition of organic materials at higher temperatures, transforms the numerous chemical compounds identified inside the cannabis plants into other different chemical molecules. The complex interactions of this large number of chemical compounds and the human body are partially elucidated.

P. Roychoudhury (✉)
Department of Anesthesia and Pain Management, Toronto General Hospital, University of Toronto, Toronto, ON, Canada

N. N. Wang
Department of Anesthesia and Pain Management, Toronto Western Hospital, University of Toronto, Toronto, ON, Canada

S. N. Narouze
Western Reserve Hospital, Center For Pain Medicine, Cuyahoga Falls, OH, USA
e-mail: narouzs@hotmail.com

S. N. Narouze (ed.), *Cannabinoids and Pain*, https://doi.org/10.1007/978-3-030-69186-8_10

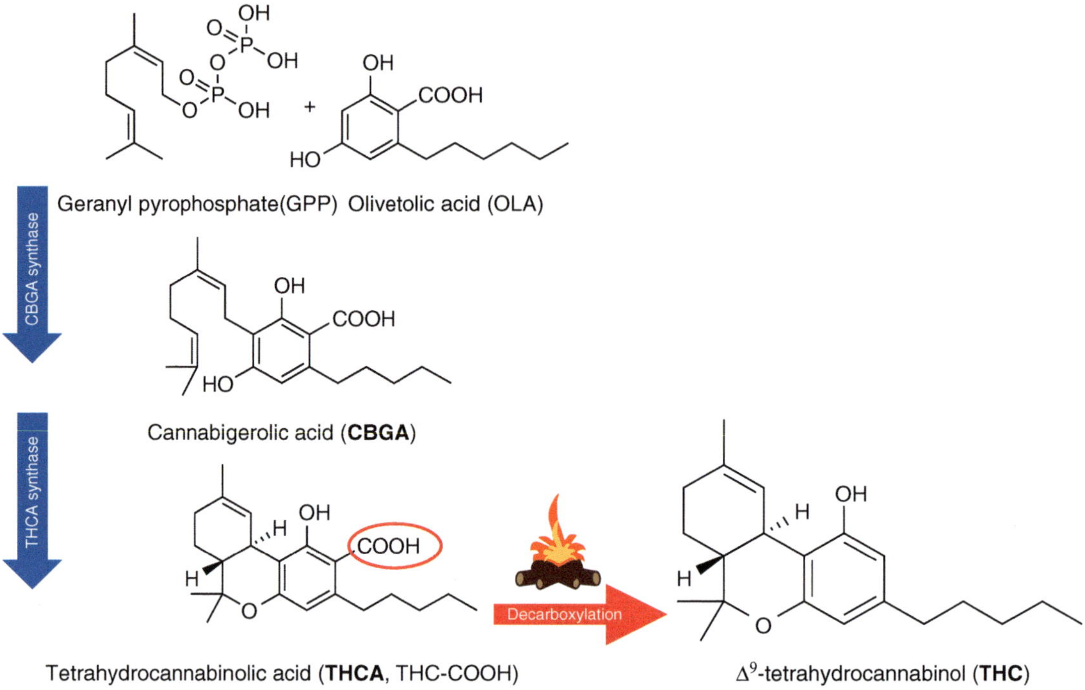

Fig. 10.1 Biosynthesis of Δ9-tetrahydrocannabinol (THC). (Reprinted with permission from Samer Narouze, MD, PhD)

Δ9-Tetrahydrocannabinol (THC)

Δ9-tetrahydrocannabinol (THC), cannabidiol (CBD), and cannabinol (CBN) are among the most studied cannabinoids. CBD was identified in 1940, while THC was first identified in 1964 [12]. THC is the main psychoactive compound of the cannabis plant. It is produced in the flowers and the leaves of the cannabis plant in varying concentrations. THC concentration varies inside different cannabis-based products ranging from 5% in marijuana to 80% in hashish oil [6]. THC produces pharmacological effects ranging from cognitive changes and psychoactive, anti-inflammatory, antipruritic, bronchodilatory, anti-spasmodic, and muscle relaxant activities [13]. It is also associated with side effects like anxiety, impaired memory, and immunosuppression [13].

Mechanism of Action of THC

THC simulates endocannabinoids like arachidonoylethanolamine (anandamide or AEA) or 2-arachidonoylglycerol (2-AG) and acts as a partial agonist at the CB1 and CB2 cannabinoid receptors [14]. Activation of the cannabinoid receptors results in a decrease in the concentration of the second messenger molecule cAMP through inhibition of adenylate cyclase.

THC exists as isomers like (+) trans-Δ9-tetrahydrocannabidiol, (−) trans-Δ9-tetrahydrocannabidiol [15], and (+) trans-Δ9-tetrahydrocannabidiol being the most abundant and well-studied isomer. Other extracted forms of THC include Δ8-THC-type [16] and the Δ 9-THC-type [17] cannabinoids, which are double-bond position isomers of THC, the former being less psychologically potent than the latter [18]. Stereochemistry of this compound is important since it influences its actions. This can be illustrated with the example of dexanabinol (HU-210): the (−)enantiomer is a potent psychotrophically active compound, while the (+)enantiomer (i.e., HU-211) has no THC-like psychotropic effects [18].

In vivo animal studies show evidence of THC acting on neuronal cannabinoid type 1 (CB1) receptors with high affinity [15]. The CB1 receptor activation mediates its psychoactive properties including changes in mood or consciousness, memory processing, and motor control [19]. In animal studies, activation of CB1R by THC produces a "tetrad" effect: (1) suppression of locomotor activity, (2) hypothermia, (3) immobility in the ring test, and (4) antinociception in the tail-flick or hot-plate test [15].

THC can both activate and inhibit neurotransmitter release on the neurons they act upon. In vivo studies by brain microdialysis confirm the CB1-mediated increase in neurotransmitter release of acetylcholine, glutamate, and dopamine in rat prefrontal cortex [20–22]. THC-mediated CB1 receptor activation can increase dopamine release in mouse and rat nucleus accumbens [21, 23]. The THC-induced dopamine release in the endocannabinoid system has been postulated as a potential mechanism of action for brain reward or specifically for animal (rat/squirrel/monkey) neural reward system [21, 23]. THC-mixed stimulatory-inhibitory effect on the central nervous system is correlated with its mixed clinical effect on cognition.

In vivo, THC can act both as a proconvulsant or an anticonvulsant [24, 25]. It also exhibits dual action as an anxiolytic as well as an anxiogenic agent in rats or mice [26, 27].

THC has many other pharmacological targets that are not related to the CB1 and CB2 receptors. It activates other receptors like GPR55 [28] and transient receptor potential cation channels (e.g., TRPV1, TRPV2, TRPA1) and the serotonin receptors 5-HT2 [29]. TRPV1 is important for detection and regulation of temperature; it provides sensation for burning, heat, and pain [30]. TRPV2 is involved in many pathological states including cancer and inflammatory response [31, 32]. Detailed mechanism of action for THC and receptor interaction are subjects of ongoing research. Please refer to Chap. 29 for details on the mechanism of antinociception.

Cannabidiol is a non-intoxicating phytocannabinoid. CBD accounts for 40% of the *Cannabis sativa* extract [33]. CBD works synergistically with THC for its analgesic effect while decreasing its psychoactive and cognitive side effects such as sedation and memory impairment of THC [34]. Despite the small number of in vivo studies, the specific THC and CBD (phytocannabinoid-phytocannabinoid) interactions and its biological or physiological effects are poorly understood. Please refer to Chap. 11 for detailed CBD pharmacology and pharmacokinetics.

Applied Pharmacology and Pharmacokinetics

A large diversity of cannabis-derived products exist in the market, and its specific use has been associated with direct health outcomes and adverse reactions. The iconic embodiment of consuming cannabis has been linked to smoking a joint. Inhalation or smoking via a joint, spliff, pipe, blunt, and water pipe/bong is the most commonly used form of consumption [35, 36]. Other routes of administration (ROA) range from vaporizing (inhalation), oral spray, edibles, tinctures (alcohol-based liquid cannabis extracts), other oromucosal/sublingual routes (e.g., capsules and lozenges), transdermal topicals (cannabis-infused lotions, balms, oils), intravenous routes (syringe) to rectal routes (suppositories) [16–37]. Their applied pharmacology and pharmacokinetics differ greatly between different ROA (Table 10.1). Refer to the Chap. 22 on dosing and titration.

Direct data comparing analgesic efficacy and safety profile of different cannabis products depending on ROA is scarce [16]. Epidemiological studies concerning the harmful effects of smoking cannabis have been reported [38]. Smoking, as the specific ROA, has been associated with many pulmonary complications.

Table 10.1 Applied pharmacology of cannabis-based products according to ROA

	Inhalation	Oral	Topical	Liquid extract	Rectal	Ophthalmic
Absorption	rapid (seconds)	1–2 h	variable, enhanced by water and oleic acid in ethanol	10–45 minutes	Variable, depends on its base formulation	1 h
Peak plasma availability	3–10 min	4–6 h	Variable, ~1.4 h	Variable	2–8 h	Several hours
Bioavailability	10–35%	Variable, 6–10%	Variable	Variable	Variable, up to 13.5%	6–40%
Duration of action	1–6 h	4–12 h	48 h steady-state	2–8 h	Variable	Variable

Absorption

Smoking

Smoking cannabis produces rapid and efficient absorption, shorter duration of action, and higher blood concentration of THC [39–42]. Absorption and bioavailability of THC depend on the depth of inhalation, the type of smoking device, the puff duration, the subjects' smoking habit (i.e., breath-holding), and the composition of cigarettes [43]. Each joint contains 500 mg–1.0 g of cannabis plant, 7.5–225 mg of THC (1–30%), and 0–180 mg CBD (0–24%) [44]. The absorption of THC through smoking is highly variable individually based on factors described above. The bioavailability of smoking THC ranges from 2 to 56% [39, 43]. In practice, systemic bioavailability ranges a maximum of 23 ± 16% [41] and 27 ± 10% [45] in plasma concentration studies. The mean plasma concentration of THC after one single inhalation of "low-dose" cannabis cigarette (1.75% THC) is 7.0 ± 8.1 ng/ml, while that of a "high-dose" cannabis cigarette (3.55% THC) is 18.1 ± 12.0 ng/m [40].

Vaporization offers a potential risk reduction tool with similar pharmacological profile as smoking cannabis [46]. It has the potential to reduce the formation of carbon monoxide, polycyclic aromatic hydrocarbon, and tar [46]. Variability in vaporized cannabis is subject to many determinants such as the type of cannabis, the amount of cannabis placed in vaporizer, the temperature, the duration of vaporization, and the type of vaporizer used. Refer to the Chap. 36 on adverse events and Chap. 37 on vaping hazards.

Oral

In contrast, oral absorption is slow, variable, and highly dependable on its associated food ingestion [45, 47]. Based on bioavailability alone, the conversion factor between inhalation and oral absorption has been estimated to be 2.5 [48].

Given that cannabinoids are lipophilic, some literature suggests that fatty meal or lipophilic formulation (cookie or oil-based) enhances cannabinoid absorption and bioavailability [49]. However, there is some controversial evidence in rats and human studies [50]. All oral ingestion undergoes first-pass metabolism in the liver. For example, dronabinol, or Marinol®, has a bioavailability of 10 to 20% of the administered dose after extensive hepatic first-pass metabolism [Marinol® FDA product monograph].

Oro-mucosal and Intranasal

Nabiximols (Sativex®) is a 50:50 THC/CBD cannabis extract in the form of buccal spray. In one single oro-mucosal administration of nabiximol (Sativex®) (four sprays totalling 10.8 mg Δ9-THC and 10 mg CBD), mean peak plasma concentrations of both THC (~5.5 ng/mL) and

CBD (~3 ng/mL) typically occur within 2 to 4 h [Sativex product monograph]. For detailed pharmacology of nabiximols, please refer to the Chap. 17 (nabiximols).

Rectal

Rectal application avoids first-pass metabolism. THC itself cannot be absorbed rectally, while its pro-drug THC-hemisuccinate is easily absorbed rectally. The suppository formulation greatly influences their absorption and bioavailability [51]. In rectal suppositories, THC-hemisuccinate formulation can offer a bioavailability of up to 13.5% [52]. Due to the lack of first-pass metabolism, the estimated relative effectiveness of the oral vs. the rectal formulation was 25–50% [51].

Transcutaneous

Transcutaneous application avoids first-pass metabolism. Transdermal cannabis-based product absorption is enhanced by using water and oleic acid in propylene glycol and ethanol [53].

Distribution

Tetrahydrocannabinol has high plasma protein binding and large volume of distribution [43]. In the blood, approximately 90% of THC is distributed to the plasma and another 10% to red blood cells [54]. The plasma concentration of THC has been described to fit two-, three-, or four-compartment models [55–58]. Given its lipophilicity, the initial volume of distribution of THC is small (2.5–3 L) compared to its steady-state volume of distribution (236 L or 3.4 L/kg assuming 70 kg bodyweight) [58, 59].

Metabolism and Elimination

THC is metabolized in the liver via microsomal hydroxylation and oxidation by cytochrome P450 enzymes CYP 2C9, 2C19, and 3A4 [6].THC is metabolized into an active form 11-OH-THC, which mimics the action of THC in the brain. Further breakdown then occurs to produce 11-nor-9-carboxy-THC, the inactive metabolite.

More than 55% of THC is excreted in the feces and ≈20% in the urine. The main metabolite in urine is the ester of glucuronic acid and THC-COOH and free THC-COOH and, in the feces, mainly 11-OH-THC [39].

Conclusion

Phytocannabinoids are natural products derived from cannabis either interacting directly with cannabinoid receptors or sharing chemical similarity with endocannabinoids. THC is the main psychoactive compound of the cannabis plant. ROA of THC range from vaporizing (inhalation), edibles, oromucosal/sublingual routes (e.g., capsules,oils, lozenges), transdermal topicals (cannabis-infused lotions, balms, oils) to rectal routes (suppositories). Their applied pharmacology and pharmacokinetics differ greatly between different ROA. THC produces pharmacological effects ranging from cognitive changes and psychoactive, anti-inflammatory, antipruritic, bronchodilatory, anti-spasmodic, and muscle relaxant activities. It is also associated with side effects like anxiety, impaired memory, and immunosuppression. Further research and human studies are required to validate medical uses of THC.

References

1. Gertsch J, Pertwee RG, Vincenzo DM. Phytocannabinoids beyond the Cannabis plant – do they exist? Br J Pharmacol. 2010;160(3):523–9.
2. Radwan MM, ElSohly MA, El-Alfy AT, Ahmed SA, Slade D, Husni AS, Manly SP, Wilson L, Seale S, Cutler SJ, et al. Isolation and pharmacological evaluation of minor cannabinoids from high-potency cannabis sativa. J Nat Prod. 2015;78(6):1271–6.
3. Lewis MA, Russo EB, Smith KM. Pharmacological Foundations of Cannabis Chemovars. Planta Med. 2018;84(4):225–33.
4. Elsohly MA, Slade D. Chemical constituents of marijuana: the complex mixture of natural cannabinoids. Life Sci. 2005;78(0024-3205; 0024-3205; 5):539–48.

5. Morales P, Hurst DP, Reggio PH. Molecular targets of the phytocannabinoids-a complex picture. Prog Chem Org Nat Prod. 2017;103:103–31. https://doi.org/10.1007/978-3-319-45541-9_4.
6. Vuckovic. Cannabinoids and pain: new insights from old molecules. Front Pharmacol. 2018;9:1259. Published online 2018 Nov 13.
7. Mehmedic Z, Chandra S, Slade D, Denham H, Foster S, Patel AS, Ross SA, Khan IA, Elsohly MA. Potency trends of delta(9)-THC and other cannabinoids in confiscated cannabis preparations from 1993 to 2008*. J Forensic Sci. 2010;55(1556–4029; 0022–1198; 5):1209–17.
8. Harrison J, Dolah V, Bauer BA, Mauck KF. Clinicians' guide to Cannabidiol and Hemp oils. Mayo Clin Proc. 2019;94(9):1840–51. Epub 2019 Aug 22
9. Taming. THC: potential cannabis synergy and phytocannabinoid-terpenoid entourage effects. Br J Pharmacol. 2011;163(7):1344–64.
10. Huestis MA. Human cannabinoid pharmacokinetics. Chem Biodivers. 2007;4(1612–1880; 1612–1872; 8):1770–804.
11. Dussy FE, Hamberg C, Luginbuhl M, Schwerzmann T, Briellmann TA. Isolation of Delta9-THCA-A from hemp and analytical aspects concerning the determination of Delta9-THC in cannabis products. Forensic Sci Int. 2005;149(0379–0738; 0379–0738; 1):3–10.
12. Gaoni Y, Mechoulam R. Isolation, structure and partial synthesis of an active constituent of hashish. J Am Chem Soc. 1964;86(8):1646–7. https://doi.org/10.1021/ja01062a046.
13. Russo EB. Taming THC: potential cannabis synergy and phytocannabinoid-terpenoid entourage effects. Br J Pharmacol. 2011;163:1344–64.
14. Howlett AC, Barth F, Bonner TI, Cabral G, Casellas P, Devane WA, Felder CC, Herkenham M, Mackie K, Martin BR, Mechoulam R, Pertwee RG. Classification of cannabinoid receptors. Pharmacol Rev. 2002;54(2):161–202. International Union of Pharmacology. XXVII.
15. Pertwee RG. The diverse CB1 and CB2 receptor pharmacology of three plant cannabinoids: Δ9-tetrahydrocannabinol, cannabidiol and Δ9-tetrahydrocannabivarin. Br J Pharmacol. 2008;153(2):199–215.
16. Russell C, Rueda S, Room R, Tyndall M, Fischer B. Routes of administration for cannabis use–basic prevalence and related health outcomes: a scoping review and synthesis. Int J Drug Policy. 2018;52:87–96.
17. Geshtakovska G, Stefkov G. Routes of cannabis administration: a brief review. Macedonian Pharm Bull. 2016;62:515–6.
18. Mazzoccanti G, Ismail OH, D'Acquarica I, Villani C, Manzo C, Wilcox M, Cavazzini A, Gasparrini F. "Cannabis through the looking glass: chemo- and enantio-selective separation of phytocannabinoids by enantioselective ultra high performance supercritical fluid chromatography" (PDF). Chem Commun. 2017;53(91):12262–5.
19. Pertwee RG. The pharmacology of cannabinoid receptors and their ligands: an overview. Int J Obes. 2006;30(Suppl 1):S13–8.
20. Pistis M, Ferraro L, Pira L, Flore G, Tanganelli S, Gessa GL, et al. Δ9-Tetrahydrocannabinol decreases extracellular GABA and increases extracellular glutamate and dopamine levels in the rat prefrontal cortex: an in vivo microdialysis study. Brain Res. 2002;948:155–8.
21. Gardner EL. Endocannabinoid signaling system and brain reward: emphasis on dopamine. Pharmacol Biochem Behav. 2005;81:263–84.
22. Pisanu A, Acquas E, Fenu S, Di Chiara G. Modulation of Δ9-THC-induced increase of cortical and hippocampal acetylcholine release by mu opioid and D-1 dopamine receptors. Neuropharmacology. 2006;50:661–70.
23. Justinova Z, Goldberga SR, Heishman SJ, Tanda G. Selfadministration of cannabinoids by experimental animals and human marijuana smokers. Pharmacol Biochem Behav. 2005;81:285–99.
24. Turkanis SA, Karler R. Electrophysiologic properties of the cannabinoids. J Clin Pharmacol. 1981;21:449S–63S.
25. Wallace MJ, Blair RE, Falenski KW, Martin BR, DeLorenzo RJ. The endogenous cannabinoid system regulates seizure frequency and duration in a model of temporal lobe epilepsy. J Pharmacol Exp Ther. 2003;307:129–37.
26. Braida D, Limonta V, Malabarba L, Zani A, Sala M. (2007). 5-HT1A receptors are involved in the anxiolytic effect of Delta9-tetrahydrocannabinol and AM 404, the anandamide transport inhibitor, in Sprague–Dawley rats. Eur J Pharmacol. 2007;555:156–63.
27. Schramm-Sapyta NL, Cha YM, Chaudhry S, Wilson WA, Swartzwelder HS, Kuhn CM. Differential anxiogenic, aversive, and locomotor effects of THC in adolescent and adult rats. Psychopharmacology. 2007;191:867–77.
28. Ryberg E, Larsson N, Sjogren S, Hjorth S, Hermansson NO, Leonova J, et al. The orphan receptor GPR55 is a novel cannabinoid receptor. Br J Pharmacol. 2007;152(7):1092–101.
29. Bukiya AN. Chapter 8. Pharmacology of medical Cannabis. In: Joshi N, Onaivi ES, editors. Recent advances in cannabinoid physiology and pathology. p. 152. Springer 2019.
30. Basbaum AI, Bautista DM, Scherrer G, Julius D. Cellular and molecular mechanisms of pain. Cell. 2009;139(2):267–84.
31. Nabissi M, Morelli MB, Amantini C, Farfariello V, Ricci-Vitiani L, Caprodossi S, et al. TRPV2 channel negatively controls glioma cell proliferation and resistance to Fas-induced apoptosis in ERK-dependent manner. Carcinogenesis. 2010;31(5):794–803.
32. Santoni G, Farfariello V, Liberati S, Morelli MB, Nabissi M, Santoni M, Amantini C. The role of transient receptor potential vanilloid type-2 ion chan-

nels in innate and adaptive immune responses. Front Immunol. 2013;4:34.
33. Campos AC, Moreira FA, Gomes FV, Del Bel EA, Guimarães FS. Multiple mechanisms involved in the large-spectrum therapeutic potential of cannabidiol in psychiatric disorders. Philos Trans R Soc Lond Ser B Biol Sci. 2012;367:3364–78.
34. Russo E, Guy GW. A tale of two cannabinoids: the therapeutic rationale for combining tetrahydrocannabinol and cannabidiol. Med Hypotheses. 2006;66(2):234–46. Epub 2005 Oct 4
35. Schauer GL, King BA, Bunnell RE, Promoff G, McAfee TA. Toking, vaping, and eating for health or fun: Marijuana use patterns in adults, U.S., 2014. Am J Prev Med. 2016;50:1–8.
36. Subritzky T, Pettigrew S, Lenton S. Issues in the implementation and evolution of the commercial recreational cannabis market in Colorado. Int J Drug Policy. 2016;27:1–12.
37. Varlet V, Concha-Lozano N, Berthet A, Plateel G, Favrat B, De Cesare M, Lauer E, Augsburger M, Thomas A, Giroud C. Drug vaping applied to cannabis: is "cannavaping" a therapeutic alternative to marijuana? Sci Rep. 2016;6:25599.
38. Hindocha C, Freeman TP, Ferris JA, Lynskey MT, Winstock AR. No smoke without tobacco: a global overview of cannabis and tobacco routes of administration and their association with intention to quit. Front Psych. 2016;7:104.
39. Huestis MA. Pharmacokinetics and metabolism of the plant cannabinoids, delta9-tetrahydrocannabinol, cannabidiol and cannabinol. Handb Exp Pharmacol. 2005;168:657–90.
40. Huestis MA, Henningfield JE, Cone EJ. Blood cannabinoids: I. absorption of THC and formation of 11-OH-THC and THCCOOH during and after smoking marijuana. J Anal Toxicol. 1992;16(5):276–82.
41. Lindgren JE, Ohlsson A, Agurell S, et al. Clinical effects and plasma levels of delta 9-tetrahydrocannabinol (delta 9-THC) in heavy and light users of cannabis. Psychopharmacology. 1981;74(3):208–12.
42. Chiang CW, Barnett G. Marijuana effect and delta-9-tetrahydrocannabinol plasma level. Clin Pharmacol Ther. 1984;36(2):234–8. https://doi.org/10.1038/clpt.1984.168.
43. Grotenhermen F. Pharmacokinetics and pharmacodynamics of cannabinoids. Clin Pharmacokinet. 2003;42(4):327–60.
44. Ridgeway G, Kilmer B. Bayesian interference for the distribution of grams of marijuana in a joint. Drug Alcohol Depend. 2016;165:175–80.
45. Ohlsson A, Lindgren JE, Wahlen A, et al. Single dose kinetics of deuterium labelled Δ1-tetrahydrocannabinol in heavy and light cannabis users. Biomed Mass Spectrom. 1982;9(1):6–10.
46. Abrams DI, Vizoso HP, Shade SB, Jay C, Kelly ME, Benowitz NL. Vaporization as a smokeless cannabis delivery system: a pilot study. Clin Pharmacol Ther. 2007;82(0009–9236; 5):572–8.
47. Harvey DJ, Samara E, Mechoulam R. Comparative metabolism of cannabidiol in dog, rat and man. Pharmacol Biochem Behav. 1991;40(3):523–32. https://doi.org/10.1016/0091-3057(91)90358-9.
48. Grotenhermen F. Harm reduction associated with inhalation and oral administration of cannabis and THC. J Cannabis Ther. 2001;1(3/4):133.
49. Zgair A, Wong JC, Lee JB, Mistry J, Sivak O, Wasan KM, Hennig IM, Barrett DA, Constantinescu CS, Fischer PM, et al. Dietary fats and pharmaceutical lipid excipients increase systemic exposure to orally administered cannabis and cannabis-based medicines. Am J Transl Res. 2016;8(8):3448–59.
50. Nadulski T, Sporkert F, Schnelle M, Stadelmann AM, Roser P, Schefter T, Pragst F. Simultaneous and sensitive analysis of THC, 11-OH-THC, THC-COOH, CBD, and CBN by GC-MS in plasma after oral application of small doses of THC and cannabis extract. J Anal Toxicol. 2005;29(8):782–9.
51. Brenneisen R, Egli A, Elsohly MA, Henn V, Spiess Y. The effect of orally and rectally administered delta 9-tetrahydrocannabinol on spasticity: a pilot study with 2 patients. Int J Clin Pharmacol Ther. 1996;34(10):446–52.
52. ElSohly MA, Stanford DF, Harland EC, et al. Rectal bioavailability of delta-9-tetrahydrocannabinol from the hemisuccinate ester in monkeys. J Pharm Sci. 1991;80(10):942–5.
53. Touitou E, Fabin B, Dany S, et al. Transdermal delivery of tetrahydrocannabinol. Int J Pharm. 1988;43:9–15.
54. Widman M, Agurell S, Ehrnebo M, et al. Binding of (+)- and (−)-Δ1- tetrahydrocannabinols and (−)-7-hydroxy-Δ1-tetrahydrocannabinol to blood cells and plasma proteins in man. J Pharm Pharmacol. 1974;26(11):914–6.
55. Wall ME, Sadler BM, Brine D, et al. Metabolism, disposition, and kinetics of delta-9-tetrahydrocannabinol, in men and women. Clin Pharmacol Ther. 1983;34(3):352–63.
56. Barnett G, Chiang CW, Perez-Reyes M, Owens SM. Kinetic study of smoking marijuana. J Pharmacokinet Biopharm. 1982;10(5):495–506. https://doi.org/10.1007/BF01059033.
57. Grotenhermen F. Pharmacokinetics and pharmacodynamics of cannabinoids. Clin Pharmacokinet. 2012;42:327–360(2003).
58. Hunt CA, Jones RT. Tolerance and disposition of tetrahydrocannabinol in man. J Pharmacol Exp Ther. 1980;215(1):35–44.
59. Sticht G, Käferstein H. Grundbegriffe, toxikokinetik und toxikodynamik. In: Berghaus G, Krüger HP, editors. Cannabis im Straßenverkehr. Stuttgart: Gustav Fischer; 1998. p. 1–11.

11 Phytocannabinoids: Cannabidiol (CBD)

Priodarshi Roychoudhury, Ning Nan Wang, and Samer N. Narouze

Phytocannabinoids

Medical use of cannabis dates back to the Neolithic times and was mentioned in the world's oldest pharmacopeia, the Pen-Ts'ao Ching [1]. Cannabis was used for diseases like rheumatic pain, constipation, and others [1]. Its medical use spread to India, the Middle East, Africa, Europe, and the Americas. It was not until the eighteenth century, when Dr. William B. O'Shaughnessy, an Irish physician, introduced cannabis for treating rheumatism, convulsions, and muscular spasms of tetanus and rabies [2]. Today, cannabis and its related products have gained broader acceptance among the public for its recreational and medical use. For the history of the cannabis use, please refer to Chap. 1.

Cannabis includes various species, the most well-known being *Cannabis sativa*, *Cannabis indica*, and *Cannabis ruderalis*. Cannabinoids are chemicals either derived from cannabis, for example, phytocannabinoids, cannabidiol (CBD) and Δ9-tetrahydrocannabinol (THC); synthetic medications like nabilone, dronabinol, and rimonabant; or endogenous chemicals that stimulate cannabinoid receptors. Phytocannabinoids consist of natural products capable of either interacting directly with cannabinoid receptors or sharing chemical similarity with endocannabinoids or both [3]. Cannabinoids consist of a promising area of interest for treatment of several disorders including neurologic diseases (seizure, multiple sclerosis, diabetic peripheral neuropathy, HIV, peripheral neuropathy), Crohn's disease, irritable bowel syndrome, generalized anxiety disorder, post-traumatic stress disorder, and chronic pain.

More than 100 active phytocannabinoids have been identified within *Cannabis sativa* plant alone [4]. The two most studied phytocannabinoids are Δ9-tetrahydrocannabinol (THC) and cannabidiol (CBD).

Cannabidiol and Its Various Clinical Effects

CBD is a non-intoxicating phytocannabinoid. It was first discovered by Dr. Roger Adams and his team at the University of Illinois in 1940; however, its chemical structure was first identified in 1963 [5] (Fig. 11.1). CBD accounts for 40% of the *Cannabis sativa* extract [6]. Its lack of psychoactivity has gained popularity and interests in its clinical use. CBD has been associated with

P. Roychoudhury (✉)
Department of Anesthesia and Pain Management, Toronto General Hospital, University of Toronto, Toronto, ON, Canada

N. N. Wang
Department of Anesthesia and Pain Management, Toronto Western Hospital, University of Toronto, Toronto, ON, Canada

S. N. Narouze
Western Reserve Hospital, Center For Pain Medicine, Cuyahoga Falls, OH, USA
e-mail: narouzs@hotmail.com

S. N. Narouze (ed.), *Cannabinoids and Pain*, https://doi.org/10.1007/978-3-030-69186-8_11

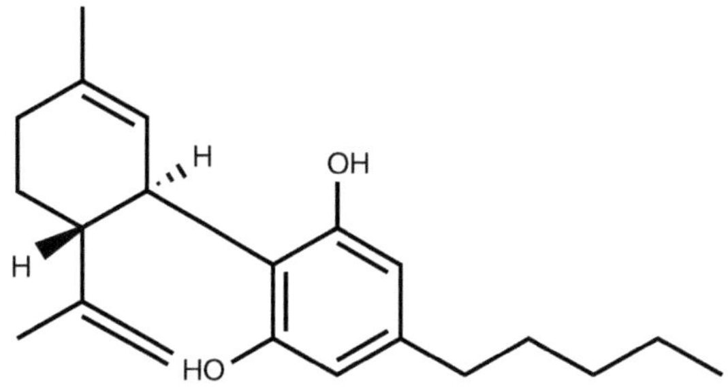

Fig. 11.1 CBD chemical structure. In public domain, https://commons.wikimedia.org/w/index.php?curid=7712509

analgesic, anti-inflammatory, anticonvulsant, anxiolytic, and antipsychotic effects [7], for example, Epidiolex®, a highly purified, plant-derived cannabidiol prescription medication that was recently approved by FDA. It is indicated for seizures associated with Lennox-Gastaut syndrome or Dravet syndrome in the USA [8]. For Epidolex's pharmacology and pharmacokinetics, please refer to the Chap. 16.

Another FDA-approved prescription medication is nabiximols or Sativex®. Nabiximols is a cannabinoid oromucosal spray containing extract of CBD and THC [9]. It is approved for multiple sclerosis-induced spasticity in Canada and many European countries but not in the USA. Multiple meta-analyses have demonstrated analgesic effects of nabiximol in the treatment of chronic neuropathic pain [10–12]. There is also some controversial evidence on the use of nabiximol for cancer pain [13, 14]. For pharmacology and pharmacokinetics of Sativex, please refer to the Chap. 16.

Pharmacodynamics of Cannabidiol

CBD has low affinity for both cannabinoid receptor 1(CB1R) and cannabinoid receptor 2 (CB2R). It acts as a partial antagonist of CB1R and as a weak inverse agonist of CB2R [15]. At the level of CB1R, it causes negative allosteric modulation of the orthosteric receptor [16–18]. CBD also interacts with other non-cannabinoid targets, including serotonin 1A receptor (or 5-TH1A), vanilloid receptor 1 (TRPV1), and adenosine A2A receptors, which regulates the perception of pain [7]. These complex CNS mechanisms can partially explain multiple clinical effects. For example, in rat models, high dose of CBD intracerebral administration activates TRPV1 receptors to produce anxiolytic effects [19]. CBD also induces antidepressant effect in mice by enhancing 5-HT and glutamate levels in the prefrontal cortex [20]. CBD acts through a positive allosteric modulation of 5-HT1A serotonin receptors and increases serotoninergic and glutamatergic transmission [20]. CBD also antagonizes alpha-1 adrenergic receptors [21, 22]. It is also an allosteric modulator of the μ- and δ-opioid receptors [23]. CBD's action as a CB2R inverse agonist may explain its anti-inflammatory properties [24]. In the presence of THC, CBD has complex physiological effects. CBD works synergistically with THC for its analgesic effect while decreasing its psychoactive and cognitive side effects such as sedation and memory impairment of THC [25].

CBD may also act as an inverse agonist of GPR3, GPR6, and GPR12 [26] and as an antagonist of the orphan receptor GPR55 which is considered a novel cannabinoid receptor [27].

For detailed mechanisms of analgesia of CBD, please refer to the Chap. 24.

Applied Pharmacology and Pharmacokinetics

A large diversity of cannabis-derived products exist in the market, and its specific use has been associated with direct health outcomes and adverse reactions. CBD-containing products range from different strains of cannabis and its derived products, "CBD oil," and prescription medications (Epidiolex® and Sativex®). First, the iconic embodiment of consuming cannabis has been linked to smoking a joint. Inhalation or smoking via a joint, spliff, pipe, blunt, and water pipe/bong is the most commonly used form of consumption [28, 29]. Other routes of administrations (ROA) range from vaporizing (inhalation), dabbing, e-cigarettes, oral spray, edibles, drinkables, tinctures (alcohol-based liquid cannabis extracts), other oromucosal/sublingual routes (e.g., capsules and lozenges), transdermal topicals (cannabis-infused lotions, balms, oils), intravenous routes (syringe) to rectal routes (suppositories) [30–32]. In addition to medical cannabis and Epidiolex®, there are many forms of "CBD oil" in the market [33]. In fact, the "cannabis oil" products can be regrouped into three subtypes: (1) hemp and seed oil, (2) hemp-based CBD oil, and (3) cannabis oil [34–36]. Their applied pharmacology and pharmacokinetics differ greatly between different ROA. Please refer to the Chaps. 18 and 21.

Smoking

Smoking cannabis produces rapid and efficient absorption, shorter duration of action, and higher blood concentration. Absorption and bioavailability depend on the depth of inhalation, the type of smoking device, the puff duration, the breath hold, and the composition of cigarettes. Little clinical data exists in literature for pharmacology of smoked CBD. It is estimated that CBD bioavailability is similar to those of THC, with a mean value of 31% (range 11–45%) [37]. Each joint contains 500 mg–1.0 g of cannabis plant, 7.5–225 mg of THC (1–30%), and 0–180 mg of CBD (0–24%) [38].

Vaporization offers a potential risk-reduction tool with similar pharmacological profile as smoking cannabis [39]. It has the potential to reduce the formation of carbon monoxide, polycyclic aromatic hydrocarbon, and tar [39]. Variability in vaporized cannabis is subject to many determinants such as the type of cannabis, the amount of cannabis placed in vaporizer, the temperature, the duration of vaporization, and the type of vaporizer used.

Oral

In contrast to smoking, oral absorption is slow, variable, and highly dependable on its associated food ingestion [40, 41]. Oral CBD bioavailability is estimated to be approximately 6% [22,42]. A double-blinded human study in 14 Huntington's disease patients for 6 weeks of oral CBD administration (10 mg/kg/day = about 700 mg/day) measured their plasma levels of cannabidiol [43]. The mean weekly plasma concentrations of CBD in treatment group ranged from 5.9 to 11.2 ng/ml over the 6 weeks of CBD administration [43]. CBD levels averaged 1.5 ng/ml 1 week after CBD was discontinued and were undetectable thereafter [43]. Administration of oral CBD (40 mg) in the form of chocolate cookie to healthy volunteer results in a mean plasma CBD levels ranged between 1.1 and 11 ng/mL (mean, 5.5 ng/mL) after 1 hour [42]. The course of CBD in the plasma over 6 hours was in the same range as the course after 20 mg THC [42].

Given that cannabinoids are lipophilic, there are a small number of animal and human studies which suggest that fatty meal or lipophilic formulation (cookie or oil-based) enhances cannabinoid absorption and bioavailability [44]. In rats, co-administration of THC and CBD (12 mg/kg) with lipid long-chain triglycerides (LCT)-based formulation (sesame oil) by oral gavage has demonstrated an absolute increase in absorption [44]. The absolute bioavailability of CBD was three times higher in the lipid-based (Cmax = 308 ng/mL; AUC = 932 h.ng/mL) versus lipid-free formulation (Cmax = 87 ng/mL; AUC = 327 h.ng/mL) [44].

Transcutaneous

Transcutaneous application of cannabinoids avoids first-pass metabolism. Cannabinoids are lipophilic, thus inhibiting the diffusion process across the aqueous layer of the skin [45]. CBD, unlike THC, is more permeable for transcutaneous absorption. In human studies for transdermal combination therapy, the permeability of CBD and CBN was found to be tenfold higher than for THC [46]. Ethanol concentrations of 30–33% also significantly increase the transdermal absorption of both THC and CBD [46]. Different formulations of CBD-related transdermal products that were investigated clinically include gel and creams [47, 48]. The CBD transdermal gel was investigated in guinea pigs in relation to their plasma concentration. The steady-state plasma concentration of CBD after transdermal gel application was 6.3 +/– 2.1 ng/mL, which was attained at 15.5 +/– 11.7 hours [48]. This steady-state plasma concentration can be increased by 3.7 times by the use of a permeation enhancer. The Cmax without the enhancer vs. with the enhancer was 9 ng/mL vs. 36 ng/mL. Time to reach maximal concentration or Tmax was reached at 38 h without enhancer and 31 h with enhancer post-application, respectively [48]. In pre-clinical studies, topical CBD cream was administered daily on experimental model of mice suffering from autoimmune encephalomyelitis (EAE) [47]. The CBD maximum concentration, or Cmax, was 8 ng/mL with a Tmax of 38 h and a steady-state plasma concentration of 6 ng/mL [47].

Direct data comparing analgesic efficacy and safety profile of different cannabis products ROA is scarce [30]. Epidemiological studies concerning the harmful effects of smoking cannabis have been reported [49]. Smoking, as the specific ROA, has been associated with many pulmonary complications. Refer to the Chaps. 36 and 37 for adverse events and vaping hazards.

Volume of Distribution

The distribution of THC and CBD is time dependent. Given their high lipophilicity, the cannabinoids rapidly penetrate the tissues and have large volume of distribution [41]. THC's volume of distribution is estimated to be around 10 L/kg [41]. Similarly, CBD has an apparent average volume of distribution of CBD of 32.7 L/kg (higher than THC) [37].

Metabolism

Similar to THC, CBD undergoes extensive hepatic first-pass metabolism in the liver [45]. It undergoes extensive phase 1 metabolism [45]. CBD is metabolized by primary oxidation and side-chain oxidation [50, 51]. CBD is metabolized predominantly by liver CYP3A4 and CYP2C19. Therefore, drugs that inhibit or induce these CYP enzymes would increase or decrease CBD levels.

Like THC, CBD plasma level decreases rapidly after smoking. The rapid decline follows a multi-phasic pattern [22]. The half-life of CBD has been estimated to be 18–33 h for intravenous administration, 27–35 h for smoking or inhalation, and 2–5 days for oral administration [43, 50].

Elimination

CBD is excreted both in urine and feces. Unlike THC, a large portion of CBD is excreted unchanged in the feces [45, 52]. More than 30 different metabolites of CBD can be identified in urine. The most abundant metabolites are hydroxylated 7 (or 11)-carboxy derivatives of CBD (inactive), with 7 (or 11)-hydroxy CBD (active) as a minor metabolite [53].

Safety Profile and Side Effects

CBD has proven to be well tolerated, with low toxicity in several studies. Common side effects of CBD include somnolence, fatigue, change in appetite, and change in sleep pattern [54]. In an animal study using rhesus monkey, the LD50 on IV administration of CBD was determined to be 212 mg/kg [55]. Rhesus monkeys were administered 150, 200, 225, 250, or 300 mg/kg intravenous (IV) CBD for 9 days [55]. The signs of toxicity were described as tremors and CNS inhibition (depression, sedation, and prostration). The oral LD50 could not be determined in that specific study [55]. To date, the exact dose of LD50 oral in human is yet to be determined. Long-term CBD safety was evaluated in children suffering from intractable seizure disorders in a multi-site, US-based program [56]. A total of 607 patients participated in the study administering oral CBD starting at 2–10 mg/kg/d, titrated to a maximum dose of 25–50 mg/kg/day for a median of 48 weeks. AEs were reported in 88% of all patients, and severe AEs such as convulsions and status epilepticus were reported for 33% of patients. A total of 146 (24%) patients withdrew; the most common reasons were lack of efficacy (89 [15%]) and AEs (32 [5%]). The severe adverse reactions of Epidiolex®, although rare, range from suicidal thoughts, suicide attempts, agitation, depression, aggression, and panic attacks [8].

Cannabidiol Interaction with Tetrahydrocannabinol

CBD and THC interactions remain poorly understood despite a few studies [57–60]. Two particular mechanisms of interaction between CBD and THC have been postulated in the literature: (1) pharmacokinetic interactions and (2) pharmacodynamic interactions. First, CBD is a known inhibitor of hepatic drug metabolism for THC through pharmacokinetic interactions [61]. In rat models, CBD pre-treatment (30 minutes) prior to the administration of THC effectively increases THC concentration in the rats' brain [62]. However, this effect is not consistently observed in simultaneous administration of THC and CBD. The additive effect was not observed in in vivo studies [Zuardi et al. 1984]. This was later explained by its pharmacodynamic interactions. Second, in rat models, THC/CBD interactions cause both antagonism or potentiation in a "rate-dependent" phenomenon due to pharmacodynamic interactions [63]. CBD exhibits a negative allosteric modulation of CB1 receptors; thus it can mitigate the negative psychotropic effects of THC. In rat models where THC and CBD were simultaneously administered, it was demonstrated that the mean dose ratio of CBD/THC was 8.1 when the antagonistic effects were observed and 1.8 when the effects of THC were potentiated [64]. These studies suggest that simultaneous administration of high-dose ratios of CBD/THC may favor a pharmacodynamic over a pharmacokinetic interaction, as what was observed in humans [64, 65].

Using functional magnetic resonance imaging (fMRI) in healthy volunteers revealed that delta-9-THC and CBD had opposite effects on regional brain function (in the striatum during verbal recall, in the hippocampus during the response inhibition task, in the amygdala when subjects viewed fearful faces, in the superior temporal cortex when subjects listened to speech, and in the occipital cortex during visual processing). Pre-treatment with CBD prevented the acute induction of psychotic symptoms by delta-9-THC [65].

Conclusion

CBD is a non-intoxicating phytocannabinoid. It acts as a partial antagonist of CB1R and as a weak inverse agonist of CB2R. CBD also interacts with other non-cannabinoid targets, including serotonin 1A receptor (or 5-TH1A), vanilloid receptor 1 (TRPV1), and adenosine A2A receptors, which regulates perception of pain. CBD has been associated with analgesic, anti-inflammatory, anticonvulsant, anxiolytic, and antipsychotic effects. CBD works synergistically with THC for its analgesic effect while decreasing its psychoactive and cognitive side effects such as sedation and memory impairment of THC. Further studies are required to validate the medicinal applications of CBD.

References

1. Zuardi AW. History of cannabis as a medicine: a review. Rev Bras Psiquiatr. 2006;28(2):153–7.
2. Fankhauser M. Chapter 4, History of cannabis in western medicine. In: Grotenhermen F, Russo E, editors. Cannabis and cannabinoids. New York: The Haworth Integrative Healing Press; 2002. p. 37–51.
3. Gertsch J. Pertwee RG, Vincenzo DM, Phytocannabinoids beyond the Cannabis plant – do they exist? Br J Pharmacol. 2010;160(3):523–9.
4. Lewis MA, Russo EB, Smith KM. Pharmacological Foundations of Cannabis Chemovars. Planta Med. 2018;84(4):225–33. https://doi.org/10.1055/s-0043-122240.
5. Mechoulam R, Shvo Y. The structure of cannabidiol. Tetrahedron. 1963;19:2073–8.
6. Campos AC, Moreira FA, Gomes FV, Del Bel EA, Guimarães FS. Multiple mechanisms involved in the large-spectrum therapeutic potential of cannabidiol in psychiatric disorders. Philos Trans R Soc Lond Ser B Biol Sci. 2012;367:3364–78.

7. Vuckovic. Cannabinoids and pain: new insights from old molecules. Front Pharmacol. 2018;9:1259. Published online 2018 Nov 13.
8. EPIDIOLEX (cannabidiol) oral solution. FDA product monograph https://www.accessdata.fda.gov/drugsatfda_docs/label/2018/210365lbl.pdf.
9. Product monograph, including patient medication information, PrSATIVEX®, consulted on June 10th 2020. https://pdf.hres.ca/dpd_pm/00054388.PDF.
10. Meng H, Johnston B, Englesakis M, Moulin DE, Bhatia A. Selective cannabinoids for chronic neuropathic pain: a systematic review and meta-analysis. Anesth Analg. 2017;125(5):1638–52.
11. Stockings E, Campbell G, Hall WD, Nielsen S, Zagic D, Rahman R, Murnion B, Farrell M, Weier M, Degenhardt L. Cannabis and cannabinoids for the treatment of people with chronic noncancer pain conditions: a systematic review and meta-analysis of controlled and observational studies. Pain. 2018;159(10):1932–54.
12. Johal H, Devji T, Chang Y, Simone J, Vannabouathong C, Bhandari M. Cannabinoids in chronic non-cancer pain: a systematic review and meta-analysis. Clin Med Insights Arthritis Musculoskelet Disord. 2020;13:1179544120906461.
13. Boland EG, Bennett MI, Allgar V, Boland JW. Cannabinoids for adult cancer-related pain: systematic review and meta-analysis. BMJ Support Palliat Care. 2020;10:14–24.
14. Häuser W, Welsch P, Klose P, et al. Efficacy, tolerability and safety of cannabis-based medicines for cancer pain: a systematic review with meta-analysis of randomised controlled trials. Schmerz. 2019;33:424–36.
15. Bruni N, Della Pepa C, Oliaro-Bosso S, Pessione E, Gastaldi D, Dosio F. Cannabinoid delivery systems for pain and inflammation treatment. Molecules. 2018;23(10):2478.
16. Laprairie RB, Bagher AM, Kelly ME, Denovan-Wright EM. Cannabidiol is a negative allosteric modulator of the cannabinoid CB1 receptor. Br J Pharmacol. 2015;172(20):4790–805.
17. McPartland JM, Duncan M, Di Marzo V, Pertwee RG. Are cannabidiol and Δ(9)-tetrahydrocannabivarin negative modulators of the endocannabinoid system? A systematic review. Br J Pharmacol. 2015;172:737–53.
18. Tham M, Yilmaz O, Alaverdashvili M, Kelly MEM, Denovan-Wright EM, Laprairie RB. Allosteric and orthosteric pharmacology of cannabidiol and cannabidiol-dimethylheptyl at the type 1 and type 2 cannabinoid receptors. Br J Pharmacol. 2018;176:1455.
19. Campos AC, Guimarães FS. Evidence for a potential role for TRPV1 receptors in the dorsolateral periaqueductal gray in the attenuation of the anxiolytic effects of cannabinoids. Prog Neuro-Psychopharmacol Biol Psychiatry. 2009;33:1517–21.
20. Linge R, Jiménez-Sánchez L, Campa L, Pilar-Cuéllar F, Vidal R, Pazos A, Adell A, Díaz Á. Cannabidiol induces rapid-acting antidepressant-like effects and enhances cortical 5-HT/glutamate neurotransmission: role of 5-HT1A receptors. Neuropharmacology. 2016;103:16–26,ISSN 0028-3908. https://doi.org/10.1016/j.neuropharm.2015.12.017.
21. Pertwee RG, Ross RA, Craib SJ, Thomas A. (−)-Cannabidiol antagonizes cannabinoid receptor agonists and noradrenaline in the mouse vas deferens. Eur J Pharmacol. 2002;456:99–106.
22. Zhornitsky S, Potvin S. Cannabidiol in humans-the quest for therapeutic targets. Pharmaceuticals (Basel). 2012;5(5):529–52.
23. Kathmann M, Flau K, Redmer A, Tränkle C, Schlicker E. Cannabidiol is an allosteric modulator at mu- and delta-opioid receptors. Naunyn Schmiedeberg's Arch Pharmacol. 2006;372(5):354–61.
24. Pertwee RG. The diverse CB1 and CB2 receptor pharmacology of three plant cannabinoids: Δ9-tetrahydrocannabinol, cannabidiol and Δ9-tetrahydrocannabivarin. Br J Pharmacol. 2008;153(2):199–215.
25. Russo E, Guy GW. A tale of two cannabinoids: the therapeutic rationale for combining tetrahydrocannabinol and cannabidiol. Med Hypotheses. 2006;66(2):234–46.
26. Laun AS, Shrader SH, Brown KJ, Song ZH. GPR3, GPR6, and GPR12 as novel molecular targets: their biological functions and interaction with cannabidiol. Acta Pharmacol Sin. 2019;40(3):300–8.
27. Ryberg E, Larsson N, Sjögren S, Hjorth S, Hermansson NO, Leonova J, Elebring T, Nilsson K, Drmota T, Greasley PJ. The orphan receptor GPR55 is a novel cannabinoid receptor. Br J Pharmacol. 2007;152(7):1092–101.
28. Schauer GL, King BA, Bunnell RE, Promoff G, McAfee TA. Toking, vaping, and eating for health or fun: Marijuana use patterns in adults, U.S., 2014. Am J Prev Med. 2016;50:1–8.
29. Subritzky T, Pettigrew S, Lenton S. Issues in the implementation and evolution of the commercial recreational cannabis market in Colorado. Int J Drug Policy. 2016;27:1–12.
30. Russell C, Rueda S, Room R, Tyndall M, Fischer B. Routes of administration for cannabis use–basic prevalence and related health outcomes: a scoping review and synthesis. Int J Drug Policy. 2018;52:87–96.
31. Geshtakovska G, Stefkov G. Routes of cannabis administration: a brief review. Macedonian Pharm Bull. 2016;62:515–6.
32. Varlet V, Concha-Lozano N, Berthet A, Plateel G, Favrat B, De Cesare M, Lauer E, Augsburger M, Thomas A, Giroud C. Drug vaping applied to cannabis: is "cannavaping" a therapeutic alternative to marijuana? Sci Rep. 2016;6:25599.
33. VanDolah HJ, Bauer B, Mauck K. Clinicians' guide to Cannabidiol and Hemp oils. Mayo Clin Proc. 2019;94(9):1840–51. Epub 2019 Aug 22
34. Russo EB. Taming THC: potential cannabis synergy and phytocannabinoid-terpenoid entourage effects. Br J Pharmacol. 2011;163(7):1344–64.

35. Callaway JC. Hempseed as a nutritional resource: an overview. Euphytica. 2004;140(1-2):65–72.
36. Grof CPL. Cannabis, from plant to pill. Br J Clin Pharmacol. 2018;84(11):2463–7.
37. Ohlsson A, Lindgren JE, Wahlen A, et al. Plasma delta-9 tetrahydrocannabinol concentrations and clinical effects after oral and intravenous administration and smoking. Clin Pharmacol Ther. 1980;28(3):409–16.
38. Ridgeway G, Kilmer B. Bayesian interference for the distribution of grams of marijuana in a joint. Drug Alcohol Depend. 2016;165:175–80.
39. Abrams DI, Vizoso HP, Shade SB, Jay C, Kelly ME, Benowitz NL. Vaporization as a smokeless cannabis delivery system: a pilot study. Clin Pharmacol Ther. 2007;82(0009-9236; 5):572–8.
40. Ohlsson A, Lindgren JE, Andersson S, Agurell S, Gillespie H, Hollister LE. Single-dose kinetics of deuterium-labelled cannabidiol in man after smoking and intravenous administration. Biomed Environ Mass Spectrom. 1986;13(2):77–83.
41. Harvey DJ. Chapter 2, Absorption, distribution and biotransformation of the cannabinoids. In: Nahas CG, Sutin KM, Harvey DJ, Agurell S, editors. Marihuana and medicine. Totowa, New Jersey: Humana Press; 1999. page 94.
42. Agurell S, Carlsson S, Lindgren JE, Ohlsson A, Gillespie H, Hollister L. Interactions of delta 1-tetrahydrocannabinol with cannabinol and cannabidiol following oral administration in man. assay of cannabinol and cannabidiol by mass fragmentography. Experientia. 1981;37(10):1090–2.
43. Consroe P, Kennedy K, Schram K. Assay of plasma cannabidiol by capillary gas chromatography/ion trap mass spectroscopy following high-dose repeated daily oral administration in humans. Pharmacol Biochem Behav. 1991;40(3):517–22.
44. Zgair A, Lee JB, Wong JCM, et al. Oral administration of cannabis with lipids leads to high levels of cannabinoids in the intestinal lymphatic system and prominent immunomodulation. Sci Rep. 2017;7(1):14542. Published 2017 Nov 6. https://doi.org/10.1038/s41598-017-15026-z.
45. Huestis MA. Human cannabinoid pharmacokinetics. Chem Biodivers. 2007;4(1612-1880; 1612-1872; 8):1770–804.
46. Stinchcomb AL, Valiveti S, Hammell DC, Ramsey DR. Human skin permeation of Delta8-tetrahydrocannabinol, cannabidiol and cannabinol. J Pharm Pharmacol. 2004;56(0022-3573; 0022-3573; 3):291–7.
47. Giacoppo S, Galuppo M, Pollastro F, Grassi G, Bramanti P, Mazzon E. A new formulation of cannabidiol in cream shows therapeutic effects in a mouse model of experimental autoimmune encephalomyelitis. Daru. 2015;23:48,015-0131-8.
48. Paudel KS, Hammell DC, Agu RU, Valiveti S, Stinchcomb AL. Cannabidiol bioavailability after nasal and transdermal application: effect of permeation enhancers. Drug Dev Ind Pharm. 2010;36(9):1088–97.
49. Hindocha C, Freeman TP, Ferris JA, Lynskey MT, Winstock AR. No smoke without tobacco: a global overview of cannabis and tobacco routes of administration and their association with intention to quit. Front Psych. 2016;7:104.
50. Agurell S, Halldin M, Lindgren JE, Ohlsson A, Widman M, Gillespie H, Hollister L. Pharmacokinetics and metabolism of delta 1-tetrahydrocannabinol and other cannabinoids with emphasis on man. Pharmacol Rev. 1986;38:21–43.
51. Harvey DJ, Martin BR, WDM P. In: Nahas GG, Paton WDM, editors. Marijuana: Biological Effects. Oxford: Pergamon Press; 1979. p. 45.
52. Wall ME, Brine DR, Perez-Reyes M. In: Braude MC, Szara S, editors. The pharmacology of marihuana. New York: Raven Press; 1976. p. 93.
53. Ujvary I, Hanus L. Human metabolites of cannabidiol: a review on their formation, biological activity, and relevance in therapy. Cannabis Cannabinoid Res. 2016;1(1):90–101.
54. Bergamaschi MM, Queiroz RH, Zuardi AW, Crippa JA. Safety and side effects of cannabidiol, a Cannabis sativa constituent. Curr Drug Saf. 2011;6(4):237–49.
55. Rosenkrantz H, Fleischman RW, Grant RJ. Toxicity of short-term administration of cannabinoids to rhesus monkeys. Toxicol Appl Pharmacol. 1981;30:118–31.
56. Szaflarski JP, Bebin EM, Comi AM, Patel AD, Joshi C, Checketts D, Beal JC, Laux LC, De Boer LM, Wong MH, Lopez M, Devinsky O, Lyons PD, Zentil PP, Wechsler R. CBD EAP study group. Long-term safety and treatment effects of cannabidiol in children and adults with treatment-resistant epilepsies: expanded access program results. Epilepsia. 2018;59:1540–8.
57. Klein C, Karanges E, Spiro A, Wong A, Spencer J, Huynh T, Gunasekaran N, Karl T, Long LE, Huang XF, et al. Cannabidiol potentiates delta(9)-tetrahydrocannabinol (THC) behavioural effects and alters THC pharmacokinetics during acute and chronic treatment in adolescent rats. Psychopharmacology. 2011;218(2):443–57.
58. Nadulski T, Pragst F, Weinberg G, Roser P, Schnelle M, Fronk EM, Stadelmann AM. Randomized, double-blind, placebo-controlled study about the effects of cannabidiol (CBD) on the pharmacokinetics of Delta9-tetrahydrocannabinol (THC) after oral application of THC versus standardized cannabis extract. Ther Drug Monit. 2005;27(0163-4356; 0163-4356; 6):799–810.
59. Zuardi AW, Shirakawa I, Finkelfarb E, Karniol IG. Action of cannabidiol on the anxiety and other effects produced by delta 9-THC in normal subjects. Psychopharmacology. 1982;76(3):245–50.
60. Karniol IG, Shirakawa I, Kasinski N, Pfeferman A, Carlini EA. Cannabidiol interferes with the effects of delta 9 - tetrahydrocannabinol in man. Eur J Pharmacol. 1974;28(0014-2999; 0014-2999; 1):172–7.

61. Paton WD, Pertwee RG. Effect of cannabis and certain of its constituents on pentobarbitone sleeping time and phenazone metabolism. Br J Pharmacol. 1972;44:250–61.
62. Jones G, Pertwee RG. A metabolic interaction in vivo between cannabidiol and 1-tetrahydrocannabinol. Br J Pharmacol. 1972;45:375–7.
63. Zuardi AW, Hallak JE, Crippa JA. Interaction between cannabidiol (CBD) and (9)-tetrahydrocannabinol (THC): influence of administration interval and dose ratio between the cannabinoids. Psychopharmacology. 2012;219(1432-2072; 0033-3158; 1):247–9.
64. Zuardi AW, Karniol IG. Pharmacological interaction between 9-tetrahydrocannabinol and cannabidiol, two active constituents of Cannabis sativa. Ciência e Cultura. 1984;36(6):386–94.
65. Bhattacharyya S, Morrison PD, Fusar-Poli P, Martin-Santos R, Borgwardt S, Winton-Brown T, Nosarti C, O' Carroll CM, Seal M, Allen P, Mehta MA, Stone JM, Tunstall N, Giampietro V, Kapur S, Murray RM, Zuardi AW, Crippa JA, Atakan Z, McGuire PK. Opposite effects of delta-9-tetrahydrocannabinol and cannabidiol on human brain function and psychopathology. Neuropsychopharmacology. 2010;35:764–74.

12 Other Phytocannabinoids

Hance Clarke, Priodarshi Roychoudhury, and Samer N. Narouze

Introduction

Cannabinoids are lipophilic molecules that interact with the human endocannabinoid system (ECS). Two cannabinoid receptor (CBR) subtypes have been identified, CB1 receptors (CB1R) (cloned in 1990) and CB2 receptors (CB2R) (cloned in 1993), which differ in signaling mechanisms, tissue distribution, agonist/antagonist sensitivity, and an amino acid sequence with CB2R sharing only 44% of amino acid sequence identity with CB1R [1–3]. Phytocannabinoids are natural products derived from cannabis either interacting directly with cannabinoid receptors or sharing chemical similarity with endocannabinoids or both. Phytocannabinoids are produced by glandular trichomes covering the cannabis plant surface. The majority of phytocannabinoids are cannabigerolic acid (CBGA) derivatives and are distinguished into classes by the way this precursor is cyclized. Most of them are insoluble in water but soluble in lipids, alcohol, and non-polar organic solvents. While Δ9-tetrahydrocannabinol (THC) and cannabidiol (CBD) are the most studied phytocannabinoids, other phytocannabinoids that require mention and can exert a physiologic action once metabolized include cannabigerol (CBG), cannabichromene (CBC), cannabinol (CBN), and tetrahydrocannabivarin (THCV).

Synthesis of Phytocannabinoids

Biosynthesis of phytocannabinoids is initiated by the combination of geranyl pyrophosphate and olivetolic acid, to form cannabigerolic acid (CBGA). CBGA is converted to either cannabigerol (CBG), tetrahydrocannabinolic acid (THCA), cannabidiolic acid (CBDA), or cannabichromenic acid (CBCA) by one of the four separate synthases, FAD-dependent dehydrogenase enzymes [4]. For the propyl homologues THCVA, CBDVA, and CBCVA, there is an analogous pathway based on CBGVA from divarinolic acid instead of olivetolic acid.

H. Clarke
Department of Anesthesia and Pain Management, Toronto General Hospital, Centre for Cannabinoid Therapeutics, University Health, Network, University of Toronto, Toronto, ON, Canada
e-mail: hance.clarke@uhn.ca

P. Roychoudhury
Department of Anesthesia and Pain Management, Toronto General Hospital, University of Toronto, Toronto, ON, Canada

S. N. Narouze (✉)
Western Reserve Hospital, Center For Pain Medicine, Cuyahoga Falls, OH, USA
e-mail: narouzs@hotmail.com
Twitter: @NarouzeMD

S. N. Narouze (ed.), *Cannabinoids and Pain*, https://doi.org/10.1007/978-3-030-69186-8_12

Cannabinoids and the Endocannabinoid System (ECS)

Cannabinoid receptors are predominantly present in cortical structures such as the hippocampus and the olfactory bulb and less densely in the basal ganglia, cerebellum, and spinal cord. This results in increased smell sensation and positive effects on memory, cognition, and movement. Historically, the most common route of administration has been inhalation. Absorption is rapid after inhalation, and the bio-availability ranges from 10% to 35%. Given the evolution of a global cannabis industry, products for oral, submucosal, sublingual, and transdermal consumption/application are widely available. There are also less relevant routes like rectal, aerosols, and eye drops available in the consumer marketplace [5, 6].

Evidence has suggested that cannabinoid-based medicines have a favorable safety profile when compared to opioid medications [7]. Due to the relative lack of receptors in the brain stem, there is minimal threat to suppress the respiratory drive. Commonly reported adverse effects are tachycardia, restlessness, excessive sedation, nausea, or vomiting as well as hallucinations.

Minor Cannabinoids

Cannabinol (CBN)

CBN was the first cannabinoid isolated from *Cannabis sativa* [8]. CBN is a nonenzymatic oxidation by-product of THC (Fig. 12.1). It was discovered accidentally due to the rampant degradation of THC to CBN due to poor quality transportation and storage conditions related to the nineteenth century [9]. It is moderately psychoactive and found in small concentrations in *Cannabis* cultivars.

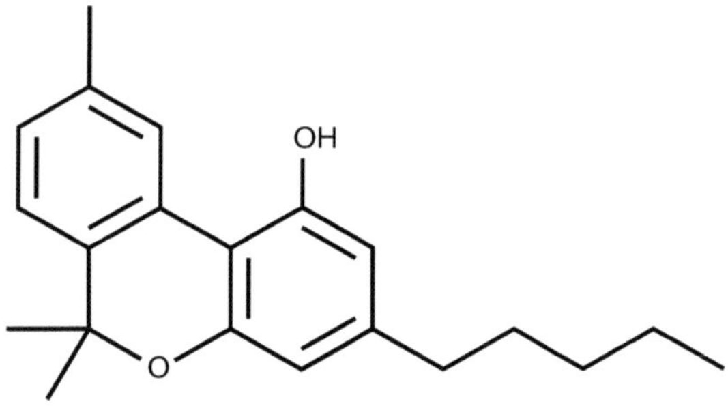

Fig. 12.1 Cannabinol (CBN)

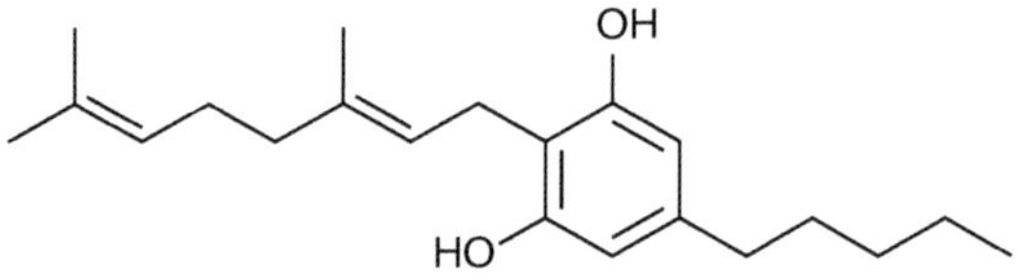

Fig. 12.2 Cannabigerol (CBG)

Though CBN has a lower affinity for CB1 (Ki 211.2 nM) and CB2 (Ki 126.4 nM) [10] and often found inactive as a sole agent, it has demonstrated greater sedative properties when combined with THC [11]. It has also demonstrated anticonvulsant [12], anti-inflammatory [13], and antibacterial properties against MRSA [14–16]. CBN is also a TRPV2 agonist with potential in the treatment of burns [17]. It inhibits keratinocyte proliferation, independent of cannabinoid receptors; thereby it may find an application in topical preparations for dermatologic conditions [18]. CBN stimulates the recruitment of quiescent mesenchymal stem cells in the bone marrow, thereby showing promise in bone formation [19]. CBN has also been found to inhibit breast cancer-resistant protein at very high concentrations (IC50 145 mM) [20].

Cannabigerol (CBG)

Cannabigerol is found in small amounts in the cannabis plant (Figs. 12.2 and 12.3). CBG was purified and isolated in the same year as THC [21], and it lacks psychotropic effects. CBG has a weak partial agonistic effect at CB1 (Ki 440 nM) and CB2 (Ki 337 nM) [22].

CBG stimulates a variety of receptors involved in pain, inflammation, and heat sensitization. It stimulates TRPV1, TRPV2, TRPA1, TRPV3, TRPV4, and α2-adrenoceptor activity [23]. CBG antagonizes TRPV8, suggesting an application in

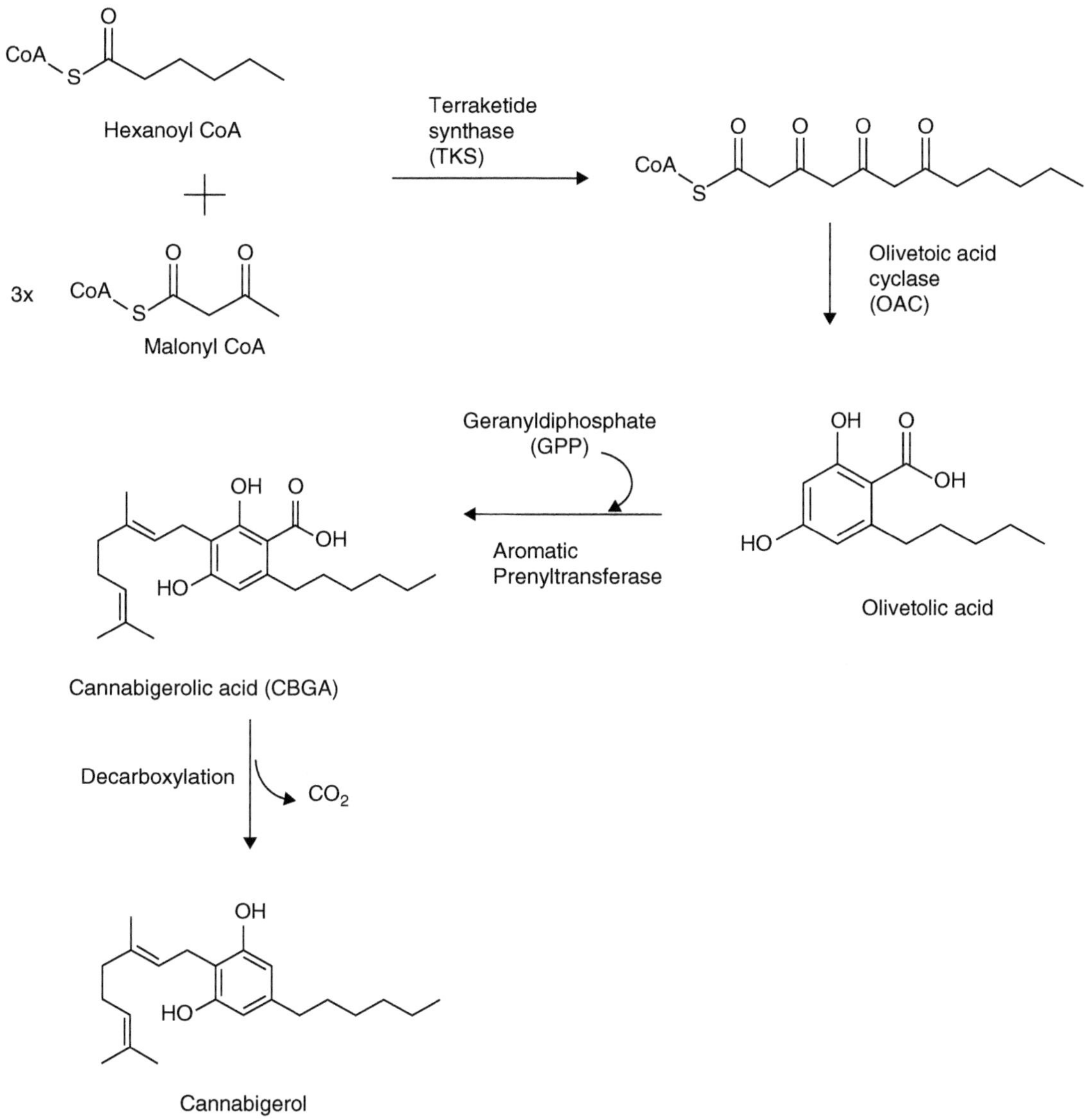

Fig. 12.3 Biosynthesis of cannabigerol. (https://commons.wikimedia.org/w/index.php?curid=61209787. By Alm7724 – Own work, CC BY-SA 4.0)

prostate cancer, detrusor overactivity, and bladder pain [24, 25], while gamma aminobutyric acid (GABA) uptake inhibition explains the muscle relaxant properties of CBG compared to CBD and THC [26].

The analgesic and anti-arrhythmic effects and lipoxygenase blocking ability were found to surpass that of THC [13]. CBG is a potent α2-adrenoreceptor agonist and moderates 5-HT1A antagonist explaining its analgesic and antidepressant properties [23, 27]. CBG was also found to have modest antifungal effects [28]. In addition, CBG has demonstrated remarkable anticancer and cytotoxic properties in high doses on human epithelioid carcinoma and breast cancer in basic research models [29, 30]. CBG inhibits keratinocyte proliferation suggesting benefits in psoriasis [18]. CBG is also a strong anandamide uptake inhibitor and has demonstrated antimicrobial effects against MRSA [14].

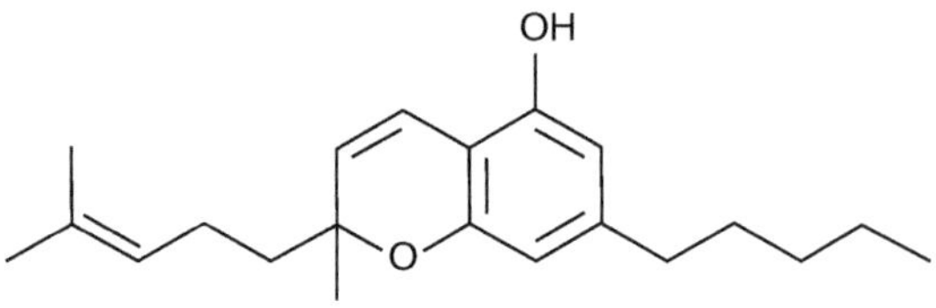

Fig. 12.4 Cannabichromene (CBC)

Cannabichromene (CBC)

CBC was isolated simultaneously by two methods, one using a hexane/florisil extraction method from hashish and the other by benzene percolation of hemp [31, 32] (Fig. 12.4).

CBC usually constitutes 0.3% of cannabis; however rich cannabis strains can be produced through extensive cross-breeding. The transient receptor potential (TRP) channels, a class of cationic channels that act as signal transducers by altering membrane potential or intracellular calcium (Ca^{2+}) concentrations, interact with the ECS, modulating inflammation and pain.

CBC interacts with TRP cation channels, inhibiting deactivation of endocannabinoids, thereby stimulating CB2 receptors (Ki 100 nm). However, it lacks significant activity at CB1 receptors (Ki > 1 μM) [32].

In animal models, CBC has demonstrated pain relief, along with potentiating the analgesic effects of THC, reducing colonic inflammation and paw edema by inhibiting macrophages and monoacylglycerol lipase (MAGL), a key enzyme involved in the hydrolysis of the endocannabinoid 2-arachidonoylglycerol (2-AG) [34, 35].

The mechanism of CBC's effects in mammals is supported by pharmacodynamic studies that have shown that CBC can stimulate TRP ankyrin type 1 (TRPA1) cation channels (EC50¼ 90 nM) and also desensitize them (IC50¼ 370 nM). CBC also interacts with TRPV3 and TRPV4 cation channels (EC50¼ 600 nM and 1.9 μM) and also desensitizes the TRPV2 and TRPV4 (IC50¼ 6.5 and 9.9 μM, respectively), thereby having an effect on reducing inflammation in animal models [33, 36, 37]. Moreover, CBC has demonstrated a positive effect on the viability of mammalian adult neural stem cell progenitor cells, thereby exhibiting a role in brain function [33].

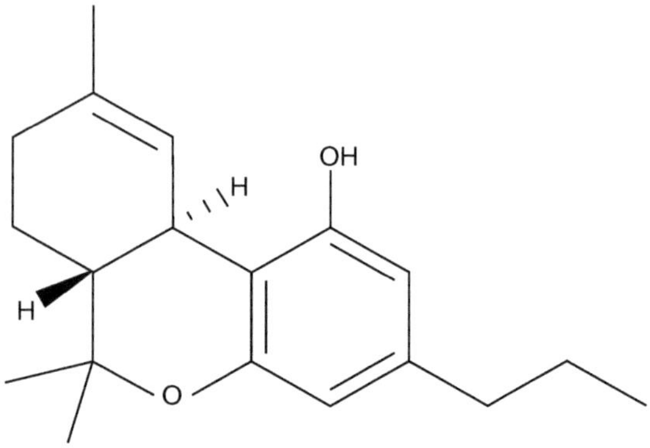

Fig. 12.5 Tetrahydrocannabivarin (THCV)

Tetrahydrocannabivarin (THCV)

THCV is a propyl analogue of THC, found in low concentrations in dried plant material (Fig. 12.5). However, concentrations as high as 16% by dry weight have been reported in certain cases [38]. THCV can exhibit dual action by behaving both as an agonist and as an antagonist at CB1 receptors depending on the concentration [39]. It has demonstrated anticonvulsant properties in rodent cerebellum and pyriform cortex [40]. There is evidence of THCV acting on CB2 receptors to suppress carrageenan-induced hyperalgesia and inflammation, as well as phases of formalin-induced pain behavior via CB1 and CB2 in animal models [41].

Through antagonizing CB1 receptors, THCV was found to suppress appetite and reverse the intoxicating effects of THC in animal models. The mechanism of neutral antagonism of THCV is free from adverse events associated with the CB1 antagonists like rimonabant (SR141716A) which led to depressive episodes and potentially worsened neurodegenerative disease outcomes, leading to withdrawal from the market for clinical uses [42].

Conclusion

While CBD and THC are the most common phytocannabinoids used clinically, the minor cannabinoids, cannabigerol (CBG), cannabichromene (CBC), cannabinol (CBN), and tetrahydrocannabivarin (THCV), have demonstrated preclinical promise as anticonvulsant, anti-inflammatory, antibacterial, and antidepressant agents. Anticancer and cytotoxic activities on human epithelioid carcinoma and breast cancer have been demonstrated in basic science models. While phytocannabinoids have demonstrated early promise, the need for further research and robust drug development in the years ahead is paramount to determine what role if any these compounds might eventually play in clinical care.

References

1. Howlett AC, Abood ME. CB1 and CB2 receptor pharmacology. Adv Pharmacol (San Diego, CA). 2017;80:169–206.
2. Munro S, Thomas KL, Abu-Shaar M. Molecular characterization of a peripheral receptor for cannabinoids. Nature. 1993;365:61–5.
3. Li X, et al. Crystal structure of the human cannabinoid receptor CB2. Cell. 2019;176:459–467.e13.
4. Carvalho Â, Hansen EH, Kayser O, Carlsen S, Stehle F. Designing microorganisms for heterologous biosynthesis of cannabinoids. FEMS Yeast Res. 2017;17(4):fox037. https://doi.org/10.1093/femsyr/fox037.
5. Ohlsson A, Lindgren JE, Andersson S, Agurell S, Gillespie H, Hollister LE. Single-dose kinetics of deuterium-labelled cannabidiol in man after smoking and intravenous administration. Biomed Environ Mass Spectrom. 1986;13(2):77–83.
6. Grotenhermen F. Pharmacokinetics and pharmacodynamics of cannabinoids. Clin Pharmacokinet. 2003;42(4):327–60.
7. Guzmán M. Cannabinoids: potential anticancer agents. Nat Rev Cancer. 2003;3(10):745–55.
8. Wood TB, Spivey WTN, Easterfield TH. III.—Cannabinol. Part I. J Chem Soc Trans. 1899;75:20–36. https://doi.org/10.1039/CT8997500020.
9. Upton R, Craker L, ElSohly M, Romm A, Russo E, Sexton M. In: Upton R, editor. Cannabis inflorescence: Cannabis spp.: standards of identity, analysis and quality control. Scotts Valley: American Herbal Pharmacopoeia; 2013.
10. Rhee MH, Vogel Z, Barg J, Bayewitch M, Levy R, Hanus L, et al. Cannabinol derivatives: binding to cannabinoid receptors and inhibition of adenylyl cyclase. J Med Chem. 1997;40:3228–33.
11. Musty RE, Karniol IG, Shirikawa I, Takahashi RN, Knobel E. Interactions of delta-9-tetrahydrocannabinol and cannabinol in man. In: Braude MC, Szara S, editors. The pharmacology of marihuana, vol. 2. New York: Raven Press; 1976. p. 559–63.
12. Turner CE, Elsohly MA, Boeren EG. Constituents of Cannabis sativa L. XVII. A review of the natural constituents. J Nat Prod. 1980;43:169–234.
13. Evans FJ. Cannabinoids: the separation of central from peripheral effects on a structural basis. Planta Med. 1991;57:S60–7.
14. Appendino G, Gibbons S, Giana A, Pagani A, Grassi G, Stavri M, et al. Antibacterial cannabinoids from cannabis sativa: a structure–activity study. J Nat Prod. 2008;71(8):1427–30. https://doi.org/10.1021/np8002673.
15. Evans FJ. Cannabinoids: the separation of central from peripheral effects on a structural basis. Planta Medica. 2007;57(S1):S60–7. https://doi.org/10.1055/s-2006-960231.
16. McPartland JM, Russo EB. Cannabis and cannabis extracts: greater than the sum of their parts? J Cannabis Ther. 2001;1(3–4):103–32. https://doi.org/10.1300/J175v01n03_08.
17. Qin N, Neeper MP, Liu Y, Hutchinson TL, Lubin ML, Flores CM. TRPV2 is activated by cannabidiol and mediates CGRP release in cultured rat dorsal root ganglion neurons. J Neurosci. 2008;28:6231–8.
18. Wilkinson JD, Williamson EM. Cannabinoids inhibit human keratinocyte proliferation through a non-CB1/CB2 mechanism and have a potential therapeutic value in the treatment of psoriasis. J Dermatol Sci. 2007;45:87–92.
19. Scutt A, Williamson EM. Cannabinoids stimulate fibroblastic colony formation by bone marrow cells indirectly via CB2 receptors. Calcif Tissue Int. 2007;80(1):50–9. https://doi.org/10.1007/s00223-006-0171-7.
20. Holland ML, Allen JD, Arnold JC. Interaction of plant cannabinoids with the multidrug transporter ABCC1 (MRP1). Eur J Pharmacol. 2008;591(1–3):128–31. https://doi.org/10.1016/j.ejphar.2008.06.079.
21. Gaoni Y, Mechoulam R. The structure and function of cannabigerol, a new hashish constituent. Proc Chem Soc. 1964;1:82.
22. Gauson LA, Stevenson LA, Thomas A, Baillie GL, Ross RA, Pertwee RG. Cannabigerol behaves as a partial agonist at both CB1 and CB2 receptors. In: Presented at the 17th annual symposium on the cannabinoids, Saint-Sauveur, Quebec. Canada: International Cannabinoid Research Society; 2007. p. 206.
23. Cascio MG, Gauson LA, Stevenson LA, Ross RA, Pertwee RG. Evidence that the plant cannabinoid can-

nabigerol is a highly potent α2-adrenoceptor agonist and moderately potent 5HT1A receptor antagonist. Br J Pharmacol. 2010;159(1):129–41. https://doi.org/10.1111/j.1476-5381.2009.00515.x.

24. De Petrocellis L, Di Marzo V. Non-CB1, non-CB2 receptors for endo-cannabinoids, plant cannabinoids, and synthetic cannabimimetics: focus on G-protein-coupled receptors and transient receptor potential channels. J Neuroimmune Pharmacol. 2010;5(1):103–21. https://doi.org/10.1007/s11481-009-9177-z.
25. Mukerji G, Yiangou Y, Corcoran SL, Selmer IS, Smith GD, Benham CD, et al. Cool and menthol receptor TRPM8 in human urinary bladder disorders and clinical correlations. BMC Urol. 2006;6:6. https://doi.org/10.1186/1471-2490-6-6.
26. Banerjee SP, Snyder SH, Mechoulam R. Cannabinoids: influence on neurotransmitter uptake in rat brain synaptosomes. J Pharmacol Exp Ther. 1975;194(1):74–81.
27. Formukong EA, Evans AT, Evans FJ. Analgesic and antiinflammatory activity of constituents of Cannabis sativa L. Inflammation. 1988;12(4):361–71.
28. ElSohly HN, Turner CE, Clark AM, Eisohly MA. Synthesis and anti- microbial activities of certain cannabichromene and cannabigerol related compounds. J Pharm Sci. 1982;71(12):1319–23.
29. Baek S, Kim YO, Kwag JS, Choi KE, Jung WY, Han DS. Boron trifluoride etherate on silica-A modified Lewis acid reagent (VII). Antitumor activity of cannabigerol against human oral epithelioid carcinoma cells. Arch Pharm Res. 1998;21(3):353–6.
30. Ligresti A, Moriello AS, Starowicz K, Matias I, Pisanti S, De Petrocellis L, et al. Antitumor activity of plant cannabinoids with emphasis on the effect of cannabidiol on human breast carcinoma. J Pharmacol Exp Ther. 2006;318(3):1375–87. https://doi.org/10.1124/jpet.106.105247.
31. Claussen U, Von Spulak F, Korte F. Zur chemischen klassifizierung von pflanzen—XXXI, haschisch—X: Cannabichromen, ein neuer haschisch-inhaltsstoff. Tetrahedron. 1966;22(4):1477–9. https://doi.org/10.1016/S0040-4020(01)99445-1.
32. Gaoni Y, Mechoulam R. Cannabichromene, a new active principle in hashish. Chem Commun (Camb). 1966;1:20–1. https://doi.org/10.1039/C19660000020.
33. Shinjyo N, Di Marzo V. The effect of cannabichromene on adult neural stem/progenitor cells. Neurochem Int. 2013;63(5):432–7. https://doi.org/10.1016/j.neuint.2013.08.002.
34. Cascio MG, Pertwee RG. Known pharmacological actions of nine non-psychotropic phytocannabinoids. In: Pertwee RG, editor. Handbook of cannabis. Oxford, UK: Oxford University Press; 2014. p. 137–56. https://doi.org/10.1093/acprof:oso/9780199662685.003.0007.
35. Maione S, Piscitelli F, Gatta L, Vita D, De Petrocellis L, Palazzo E, et al. Non- psychoactive cannabinoids modulate the descending pathway of antinociception in anaesthetized rats through several mechanisms of action. Br J Pharmacol. 2011;162(3):584–96. https://doi.org/10.1111/j.1476-5381.2010.01063.x.
36. Romano B, Borrelli F, Fasolino I, Capasso R, Piscitelli F, Cascio M, et al. The cannabinoid TRPA1 agonist cannabichromene inhibits nitric oxide production in macrophages and ameliorates murine colitis. Br J Pharmacol. 2013;169(1):213–29. https://doi.org/10.1111/bph.12120.
37. De Petrocellis L, Orlando P, Moriello AS, Aviello G, Stott C, Izzo AA, et al. Cannabinoid actions at TRPV channels: effects on TRPV3 and TRPV4 and their potential relevance to gastrointestinal inflammation. Acta Physiol. 2012;204(2):255–66. https://doi.org/10.1111/j.1748-1716.2011.02338.x.
38. Meijer EPM, Hammond KM. The inheritance of chemical phenotype in Cannabis sativa L. (II): Cannabigerol predominant plants. Euphytica. 2005;145(1–2):189–98. https://doi.org/10.1007/s10681-005-1164-8.
39. Pertwee RG. The diverse CB1 and CB2 receptor pharmacology of three plant cannabinoids: Delta9-tetrahydrocannabinol, cannabidiol and delta9- tetrahydrocannabivarin. Br J Pharmacol. 2008;153(2):199–215. https://doi.org/10.1038/sj.bjp.0707442.
40. Hill AJ, Weston SE, Jones NA, Smith I, Bevan SA, Williamson EM, et al. Delta-Tetrahydrocannabivarin suppresses in vitro epileptiform and in vivo seizure activity in adult rats. Epilepsia. 2010;51(8):1522–32. https://doi.org/10.1111/j.1528-1167.2010.02523.x.
41. Bolognini D, Costa B, Maione S, Comelli F, Marini P, Di Marzo V, et al. The plant cannabinoid Delta9-tetrahydrocannabivarin can decrease signs of inflammation and inflammatory pain in mice. Br J Pharmacol. 2010;160(3):677–87. https://doi.org/10.1111/j.1476-5381.2010.00756.x.
42. McPartland JM, Duncan M, Di Marzo V, Pertwee RG. Are cannabidiol and Delta(9)-tetrahydrocannabivarin negative modulators of the endocannabinoid system? A systematic review. Br J Pharmacol. 2015;172(3):737–53. https://doi.org/10.1111/bph.12944.

Cannabis Drug Interactions

13

George Polson, Matthew Chung, Salman Hirani, and Christina Le-Short

Introduction

Roughly 70% of Americans take at least one prescription drug, with 50% of the population taking at least two and 20% taking five or more prescription drugs [1]. In addition, up to 80% of Americans use some form of over-the-counter medication, while 25% of Americans are regular consumers of herbal remedies [2]. With such widespread use of prescription and non-prescription medications, and the increasing availability of cannabis-derived products available over the counter, it is imperative health-care providers understand the potential drug-drug interactions and mechanisms of interaction that prescription, over-the-counter, and herbal medications have with cannabis.

While cannabinoids can be a promising treatment modality for pain, favored for its relatively benign side effect profile, the risks associated with its use should be seriously taken into account. In this chapter we will delve into cannabis drug interactions that providers should be aware of in order to ensure patient safety.

G. Polson (✉)
Department of Pain Medicine, Division of Anesthesiology, Critical Care and Pain Medicine, The University of Texas MD Anderson Cancer Center, Houston, TX, USA

Department of Physical Medicine and Rehabilitation, Baylor College of Medicine, Houston, TX, USA
e-mail: george.polson@bcm.edu

M. Chung · S. Hirani · C. Le-Short
Department of Pain Medicine, Division of Anesthesiology, Critical Care and Pain Medicine, The University of Texas MD Anderson Cancer Center, Houston, TX, USA

Routes of Administration

Cannabis and cannabinoids can be consumed in a variety of ways, including inhalation, ingestion, mucosal, topical, and rectal administration. Each method has unique characteristics that make it more or less appropriate for consumers. The pharmacokinetics and effects observed should be taken into consideration during selection of a route of administration [3]. Pertaining to the pharmacokinetics of the two most common ingredients of THC and CBD, studies thus far have considerable variation and are far too heterogenous to report specifically beyond what is mentioned in the administration routes that follow.

Inhalation through combustion is the primary method of delivery chosen by the majority of cannabis users due to its rapid delivery, quick onset of effects, and ease in titrating the dose to the desired degree [4]. Smoking cannabis involves burning the *Cannabis sativa* flower (including its stems and seeds) and inhaling the active components released. Methods for smoking have included joints, bowls, variations of pipes (including water pipes), hookahs, or blunts (cannabis rolled into tobacco-leaf wrapper from a

S. N. Narouze (ed.), *Cannabinoids and Pain*, https://doi.org/10.1007/978-3-030-69186-8_13

cigar). Bioavailability of tetrahydrocannabinol (THC) through this route has been reported to be as high as 30% [5]. Cannabidiol (CBD) has a similar bioavailability to THC at approximately 31% [6]. Alternatively, vaporization requires heating the flower to a temperature at which active ingredients of the plant are released for inhalation. This method is perceived to be a safer alternative to smoking due to the absence of combustible irritants although potentially toxic levels of elevated ammonia and heavy metals have also been found [7]. Oil-based vaporizers place users at risk for consumption of higher concentrations of THC and CBD. Much like its combustion counterpart, vaporization has various limitations given its lack of testing and inconsistencies with surrounding content including additive residues.

With oral consumption, absorption is slower with a delayed peak THC concentration. In this format, bioavailability of THC is much lower than its smoking counterpart, ranging from 4% to 20%, due to variable absorption rates and significant first-pass metabolism. Available oral formulations include hashish resins or oil concentrates (in the form of hash, butane honey, or butane hash oils). Due to the low bioavailability of cannabinoid formulations, alternative routes have largely been developed to improve the amount of delivered cannabinoids [8].

Oromucosal formulations in the form of dissolvable strips, sprays, medicated lozenges, or tinctures were developed to avoid first-pass metabolism by the liver. This route is more commonly used by patients who are in need of a continually high level of cannabinoid concentration, with THC and CBD content comprising as much as 70% of some products. In comparison to inhalation, this route has an increased time to effect and increased duration of effect and has lower potency at an equivalent dose (due to a lower bioavailability). In essence, there are no significant differences among oral and oromucosal routes (including sublingual forms) [8].

Topical administration, including ointments, creams, and dermal patches, innately serves to produce an extended effect as it avoids exposure to first-pass metabolism. Cannabinoids are highly hydrophobic, making transport across the dermal barrier the rate-limiting step [8]. No controlled studies to date have been conducted on topical ointments and creams. Dermal patches are limited to preclinical data which suggest low absorption with max peak plasma levels at 1.5 hours.

Rectal administration poses as an attractive alternative in cases of significant comorbidity with its potentially higher absorption and lower first-pass metabolism [8]. However current knowledge surrounding rectal administration of cannabis is limited. Despite the paucity of data, there are increasing reports of its use as this route allows for high concentrations, especially of THC, without their associated psychotropic effects as it avoids initial metabolism by the liver.

Cannabinoid Drug Interactions

The most clinically relevant cannabinoid drug interactions are additive pharmacodynamic interactions when co-administered with other agents that have similar physiological effects. Sedation may be increased with other CNS depressants, opioids, alcohol, and antihistamines, while tachycardia may increase with tricyclic antidepressants, stimulants, and sympathomimetics [9]. THC is metabolized by liver cytochrome P450 enzymes, predominantly CYP3A4 and CYP2C9, while CBD is metabolized predominantly by CYP3A4 and CYP2C19. Therefore, drugs that inhibit or induce these CYP enzymes would increase or decrease THC and CBD levels [8, 9].

Specific Drug Interactions

Over-the-Counter (OTC) Analgesics

Over-the-counter analgesics consistently are prescribed as first-line treatment for a variety of pain syndromes. As a significant number of medications fall under this category, studies into their potential interactions with cannabis derivatives are quite fragmented. Despite this challenge, it remains imperative to raise awareness of potential interactions due to the ubiquitous presence of these medications throughout the general public.

Nonsteroidal anti-inflammatory drugs (NSAID) such as ibuprofen, naproxen, or aspirin serve to reduce inflammation as a means of managing increased systemic pain. NSAIDs work by selectively or broadly inhibiting COX-1 and COX-2 enzymes, which in turn decreases prostaglandin synthesis that is involved in inflammation [10]. While CBD and THC also display anti-inflammatory effects, this is accomplished by a separate mechanism involving endocannabinoids and T-cell regulation [11]. It has been shown that even at physiologic doses, THC and CBD do not appear to affect COX inhibition [12]. Despite this finding, providers should exhibit caution as there is insufficient evidence to draw any specific conclusions from.

Of particular interest is aspirin, formally known as acetylsalicylic acid, as it is not only used as an analgesic but also as an anti-thrombotic for those with extensive cardiac history. Aspirin serves as an irreversible inhibitor of COX-1, which can decrease levels of thromboxane A2 leading to decreased platelet aggregation [4]. This anti-thrombotic effect helps to decrease the risk of cardiovascular events, and thus aspirin is a globally prescribed medication. As mentioned above, while no direct drug-drug interactions have been found between NSAIDs and cannabis derivatives, one study did show that THC demonstrated an anti-inflammatory effect that was nearly 20 times greater than that of aspirin [13]. However providers should be aware of the limits of current knowledge.

Another common over-the-counter agent is paracetamol or acetaminophen, which displays both analgesic and antipyretic effects. While the exact mechanism of action has yet to be elucidated, current understanding includes mediation of analgesia through descending serotonergic pathways with a peripheral site of activation either occurring through prostaglandin inhibition or the activation of cannabinoid receptors [14]. Where practitioners should exhibit caution with paracetamol and cannabis-derived medications is the potential for liver injury due to the overload of drugs that are predominantly metabolized through the hepatic P450 system. CBD and acetaminophen share the CYP2E1 and CYP1A2, and potential concomitant use of both medications increases the risk for drug-induced hepatotoxicity [15]. Practitioners should advise of cautious and measured use of paracetamol in the context of associated use of cannabis or its derivatives.

Neuropathic Agents

Classically, pain symptoms are categorized as either nociceptive or neuropathic in origin. Neuropathic analgesics acting directly on the somatosensory system have continued to grow in usage. While there have been minimal studies involving interactions between neuropathic agents and cannabis, preliminary evidence has shown potential for likely associations that can alter pain management decision making.

Gabapentin is an anticonvulsant that is frequently used for neuropathic pain that displays a mechanism of action that is primarily based on voltage-dependent calcium channels [16]. Cannabinoid agonists alter voltage-dependent calcium channel (VDCC) function by both cannabinoid (CB) receptor-mediated G-protein activation and modulation by CB ligands [17, 18]. As it pertains to specific cannabis derivatives, it has been shown that THC given in combination with gabapentin can increase the potency of anti-allodynic effects of both drugs without significantly increasing the risk for negative side effects [19]. The ability for gabapentin and cannabinoids to have overlapping effects also allows for gabapentin to be used as an agonist replacement for substance use disorders, including cannabis [20].

Pregabalin is another anticonvulsant agent that can be considered first-line treatment for neuropathic pain alongside gabapentin. One preclinical study showed that pregabalin, another VDCC ligand, was able to curb physical and mental responses that occur during cannabinoid agonist cessation likely as it works on similar metabolites [21]. There is evidence to suggest that cannabinoid direct agonists, endogenous cannabinoids, and gabapentinoids such as gabapentin and pregabalin share pain systems [20]. Practitioners should monitor for potential overlapping effects when both agents are used in combination with cannabis.

While not as widely used as gabapentinoids, tricyclic antidepressants (TCA) also provide neuropathic analgesia albeit through unclear mechanisms. As best understood, TCAs appear to indirectly affect endogenous opioid receptors within the central nervous system [22]. While not as delineated as other medications, TCAs are assumed to be processed by hepatic cytochrome P450 isozymes that are also shared by THC [23]. There are multiple reports of cardiac side effects when TCAs are administered in the context of recreational cannabis use [23–25]. Due to the significant cardiac profile that tricyclic depressants display on its own, the possibility of increased risk due to additional use of cannabis or its derivatives should caution providers.

Opiates

With recent increased public scrutiny on overuse of opioid medications for both acute and chronic pain, there have been introductory efforts examining how cannabis derivatives and opioids interact with one another. In 2018, approximately 2/3 of all drug overdose deaths (46,802 deaths) in the USA were attributed to opioid use [26]. Despite this statistic, the CDC reported that in 2018 there were still 170 million opioid prescriptions written that year. As there is continued legalization at the state level of recreational and medicinal cannabis within the USA, practitioners should closely examine for potential interactions with concomitant use of both agents.

Various efforts have begun to describe a connection between cannabinoids and opioid medications as it pertains to pain signaling pathways as well as general cytochrome P450 metabolism. While limited in overall scope, current literature has been able to demonstrate rudimentary associations between opioids and cannabis derivatives such as THC and CBD.

Studies have shown that the previously accepted THC stimulation of kappa and delta opioid receptors may also enhance the analgesic effect that morphine displays through mu opioid receptors. There is also evidence that both classes of drugs share signal transduction mechanisms through decreases of cyclic adenosine monophosphate production by G-protein activation [27]. Both mu opioid and cannabinoid receptors share use of these G-protein-related activation systems and are found to be in close proximity to one another in areas such as the nucleus accumbens and dorsal striatum [28]. Furthermore, THC leads to release of dynorphin A which is metabolized into opioid metabolites, possibly leading to a synergistic effect [29].

One study showed that buprenorphine, a partial mu opioid agonist, had interactions with multiple cytochrome P450 isozymes, with the most significant being CYP3A4, as well as to a lesser extent with CYP2C8 and UGT2B7 pathways [30]. In vitro data demonstrated that CBD (but not THC) served as an inhibitor for the CYP3A4 system. Both buprenorphine and CBD serve as competitive substrates for UGT2B7. This inhibitory combination could lead to elevations of serum buprenorphine levels [31].

It has been shown that vaporized cannabis can enhance the antinociception of morphine and oxycodone without significant increased risk of adverse effects [27]. An appropriate oral dose of THC can augment the analgesic potential of acute oral doses of morphine, codeine, and other opioid analgesics [29]. Animal models have shown that CBD does not affect brain concentrations of morphine or methadone [28]. This same study also showed that CBD co-administration with fentanyl did not worsen respiratory depression or cardiovascular complication and, in general, was safe and well tolerated [28]. Vierke et al. however did show that CBD increased blood concentration levels of buprenorphine, a common medication used for opioid maintenance therapy [30].

Despite these potential interactions, there is continued evidence of synergistic analgesic effects that cannabis has with opioids as well as reduction in complications and withdrawal symptoms [9]. Furthermore, there has been evidence to show that prescribed cannabis use has led to lower opioid overdose mortality rates in areas with access to medical marijuana as well as decreased use of opioids all together [1, 9]. One study revealed that patients with terminal cancer refractory to optimal opioid treatment achieved significant pain improvement with a THC/CBD oromucosal spray (nabiximols) without the need for increasing pain medication use later on [30]. Overall, with current widespread use of opioid medications, there is a need for continued work to examine its interactions with cannabis and cannabinoid derivatives.

Antiepileptics

There has been growing consumer interest with cannabis derivatives, specifically CBD, as it pertains to seizure management. While multiple studies show promising benefits of cannabis for refractory syndromes, there remains a significant lack of data before it can be considered standard of care [32]. Further complicating the prescribing of medications is the preponderance of CBD-derived agents labeled as "natural plant-based product" that is outside the purview of many practitioners [33]. Despite these barriers, most providers whose management includes the use of antiepileptic drugs (AEDs) recognize that counseling and education as it pertains to the risks and benefits of medical marijuana will continue to become more commonplace [34].

While CBD is recognized as having a larger role in seizure control compared to THC, its exact mechanism of action has yet to be fully delineated. Various proposals for CBD include indirect activation of the endocannabinoid system by blocking anandamide (ANA) uptake, modulation of calcium channels of TRPV1 receptors, antagonism of G-protein-coupled receptor GPR55, or possibly even target abnormal sodium channels [35]. THC, on the other hand, has weak agonist activity of endocannabinoid receptors CB1 and CB2 [35]. In addition, the cytochrome P450 system is shared between cannabis derivatives and antiepileptic drugs such as CBD, clobazam, and topiramate, which all serve as substrates for the CYP2C19 isozyme system [35].

One open-label safety study showed that increasing levels of Epidiolex (cannabidiol) demonstrated significantly increased serum levels of clobazam, rufinamide, topiramate, zonisamide, and eslicarbazepine [36]. This same study showed consistent transaminitis as an adverse effect when there was concomitant use of Epidiolex and valproate. In a different animal study, CBD was shown to potentiate the antiepileptic effects of phenytoin and phenobarbital while reducing the effects of chlordiazepoxide, clonazepam, and ethosuximide [37]. A small pediatric study found that CBD raised clobazam levels and adjustments of clobazam were required to avoid side effects [38]. Adverse effects such as sedation or altered mental status due to increased levels of AEDs have been reported in these studies. While use of most antiepileptic medications should be managed under the care of an experienced neurologist, practitioners of all backgrounds should be aware of potential drug-drug interactions that arise due to use of cannabis derivatives alongside antiepileptics.

Psychotropics

Typically used as an umbrella term for medications predominantly prescribed by a psychiatrist, psychotropic drugs can be broadly defined as any agent that affects the mind, emotions, or behaviors [39]. Antidepressants, anxiolytics, and antipsychotics are among the most commonly prescribed medications in the USA with an increasing percentage of the population prescribed with these medications for a longer duration of time [40]. Evidence has shown that illicit cannabis use leads to an increased likelihood of treatment failure and subsequent psychotic relapse, which unfortunately is often further treated with the introduction of additional psychotropic agents [41]. Due to the sheer volume and variety of drugs under the classification of psychotropic medications, there are limited studies that explore the possible drug-drug interactions as it pertains to cannabis.

One overarching assumption is that within the central nervous process, cannabinoids may interfere with the efficacy of various antipsychotics or antidepressants by interfering with dopaminergic and serotonergic systems [42]. Psychotropic agents share various hepatic CYP450 isozymes with both CBD and THC. Antipsychotics, benzodiazepines, and antidepressants all serve as CYP3A4 substrates, leading to potential increases or decreases of systemic CBD bioavailability [43]. THC has been found to be an inducer of CYP1A2; therefore THC can potentially decrease serum concentrations of clozapine, duloxetine, olanzapine, haloperidol, and chlorpromazine [44, 45]. Additional pathways that CBD, THC, and psychotropics share include CYP2C9 and CYP2C19, all of which emphasize the need for providers to be observant of potential, negative drug-drug interactions [40].

Drug-specific studies between psychotropics are also limited in number. One in vivo study found that THC decreased the neurobehavioral efficacy of risperidone but not clozapine [42]. Researchers attributed this finding to a specific P-glycoprotein (P-gp) at the blood-brain barrier whose expression is upregulated by THC. Risperidone has a greater affinity for this P-gp compared to clozapine; thus THC exposure can lead to lower brain concentrations of risperidone compared to clozapine. This possibly can explain why clozapine is the typical agent of choice once first-line antipsychotics fail. CBD has also consistently been shown to display anxiolytic effects regardless of dose, while THC also displays these same properties albeit at controlled doses. Researchers used this finding as it pertained to prescribing cannabis replacement therapy to wean patients off of benzodiazepines and, in doing so, did not find significant side effects with use of both agents concomitantly [46]. Introductory research has also demonstrated that CBD has limited effects on certain barbiturate medications [47].

Anticoagulants and Antiplatelets: "Blood Thinners"

While cannabis has many assumed or theoretical interactions with a variety of prescribed medications, the most pervasive in the literature is the interaction that THC, CBD, and, to a lesser extent, cannabinol (CBN) may have with various anticoagulant and antiplatelet agents. Precautions should be taken to closely monitor patients with concomitant use of cannabis-derived medications. It has been shown through in vitro studies that THC and CBN display anti-thrombotic activity and inhibit clot formation [48].

Warfarin

Warfarin shares many of the same cytochrome P450 enzymes that cannabis serves as a substrate for, including CYP2C9, CYP2C19, and CYP3AA4 [49]. Yamaori et al. demonstrated through in vitro studies that the three major components of cannabis, THC, CBD, and CBN, all showed competitive inhibition of CYP2C9 of the S-warfarin isomer [50]. As such, there are multiple reported cases where the addition of a cannabis-derived medication led to supratherapeutic INR levels in patients using warfarin for various comorbidities [51, 52]. As warfarin dosages fall within a narrow therapeutic window, close and regular monitoring of INR should be performed to enable proper titration of this anticoagulant while a patient is also on drugs that contain THC, CBD, or CBN.

Direct Oral Anticoagulants

Increasing in prevalence are direct Xa and thrombin inhibitors, all of which are grouped together as direct oral anticoagulants (DOACs). DOACs serve as substrates for P-glycoproteins and, to a lesser extent, the CYP3A system, both of which can be affected by cannabis [49]. DOAC absorption occurs through the gastrointestinal tract, specifically through P-gp efflux transporter, for which CBD is a substrate [53]. This inhibitory effect could theoretically lead to unintentional accumulation of DOACs. As these drugs are unable to be measured regularly by any serum marker, precautions should be made with use of these novel anticoagulants in combination with cannabis-derived medications. While there are no specific reported cases of such adverse reactions, both apixaban and rivaroxaban warn against interactions with CYP3A and P-gp inhibitors on its product labels, due to the increased bleeding risk [49].

Clopidogrel

Antiplatelet agents also have widespread utility for a variety of medical conditions. Clopidogrel, formally known as Plavix, prevents platelet activation and aggregation by inhibiting the $P2Y_{12}$ [49]. While the exact mechanism of metabolism has yet to be elucidated, CYP2C19 has been found to be one pathway that is used by clopidogrel during its inactive prodrug form [54]. CBD serves as an inhibitory substrate of CYP2C19, thus could lead to increased serum levels of clopidogrel due to decreased metabolism [55].

Heparin/Fondaparinux

Neither heparin nor fondaparinux is expected to have interactions with cannabis or its derivatives [49]. Neither has been associated with the cytochrome P450 system, UDP glucuronosyltransferases, or P-glycoprotein. Heparin is cleared either through saturation by endothelial cells or renal excretion, while fondaparinux is also cleared by the renal system [56] (Table 13.1).

Table 13.1 Summary of cannabis drug interactions found in literature

Drug class	Specific medication	Potential interaction
Over-the-counter analgesics	NSAID	No demonstrable effect that THC or CBD has on COX inhibition
	Aspirin	No distinct drug-drug interaction; THC may potentiate anti-inflammatory effects of aspirin
	Paracetamol	In theory, concern for hepatic overload with concomitant use of THC and CBD
[a]Neuropathic agents	Gabapentin	Overlapping effects on cannabinoid receptors leading to increase anti-allodynic effects
	Pregabalin	Possibility of sharing similar metabolites and pain systems as cannabinoids
	TCA	Case reports of recreational cannabis use increasing the risk of cardiac side effects
[a]Opioids	Morphine	Enhanced antinociception without significant increase in adverse effects
	Codeine	THC shown to augment analgesic potential when both administered orally
	Fentanyl	Co-administration with CBD did not worsen respiratory or cardiovascular function and was well tolerated
	Buprenorphine	Combination with CBD may increase serum buprenorphine levels
[a]Antiepileptics	Clobazam, rufinamide, topiramate, zonisamide, eslicarbazepine	CBD-derived anticonvulsant raised serum levels of these medications
	Valproate	Persistent transaminitis with adjacent use of CBD derivatives
	Phenytoin, phenobarbital	CBD may increase anticonvulsant effects
	Chlordiazepoxide, clonazepam, ethosuximide	CBD may decrease anticonvulsant effects
[a]Psychotropics	Duloxetine, clozapine, olanzapine, haloperidol, chlorpromazine, risperidone	THC potentially decreases serum concentrations and neurobehavioral efficacy
Blood thinners	Warfarin	Cannabis derivatives lead to supratherapeutic INR levels
	DOAC	CBD shares cytochrome P450 isozymes that theoretically can increase DOAC serum levels
	Clopidogrel	CBD can decrease metabolism of clopidogrel due to competitive inhibition of shared substrates
	Heparin/fondaparinux	No known interaction as these agents are processed by endothelial and renal cells

[a]Co-administered cannabinoids with these medications may lead to additive pharmacodynamic interactions and increased sedation with other CNS depressants, opioids, benzodiazepines, and alcohol. Tachycardia may increase with tricyclic antidepressants and stimulants

Acknowledgments No financial disclosures to report.

References

1. Haroutounian D, Ratz Y, Ginosar Y, Furmanov K, Saifi F, Meidan R, Davidson E. The effect of medicinal cannabis on pain and quality-of-life outcomes in chronic pain. Clin J Pain. 2016;32(12):1036–43.
2. Castleman M. The new healing herbs: the classic guide to nature's best medicines; 2001. p. IX; ISBN 1-57954-304-9.
3. Lucas CJ, Galettis P, Schneider J. The pharmacokinetics and pharmacodynamics of cannabinoids. Br J Clin Pharmacol. 2018;84:2477–82.
4. Toghi H, Konno S, Tamura K, Kimura B, Kawano K. Effects of low-to-high doses of aspirin on platelet aggregability and metabolites of thromboxane A2 and prostacyclin. Stroke. 1992;23(10):1400–3.
5. McGilveray I. Pharmacokinetics of cannabinoids. Pain Res Manag. 2005;10(Suppl A):15A–22A.
6. Millar S, Stone N, Yates A, O'Sullivan S. A systematic review on the pharmacokinetics of cannabidiol in humans. Front Pharmacol. 2018;9(1365):1–13.
7. Ghasemiesfe M, Barrow B, Leonard S. Association between marijuana use and risk of cancer: a systematic review and meta-analysis. Subst Use Addict. 2019;2(11):e1916318. https://doi.org/10.1001/jamanetworkopen.
8. Huestis MA. Human cannabinoid pharmacokinetics-review. Chem Biodivers. 2007;4:1770–99.
9. MacCallum C, Russo E. Practical consideration in medicinal cannabis administration and dosing. Eur J Intern Med. 2018;49:12–9.
10. Russo E. Current therapeutic cannabis controversies and clinical trial design issues. Front Pharmacol. 2016;7(309):1–19.
11. Nagarkatti P, Pandey R, Rieder S, Hegde V, Nagarkatti M. Cannabinoids as novel anti-inflammatory drugs. Future Med Chem. 2009;1(7):1333–49.
12. Stott C, Guy G, Wright S, Whittle B. The effects of cannabis extracts Tetranabinex and Nabidiolex on human cytochrome P450-mediated metabolism. In: Symposium on the cannabinoids; 2005. p. 163.
13. Russo E. Cannabinoids in the management of difficult to treat pain. Ther Clin Risk Manag. 2008;4(10):245–59.
14. Anderson B. Paracetamol (acetaminophen): mechanisms of action. Pediatr Anesth. 2008;18(10):915–21.
15. Ewing L, McGill M, Yee E, Quick C, Skinner C, Kennon-McGill S, Clemens M, Vazquez J, McCullough S, Williams D, Kutanzi K, Walker L, ElSholy M, James L, Gurley B, Koturbash I. Paradoxical patterns of sinusoidal obstruction syndrome-like liver injury in aged female CD-1 mice triggered by cannabidiol-rich cannabis extract and acetaminophen co-administration. Molecules. 2019;24(2256):1–12.
16. Sills G. The mechanism of action of gabapentin and pregabalin. Curr Opin Pharmacol. 2006;6(1):108–13.
17. Howlett A, Blume L, Dalton G. CB(1) cannabinoid receptors and their associated proteins. Curr Med Chem. 2010;17:1382–93.
18. Lozovaya N, Min R, Tsintsadze V, Burnashev N. Dual modulation of CNS voltage-gated calcium channels by cannabinoids: focus on CB1 receptor-independent effects. Cell Calcium. 2009;46:154–62.
19. Atwal N, Case S, Mitchell V, Vaughan C. THC and gabapentin interactions in mouse neuropathic pain model. Neuropharmacology. 2019;144:115–21.
20. Lile J, Wesley M, Kelly T, Hays L. Separate and combined effects of gabapentin and delta-THC in humans discriminating delta THC. Behav Pharmacol. 2017;27(2–3):215–24.
21. Aracil-Fernández A, Almela P, Manzanares J. Pregabalin and topiramate regulate behavioural and brain gene transcription changes induced by spontaneous cannabinoid withdrawal in mice. Addict Biol. 2013;18:252–62.
22. Benbouzid M, Gaveriaux-Ruff C, Yalcin I, Waltisperger E, Tessier L, Muller A, Kieffer B, Freund-Mercier M, Barrot M. Delta-opioid receptors are critical for tricyclic antidepressant treatment of neuropathic allodynia. Biol Psychiatry. 2008;63(6):633–6.
23. Wilens T, Bierderman J, Spencer T. Case study: adverse effects of smoking marijuana while receiving tricyclic antidepressants. J Acad Child Adolesc Psychiatry. 1997;36(1):45–8.
24. Kizer K. Possible interaction of TCA and marijuana. Ann Emerg Med. 1980;9(8):444.
25. Mannion V. Case report: adverse effects of taking tricyclic antidepressant and smoking marijuana. Can Fam Physician. 1999;45:2683–4.
26. Wilson N, Kariisa M, Seth P, Smith H, Davis N. Drug and opioid-involved overdose deaths – United States 2017–2018. Weekly. 2020;69(11):290–7.
27. Abrams D, Couey P, Shade S, Kelly M, Benowitz N. Cannabinoid-opioid interaction in chronic pain. Clin Pharmacol Ther. 2011;90(6):844–51.
28. Manini A, Yiannoulos G, Bergamaschi M, Hernandez S, Olmedo R, Barnes S, Jutras-Aswad D, Huestis M. Safety and pharmacokinetics of oral cannabidiol when administered concomitantly with intravenous fentanyl in humans. J Addict Med. 2015;9(3):204–10.
29. Cichewicz D. Synergistic interactions between cannabinoid and opioid analgesics. Life Sci. 2004;74:1317–24.
30. Vierke C, Marxen B, Boettcher M, Hiemke C, Havemann-Reinecke U. Buprenorphine-cannabis interaction in patients undergoing opioid maintenance therapy. Eur Arch Psychiatry Clin Neurosci. 2020. https://doi.org/10.1007/s00406-019-01091-0.
31. Johnson J, Lossignol D, Burnell-Nugent M, Fallon M. An open-label extension study to investigate the long-term safety and tolerability of THC/CBD oromucosal spray and oromucosal THC spray in patient with terminal cancer related pain refractory

to strong opioid analgesics. J Pain Symptom Manag. 2013;46:207–18.
32. Friedman D, Devinsky O. Cannabinoids in the treatment of epilepsy. N Engl J Med. 2015;373:1048–58.
33. O'Connell B, Gloss D, Devinsky O. Cannabinoids in treatment-resistant epilepsy: a review. Epilepsy Behav. 2017;70:341–8.
34. Chang B. Cannabidiol and serum antiepileptic drug levels: The ABCs of CBD with AEDs. Epilepsy Curr. 2018;18(1):33–4.
35. Gaston T, Szaflarksi J. Cannabis for the treatment of epilepsy: an update. Curr Neurol Neurosci Rep. 2018;18(73):1–9.
36. Gaston T, Bebin E, Cutter G, Liu Y, Szaflarski J. Interactions between cannabidiol and commonly used antiepileptic drugs. Epilepsia. 2017;58(9):1586–92.
37. Consroe P, Wolkin A. Cannabidiol–antiepileptic drug comparisons and interactions in experimentally induced seizures in rats. J Pharmacol Exp Ther. 1977;201:26–32.
38. Geffrey A, Pollack S, Bruno P, Thiele E. Drug-drug interaction between clobazam and cannabidiol in children with refractory epilepsy. Epilepsia. 2015;56(8):1246–51.
39. Rao T, Andrade C. Classification of psychotropic drugs: problems, solutions, and more problems. Indian J Psychiatry. 2016;58(2):111–3.
40. Rong C, Carmona N, Lee Y, Ragguett R, Pan Z, Rosenblat J, Subramaniapillai M, Shekotikhina M, Almatham F, Alageel A, Mansur R, Ho R, McIntyre R. Drug-drug interactions as a result of co-administering delta-THC and CBD and other psychotropic agents. Expert Opin Drug Saf. 2018;17(1):51–4.
41. Patel R, Wilson R, Jackson R, Ball M, Shetty H, Broadbent M, Stewart R, McGuire P, Bhattacharyya S. Association of cannabis use with hospital admission and antipsychotic treatment failure in first episode psychosis: an observational study. Br Med J. 2016;6(3):1–9.
42. Brzozowska N, Tonnerre E, Li K, Wang X, Boucher A, Callaghan P, Kuligowski M, Wong A, Arnold J. The differential binding of antipsychotic drugs to the ABC transporter P-glycoproteins predicts cannabinoid-antipsychotic drug interactions. Neuropyschopharmacology. 2017;42:2222–31.
43. Brown J. Potential adverse drug events and drug-drug interactions with medical consumer cannabidiol (CBD) use. J Clin Med. 2019;8(989):1–14.
44. Flockhart DA. Drug interactions: cytochrome P450 drug interaction table. Indiana University School of Medicine; 2007.
45. Watanabe K, Yamaori S, Funahashi T, Kimura T, Yamamoto I. Cytochrome P450 enzymes involved in the metabolism of tetrahydrocannabinols and cannabinol by human hepatic microsomes. Life Sci. 2007;80(15):1415–9.
46. Purcell C, Davis A, Moolman N, Taylor S. Reduction of benzodiazepine use in patients prescribed medical cannabis. Cannabis Cannabinoid Res. 2019;4(3):214–8.
47. Benowitz N, Nguyen T, Jones R, Heming R, Bachman J. Metabolic and psychophysiologic studies of cannabidiol-hexobarbital interaction. Clin Pharmacol Ther. 1980;28(1):115–20.
48. Coetzee C, Levendal R, Van De Venter M, Frost C. Anticoagulant effects of a Cannabis extract in an obese rat model. Phytomedicine. 2007;14:333–7.
49. Greger J, Bates V, Mechtler L, Gengo F. A review of cannabis and interactions with anticoagulant and antiplatelet agents. J Clin Pharamcol. 2020;60(4):432–8.
50. Yamaori S, Koeda K, Kushihara M, Hada Y, Yamamoto I, Watanabe K. Comparison in the in vitro inhibitory effects of major phytocannabinoids and polycyclic aromatic hydrocarbons contained in marijuana smoke on cytochrome P450 2C9 activity. Drug Metab Pharmacokinet. 2012;27(3):294–300.
51. Damkier P, Lassen D, Christensen M, Madsen K, Hellfritzsch M, Pottegard A. Interaction between warfarin and cannabis. Basical Clin Pharmacol Toxicol. 2019;124:28–31.
52. Grayson L, Vines B, Nichol K, Szaflarski J. An interaction between warfarin and cannabidiol, a case report. Epilepsy Behav Case Rep. 2018;9:10–1.
53. Zhu H, Wang J, Markowitz J, Donovan J, Gibson B, Gefroh H, Devane C. Characterization of P-glycoprotein inhibition by major cannabinoids from marijuana. J Pharmacol Exp Ther. 2006;317(2):850–7.
54. Ford N. The metabolism of clopidogrel: CYP2C19 is a minor pathway. J Clin Pharmacol. 2016;56(12):1474–83.
55. Jiang R, Yamaori S, Okamoto Y, Yamamoto I, Watanabe K. Cannabidiol is a potent inhibitor of the catalytic activity of cytochrome P450 2C19. Drug Metab Pharmacokinet. 2013;28(4):332–8.
56. Stout S, Cimino N. Exogenous cannabinoids as substrates, inhibitors, and inducers of human drug metabolizing enzymes: a systemic review. Drug Metab Rev. 2014;46(1):86–95.

Part III

Pharmaceutical Cannabinoids

Dronabinol (Marinol®)

14

Juliet Gaisey and Samer N. Narouze

Introduction

Dronabinol, the active ingredient in Marinol® capsules, is synthetic delta-9-tetrahydrocannabinol (delta-9-THC). Delta-9-tetrahydrocannabinol is a naturally occurring component of *Cannabis sativa L.* Dronabinol is a cannabinoid designated chemically as (6aR-trans)-6a,7,8,10a-tetrahydro-6,6,9-trimethyl-3-pentyl-6H-dibenzo[b,d]pyran-1-ol (Fig. 14.1).

Dronabinol is insoluble in water and is formulated in sesame oil. Marinol (Solvay Pharmaceuticals, Belgium) is an oral soft gelatin capsule that is available in 2.5 mg, 5 mg, and 10 mg doses [1].

The Drug Enforcement Administration (DEA) maintains FDA-approved products of oral solutions containing dronabinol in Schedule II of the Controlled Substances Act [2].

Marinol is indicated for the treatment of:

1. Anorexia associated with weight loss in patients with AIDS
2. Nausea and vomiting associated with cancer chemotherapy in patients who have failed to respond adequately to conventional antiemetic treatments

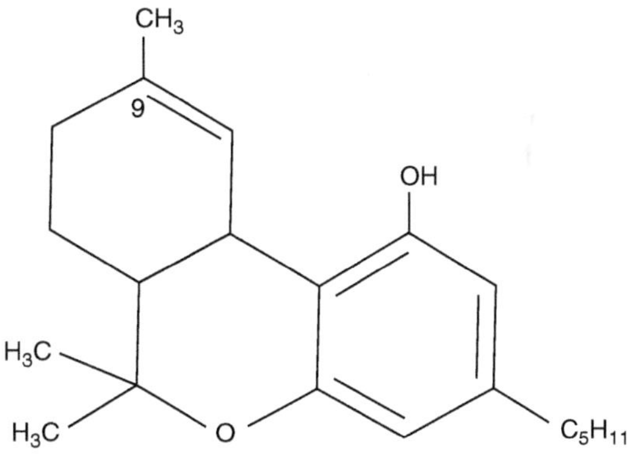

$CH_{21}H_{30}O_2$ (Molecular weight = 314.47)

Fig. 14.1 Empirical and structural formulas for dronabinol [1]

Mechanism of Action

All cannabinoids act on CB_1 and CB_2 receptors in the central nervous system and peripheral organs and tissues including the immune cells, liver, and lungs [3, 4]. Dronabinol has equal affinity for CB_1 and CB_2 receptors, but efficacy is less at CB_2 receptors. Cannabinoid receptors found in neural tissues are thought to be responsible for dronabinol's therapeutic effects. CB_1 likely mediates its anti-emetic and appetite-stimulating effects [5].

J. Gaisey
Department of Physical Medicine and Rehabilitation, Johns Hopkins Hospital, Baltimore, MD, USA

S. N. Narouze (✉)
Western Reserve Hospital, Center For Pain Medicine, Cuyahoga Falls, OH, USA
e-mail: narouzs@hotmail.com
Twitter: @NarouzeMD

S. N. Narouze (ed.), *Cannabinoids and Pain*, https://doi.org/10.1007/978-3-030-69186-8_14

Pharmacokinetics

The pharmacokinetics of dronabinol is very different from smoked or vaporized cannabis which enters the bloodstream and brain in seconds. The onset of action of dronabinol is 30–60 minutes after ingestion [6]. The maximal plasma concentration is reached 60–120 minutes after oral ingestion, but may take up to 6 hours [3]. The half-life of dronabinol is 25–36 hours [1].

Of the ingested dose, 90–95% is absorbed from the gastrointestinal tract, but due to the first-pass hepatic metabolism and high lipid solubility, only 10 to 20% of the dose reaches the systemic circulation [6]. The volume of distribution is large, 10 L/kg, resulting in low levels of excretion for prolonged periods of time [1]. The drug is predominately metabolized by the liver and excreted predominately in feces (50%) and some in the urine (10–15%) [7, 8].

Therapeutic Use

Dronabinol is FDA approved to treat anorexia in patients with HIV/AIDS and chemotherapy-induced nausea and vomiting unresponsive to more conservative antiemetics. It has also been used off label in moderate to severe obstructive sleep apnea [9]. The recommended starting dose for HIV associated anorexia is 2.5 mg twice a day, 1 hour before lunch and dinner [10]. For chemotherapy-induced nausea and vomiting, the recommended starting dose is 5 mg 1–3 hours prior to chemotherapy followed by 5 mg every 2–4 hours [10].

Although dronabinol is not FDA approved for pain, there are few reports suggesting a potential role. Cooper et al. [11] conducted a randomized, placebo-controlled, double-blind study comparing the magnitude and duration of analgesic effects of smoked marijuana and dronabinol using a validated experimental pain model. Both marijuana and dronabinol decrease pain severity, with dronabinol provided longer-lasting pain relief while having less abuse potential.

A number of other studies have shown some analgesic effect in chronic pain when compared to placebo, but more evidence is necessary [3]. Narang et al. [12] found that dronabinol can provide additional analgesia for patients taking opioids for chronic noncancer pain. Another randomized double-blind placebo-controlled crossover trial showed that dronabinol has a modest but clinically relevant analgesic effect on central pain in patients with multiple sclerosis [13].

Safety, Toxicity, and Adverse Effects

Several studies have shown no major safety issues and good tolerability of dronabinol [4]. However, due to its psychotropic effects and drug abuse potential, its therapeutic use is controversial. Substance use disorder is actually uncommon and only seen in prolonged use of high doses [1]. The most common adverse effects include headache, dizziness, tiredness, myalgia, and muscle weakness [4, 13]. The side effects are dose dependent and rarely cause discontinuation of therapy [14, 15]. Caution should be used in the elderly population as they are more susceptible to the CNS sedative side effects [10]. Common drug-drug interactions are summarized in Table 14.1 [1].

Table 14.1 Dronabinol drug-drug interactions

Drug	Clinical effect
Opioids, barbiturates, benzodiazepines, ethanol, lithium, antihistamines, muscle relaxants, other CNS depressants	Additive drowsiness and CNS depression
Amphetamines, cocaine, other sympathomimetic agents	Additive hypertension, tachycardia, possibly cardiotoxicity
Atropine, scopolamine, antihistamines, other anticholinergic agents	Additive tachycardia, drowsiness
Amitriptyline, amoxapine, desipramine, other tricyclic antidepressants	Additive tachycardia, hypertension, drowsiness
Fluoxetine, disulfiram	Hypomanic reaction
Barbiturates, antipyrine	Decreased clearance of these medications due to competitive inhibition of metabolism
Theophylline	Increased theophylline metabolism (similar effect to that reported with smoking of marijuana)

References

1. Marinol (Dronabinol). U.S. Food and Drug Administration. https://www.accessdata.fda.gov/drugsatfda_docs/label/2005/018651s021lbl.pdf. Accessed 11/7/2020.
2. Department of Justice. Drug Enforcement Administration. Schedules of controlled substances: placement of FDA-approved products of oral solutions containing dronabinol [(-)-delta-9-trans-tetrahydrocannabinol (delta-9-THC)] in schedule II. Fed Regist;82(224) (Wednesday, November 22, 2017). https://www.deadiversion.usdoj.gov/fed_regs/rules/2017/fr1122_6.htm. Accessed on 11/4/2021.
3. De Vries M, Van Rijckevorsel DC, Wilder-Smith OH, Van Goor H. Dronabinol and chronic pain: importance of mechanistic considerations. Expert Opin Pharmacother. 2014;15:1525–34.
4. Schimrigk S, Marziniak M, Neubauer C, Kugler EM, Werner G, Abramov-Sommariva D. Dronabinol is a safe long-term treatment option for neuropathic pain patients. Eur Neurol. 2017;78(5–6):320–9.
5. Badowski ME. A review of oral cannabinoids and medical marijuana for the treatment of chemotherapy-induced nausea and vomiting: a focus on pharmacokinetic variability and pharmacodynamics. Cancer Chemother Pharmacol. 2017;80(3):441–9.
6. Milman G, Bergamaschi MM, Lee D, Mendu DR, Barnes AJ, Vandrey R, et al. Plasma cannabinoid concentrations during dronabinol pharmacotherapy for cannabis dependence. Ther Drug Monit. 2014;36(2):218–24.
7. Grotenhermen F. Pharmacokinetics and pharmacodynamics of cannabinoids. Clin Pharmacokinet. 2003;42(4):327–60.
8. Lucas CJ, Galettis P, Schneider J. The pharmacokinetics and the pharmacodynamics of cannabinoids. Br J Clin Pharmacol. 2018;84(11):2477–82.
9. Carley DW, Prasad B, Reid KJ, Malkani R, Attarian H, Abbott SM, et al. Pharmacotherapy of apnea by cannabimimetic enhancement, the PACE clinical trial: effects of dronabinol in obstructive sleep apnea. Sleep. 2018;41(1):zsx184. https://doi.org/10.1093/sleep/zsx184.
10. Bar-Sela G, Zalman D, Semenysty V, Ballan E. The effects of dosage-controlled cannabis capsules on cancer-related cachexia and anorexia syndrome in advanced cancer patients: pilot study. Integr Cancer Ther. 2019;18:1534735419881498.
11. Cooper ZD, Comer SD, Haney M. Comparison of the analgesic effects of dronabinol and smoked marijuana in daily marijuana smokers. Neuropsychopharmacology. 2013;38(10):1984–92.
12. Narang S, Gibson D, Wasan AD, Ross EL, Michna E, Nedeljkovic SS, et al. Efficacy of dronabinol as an adjuvant treatment for chronic pain patients on opioid therapy. J Pain. 2008;9(3):254–64.
13. Svendsen KB, Jensen TS, Bach FW. Does the cannabinoid dronabinol reduce central pain in multiple sclerosis? Randomised double blind placebo controlled crossover trial. BMJ. 2004;329(7460):253.
14. Beal JE, Olson R, Laubenstein L, Morales JO, Bellman P, Yangco B, et al. Dronabinol as a treatment for anorexia associated with weight loss in patients with AIDS. J Pain Symptom Manag. 1995;10(2):89–97.
15. Plasse TF, Gorter RW, Krasnow SH, Lane M, Shepard KV, Wadleigh RG. Recent clinical experience with dronabinol. Pharmacol Biochem Behav. 1991;40(3):695–700.

15 Nabilone (Cesamet)

Nathan J. Harrison and Hunter Simpson

Introduction

Chemotherapy remains one of the mainstay treatments for many forms of cancer. Unfortunately, chemotherapy-induced nausea and vomiting (CINV) is a common side effect that can present significant challenges to continuing treatment. For example, patients may experience inability to perform activities of daily living, difficulty maintaining weight, and interference with socializing and rest. Without a prophylactic antiemetic, approximately 70–80% of cancer patients receiving chemotherapy will experience nausea and vomiting [1, 2]. Up to 30% of patients actually consider discontinuing chemotherapy because of CINV's disruptive effects [3].

In the 1970s, some younger cancer patients smoking marijuana reported improvement in their CINV symptoms [4]. As a result, academic- and industry-sponsored studies began investigating Δ^9-tetrahydrocannabinol (Δ^9-THC) and synthetic analogues, including nabilone, for CINV [5, 6]. Nabilone is a synthetic cannabinoid whose structure mimics Δ^9-THC (Fig. 15.1). Initially developed by Eli Lilly and Company, it received FDA approval in 1985 but was withdrawn prior to marketing. Valeant Pharmaceuticals

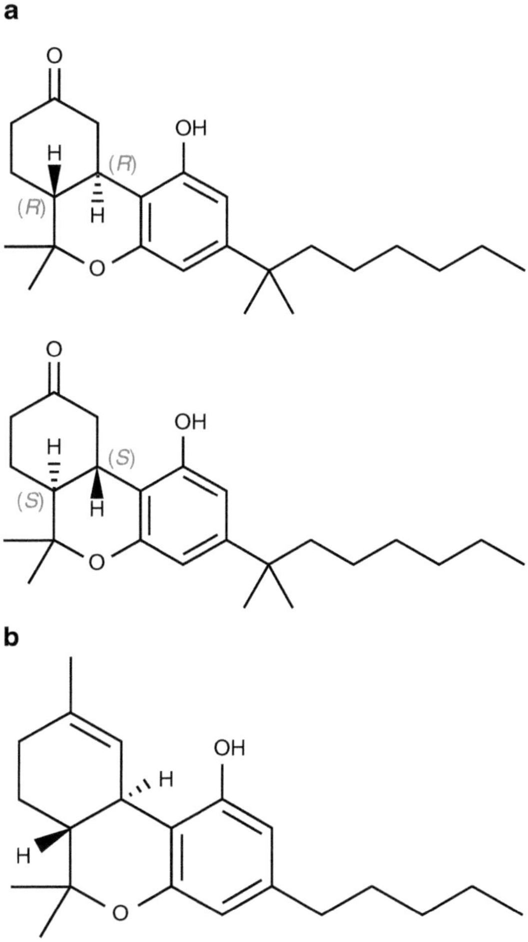

Fig. 15.1 Comparison of chemical structures of nabilone (**a**) and Δ^9-THC (**b**)

N. J. Harrison (✉) · H. Simpson
Ochsner Health Systems, Department of Anesthesiology and Critical Care Medicine, New Orleans, LA, USA
e-mail: nharrison@ochsner.org

S. N. Narouze (ed.), *Cannabinoids and Pain*, https://doi.org/10.1007/978-3-030-69186-8_15

then acquired the product, secured FDA approval, and marketed it under the name Cesamet. It is approved by the FDA for the treatment of chemotherapy-induced nausea and vomiting.

While earlier studies of nabilone showed promise compared to older antiemetics such as prochlorperazine, the advent of serotonin antagonists and their superior efficacy has supplanted these older antiemetics [7]. Nonetheless, Cesamet remains an option for breakthrough CINV resistant to the conventional treatments. Due to its role in modulation of the endocannabinoid system, clinical trials have investigated the use of nabilone as an analgesic. However, results are inconclusive, and its use for pain control is not currently FDA approved nor widely recommended [8–17].

Clinical Trials

Nabilone was developed in the 1970s, when interest was rising in non-Δ^9-THC cannabinoids that could produce therapeutic effects without the side effects that accompany botanical marijuana [5]. In one of the earliest clinical trials of CINV, patients received 2 mg of nabilone or 10 mg prochlorperazine during the first cycle of chemotherapy for various cancers. Patients were then crossed over to receive the opposite antiemetic for the second cycle of chemotherapy [6]. Nabilone was more effective for providing complete relief of nausea and vomiting (8% vs. 0%) and more effective for partial response (72% vs. 32%) [6]. In a similar study of patients receiving cisplatin, a highly emetogenic agent, Einhorn et al. performed a double-blind crossover trial of 2 mg nabilone or 10 mg prochlorperazine for the first cycle of chemotherapy. The patients were crossed over to the other antiemetic for the second cycle. Nabilone significantly reduced severity and duration of nausea and frequency of vomiting [18]. Several more studies reported nabilone's superiority as an antiemetic compared to prochlorperazine but, not surprisingly, also noted numerous side effects including dizziness and disorientation, which suggested a need for close monitoring of this THC analogue [19, 20].

With the advent of more effective antiemetic categories including serotonin antagonists such as ondansetron and substance P/neurokinin 1 (NK-1) antagonists such as aprepitant, older agents like prochlorperazine and nabilone are less often used. In fact, current guidelines by the National Comprehensive Cancer Network recommend dexamethasone, serotonin receptor antagonists, and aprepitant for medium- and high-emetic-risk chemotherapy [21]. Nabilone is not listed as a first-line antiemetic but instead is suggested as a rescue for breakthrough nausea and vomiting [21].

While not an approved FDA use, numerous clinical trials have investigated the use of nabilone as an analgesic. Some of these trials report small yet significant improvements in perceived pain [8–14, 22]. Specific studies suggest its efficacy in the treatment of various subtypes of chronic pain including neuropathic pain, fibromyalgia, non-cancer pain, and spasticity associated with multiple sclerosis [8–14, 22]. Interestingly, one observational study on the use of nabilone as an adjunct in palliative cancer pain found that nabilone was associated with an overall decrease in the use of opioids and other drugs (e.g., NSAIDs, TCAs, gabapentin, dexamethasone, metoclopramide, ondansetron) [22]. Finally, two studies on the use of nabilone in pain associated with fibromyalgia found significant improvements in sleep when compared to placebo [11] and amitriptyline [16].

Unfortunately, other studies on the analgesic effects of nabilone have found virtually no improvement [15–17]. Furthermore, more recent systematic reviews of the current literature on nabilone have concluded that the quality of evidence to support the use of nabilone as an analgesic is rather weak [23–25].

Pharmacology and Pharmacokinetics

Nausea and vomiting are largely regulated in the area postrema to the nucleus tractus solitarius. The neurotransmitters involved include serotonin, dopamine, substance P, and NK-1. CB2 receptors are primarily found on immune cells, whereas the CB1 receptors are found throughout the central and peripheral neurons [26]. CB1 is an inhibitory receptor that reduces neuronal excitability and neurotransmitter release and is found in large numbers in the central nervous system, in areas known to be involved in CINV [27]. Nabilone is an orally active synthetic cannabinoid, and an analog of THC and its mechanism of action appears to be its agonism at CB1 receptors and indirect modulation of the other neurotransmitters involved in nausea and vomiting [5, 27–29]. The analgesic properties of nabilone derive from stimulation of both CB1 and CB2, known to be found throughout regions involved in nociception in the CNS and spinal cord [30, 31].

Nabilone is rapidly and completely absorbed in the GI tract [5] and has 95–100% bioavailability [16]. Food has not been shown to affect its absorption [32]. Time to reach peak plasma concentration is within 2 hours [32]. The apparent volume of distribution is 12.5 L/kg [32], and it displays extensive and rapid tissue distribution [16]. Nabilone is extensively metabolized, but the activity of its metabolites is not established [32]. In vitro, it has been shown to only be a weak inhibitor of the cytochrome P450 system and thought to not interfere with the metabolism of other P450-mediated medications [32]. Nabilone is excreted primarily in the feces (~60%) [32]. It has not been determined how age, gender, and hepatic and renal function may affect the metabolism and elimination of nabilone [32].

Dosage and Administration

Cesamet is supplied as 1 mg capsules, and the usual adult dosage is 1 or 2 mg twice daily with the lowest effective dosage tried first. The maximum recommended daily dose is 6 mg divided in three doses daily. Cesamet can be given two to three times daily during the cycle of chemotherapy and up to 48 hours after the cycle ends.

Monitoring, Adverse Events, Drug Interactions, and Abuse Potential

The effect of renal and hepatic dysfunction on Cesamet metabolism is not known. Currently there is no recommendation for renal or hepatic function testing prior to starting treatment. Cesamet is a Schedule II controlled substance with abuse potential and psychoactive effects, so it should be cautiously monitored in patients with a personal or family history of substance abuse or mental health disorders. Safety and efficacy for patients under 18 years of age have not yet been established, so caution should be taken regarding its psychoactive effects.

Adverse Effects

Common central nervous system side effects from nabilone include drowsiness, dizziness, vertigo, euphoria, ataxia, depression, lack of concentration, and somnolence [32]. Due to these CNS effects, patients should be instructed not to drive, operate machinery, or engage in any hazardous activity while receiving nabilone. In addition to CNS effects, xerostomia is the second most encountered adverse effect [32]. Patients may also experience cardiovascular effects such as tachycardia and hypotension [32].

Drug Interactions

Currently, there is limited data on potential drug interactions with nabilone. However, there are additive CNS depressant effects when combined with benzodiazepines, alcohol, and codeine, so caution should be used when patients using these medications are being started on nabilone treatment [32].

Abuse Potential

Nabilone can produce euphoria or marijuana-like "high" effects in some patients, so similar to marijuana, the potential for abuse exists [32]. There does not appear to be any withdrawal symptoms after discontinuation of clinical trials of 5 days duration [32]. Longer-term studies on nabilone have not been conducted, but abstinence syndrome has been demonstrated with high-dose Δ^9-THC after duration of greater than 12 days [32].

References

1. Morran C, Smith DC, Anderson DA, et al. Incidence of nausea and vomiting with cytotoxic chemotherapy: a prospective randomized trial of antiemetics. BMJ. 1979;(1):1323–4.
2. Jenss K. Importance of nausea. Cancer Nurs. 1994;17:488–93.
3. Wiser W, Berger A. Practical management of chemotherapy-induced nausea and vomiting. Oncology. 2005;19:637–45.
4. Darmani NA. Δ^9-Tetrahydrocannabinol and synthetic cannabinoids prevent emesis produced by the cannabinoid CB1 receptor antagonist/inverse agonist SR 141716A. Neuropsychopharmacology. 2001;24(2):198–203.
5. Lemberger L, Rowe H. Clinical pharmacology of nabilone, a cannabinol derivative. Clin Pharmacol Ther. 1975;18(6):720–6.
6. Herman TS, Einhorn LH, Jones SE, et al. Superiority of nabilone over prochlorperazine as an antiemetic in patients receiving cancer chemotherapy. N Engl J Med. 1979;300:1295–7.
7. Pergolizzi JV, Taylor R, LeQuang JA, et al. Concise review of the management of iatrogenic emesis using cannabinoids: emphasis on nabilone for chemotherapy-induced nausea and vomiting. Cancer Chemother Pharmacol. 2017;79:467–77.
8. Turcotte D, Doupe M, Torabi M, et al. Nabilone as an adjunctive to gabapentin for multiple-sclerosis-induced neuropathic pain: a randomized controlled trial. Pain Med. 2015;16:149–59.
9. Toth C, Mawani S, Brady S, et al. An enriched-enrolment, randomized withdrawal, flexible-dose, double-blind, placebo controlled, parallel assignment efficacy study of nabilone as adjuvant in the treatment of diabetic peripheral neuropathic pain. Pain. 2012;153:2073–82.
10. Bestard J, Toth C. An open-label comparison of nabilone and gabapentin as adjuvant therapy or monotherapy in the management of neuropathic pain in patients with peripheral neuropathy. Pain Pract. 2011;11:353–68.
11. Skrabek R, Galimova L, Ethans K, Perry D. Nabilone for the treatment of pain in fibromyalgia. J Pain. 2008;9:164–73.
12. Pooyania S, Ethans K, Sztum T, Casey A, Perry D. A randomized, double-blinded, crossover pilot study assessing the effect of nabilone on spasticity in persons with spinal cord injury. Arch Phys Med Rehabil. 2010;91:703–7.
13. Wissel J, Haydn T, Muller J, et al. Low dose treatment with the synthetic cannabinoid nabilone significantly reduces spasticity-related pain: a double-blind placebo-controlled crossover trial. J Neurol. 2006;253:1337–41.
14. Pinsger M, Schimetta W, Volc D, et al. Benefits of an add-on treatment with the synthetic cannabinomimetic nabilone on patients with chronic pain—a randomized controlled trial. Wien Klin Wochenschr. 2006;118:327–35.
15. Frank B, Serpell M, Hughes J, Matthews J, Kapur D. Comparison of analgesic effects and patient tolerability of nabilone and dihydrocodeine for chronic neuropathic pain: randomised, crossover, double blind study. BMJ. 2008;336:199–201.
16. Ware M, Fitzcharles M, Joseph L, Shir Y. The effects of nabilone on sleep in fibromyalgia: results of a randomized controlled trial. Anesth Analg. 2010;110:604–10.
17. Berlach D, Shir Y, Ware M. Experience with the synthetic cannabinoid nabilone in chronic noncancer pain. Pain Med. 2006;25–9(25):7.
18. Einhorn LH, Nagy C, Furnas B. Nabilone: an effective antiemetic in patients receiving cancer chemotherapy. J Clin Pharmacol. 1981;21(suppl):64–9.
19. Ahmedzai S, Carlyle DL, Calder IT, et al. Anti-emetic efficacy and toxicity of nabilone, a synthetic cannabinoid, in lung cancer chemotherapy. Br J Cancer. 1983;48(5):657–63.
20. Niiranen A, Mattson K. A cross-over comparison of nabilone and prochlorperazine for emesis induced by cancer chemotherapy. Am J Clin Oncol. 1985;8:336–40.
21. Ettinger DS, Armstrong DK, Barbour S, et al. Antiemesis: clinical practice guidelines in oncology. J Natl Compr Cancer Netw. 2009;7(5):572–95.
22. Maida V, Ennis M, Irani S, et al. Adjunctive nabilone in cancer pain and symptom management: a prospective observational study using propensity scoring. J Support Oncol. 2008:6119–24.
23. Hill K. Medical use of cannabis in 2019. JAMA. 2019;332(10):974–5.
24. Whiting P, Wolff RF, Deshpande S, et al. Cannabinoids for medical use: a systematic review and meta-analysis. JAMA. 2015;313(24):2456–73.
25. Meng H, Johnston B, Englesakis M, et al. Selective cannabinoids for chronic neuropathic pain: a systematic review and meta-analysis. Anesth Analg. 2017;125(5):1638–52.
26. Wilcock A, Twycross R. Therapeutic reviews: cannabinoids. J Pain Symptom Manag. 2013;46(1):142–9.
27. Martin BR, Wiley JL. Mechanism of action of cannabinoids: how it may lead to treatment of cachexia, emesis, and pain. J Support Oncol. 2004;2:305–14.
28. Davis MP. Oral nabilone capsules in the treatment of chemotherapy-induced nausea and vomiting and pain. Expert Opin Investig Drugs. 2008;17(1):85–95.
29. Hornby P. Central neurocircuitry associated with emesis. Am J Med Genet. 2001;111(Suppl 8 A):106S–12S.
30. Herkenham M, Lynn AB, Little MD, et al. Cannabinoid receptor localization in brain. Proc Natl Acad Sci U S A. 1990;87:1932–6.
31. Hohmann AG, Briley EM. Herkenhamm. Pre- and postsynaptic distribution of cannabinoid and mu opioid receptors in rat spinal cord. Brain Res. 1999;822:17–25.
32. Cesamet® (nabilone) capsules for oral administration [package insert]. Valeant Pharmaceuticals: Costa Mesa; 2006.

16 Cannabidiol (Epidiolex)

Nathan J. Harrison

Introduction

Lennox-Gastaut syndrome (LGS) and Dravet syndrome (DS) are two rare, treatment-resistant seizure disorders in the category of childhood-onset epileptic encephalopathies [1, 2]. These disorders can lead to developmental slowing, cerebral and cognitive dysfunction, and behavioral disturbances due to epileptogenic activity during brain maturation [3–5]. DS produces convulsive seizures, while LGS causes drop seizures, both of which can lead to significant traumatic injuries. The first-line antiepileptic drugs (AEDs) for these syndromes include valproate, lamotrigine, and topiramate but can often be poorly tolerated and ineffective and usually require multiple alternative AEDs in combination, yet still may not completely control the seizures. This leaves patients, parents, and clinicians seeking alternative treatments [4].

The use of *Cannabis sativa* plant as medicine dates back as far as 2700 B.C. in China [6]. The first mention of cannabis used as an anticonvulsant dates back to 1843 when the physician and chemistry professor W.B. O'Shaughnessy in Calcutta, India, tested a preparation of *Cannabis indica* on multiple animal species and humans to determine benefit to various conditions. Among his most pertinent results, he reported a 4-day, seizure-free period after administering a preparation *Cannabis indica* to a 40-day-old girl with recurrent seizures previously resistant to any of the typical treatments of the day [7].

Approximately 100 different phytocannabinoids have been identified in *Cannabis sativa* and *C. indica*, with Δ^9-tetrahydrocannabinol (Δ^9-THC) and cannabidiol (CBD) being the two most studied pharmacologically active cannabinoids [8] Fig. 16.1. In contrast to Δ^9-THC, CBD lacks the psychotropic and intoxicating effects but remains pharmacologically active through a different mechanism of action than Δ^9-THC and therefore presents a promising option for treatment-resistant epilepsy (TRE) [9]. Several small human trials examining CBD were performed in the 1980s and 1990s that suggested its possible benefit as an anticonvulsant [10–12].

Greenwich Biosciences, a branch of GW Pharmaceuticals, began developing a plant-derived pharmaceutical grade liquid CBD which was utilized in an Expanded Access Program (EAP) to treat TREs [13]. This EAP evolved into three pivotal human studies that eventually led to a 2018 FDA approval of this liquid CBD under the brand name Epidiolex and in 2019 under the name Epidyolex in Europe.

N. J. Harrison (✉)
Ochsner Health Systems, Department of Anesthesiology and Critical Care Medicine, New Orleans, LA, USA
e-mail: nharrison@ochsner.org

S. N. Narouze (ed.), *Cannabinoids and Pain*, https://doi.org/10.1007/978-3-030-69186-8_16

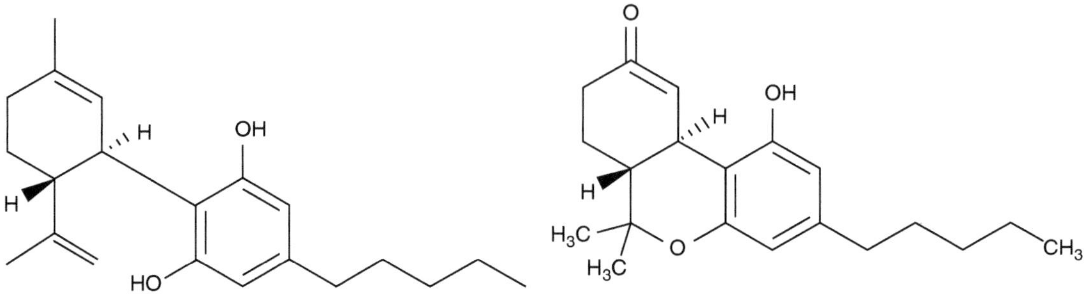

Cannabidiol (CBD) $\varnothing^9$-tetrahydrocannabinal ($\varnothing^9$-THC)

Fig. 16.1 Chemical structure of cannabidiol (CBD) compared to tetrahydrocannabinol (THC)

Clinical Trials

The first open-label EAP trial with CBD included 162 patients aged 1–30 with greater than 17 different seizure disorders, of which DS and LGS were the most common (23% and 22%, respectively) [13]. The promising results led to three robust trials named GWPCARE 1, 3, and 4.

GWPCARE 1 Devinsky et al. examined the effects of CBD on Dravet syndrome at 20 mg/kg/day divided twice daily against placebo [14]. Both the placebo and the CBD group had similar demographics, concomitant AEDs, and seizure frequency. They found an adjusted median difference of 22.8% fewer monthly seizures in the CBD group and a 19.2% reduction in total seizures. As a determination of how the caregiver perceived benefits with treatments, the Caregiver Global Impression of Change (CGIC) scale demonstrated 62% reporting improvement in the CBD group compared to 34% in the placebo group [14].

GWPCARE 4 Thiele et al. conducted a similar study with CBD 20 mg/kg/day divided BID compared to placebo for LGS and found 17.2% decrease in monthly drop seizure frequency in the CBD group and a CGIC improvement of 58% in the CBD group compared to 34% in the placebo group [15].

GWPCARE 3 Devinsky et al. compared the reduction in drop seizures in LGS patients using 10 mg/kg/day BID vs. 20 mg/kg/day BID against placebo in order to determine if a lower dosing retained effectiveness [16]. The reduction in monthly drop seizure frequency was 41.9%, 37.2%, and 17.2% in the 20 mg/kg/day, 10 mg/kg/day BID, and placebo group, respectively [16]. Adverse effects had been noted in GWPCARE 1 and GWPCARE 4 including somnolence, diarrhea, decreased appetite, and elevated LFTs [14, 15]. In GWPCARE 3, there were adverse effects in 94% of the 20 mg/kg/day BID group compared to a lower rate of 84% in the 10 mg/kg/day BID group and 72% in the placebo group. Correspondingly, this reduction in side effects but continued seizure reduction may account for the CGIC score of 66% in the 10 mg/kg/day BID group compared to only 57% in the 20 mg/kg/day BID group. Fortunately, while each of the three studies noted adverse effects in CBD treatment arms, these adverse effects largely resolved with time or dose reduction [16]. These studies collectively demonstrated that CBD could reduce seizure frequency compared to placebo in LGS and DS and dose reduction decreased the incidence of side effects [14–16].

Pharmacology and Pharmacokinetics

CBD's anticonvulsant exact mechanism of action is not known but seems to be unrelated to direct agonism of receptors CB1 and CB2 of the endocannabinoid system in contrast to how Δ^9-THC functions [9]. Instead, CBD's anticonvulsant effect appears to occur from its action at numerous other receptors, ion channels, and neurotransmitter transporters that may be part of the endocannabinoid system and whose overall downstream effect is to decrease neuronal excitability. For instance, CBD appears to antagonize G protein-coupled receptor 55 (GPR55) and transient receptor potential cation channel (TRPM8) and acts as an agonist at 5HT-1a and 5HT-2a, TRPV1-3, and TRPV4 [17]. CBD also inhibits anandamide reuptake which could play a beneficial role as anandamide can antagonize epileptic discharges in the hippocampus. Anandamide levels have been found to be low in the cerebrospinal fluid of new-onset temporal lobe epilepsy patients suggesting its presence in greater amounts has an antiepileptic effect [18].

CBD is metabolized mainly by the enzymes CYP3A4 and CYP2C19. Therefore, when coadministering an inhibitor of these enzymes, the plasma levels of Epidiolex may increase, and a reduction in dose may be necessary to avoid adverse reactions. Similarly, coadministration of other medications metabolized by CYP3A4 and CYP2C19 will result in elevated levels of that medication [19]. For example, a threefold increase in the CYP2C19 substrate N-desmethylclobazam (norclobazam) was observed when coadministering Epidiolex and clobazam which can lead to clobazam-related side effect. Clobazam is commonly used as a concomitant antiepileptic drug (AED) for treatment-resistant epilepsy, so caution should be observed when coadministering Epidiolex and clobazam [20]. Another commonly used AED, valproic acid, is an inhibitor of CYP2C9 and when coadministered with Epidiolex can elevate liver enzymes [21].

Epidiolex has a time to maximum plasma concentration of 2.5–5 hours at steady state. Coadminstration of Epidiolex with a high-calorie/high-fat meal can increase the maximum serum concentration by fivefold versus healthy volunteers who fasted. It is recommended that a high-calorie/high-fat meal accompany each dosing to reduce dose variability. The half-life of cannabidiol is 56–61 hours after twice-daily administration for 1 week. Cannabidiol is primarily metabolized by the liver with a minor contribution of the gut by the enzymes CYP3A4 and CYP2C19. Cannabidiol is converted to an active metabolite, 7-OH-CBD, at a 39% lower dosage than the parent drug and then further converted to an inactive metabolite, 7-COOH-CBD. Cannabidiol is excreted in the feces with a small contribution of renal clearance [19].

Dosage and Administration

Epidiolex is supplied as 100 ml of a colorless, strawberry flavored oil in a 100 mg/ml bottle and includes a calibrated syringe for dosing. Weekly titration is recommended to reach the minimal effective dose and monitor for any adverse effects (Table 16.1). Initial dosing of Epidiolex starts at 2.5 mg/kg twice daily (5 mg/kg/day) for the first week. Titration can continue by 5 mg/kg/day weekly (2.5 mg/kg BID) up to a maximum dosage of 20 mg/kg/day (10 mg/kg BID) [19]. While the recommended maintenance dose is 10 mg/kg/day, 20 mg/kg/day did produce a greater reduction in seizure frequency, albeit with increased adverse effects [16]. While the pediatric population is the primary consumer of Epidiolex, the drug's safety and efficacy have not been established in patients less than 2 years old [19].

Table 16.1 Initiation, titration, and monitoring of Epidiolex

Approved for treatment of seizures associated with Lennox-Gastaut syndrome or Dravet syndrome in patients 2 years old or older
Obtain serum transaminases (AST, ALT) and total bilirubin prior to initiating treatment
Dose adjustment needed for moderate to severe hepatic impairment
Recommend starting dose of 2.5 mg/kg BID and can titrate upward weekly by 2.5 mg/kg BID to minimum effective dose up to maximum of 10 mg/kg BID
Monitor AST, ALT, and total bilirubin at 1, 3, and 6 months

Monitoring, Adverse Events, and Drug Interactions

Prior to starting treatment with Epidiolex, serum liver transaminases (AST and ALT) and total bilirubin should be obtained because there is potential for cannabidiol to cause hepatocellular injury [14, 15, 19]. Patients with elevated baseline transaminase levels three times above the upper limit of normal and elevations of bilirubin twice the upper limit of normal (ULN) should be evaluated for causes prior to initiating treatment with Epidiolex. After initiating treatment of Epidiolex, repeat serum transaminases and total bilirubin should be monitored at 1 month, 3 months, 6 months, and thereafter if any symptoms arise suggesting hepatic dysfunction. In clinical trials, elevated transaminases greater than 3 times the ULN occurred most commonly when Epidiolex was administered with valproic acid and clobazam combined (30%), followed by valproic acid only (21%) and then clobazam alone (4%), which was only slightly greater than Epidiolex alone (3%) [19].

If the patient has mild hepatic impairment (Child-Pugh A), no dose adjustments are necessary. If moderate hepatic impairment exists (Child-Pugh B), start titration at 2.5 mg/kg/day gradually increasing as necessary to a maximum of 10 mg/kg/day. When the patient has severe hepatic impairment (Child-Pugh C), initiate at 1 mg/kg/day titrating to a maximum of 4 mg/kg/day [19].

Adverse Effects

The most common side effects of CBD include gastrointestinal effects such as diarrhea, abdominal pain, decreased appetite/weight loss, and increased LFTs. Central nervous system adverse effects include somnolence and fatigue. The incidence of somnolence and fatigue was related to dose, with a higher incidence of patients experiencing sedation with 20 mg/kg/day than with 10 mg/kg/day [16]. Patients receiving clobazam in addition to cannabidiol also experienced a significantly higher incidence of somnolence and fatigue than patients only using cannabidiol [19].

Antiepileptic drugs are known to increase the risk of suicidal ideations and behavior, so it is recommended to consider these same risks when prescribing Epidiolex. While there were no reports of suicidal thoughts or events in any of the landmark trials GWPCARE 1, GWPCARE 3, or GWPCARE 4, the manufacturer recommends close monitoring for changes in behavior or mood, worsening depression, or any suicidal ideation.

Abuse Potential

While cannabidiol is derived from the *Cannabis sativa* plant, it appears to lack the euphoric effects of the other neuroactive cannabinoid, Δ^9-THC [6]. In order to test if the same was true of Epidiolex, a study was conducted with therapeutic and even supratherapeutic doses of Epidiolex in recreational polydrug users [22]. After approval by the FDA in 2018, the DEA classified Epidiolex as a Schedule V controlled substance.

References

1. Jahngir MU, Ahmad MQ, Jahangir M. Lennox-Gastaut syndrome: in a nutshell. Cureus. 2018;10(8):e3134. https://doi.org/10.7759/cureus.3134.
2. Guerrini R. Dravet syndrome: the main issues. Eur J Paediatr Neurol. 2012. https://doi.org/10.1016/j/ejpn.2012.04.006.
3. Wolff M, Casse-Perrot C, Dravet C. Severe myoclonic epilepsy of infants (Dravet syndrome): natural history and neuropsychological finding. Epilepsia. 2006;47(Suppl. 2):45–8.
4. Asadi-Pooya AA. Lennox-Gastaut syndrome: a comprehensive review. Neurol Sci. 2018;39:403–14.
5. Khan S, Al Baradie R. Epileptic encephalopathies: an overview. Epilepsy Res Treat. 2012;403592. https://doi.org/10.1155/2012/403592.
6. Devinsky O, Cilio MR, Cross H, et al. Cannabidiol: pharmacology and potential therapeutic role in epilepsy and other neuropsychiatric disorders. Epilepsia. 2014;55(6):791–802.

7. O'Shaughnessy WB. On the preparations of the Indian hemp, or Gunjah: Cannabis indica their effects on the animal system in health, and their utility in the treatment of tetanus and other convulsive diseases. Prov Med J Restrosp Med Sci. 1843;5:362–9.
8. Pertwee RG. The diverse CB1 and CB2 receptor pharmacology of three plant cannabinoids: Delta9-tetrahydrocannabinol, cannabidiol and delta9-tetrahydrocannabivarin. Br J Pharmacol. 2008;153:199–215.
9. Gaston TE, Friedman D. Pharmacology of cannabinoids in the treatment of epilepsy. Epilepsy Behav. 2017;70:313–8.
10. Cunha JM, Carlini EA, Pereira AE, et al. Chronic administration of cannabidiol to healthy volunteers and epileptic patients. Pharmacology. 1980;21:175–85.
11. Trembly B, Sherman M. Double-blind clinical study of cannabidiol as a secondary anticonvulsant. Presented at the Marijuana '90 International Conference on Cannabis and Cannabinoids, Kolympari, Crete, July 8–11, 1990.
12. Ames FR, Cridland EA. Toward drugs derived from cannabis. Naturwissen of cannabidiol. S Afr Med J. 1986;69:14.
13. Devinsky O, Marsh E, Friedman D, et al. Cannabidiol in patients with treatment-resistant epilepsy: and open-label interventional trial. Lancet Neurol. 2016;15:270–8.
14. Devinsky O, Cross JH, Laux L, et al. Trial of cannabidiol for drug-resistant seizures in the Dravet syndrome. N Engl J Med. 2017;376:2011–20.
15. Thiele EA, Marsh ED, French JA, et al. Cannabidiol in patients with seizures associated with Lennox-Gastaut syndrome (GWPCARE4): a randomized, double-blind, placebo-controlled phase 3 trial. Lancet. 2018;391:1085–96.
16. Devinsky O, Patel AD, Cross JH, et al. Effect of cannabidiol on drop seizures in the Lennox-Gastaut syndrome. N Engl J Med. 2018;378:1888–97.
17. Jones NA, Hill AJ, Smith I, et al. Cannabidiol displays antiepileptiform and antiseizure properties in vitro and in vivo. J Pharmacol Exp Ther. 2010;332(2):569–77.
18. Romigi A, Bari M, Placidi F. Cerebrospinal fluid levels of the endocannabinoid anandamide are reduced in patients with untreated newly diagnosed temporal lobe epilepsy. Epilepsia. 2010;51:768–72.
19. Greenwich Biosciences, Inc. EPIDIOLEX® (cannabidiol) oral solution. Highlights of prescribing information; 2018.
20. Geffrey AL, Pollak SF, Bruno PL, et al. Drug-drug interaction between clobazam and cannabidiol in children with refractory epilepsy. Epilepsia. 2015;56:1246–51.
21. Wen X, Wang JS, Kivisto KT, et al. In vitro evaluation of valproic acid as an inhibitor of human cytochrome P450 2C9 (CYP2C9). Br J Clin Pharmacol. 2001;52:547–53.
22. Schoedel KA, Szeto I, Setnik B, et al. Abuse potential assessment of cannabidiol (CBD) in recreational polydrug users: a randomized, double-blind, controlled trial. Epilepsy Behav. 2018;88:162–71.

Nabiximols (Sativex®)

17

Michael Boivin

Introduction

Nabiximols (Sativex®) is a prescription cannabinoid approved in 29 countries outside of the United States [1]. Like other prescription cannabinoids (nabilone, dronabinol), nabiximols meets all the standards for efficacy, safety, and consistency required for approval of any pharmaceutical [1]. Unlike prescription cannabinoids, nabiximols is formulated from extracts from the *Cannabis sativa* plant versus being synthetically produced [2]. Although this medication has been consistently approved as an adjunct for the symptomatic relief of MS spasticity, some countries have approved it as an adjunct for the management of MS-related neuropathic pain and cancer-related pain unresponsive to opioid therapy [2]. This chapter will review this cannabinoid, the evidence to support its use, and key considerations when being used for chronic pain.

Nabiximols Production

GW Pharmaceuticals was founded in 1998 in the UK [3]. It has grown millions of cannabis plants in a sophisticated glasshouse environment to allow for control over the many factors that impact cannabis plant development [3]. The uniformity of this facility allows for the production of cannabis that meets the pharmaceutical industry's demand for quality, safety, and efficacy [3]. Even with control of the plant's environment, growth medium, genetics, and processing, it is important to remember that product of the cannabis plant can be highly variable [3].

Once grown, the manufacturer harvests and extracts the cannabinoids from the plant material. The manufacturer immerses batches of dried plant material into liquid carbon dioxide at extremely high pressure to extract ingredients into the solvent [3]. These ingredients are then separated and purified [3].

To produce a uniform pharmaceutical product, the manufacturer produces two types of botanical drug substances (BDS) [4]. The first BDS (Tetranabinex®) is an extract of a cannabis plant containing delta-9-tetrahydrocannabinol (THC) as the principle cannabinoid [4]. The second BDS (Nabidiolex®) is an extract of a cannabis plant containing cannabidiol (CBD) as the principle cannabinoid [4]. Other BDS may be generated from extracts high in other cannabinoids (CBC, CBG, THC-V, CBD-V) [4]. The different BDS are blended to ensure that the ratio of THC/CBD is consistent across each batch and each ml contains 27 mg of THC and 25 mg of CBD [2]. Each BDS also contains a proprietary blend of non-cannabinoid ingredients seen with whole-plant extracts such as terpenoids, sterols, fatty acids, carotenoids, and flavonoids [4].

M. Boivin (✉)
CommPharm Consulting, Barrie, ON, Canada
e-mail: mike@commpharm.com

S. N. Narouze (ed.), *Cannabinoids and Pain*, https://doi.org/10.1007/978-3-030-69186-8_17

Nabiximols Approval and Indications

Nabiximols has attained regulatory approval in 29 countries for the adjunctive treatment of spasticity related to multiple sclerosis (MS) [1].

It was approved in Canada in 2005. In this country, it also has received indication for adjunctive treatment for neuropathic pain due to MS and as adjunctive treatment for moderate to severe persistent background cancer pain not responsive to the highest tolerated dose of strong opioid therapy [2].

Nabiximols has been used off-label for a variety of conditions. Case reports and studies have evaluated its role in neuropathic pain [5–8], pain associated with rheumatoid arthritis [9], treating cannabis dependence [10, 11], and tic reduction [12].

Nabiximols Contraindication

The Canadian product monograph lists that nabiximols is contraindicated in [2]:

- Patients with known or suspected allergy to cannabinoids, propylene glycol, ethanol, or peppermint oil
- Patients with serious cardiovascular disease, such as ischemic heart disease, arrhythmias, poorly controlled hypertension, or severe heart failure
- Patients with a history of schizophrenia or any other psychotic disorder
- Children under 18 years of age
- Women of child-bearing potential not on a reliable contraceptive or men intending to start a family
- Pregnant or nursing women

Nabiximols Evidence

Nabiximols for MS-Related Spasticity

Spasticity is common in people with MS [13]. Over 85% of people with MS have some spasticity, 50% have at least mild spasticity, and up to 17% have severe spasticity [13]. Although medications such as baclofen, tizanidine, benzodiazepines, and botulinum toxin are used to manage MS-related spasticity, they may not be effective or are limited due to adverse effects [13].

There have been a number of studies exploring the role of nabiximols in reducing MS-related spasticity (Table 17.1). These studies reported improvement in self-reported spasticity severity, and some reported improvement in sleep quality/disruption. One observational study reported that people with MS-related spasticity will normally respond within the first 6 weeks of treatment [14]. This provides guidance when starting this therapy, as poor response by 6 weeks may be a strong indicator of a poor responding patient [14].

Nabiximols for MS-Related Neuropathic Pain

Pain has been reported to occur in up to 86% of people with MS [19]. One study found that 61% of people with MS reported a painful condition with an intensity on a visual analogue scale of at least 4/10 [19]. MS-related pain includes headache (43%), neuropathic pain in the arms or legs (26%), back pain (20%), painful spasms (15%), and trigeminal neuralgia (3.8%) [13]. Of note, 68% of the people in one study reported dissatisfaction with care received and that clinicians often underestimate the pain problem [19].

Most of the pain experience by people with MS is neuropathic in origin [13]. There has been interest in the potential role of cannabinoids in managing neuropathic pain as many individuals do not experience significant pain reduction or cannot tolerate current treatment options [20].

Two studies have evaluated the role of nabiximols in the management of MS-related neuropathic pain (Table 17.2). These studies demonstrate that there may be a potential role for nabiximols in the management of MS-related neuropathic pain and sleep quality/duration.

Table 17.1 Nabiximols for MS-related spasticity

Reference	Type	Participants	Intervention	Duration	Discussion and results
[15]	RCT	160 (80 placebo)	Nabiximols adjustable dose versus placebo	6 weeks	A 100 mm visual analogue scale was used to assess the improvement in the participant's symptoms Significant improvements in: Spasticity Quality of sleep
[16]	RCT	189 (65 placebo)	Nabiximols adjustable dose versus placebo	6 weeks	Numerical rating scale (0–10) to assess spasticity severity Significant improvement in patient self-reported spasticity severity No significant change in Ashworth scale
[17]	RCT	337 (170 placebo)	Nabiximols adjustable dose versus placebo	15 weeks	Numerical rating scale (0–10) to assess spasticity severity Significant chance in self-reported spasticity severity
[18]	RCT	241 (117 placebo)	Nabiximols adjustable dose versus placebo	19 weeks	572 patients given nabiximols for 4 weeks run-in, participants who responded to nabiximols in run-in were then randomized to nabiximols (n = 124) or placebo (n = 117) Numerical rating scale (0–10) to assess spasticity severity Compared to placebo, there was a significant improvement in self-reported spasticity severity and frequency. There was also an improvement in sleep disruption

Table 17.2 Studies evaluating nabiximols for MS-related neuropathic pain

Reference	Type	Participants	Intervention	Duration	Discussion and results
[21]	RCT	339 (172 placebo)	Nabiximols adjustable dose versus placebo	14-week initial phase to determine responders 14-week open-label randomized withdrawal	Numerical rating scale (0–10) to assess pain intensity Non-significant reduction in pain at 14 weeks. 50% of those receiving nabiximols and 45% of those receiving placebo reached a 30% reduction in NRS score During withdrawal phase of nabiximols responders, there was a significant difference in 30% reduction in pain intensity, sleep quality, and change in pain intensity from baseline versus placebo
[22]	RCT	66 (32 placebo)	Nabiximols adjustable dose versus placebo	5 weeks	Numerical rating scale (0–10) to assess to assess symptom intensity Nabiximols was associated with a significant improvement in mean intensity of pain and sleep disturbances versus placebo A 2-year open-label extension of the study found that there was no evidence of tolerance in responders to nabiximols treatment [23]

Nabiximols for Cancer-Related Pain

Individuals with cancer will often present with chronic pain which may be related directly from tumor involvement or due to an adverse effect from chemotherapy [24]. Traditionally, opioids have been relied upon to manage cancer-related pain [24]. This treatment option can be problematic for many people [24]. There has been increased interest in opioid alternatives or adjunctive treatment to help to improve pain control and reduce opioid-related harm.

Several studies have evaluated nabiximols as adjunctive treatment in the management of cancer-related pain (Table 17.3). Overall, the results are mixed with some studies finding the addition of nabiximols leading to significant improvement in pain intensity, where others have not.

Another trial evaluated nabiximols for chemotherapy-related neuropathic pain [25]. This small study ($n = 16$) did not find a statistical significant difference between placebo and nabiximols [25]. There were five participants who reported a 2/10 or greater reduction in pain intensity [25]. This trended toward statistical sig-

Table 17.3 Studies evaluating nabiximols for advanced cancer pain

Reference	Type	Participants	Intervention	Duration	Discussion and results
[26]	RCT	360 (59 placebo)	Nabiximols adjustable dose versus placebo Also compared THC extract	2 weeks	Numerical rating scale (0–10) to assess pain intensity Statistical reduction in pain intensity with nabiximols, compared to placebo THC extract was associated with a non-significant reduction in pain intensity compared to placebo Twice as many patients taking nabiximols showed a reduction of more than 30% from baseline pain NRS score when compared with placebo No change in the median dose of opioid background medication, breakthrough doses, sleep quality, or nausea scores
[27]	RCT	360 (91 placebo)	3 nabiximols treatment groups (1–4 sprays, 6–10 sprays, 11–16 sprays) and placebo	9 weeks	Numerical rating scale (0–10) to assess pain intensity The 30% responder rate primary analysis was not significant for nabiximols versus placebo A secondary continuous responder analysis of average daily pain from baseline to end of study demonstrated that the proportion of patients reporting analgesia was greater for nabiximols than placebo overall and specifically in the low-dose and medium-dose groups
[28]	RCT	399 study 1 404 study 2	Nabiximols adjustable dose versus placebo	5 weeks	Numerical rating scale (0–10) to assess pain intensity The primary efficacy endpoint (percent improvement (study 1) and mean change (study 2) in average daily pain NRS scores) was not met in either study Post hoc analyses of the primary endpoints identified statistically favorable treatment effect for nabiximols in US participants <65 years that was not observed in patients <65 years from the rest of the world
[29]	RCT	397 (198 placebo)	Nabiximols adjustable dose versus placebo	5 weeks	Numerical rating scale (0–10) to assess pain intensity Non-significant reduction in average pain with nabiximols compared to placebo Nabiximols was statistically superior to placebo on two of three quality-of-life instruments at week 3 and on all three at week 5 In exploratory post hoc analyses, US patients, but not patients from the rest of the world, experienced significant benefits from nabiximols on multiple secondary endpoints

nificance, and the authors reported a number needed to treat as five [25].

Nabiximols for Chronic Pain

Nabiximols has also been studied for the management of chronic pain (Table 17.4). The current studies evaluated nabiximols for neuropathic pain and pain associated with rheumatoid arthritis. Studies conducted to date demonstrate that some individuals with chronic neuropathic pain or rheumatoid arthritis may benefit from the use of nabiximols.

Nabiximols Tolerability

Like other cannabinoid medications, nabiximols is associated with an increased risk of central nervous system (CNS) adverse effects and a potential for dependence [2]. In placebo-controlled

Table 17.4 Studies evaluating nabiximols for chronic pain

Reference	Type	Participants	Intervention	Duration	Discussion and results
[6]	RCT	125 (62 placebo) with neuropathic pain characterized by allodynia	Nabiximols adjustable dose versus placebo	5 weeks	Numerical rating scale (0–10) to assess symptom change The mean reduction in pain intensity scores (primary outcome measure) was greater in patients receiving nabiximols than placebo Improvements in Neuropathic Pain Scale composite score, sleep NRS, dynamic allodynia, punctate allodynia, Pain Disability Index, and Patient Global Impression of Change were greater on nabiximols vs. placebo
[7]	RCT	303 (118 placebo) with peripheral neuropathic pain with allodynia	Nabiximols adjustable dose versus placebo	15 weeks	Numerical rating scale (0–10) to assess symptom change At the 30% responder level, there were statistically significant treatment differences in favor of nabiximols There was also a reduction in mean peripheral neuropathic pain 0–10 NRS scores in both treatment groups that was numerically higher in the nabiximols group but which failed to reach statistical significance Sleep quality 0–10 NRS score and Subject Global Impression of Change (SGIC) also demonstrated statistically significant treatment differences in favor of nabiximols An open-label 9-month extension of the study found that efficacy was maintained with no evidence of tolerability developing [8]
[5]	RCT	48 crossover trial in patients with neuropathic pain due to brachial plexus avulsion	Nabiximols adjustable dose THC spray with adjustable dose	14–20 days on each treatment	Numerical rating scale (0–10) to assess symptom change The primary outcome measure was the mean pain severity score during the last 7 days of treatment Secondary outcome measures included pain-related quality of life assessments The differences in pain diary scores were clinically significant Measures of sleep showed statistically significant improvements

(continued)

Table 17.4 (continued)

Reference	Type	Participants	Intervention	Duration	Discussion and results
[9]	RCT	58 (27 placebo)	Nabiximols adjustable dose versus placebo	5 weeks	Numerical rating scale (0–10) to assess symptom change In comparison with placebo, the nabiximols produced statistically significant improvements in pain on movement, pain at rest, quality of sleep, DAS28, and the short-form McGill Pain Questionnaire at present component

Table 17.5 Most common nabiximols-related adverse effects [2]

	Nabiximols (%)	Placebo (%)
Dizziness	25.0	8.2
Fatigue	12.5	8.4
Nausea	9.6	5.7
Vertigo	6.5	2.0
Dry mouth	6.1	3.1
Asthenia	5.6	3.1
Diarrhea	5.5	3.9
Disorientation (includes confusion)	4.1	0.8
Disturbances in attention	3.9	0.1

Note: The lists of adverse effects in this table are not complete. Clinicians are encouraged to review the nabiximols product information for a complete list of adverse effects

trials in MS, adverse events have usually been mild or moderate in severity with discontinuation rates from treatment due to undesirable effects of 9.8% of patients on nabiximols compared to 4.7% on placebo [2]. With nabiximols being self-titrated to effect, patients are likely to experience a higher incidence of adverse events during the titration period than when the optimal dose is established [2].

The most prevalent adverse effects from the Canadian nabiximols product monograph are listed in Table 17.5.

Nabiximols Dosage and Administration

Administration

Nabiximols is for buccal use only. The spray should be directed to below the tongue or toward the inside of the cheeks [2]. The site should be varied, and the patient should be advised not to direct the spray towards the pharynx and not to inhale the spray. It must not be sprayed into the nose [2].

Dosing

Nabiximols is normally dosed using a self-titration method [2]. The treatment initiation and titration commonly involves [2]:

- On day 1 of treatment, patients should take one spray during the morning and one spray during the afternoon/evening. The morning dose can be taken at any time between waking up and 12 noon and, the afternoon dose can be taken at any time between 4 pm and bedtime.
- On subsequent days, the patient may gradually increase the total number of sprays, by one spray each day, as needed and tolerated. There should be at least a 15-minute gap between sprays. During initial titration, sprays should be evenly spread out over the day.
- If unacceptable adverse reactions such as dizziness or other CNS-type reactions develop at any time, dosing should be suspended until they have resolved. Some patients may be able to continue therapy at the dose reached by increasing the interval between doses; others may require their subsequent doses reduced. Patients should then carefully re-titrate to a tolerated dosage regimen that gives acceptable symptom relief.

The usual dose ranges between 4 and 8 sprays daily. The majority of patients require 12 sprays or less, and the dosage should be adjusted as needed and tolerated. There is limited experience with doses higher than 12 sprays per day. Some patients may require and may tolerate a higher number of sprays [2].

Storage, Stability, and Dosage Form

Storage and Stability

Once opened and in use, nabiximols should be used within 28 days (5.5 ml vial) or 42 days (10 ml vial). Prior to opening, nabiximols should be stored upright in a refrigerator (2–8 °C). Once opened, the spray may be stored at room temperature (15–25 °C) [2].

Dosage Form

Nabiximols is provided in a buccal spray [2]. Each 100 microliter spray contains 2.7 mg THC and 2.5 mg CBD [2]. The extract contains 50% v/v ethanol [2]. It also contains the non-medicinal ingredients of propylene glycol and peppermint oil [2].

Summary

Nabiximols is a prescription cannabinoid that matches all the regulatory requirements for other pharmaceutical medications. It is approved in many regions of the world for the adjunctive management of MS-related spasticity, MS-related pain, and advanced cancer pain not responding to opioid therapy [2]. Unlike other prescription cannabinoids (nabilone, dronabinol), nabiximols is a whole plant derivative that contains additional ingredients including terpenoids, fatty acids, and flavonoids. Although there is some conflicting efficacy data, there is evidence to support the use of nabiximols for a variety of different neuropathic pain conditions. Overall, nabiximols is well tolerated, and tolerance to adverse effects normally occurs with continued use. The buccal administration and proper storage are important to ensure a patient achieves the most benefit from this product.

References

1. MacCallum CA, Russo EB. Practical considerations in medical cannabis administration and dosing. Eur J Intern Med. 2018;49:12–9.
2. GW Pharma. Sativex product monograph. Toronto; 2012.
3. Potter DJ. A review of the cultivation and processing of cannabis (Cannabis sativa L.) for production of prescription medicines in the UK: cultivation and processing of cannabis for production of prescription medicines. Drug Test Anal. 2014;6:31–8.
4. Guy GW, Stott CG. The development of Sativex® – a natural cannabis-based medicine. In: Raphael Mechoulam, ed. Cannabinoids as Therapeutics. 1st ed. Birkhäuser; 2005:34.
5. Berman JS, Symonds C, Birch R. Efficacy of two cannabis based medicinal extracts for relief of central neuropathic pain from brachial plexus avulsion: results of a randomised controlled trial. Pain. 2004;112:299–306.
6. Nurmikko TJ, Serpell MG, Hoggart B, Toomey PJ, Morlion BJ, Haines D. Sativex successfully treats neuropathic pain characterised by allodynia: a randomised, double-blind, placebo-controlled clinical trial. Pain. 2007;133:210–20.
7. Serpell M, Ratcliffe S, Hovorka J, Schofield M, Taylor L, Lauder H, Ehler E. A double-blind, randomized, placebo-controlled, parallel group study of THC/CBD spray in peripheral neuropathic pain treatment: efficacy of THC/CBD spray in peripheral neuropathic pain. Eur J Pain. 2014;18:999–1012.
8. Hoggart B, Ratcliffe S, Ehler E, Simpson KH, Hovorka J, Lejčko J, Taylor L, Lauder H, Serpell M. A multicentre, open-label, follow-on study to assess the long-term maintenance of effect, tolerance and safety of THC/CBD oromucosal spray in the management of neuropathic pain. J Neurol. 2015;262:27–40.
9. Blake DR, Robson P, Ho M, Jubb RW, McCabe CS. Preliminary assessment of the efficacy, tolerability and safety of a cannabis-based medicine (Sativex) in the treatment of pain caused by rheumatoid arthritis. Rheumatology. 2006;45:50–2.
10. Lintzeris N, Bhardwaj A, Mills L, et al. Nabiximols for the treatment of cannabis dependence: a randomized clinical trial. JAMA Intern Med. 2019;179:1242–53.
11. Trigo JM, Soliman A, Quilty LC, et al. Nabiximols combined with motivational enhancement/cognitive behavioral therapy for the treatment of cannabis dependence: a pilot randomized clinical trial. PLoS One. 2018;13:e0190768.
12. Kanaan AS, Jakubovski E, Müller-Vahl K. Significant tic reduction in an otherwise treatment-resistant

patient with Gilles de la Tourette syndrome following treatment with nabiximols. Brain Sci. 2017;7:47.
13. Rice J, Cameron M. Cannabinoids for treatment of MS symptoms: state of the evidence. Curr Neurol Neurosci Rep. 2018;18:50.
14. Messina S, Solaro C, Righini I, et al. Sativex in resistant multiple sclerosis spasticity: discontinuation study in a large population of Italian patients (SA.FE. study). PLoS One. 2017;12:e0180651.
15. Wade DT, Makela P, Robson P, House H, Bateman C. Do cannabis-based medicinal extracts have general or specific effects on symptoms in multiple sclerosis? A double-blind, randomized, placebo-controlled study on 160 patients. Mult Scler. 2004;10:434–41.
16. Collin C, Davies P, Mutiboko IK, Ratcliffe S, for the Sativex Spasticity in MS Study Group. Randomized controlled trial of cannabis-based medicine in spasticity caused by multiple sclerosis: Cannabis-based medicine in spasticity by multiple sclerosis. Eur J Neurol. 2007;14:290–6.
17. Collin C, Ehler E, Waberzinek G, et al. A double-blind, randomized, placebo-controlled, parallel-group study of Sativex, in subjects with symptoms of spasticity due to multiple sclerosis. Neurol Res. 2010;32:451–9.
18. Novotna A, Mares J, Ratcliffe S, et al. A randomized, double-blind, placebo-controlled, parallel-group, enriched-design study of nabiximols* (Sativex ®), as add-on therapy, in subjects with refractory spasticity caused by multiple sclerosis: Sativex for refractory spasticity in MS. Eur J Neurol. 2011;18:1122–31.
19. Pöllmann W, Feneberg W. Current management of pain associated with multiple sclerosis. CNS Drugs. 2008;22:291–324.
20. Moulin D, Boulanger A, Clark A, et al. Pharmacological management of chronic neuropathic pain: revised consensus statement from the Canadian Pain Society. Pain Res Manag. 2014;19:328–35.
21. Langford RM, Mares J, Novotna A, Vachova M, Novakova I, Notcutt W, Ratcliffe S. A double-blind, randomized, placebo-controlled, parallel-group study of THC/CBD oromucosal spray in combination with the existing treatment regimen, in the relief of central neuropathic pain in patients with multiple sclerosis. J Neurol. 2013;260:984–97.
22. Rog DJ, Nurmikko TJ, Friede T, Young CA. Randomized, controlled trial of cannabis-based medicine in central pain in multiple sclerosis. Neurology. 2005;65:812–9.
23. Rog D, Nurmikko T, Young C. Oromucosal Δ9-tetrahydrocannabinol/cannabidiol for neuropathic pain associated with multiple sclerosis: an uncontrolled, open-label, 2-year extension trial. Clin Ther. 2007;29:2068–79.
24. Blake A, Wan BA, Malek L, DeAngelis C, Diaz P, Lao N, Chow E, O'Hearn S. A selective review of medical cannabis in cancer pain management. Ann Palliat Med. 2017;6:S215–22.
25. Lynch ME, Cesar-Rittenberg P, Hohmann AG. A double-blind, placebo-controlled, crossover pilot trial with extension using an oral mucosal cannabinoid extract for treatment of chemotherapy-induced neuropathic pain. J Pain Symptom Manag. 2014;47:166–73.
26. Johnson JR, Burnell-Nugent M, Lossignol D, Ganae-Motan ED, Potts R, Fallon MT. Multicenter, double-blind, randomized, placebo-controlled, parallel-group study of the efficacy, safety, and tolerability of THC:CBD extract and THC extract in patients with intractable cancer-related pain. J Pain Symptom Manag. 2010;39:167–79.
27. Portenoy RK, Ganae-Motan ED, Allende S, Yanagihara R, Shaiova L, Weinstein S, McQuade R, Wright S, Fallon MT. Nabiximols for opioid-treated cancer patients with poorly-controlled chronic pain: a randomized, placebo-controlled, graded-dose trial. J Pain. 2012;13:438–49.
28. Fallon MT, Albert Lux E, McQuade R, Rossetti S, Sanchez R, Sun W, Wright S, Lichtman AH, Kornyeyeva E. Sativex oromucosal spray as adjunctive therapy in advanced cancer patients with chronic pain unalleviated by optimized opioid therapy: two double-blind, randomized, placebo-controlled phase 3 studies. Br J Pain. 2017;11:119–33.
29. Lichtman AH, Lux EA, McQuade R, Rossetti S, Sanchez R, Sun W, Wright S, Kornyeyeva E, Fallon MT. Results of a double-blind, randomized, placebo-controlled study of nabiximols oromucosal spray as an adjunctive therapy in advanced cancer patients with chronic uncontrolled pain. J Pain Symptom Manag. 2018;55:179–188.e1.

Part IV

Medical Cannabis

Cannabis Strains to Chemovars

18

Michael Boivin

Introduction

Cannabis is one of the world's oldest cultivated plants [1]. It originated in Central Asia and has been grown and used as food, for its fiber, and as a drug plant [2, 3]. With the wide number of uses, the plant was widespread by man to different regions of the world [1].

The medical use of cannabis dates back over 5000 years, where it was considered for the management of fatigue, rheumatism, and malaria [4]. Although used for millennia for the management of pain, it was strongly prohibited in the twentieth century due to its psychoactivity and recreational use. Its use was highly restricted based in international regulations [4].

This chapter will provide a quick review on the cannabis plant growth, plant components, cannabis classification, and the implication of chemovars on medical cannabis use.

Cannabis sativa L.

Cannabis sativa L. is a dioecious (containing male and female productive organs) annual plant [4]. It is found in a wide variety of regions around the world [5]. It can be found in all temperate and tropical climates, except humid tropical rainforests [3]. It is estimated that close to one-third of the earth's land mass would be suitable for outdoor cannabis cultivation in some form [6].

There has been significant debate on the taxonomy of the cannabis plant [3]. Some view cannabis as a single species with multiple varieties or up to four different species: *Cannabis sativa*, *Cannabis indica*, *Cannabis ruderalis*, and *Cannabis afghanica* [7].

Cannabis sativa and *Cannabis indica* are the most relevant for medical cannabis use [5]. *Cannabis ruderalis* is a hardier variety of cannabis that is characterized by sparse growth and rarely used as a source for medical cannabis [5]. *Cannabis sativa* is a tall plant (2.5 m to 3.5 m) with thin leaves, whereas *Cannabis indica* tends to be shorter (1.8 m), bushier, and with broader and darker green leaves [5].

Cannabis Cultivation and Trichomes

Cannabis cultivation and processing have a significant impact on the cannabinoid and constituents within the plant. The plant genetics, growth medium, environmental conditions, nutrition, and processing can impact the yields of different constituents [8]. Even small changes in any of these factors can lead to changes in cannabis products produced. This is important from a clinician's perspective as unlike pharmaceutical products, which are synthesized to be identical for each batch, there

M. Boivin (✉)
CommPharm Consulting, Barrie, ON, Canada
e-mail: mike@commpharm.com

S. N. Narouze (ed.), *Cannabinoids and Pain*, https://doi.org/10.1007/978-3-030-69186-8_18

can be some variance between cannabinoids and other constituents between similar plants and growing conditions.

Importance of Trichomes

A key area of focus for medical cannabis is the trichomes on the cannabis plant. These trichomes (hair-like outgrowths) cover the leaves, bracts, and stems of the cannabis plant [4]. The trichomes are also concentrated on the female flower [3].

These trichomes secrete resin that contains pharmacologically compounds [3]. The ones of most interest are cannabinoids and terpenoids [3]. These compounds are secondary metabolites which are not used by the plant in normal structural growth, development, or reproduction of the organism [8]. It is thought that these compounds play an important role in the defense of the plant from herbivores and environmental stresses [8]. The trichomes are designed to protect the vital areas of plant structure for species survival [8]. Like other plants, the most vital area for plant survival is in the reproductive areas such as the flower, and thus it contains a large portion of these trichomes and cannabinoids [8].

Cannabis Constituents

Although the focus of patients and research tends to be on the cannabinoids delta-9-tetrahydrocannabinol (Δ^9-THC, THC) and cannabidiol (CBD) concentration of a cannabis product, there are over 500 distinct compounds in cannabis. This includes constituents from 18 different chemical classes and over 100 different phytocannabinoids [9].

Cannabinoids

There have been more than 100 different cannabinoids that have been identified in cannabis [10]. In *C. sativa*, cannabinoids are biosynthesized and accumulated as cannabinoid acids and subsequently decarboxylated into their active forms [4]. The most prominent phytocannabinoids in the cannabis plant are tetrahydrocannabinolic acid (THCA) and cannabidiolic acid (CBDA), which are converted to THC and CBD when heated [11]. The cannabinoids in cannabis are divided into ten subclasses [4, 12]:

- THC – Δ^9-Tetrahydrocannabinol
- CBD – Cannabidiol
- THCV – Δ^9-Tetrahydrocannabivarin
- CBC – Cannabichromene
- CBDV – Cannabidivarin
- CBL – Cannabicyclol
- CBN – Cannabinol
- CBG – Cannabigerol

Although the cannabinoid focus has been primarily on THC and CBD, there is increased interest in the role of other cannabinoids. In a typical cannabis plant, there are low concentrations of these other cannabinoids, but through plant genetics and breeding, cannabis plants are being grown with significantly higher levels. This will hopefully increase the number of studies being conducted to evaluate their role in chronic disease management.

The pharmacology and evidence of the different cannabinoids in the management of chronic pain will be reviewed in more detail in later chapters.

Terpenoids

Terpenoids (terpenes) are essential oils and are part of the largest group of plant chemicals with 15,000–20,000 fully characterized [12]. Terpenes are not unique to the cannabis plant, and there are more than 150 different types in the cannabis plant [13]. Terpenoid concentrations in cannabis flowers can range from up to 10% within trichomes, and with selective breeding, there are cannabis plants with terpenoids making up to 3.5% of the flower concentration [14]. Terpenoids, and not the cannabinoids, are responsible for the aroma of cannabis [12].

There has been increasing interest in terpenoids for their pharmacological properties. Table 18.1 reviews the different key terpenoids of interest in the cannabis plant.

Table 18.1 Terpenoids of interest in cannabis [4, 12, 14]

Terpenoid	Commonly found in	Key points
ß-Myrcene	Hops	Widespread in *C. sativa* May provide analgesia and muscle relaxation May reduce inflammation When combined with THC, it is thought to cause the "couch-lock" seen with recreational cannabis use
α-Pinene	Pine	May reduce inflammation Bronchodilation effects Acetylcholinesterase inhibitor which may counteract the short-term memory deficits from THC
Limonene	Lemon	Anxiolytic and antidepressant actions May improve gastroesophageal reflux Promotes apoptosis of breast cancer cells
Linalool	Lavender	May reduce anxiety May promote sedation May provide analgesia and local anesthetic effects Anticonvulsant/anti-glutamate properties
ß-Caryophyllene	Pepper	Anti-inflammatory action May be cytoprotective on gastric tissues May have anti-malarial action
Caryophyllene oxide	Lemon balm	Antifungal properties May be associated with decreased platelet aggregation

Like phytocannabinoids, selective cannabis breeding can allow for higher concentrations of specific terpenoids. This will hopefully provide clear guidance on the ideal concentrations of cannabinoids and terpenoids to reduce specific patient symptoms.

Other Cannabis Compounds

Along with cannabinoids and terpenoids, there are a large number of other compounds found in cannabis. There is currently not a significant amount of evidence on the potential role of these compounds when consumed with cannabis [9]. These compounds include [9]:

- Nitrogenous compounds
- Amino acids
- Proteins
- Enzymes
- Glycoproteins
- Hydrocarbons
- Simple alcohols
- Aldehydes
- Ketones
- Fatty acids
- Simple esters and lactones
- Steroids
- Non-cannabinoid phenols
- Flavonoids
- Vitamins
- Pigments

Entourage Effect of Cannabis Constituents

The focus to date has generally been on the selection of cannabis varieties based on the level of THC and CBD in the product. Originally, it was thought that the main actions of cannabis were only dependent on the levels of these specific cannabinoids. Besides cannabinoids, there are hundreds of other potentially pharmacologically active compounds that are consumed when cannabis is used by an individual.

The "entourage effect" is the belief that the pharmacological benefits of medical cannabis are not associated with the cannabinoids alone, but are also associated with the terpenoids and other constituents in the plant [12]. This is supported by the response to botanical cannabis often being more effective than when an isolated cannabinoid is used alone [15].

Cannabis Classification: Strains Versus Chemovars

Herbal cannabis is unique from traditional medicine as the latter tends to focus on a single medication that targets a specific site [16]. Although the THC and CBD within cannabis were once thought to be the only active ingredients, it is now believed that the range of constituents contribute to the therapeutic effects of cannabinoids [16].

There are thousands of different cannabis varieties available for both recreational and medical users. This can seem overwhelming for clinicians and patients to select the optimal product for their specific condition or symptoms. There have been a number of different classification systems to help to differentiate between the wide number of products.

Strains

Cannabis strain terminology was adapted to identify different varieties of cannabis. While the strain term is used in microbiology to describe bacteria or viruses with certain attributes, it has no official standing in botany [17]. The use of the term strain is not recommended when selecting medical cannabis.

Due to the illicit growth and use of cannabis, there has been the creation of a wide number of names associated with specific cannabis varieties [16]. Names such as *Pink kush*, *AK-47*,and *Bubba Kush* are commonly used by recreational users and producers [16]. These names are picked based on the plant morphology, leaf shape, plant height, color, smell, and speed of growth [16]. They are also classified based on the plant origin as being either "*indica*-based" or "*sativa*-based" [16]. There is a belief that the sativa-based products tend to be uplifting, energetic, and causing more cerebral effects whereas *indica*-based products are promoted as being more calming and grounding [16].

Unfortunately, there are significant issues with this classification system, such as the following [16]:

- The vast majority of current cannabis varieties available for purchase are hybrids of *indica* and *sativa* plants. The use of *indica* versus *sativa* is discouraged by many experts for medical cannabis use [7].
- There is no consistency in the naming convention of cannabis. A *Pink kush* from one producer can vary significantly in constituents from a product with the same name from another producer.
- There is no link between this labelling and classification and how it relates to the management of patients with specific symptoms.

Chemovar

When referring to a specific cannabis variety, the preferred term is chemovar [11]. This term is used as it refers to not only the cannabinoid components but also the other constituents in the product that contribute to the pharmacological effects of cannabis [11].

Practical Chemovar Selection for Clinicians

Currently, there is not strong evidence to support the selection of one specific chemovar for the management of patients with chronic pain. Some clinicians find chemovar selection challenging. It is important to remember that chemovar selection is guided based on primarily on expert opinion. Table 18.2 provides some key considerations to aid clinicians when selecting chemovars.

Table 18.2 Practical guidance when selecting chemovars

Guidance	Rationale
Consider dividing chemovars based on THC/CBD ratio	Cannabis is commonly divided into three categories based on cannabinoid content [17]: Type I – THC predominant which is high in THC and low in CBD Type II – Balanced which contains an approximately equal amount of THC and CBD Type III – CBD predominant which is low in THC and high in CBD This simple categorization is commonly used to narrow down thousands of potential products into several chemovars that can be considered for a specific patient
There is no perfect chemovar selection	There is limited data to support the use of a specific chemovar It is common to experience some trial and error to find the chemovar which reduces symptoms with a low incidence of adverse effects
There are interpatient differences	Although one chemovar may work very well for one patient, it can be ineffective or intolerable in another
CBD-predominant chemovars are better tolerated	In patients who are at an elevated risk of adverse effects, consider starting with a CBD-predominant chemovar as they tend to be better tolerated [11]
Poor response to one chemovar should not be viewed as a poor response to cannabis	It is common for a patient to not respond well to a specific chemovar but do well on another If the patient does not respond to or cannot tolerate a specific chemovar, consider selecting another chemovar before assessing response to cannabis
Select chemovars with a complete constituent profile	As more research is being conducted on the other constituents in cannabis, it will be important to know their concentration in cannabis chemovars An increasing number of producers are providing detailed lists of the concentrations of cannabinoids and terpenoids in their chemovars
Avoid recommending indica or sativa 'strains'	This terminology is not applicable for medical cannabis use as most products are hybrids and may not be reflective of the intended effects
Medical versus recreational chemovar selection	Recreational cannabis users tend to prefer cannabis chemovars high in THC, low in CBD, and high in the terpenoid myrcene For medical cannabis users, they frequently use CBD predominant chemovars with the smallest amount of THC to provide the greatest symptom control and the lowest risk of adverse effect [11]
Titrate appropriately regardless of the chemovar	Dosing and titration will be reviewed in a later chapter Fundamentally, dosing is highly patient-specific, and most patients are initiated on a low dose and increased slowly to the lowest dose required to reach the patient's treatment goal High dose initiation and rapid titration may decrease the tolerability of the product

Summary

Cannabis has been used medically for thousands of years. Although the taxonomy of the plant is a topic of debate, the use of chemovars aims to highlight the role of different constituents in the pharmacological effects of medical cannabis. Clinicians must remember that cannabis is a plant-based medicine. This can lead to differing levels of active compounds based on how the plant is grown and processed.

Currently, there are no absolute recommendations on which chemovar to use for a specific patient. As more research is published on the role of the different constituents, it will become increasingly a more precise chemovar selection process for a specific patient with a medical condition.

References

1. ElSohly M, Gul W. Constituents of Cannabis sativa. In: Handbook of cannabis. Oxford: Oxford University Press; 2014.
2. Pisanti S, Bifulco M. Medical Cannabis: a plurimillennial history of an evergreen. J Cell Physiol. 2019;234:8342–51.

3. Klumpers LE, Thacker DL. A brief background on cannabis: from plant to medical indications. J AOAC Int. 2019;102:412–20.
4. Bonini SA, Premoli M, Tambaro S, Kumar A, Maccarinelli G, Memo M, Mastinu A. Cannabis sativa: a comprehensive ethnopharmacological review of a medicinal plant with a long history. J Ethnopharmacol. 2018;227:300–15.
5. ElSohly MA, Radwan MM, Gul W, Chandra S, Galal A. Phytochemistry of Cannabis sativa L. In: Kinghorn AD, Falk H, Gibbons S, Kobayashi J, editors. Phytocannabinoids. Cham: Springer International Publishing; 2017. p. 1–36.
6. Potter DJ. Cannabis horticulture. In: Handbook of cannabis. 1st ed. Oxford, UK/New York: Oxford University Press; 2014. p. 65–88.
7. Piomelli D, Russo EB. The Cannabis sativa versus Cannabis indica debate: an interview with Ethan Russo, MD. Cannabis Cannabinoid Res. 2016;1: 44–6.
8. Potter DJ. A review of the cultivation and processing of cannabis (Cannabis sativa L.) for production of prescription medicines in the UK: cultivation and processing of cannabis for production of prescription medicines. Drug Test Anal. 2014;6:31–8.
9. Health Canada. Information for Health Care Professionals: cannabis (marihuana, marijuana) and the cannabinoids. In: AEM; 2018. https://www.canada.ca/en/health-canada/services/drugs-medication/cannabis/information-medical-practitioners/information-health-care-professionals-cannabis-cannabinoids.html. Accessed 20 June 2020.
10. National Academies of Sciences, Engineering, and Medicine, Health and Medicine Division, Board on Population Health and Public Health Practice, Committee on the Health Effects of Marijuana: An Evidence Review and Research Agenda. The health effects of cannabis and cannabinoids: the current state of evidence and recommendations for research. Washington, DC: National Academies Press; 2017.
11. MacCallum CA, Russo EB. Practical considerations in medical cannabis administration and dosing. Eur J Intern Med. 2018;49:12–9.
12. Russo EB. Taming THC: potential cannabis synergy and phytocannabinoid-terpenoid entourage effects. Br J Pharmacol. 2011;163:1344–64.
13. Booth JK, Bohlmann J. Terpenes in Cannabis sativa – from plant genome to humans. Plant Sci. 2019;284:67–72.
14. Russo EB, Marcu J. Cannabis pharmacology: the usual suspects and a few promising leads. In: Advances in pharmacology. 1st ed. Cambridge, MA: Elsevier; 2017. p. 67–134.
15. Russo EB. The case for the entourage effect and conventional breeding of clinical cannabis: no "strain," no gain. Front Plant Sci. 2019. https://doi.org/10.3389/fpls.2018.01969.
16. Hazekamp A, Tejkalová K, Papadimitriou S. Cannabis: from cultivar to chemovar II—a metabolomics approach to Cannabis classification. Cannabis Cannabinoid Res. 2016;1:202–15.
17. Lewis M, Russo E, Smith K. Pharmacological foundations of cannabis chemovars. Planta Med. 2018;84:225–33.

19 The Model of a Medical Cannabis Clinic

Maria Fernanda Arboleda and Erin Prosk

Introduction

Despite its long and complex history, the most common medical reasons for cannabinoid use have remained consistent. Most patients are using medical cannabis for mental health conditions such as anxiety, depression, or post-traumatic stress disorder (PTSD), chronic pain management, and sleep improvement [1]. Due to persistent social stigma and patients' fear to discuss current cannabis use with their physician, most are not receiving any professional guidance or supervision [2].

Additional barriers may contribute to access challenges to cannabinoid treatments such as limited medical education, variable regulatory restrictions, and lack of high-quality evidence to support its clinical safety and efficacy [3].

Although cannabis has been legally approved for medical purposes in various countries, patients are still accessing to illicit medical cannabis products [4, 5]. Unfortunately, many patients are taking cannabis products without any knowledge of dosage, actual indications, specific contraindications, potential drug-drug interactions, risks of some methods of administration, and possible side effects. The vast majority are not familiar with the importance of consuming only standardized and compliant cannabis-based treatments versus illicit cannabis products [6]. Consequently, establishment of supportive educational programs for patients [7] is also key to promote a responsible use of cannabinoids for medical purposes.

The ongoing development and expansion of recognized medical cannabis clinics have been significant throughout the last decade in most countries where cannabis for medical purposes has been approved. In many cases, the emergence of medical cannabis clinics followed the development of compassion clubs or medical cannabis dispensaries throughout the 1990s and 2000s in North America. The focus on clinical support led to care models utilizing multidisciplinary teams to provide medical assessment and professional advice regarding medical cannabis use. Medical cannabis advocates or education specialists may support integration of cannabis and clinical knowledge within the care model. The support of cannabis educators may be important for knowledge transfer to healthcare professionals within a medical cannabis clinic and to bridge care and education to patients who are already using illicit or unregulated cannabis and seek to transition to cannabis-based medicines. Furthermore, within the multidisciplinary approach, standardized protocols, and implementation of effective models, ongoing development and expansion of care are necessary to deliver consistent service and education, to ensure best practice care and positively impact health-related quality of life [8].

M. F. Arboleda (✉) · E. Prosk
Research Department, Santé Cannabis Clinic, Montreal, QC, Canada
e-mail: mfarboleda@santecannabis.ca

S. N. Narouze (ed.), *Cannabinoids and Pain*, https://doi.org/10.1007/978-3-030-69186-8_19

Notably, a medical cannabis clinic should focus on patient-centered interventions [9] and prescription of individualized cannabinoid-based treatments based on available clinical evidence [10]. The clinic model must make clear distinction between medical and non-medical use of cannabis, and personnel should avoid recommendations for the use of cannabis for non-medical or recreational purposes.

The aim of this chapter is to describe a sustainable, adaptive way to deliver healthcare services to patients that might be candidates for cannabinoid therapy. While initially the establishment of the best model of care is a critical focus, the implementation of continuing medical education and clinical research development should also be relevant and a high priority. In order to support the recommendations and enrich the discussion, we share the experience from a leading medical cannabis clinic, Santé Cannabis, located in Québec, Canada. Santé Cannabis has operated four clinical sites since 2014 and has assessed more than 8000 patients for cannabinoid-based treatments.

Description of a Medical Cannabis Clinic

As occurs in other ambulatory clinics such as chronic pain clinics, the creation of a comprehensive and multidisciplinary team [11] is crucial for optimal patients' care [12]. When establishing the clinic model, it is essential to determine the clinic objectives and assess available resources, whether the clinic will serve institutional or community needs. These objectives should inform clinic protocols in accordance with the goals and in consideration of regulatory framework, needs of the medical community, and resource limitations, including trained healthcare professionals and support personnel.

For a dedicated medical cannabis clinic, integration with the healthcare community will be an initial challenge. Importantly, cannabinoid-based treatments must always be considered as an adjunct to conventional therapies so communication with a patient's healthcare team is always necessary.

During the development of Santé Cannabis in 2014, the medical cannabis regulations were evolving to introduce regulated commercial production; however, distribution was limited to direct mail order from producers rather than via pharmacies. This meant that medical cannabis patients would require significant education to support the initiation and titration of medical cannabis treatments. Additionally, conservative medical community and limited guidelines for physicians emphasized the need for peer support among medical cannabis prescribing physicians. Patient care and education were established as the key pillars for the model development.

The initial process involved in this model of care is presented in Fig. 19.1. Importantly, patients were established and remain at the center of the model. With a diverse group of physicians, all practicing part-time, this model relies on the core team of trained, expert registered nurses. Standards of care must be adapted to each particular healthcare system, medical cannabis regulations, and country-specific community challenges [13].

The model of this community-based clinic has rapidly evolved to offer diverse services such as:

1. *Medical cannabis clinic* with a referral model for institutional and community-based physicians and nurse practitioners. After screening, eligible patients receive assessment, prescription and treatment initiation, and follow-up until stable. Once patients are stable, they may be transferred back to the referring physician to continue the medical cannabis treatment.

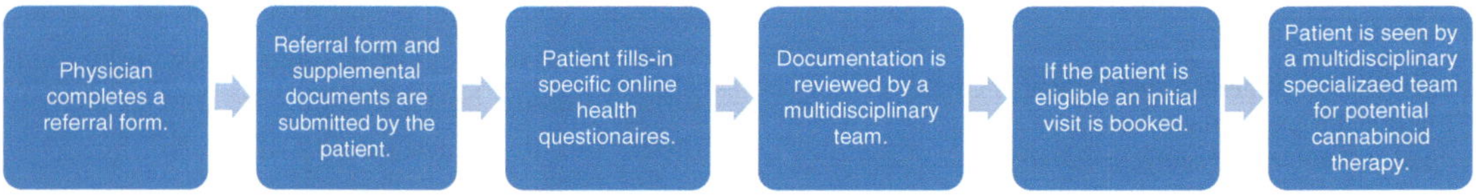

Fig. 19.1 Initial process at a medical cannabis clinic

2. *Training and resource center* for healthcare practitioners; Santé Cannabis shares its treatment protocols, procedures, and guidelines with interested physicians. A continuing medical education series of webinars, CMEs, and preceptorships is available. Support services are available for medical cannabis patients and their families.
3. *Contract research organization* offering a full suite of research services to public and private partners. Unique patient database may be accessed for the development of randomized-controlled trials with cannabis industry partners.

Referral and Screening

Generally, there are two ways in which a patient may access a medical cannabis clinic:

1. *Referral initiated by a physician*

   A referral for medical cannabis consultation may be received internally at a large clinical center, hospital, or other institution or from other external physicians in a community-based setting. Referral is often necessary as many physicians are not prepared to assess patients for medical cannabis, for reasons of limited medical education, lack of resources, or an organizational policy. The referral may have been generated by the patient request, but to be considered valid must be authorized by a licensed physician or other authorized healthcare professional.
2. *Direct access or self-referral*

   A medical cannabis clinic may consider admitting patients who are unable to receive a referral from a treating physician. In the early days of a medical cannabis clinic establishment, or a new regulatory framework, direct access may be necessary to support patient needs. It is also common that patients do not have access to a family or primary care physician at all.

   Medical cannabis clinics must consider their own resource limitations, liability, and credibility when considering whether to accept self-referral patients. In all cases, it is recommended to encourage patient referral if possible, to support integration of medical cannabis treatments with primary care. In the event that a referral is not possible, a patient may still consent to communication with their primary care physicians and healthcare providers such that information about the medical cannabis treatment may be communicated.

   In both cases, the referral form must be attached to supporting documents such as a summary of the medical record, list of current and previous medications, relevant laboratory test results, and diagnostic and imagery reports.

A referral form may follow a standard consultation request template but ideally should at least include the following information:

- Patient's personal information (name, date of birth, contact information)
- Primary diagnosis
- Secondary diagnoses
- Medical summary
- Previous and current pharmacological treatments
- Healthcare professional contact information

And detail about the specific relative contraindications for cannabinoids:

- Cardiovascular status
- History of substance use
- Mental health, especially personal or family history of schizophrenia, bipolar disorder, or psychotic episodes

Once the patient's referral and documentation are received, a screening review for eligibility should be completed prior to booking an initial visit. If possible, the review should be completed or at least verified by a healthcare professional such as a trained nurse.

Some of the main aspects to be considered during screening are the following:

- The patient has a chronic condition for which clinical evidence has shown a potential benefit for cannabinoid-based treatment:
  - Neurological disorders (i.e., multiple sclerosis, drug-resistant epilepsy, Parkinson's disease)
  - Chronic pain (of various etiologies)
  - Mental health illness (i.e., social anxiety disorder, PTSD)
  - Symptoms associated to cancer and its treatments (i.e., chemotherapy-induced nausea and vomiting, cancer pain, anorexia, etc.)
- Previous trial of conventional pharmacological treatments has failed to relieve symptoms.
- Patient is not pregnant, breastfeeding, or planning to become pregnant.
- Patient age and risk-benefit of cannabinoid-based treatments considering the severity of symptoms and the patient's trial of conventional pharmacological treatments.
- No uncontrolled or unstable cardiovascular disease.
- No history of substance use disorder or cannabis use disorder.
- No personal history of psychosis, unstable schizophrenia, and bipolar disorder.

If any complication or missing information is identified, the patient file may be considered a screening failure. The referring physician or other physician or specialist may be required to provide further information in order to complete the screening. Patients should be made aware of the status of their file during the review process.

If the patient fulfills this screening criteria, allocation to a specific physician should follow according to the primary symptom or medical condition. Where possible, an interdisciplinary team of pain specialist, neurologist, psychiatrist, and palliative care specialist is ideal to support the vast majority of patient needs.

Initial Visit

The role of clinic support staff is critical to explain clinic policies and set reasonable expectations with admitted patients. Patients should be advised that coming for an initial visit does not mean that they will certainly be prescribed with cannabinoid-based treatments. They might not be candidates for this specific therapy. At the initial visit, further discussion with the healthcare provider will determine final treatment decisions.

Finally, in most countries more than 90% of patients do not have insurance coverage for their medical cannabis treatment. Generally, patients spend approximately $85 USD per month [5]. Costs could be an important barrier to access cannabinoid therapy [14]. Having this conversation with patients and/or family is also necessary.

At initial visit, patients should complete specific health questionnaires or validated scales related to their main symptom [15]. Other measurement tools to support assessment of other symptoms and for health-related quality of life assessment are also suggested such as the revised Edmonton Symptom Assessment System (ESAS-r) and the EQ-5D tool [16, 17]. In order to assist this process, support staff may orient patients and answer any questions that they might have.

Where possible, the assessment may be initiated by a registered nurse in order to improve clinic efficiency and continuity of care for patients. The nurse completes a standardized evaluation to confirm all information from the referral process and reviews the baseline measurement tools in detail as well as clinical data such as vital signs, weight, etc.

This detailed medical history and customized information about medical cannabis risk factors are essential to confirm eligibility and to design the appropriate treatment plan. Selection of specific chemovar such as THC-predominant, THC-CBD balanced or CBD-predominant products, as well as presence of other cannabinoids and certain terpenes will always require a complete clinical assessment. [18, 19].

Finally, the patient will be seen by the physician specialist. Certain cases must be discussed between the multidisciplinary team of the registered nurse and physician before deciding if the patient is a candidate for cannabinoid therapy.

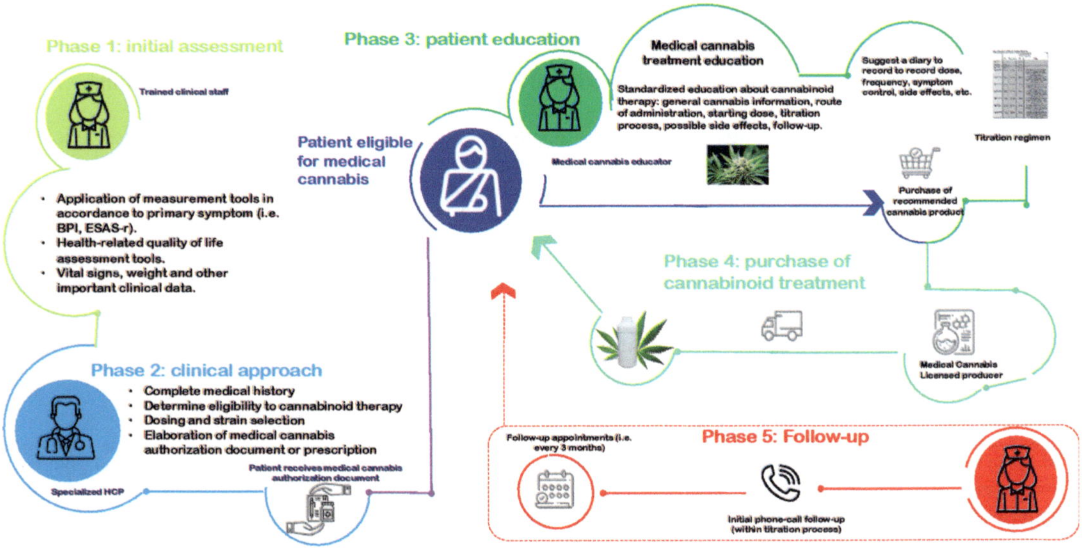

Fig. 19.2 Phases for medical cannabis treatment and safe access

This conversation will also help to establish appropriate chemovar selection, starting dose, and titration regimen [20].

If incorporation of cannabinoid treatment is considered, complete medical cannabis education is provided to patient and/or family (caregivers). Professional guidance for safe access to standardized cannabinoid-based products should be carefully delivered. Patients will then purchase the recommended medical cannabis treatment and initiate treatment.

Follow-Up and Monitoring

Throughout the titration process, a close monitoring and supervision by clinical staff are critical. Close monitoring of medical cannabis treatments improves adherence and could identify the emergence of possible adverse effects. If possible, monthly phone follow-up is highly recommended until a stable dose is met. Vulnerable patients may benefit from an in-person follow-up visit at 4–6 weeks post treatment initiation. Generally, follow-up at 3-month intervals is recommended until treatment is stable. If required, refer patients back to the treatment agreement to confirm their commitment agreed upon program [21].

Figure 19.2 illustrates a proposed patient-centered pathway for clinical assessment, medical cannabis prescription, and follow-up.

Patient Education and Physician Communication

Standardized patient education is essential to offer reliable medical cannabis information, manage patient's expectations, clarify frequent misconceptions, and review treatment objectives.

A medical cannabis educator may be a trained nurse or in some cases clinic support staff. Table 19.1 includes the main subjects to be discussed with the patient and/or family. Elaboration and delivery of educational material, handouts, and patient leaflets are highly recommended.

To ensure best ongoing care, a referral report of communication letter should be sent to the referring physician or healthcare professional within 1–2 days of treatment initiation. The communication should indicate the recommended treatment and follow-up frequency for the medical cannabis treatment as well as specific recommendations such as monitoring of potential risk

Table 19.1 Medical cannabis patient education

Main subject	Description
Medical cannabis general information	• Medical cannabis is not an approved medical treatment and is therefore not a first-line treatment • As a complementary or adjunct treatment, patient should not stop concomitant medications • Medical cannabis is a personalized treatment and response is individual • Difference between medical and non-medical cannabis use • General and basic concepts about the cannabis plant and its main components • THC versus CBD general characteristics
Treatment objectives	• Specify primary and secondary symptoms for medical cannabis treatment • Reduction of pharmaceutical medications with physician support may be possible once cannabinoid-based treatments are stable • Review and manage treatment expectations • Ensure the importance of ongoing communication and follow-up is understood • Highlight treatment agreement and patient's commitment to follow treatment plan • Eliminate the use of illicit products (whenever applicable)
Cannabinoid-based treatment administration	• Explain the recommended route of administration (i.e., oral, inhaled, combined) and give specific and detailed instructions • Starting dose and titration regimen instructions • Importance of treatment adherence and compliance • Use of a journal to record complete treatment information
Potential side effects	• Always mention possible side effects related to THC and/or CBD • Explain that most side effects can often be avoided with patient, careful titration, and close follow-up • Offer a strategy to stay in close contact with patient and family to report any adverse effects and to answer any questions related to their treatment
Support access to safe cannabinoid products	• Recommend safe and consistent products with certified laboratory testing • Encourage purchase of cannabinoid products from licensed providers only
Warnings and precautions	• Risk of impairment, especially with THC products • Patient to be aware of legal requirements, travel restrictions, and any home- or work-based limitations • Patient to ensure products are stored securely and discretely • Caution against concomitant use of alcohol or other recreational drugs

factors, potential adverse effects, or down-titration of pharmaceutical medication.

Protocols and Procedure Guidelines

One of the key projects for the establishment of a medical cannabis clinic is the development of guidelines and protocols. The development, training and implementation, and ongoing improvement of clinic protocols are crucial to assure best practice of care.

First, the profile, role, and responsibly of each clinic team member should be determined in accordance to the proposed clinic model. Administrative support staff complement the clinic team to ensure efficiency and continuous care. Roles of the clinical care team must consider the specific regulations and healthcare training of each member. Registered nurses, physicians, and medical cannabis educators must all receive effective training on clinic protocols, related not only to cannabinoid therapy but also to the specific model of care.

Protocols and procedure guidelines should be aligned with the mission of the clinic. Generally, a medical cannabis clinic should strive to be a center of excellence that provides best clinical practice for medical cannabis treatments.

Detailed protocols must be developed and could be adapted to different clinical environments mainly for:

- Clinical indications for medical cannabis treatments based on available evidence and the expertise of the physician team

- Proper screening for cannabinoid contraindications and precautions
- Collection of clinical data, patient sociodemographic information, complete medical history, and validated symptom measures
- Identification of problematic cannabis use
- Standardized treatment plan development
  - Method of administration and chemovar selection according to primary and secondary treatment objectives
  - Starting dose and titration regimen according to patient's medical condition and health status
  - Follow-up and monitoring schedule
- Patient treatment agreement, including expectations for compliance, warnings, and precautions
- Standards of medical cannabis patient education, including prepared documentation to provide to patients, caregivers, and family
- Processes for ongoing communication with patients, family, and referral physicians
- Methods for the clinic to maintain compliance with regulatory requirements, such as documentation templates and a process to review regulation changes regularly

Continuing Medical Education

Among the greatest challenges to the understanding and recommendation of cannabinoid-based treatments is the limited access to medical cannabis education [22, 23]. Medical cannabis education of healthcare professionals through medical cannabis clinics has emerged upon development with recognized academic institutions. Such partnerships between medical cannabis clinics and academic centers facilitate changes in medical training which are generally long-term multi-year projects. Initially, programs may be developed via elective opportunities for medical trainees that enhance the knowledge level and understanding of practical considerations for cannabinoid prescription upon graduation.

The development of complementary, continuing medical education programs for visiting physicians, residents, nurses, and pharmacists provides outstanding opportunities to acquire practical skills on cannabinoid prescription. Beyond the theoretical and pharmacological education, practical training programs have been developed by Santé Cannabis including physician and healthcare professional mentorship and preceptorships to observe clinical activity in action [24]. Such methods allow physicians to become more confident about recommending and prescribing cannabinoid-based treatments for specific conditions. Nurse and pharmacist education is also critical to provide complementary education and support to medical cannabis patients [25].

Provision of educational resources to medical professionals may also serve as supplemental funding opportunity for medical cannabis clinics. Moreover, community-based education and support services for medical cannabis patients should be encouraged at every opportunity.

Finally, as more countries adopt medical cannabis regulations, the creation of international training programs and preceptorships is also possible through medical cannabis centers. This certainly contributes to improve patient access and education to highly trained physician leaders worldwide.

Research Development

As part of the clinical experience at a medical cannabis clinic, accurate data collection requires specific commitment and resource allocation under precise protocols and data monitoring requirements. Initially, this allows the development of real-world evidence via prospective observational studies, registries, and patient surveys. Real-world evidence has gained significant attention as a complement to medical cannabis randomized controlled trials (RCTs). Real-world data may be more reflective of actual clinical practice and offers valuable insights on adverse effects and therapeutic benefits of medical cannabis.

As RCTs to assess safety and efficacy of medical cannabis treatments continue to develop slowly, observational studies and real-world evidence that emerge from medical cannabis clinics may complement findings and bridge gaps to clinical practice and social realities. However, real-world evidence does not substitute evidence of RCTs on safety and efficacy of cannabinoid-based treatments [26].

A medical cannabis clinic might be a suitable site for the completion of well-designed clinical trials. Development of clinical trials might open an opportunity to strengthen the clinical revenue model via partnerships with pharmaceutical companies and industry leaders to support the development of new cannabis-based therapeutic drugs. This requires a team of experts, research staff, good clinical practice training and certification, and authorization from regulatory bodies. After several years of real-world evidence collection and subsequent protocol improvements, Santé Cannabis began developing services as a cannabis-focused contract research organization in 2018, now offering CRO services to several sponsors.

Conclusion

The establishment of a medical cannabis clinic first requires a detailed assessment of the regulatory system for medical cannabis products and the needs of the medical and patient communities. Once understood, the clinic model should be built upon specific protocols and guidelines to ensure standards of care. A multidisciplinary team is always required to provide patient-centered interventions aligned with medical cannabis treatment objectives. Patient education must be a key pillar of the clinic model and may evolve over time as the needs of patients change. There is a significant need and, therefore, an opportunity to develop medical cannabis education programs for healthcare professionals. Such programs provide key leadership to the medical community and support the validation of clinical practice guidelines, including elements for safe and responsible cannabinoid prescription. Research development has been hindered by limited resources and regulatory restrictions. However, clinical experience and observational studies have opened up many possibilities to advance in the deployment of RCTs. Medical cannabis clinics might operate as training and resource centers for the establishment of clinical practice guidelines and as research centers to support collection of real-world evidence and the development of investigational cannabinoid-based drugs. Established medical cannabis clinics such as Santé Cannabis in Quebec, Canada, offer invaluable knowledge transfer and can serve as a model for development and adaptation of focused medical cannabis practices and clinics across many international countries.

References

1. Azcarate PM, Zhang AJ, Keyhani S, Steigerwald S, Ishida JH, Cohen BE. Medical reasons for marijuana use, forms of use, and patient perception of physician attitudes among the US population. J Gen Intern Med. 2020;35:1979–86.
2. Lintzeris N, Mills L, Suraev A, Bravo M, Arkell T, Arnold JC, et al. Medical cannabis use in the Australian community following introduction of legal access: the 2018-2019 Online Cross-Sectional Cannabis as Medicine Survey (CAMS-18). Harm Reduct J. 2020;17(1):37.
3. Glickman A, Sisti D. Prescribing medical cannabis: ethical considerations for primary care providers. J Med Ethics. 2020;46(4):227–30.
4. Arboleda MF, Prosk E, Cyr C, Gamaoun R, Vigano A. Medical cannabis in supportive cancer care: lessons from Canada. Support Care Cancer. 2020;28:2999–3001.
5. Health Canada. Canadian cannabis survey 2019 – summary. 2019. Available from: https://www.canada.ca/en/health-canada/services/publications/drugs-health-products/canadian-cannabis-survey-2019-summary.html.
6. Wheeler M, Merten JW, Gordon BT, Hamadi H. CBD (cannabidiol) product attitudes, knowledge, and use among young adults. Subst Use Misuse. 2020;55(7):1138–45.
7. Joypaul S, Kelly F, McMillan SS, King MA. Multidisciplinary interventions for chronic pain involving education: a systematic review. PLoS One. 2019;14(10):e0223306.
8. Davy C, Bleasel J, Liu H, Tchan M, Ponniah S, Brown A. Effectiveness of chronic care models: opportunities for improving healthcare practice and health outcomes: a systematic review. BMC Health Serv Res. 2015;15:194.

9. Scholl I, Zill JM, Härter M, Dirmaier J. An integrative model of patient-centeredness - a systematic review and concept analysis. PLoS One. 2014;9(9):e107828.
10. Abrams DI. The therapeutic effects of cannabis and cannabinoids: an update from the National Academies of Sciences, Engineering and Medicine report. Eur J Intern Med. 2018;49:7–11.
11. Mahrer NE, Gold JI, Luu M, Herman PM. A cost-analysis of an interdisciplinary pediatric chronic pain clinic. J Pain. 2018;19(2):158–65.
12. Joypaul S, Kelly FS, King MA. Turning pain into gain: evaluation of a multidisciplinary chronic pain management program in primary care. Pain Med Malden Mass. 2019;20(5):925–33.
13. Reynolds HW, Sutherland EG. A systematic approach to the planning, implementation, monitoring, and evaluation of integrated health services. BMC Health Serv Res. 2013;13:168.
14. Zylla D, Steele G, Eklund J, Mettner J, Arneson T. Oncology clinicians and the Minnesota Medical Cannabis Program: a survey on medical cannabis practice patterns, barriers to enrollment, and educational needs. Cannabis Cannabinoid Res. 2018;3(1):195–202.
15. Atkinson TM, Rosenfeld BD, Sit L, Mendoza TR, Fruscione M, Lavene D, et al. Using confirmatory factor analysis to evaluate construct validity of the Brief Pain Inventory (BPI). J Pain Symptom Manag. 2011;41(3):558–65.
16. Hui D, Bruera E. The Edmonton symptom assessment system 25 years later: past, present, and future developments. J Pain Symptom Manag. 2017;53(3):630–43.
17. Matter-Walstra K, Klingbiel D, Szucs T, Pestalozzi BC, Schwenkglenks M. Using the EuroQol EQ-5D in Swiss cancer patients, which value set should be applied? PharmacoEconomics. 2014;32(6):591–9.
18. Russo EB. Taming THC: potential cannabis synergy and phytocannabinoid-terpenoid entourage effects. Br J Pharmacol. 2011;163(7):1344–64.
19. Russo EB. Beyond cannabis: plants and the endocannabinoid system. Trends Pharmacol Sci. 2016;37(7):594–605.
20. MacCallum CA, Russo EB. Practical considerations in medical cannabis administration and dosing. Eur J Intern Med. 2018;49:12–9.
21. Wilsey B, Atkinson JH, Marcotte TD, Grant I. The medicinal cannabis treatment agreement: providing information to chronic pain patients through a written document. Clin J Pain. 2015;31(12):1087–96.
22. St Pierre M, Matthews L, Walsh Z. Cannabis education needs assessment among Canadian physicians-in-training. Complement Ther Med. 2020;49:102328.
23. Ware MA, Ziemianski D. Medical education on cannabis and cannabinoids: perspectives, challenges, and opportunities. Clin Pharmacol Ther. 2015;97(6):548–50.
24. Prescriber Training Program | Santé Cannabis. Available from: https://www.santecannabis.ca/en/physicians/to-prescribe-medical-cannabis/.
25. Clark CS. Medical cannabis: the oncology nurse's role in patient education about the effects of marijuana on cancer palliation. Clin J Oncol Nurs. 2018;22(1):E1–6.
26. Graham M, Lucas CJ, Schneider J, Martin JH, Hall W. Translational hurdles with cannabis medicines. Pharmacoepidemiol Drug Saf. 2020;29:1325–30.

Barriers for the Prescription of Cannabinoid-Based Medicines

20

Maria Fernanda Arboleda and Erin Prosk

Introduction

The clinical use of cannabinoid-based medicines as a complement for the treatment of different medical conditions, including chronic pain, is becoming more frequent worldwide. More than 70% of patients report seeking professional advice regarding potential therapeutic benefits of medical cannabis [1]. However, several challenges and limitations have been encountered which prevent healthcare professionals from providing informed recommendations concerning the use of cannabinoid therapy [2]. A recent survey showed that more than 80% of healthcare practitioners are not sufficiently prepared and knowledgeable about medical cannabis. Thus, more than 50% do not feel comfortable discussing about this possible treatment with their patients [3].

While these challenges remain, many developments are underway to find appropriate solutions and to meet the needs of patients. The aim of this chapter is to review the main barriers for the safe and responsible prescription of medical cannabis and to present an overview of strategies to meet or mitigate the present challenges.

M. F. Arboleda (✉) · E. Prosk
Research Department, Santé Cannabis Clinic, Montreal, QC, Canada
e-mail: mfarboleda@santecannabis.ca

Barriers for Cannabinoid Prescription

The growing patient's interest in the potential benefits of cannabinoid-based medicines is often at odds with the concerns among physicians and other healthcare professionals [4]. Diverse barriers have been identified for the prescription of cannabinoid-based treatments, and these are summarized in Fig. 20.1. The most significant hurdles are discussed in more details below.

Social Stigma for the Use of Cannabis

Most people have grown up in an era where cannabis has been prohibited. Previously, the use of cannabis as a medical tool has been recorded as early as 2700 B.C. [5]. It was used by Chinese physicians to treat malaria, constipation, and rheumatic pains and as an analgesic in childbirth, among others. During the nineteenth century, cannabis was introduced to Western medicine by Dr. O'Shaughnessy and was widely used and accepted by recognized European physicians for its anticonvulsant, anti-inflammatory, and analgesic effects [6]. In fact, cannabis was classified as a legitimate medical compound by the United States Pharmacopeia in 1851. Unfortunately, with rising concerns over its psychotropic effects, association with various crimes, and political interests, it was removed during the 1940s from this list. Furthermore, cannabis was prohibited in

S. N. Narouze (ed.), *Cannabinoids and Pain*, https://doi.org/10.1007/978-3-030-69186-8_20

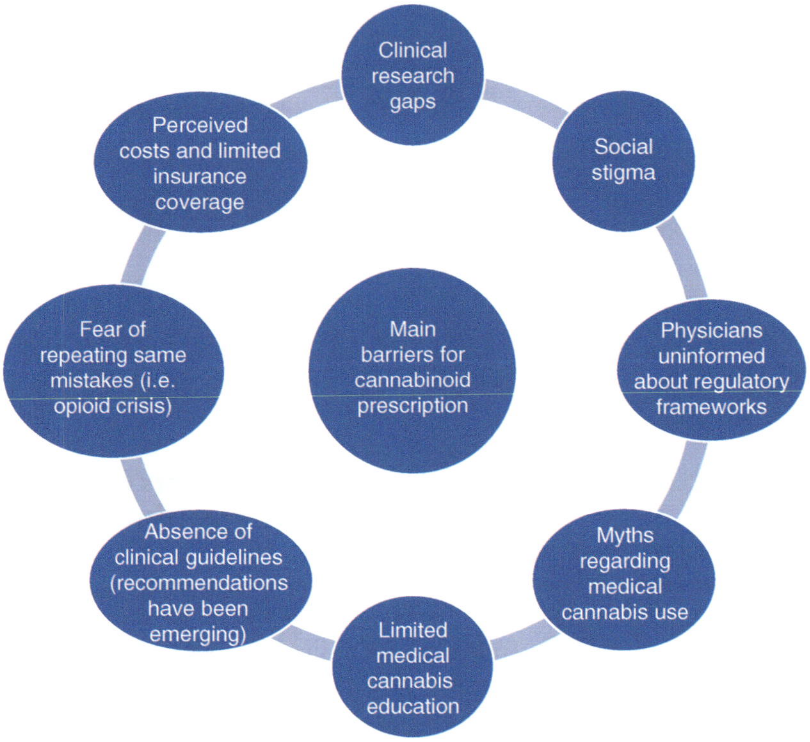
Clinical research gaps
Social stigma
Physicians uninformed about regulatory frameworks
Myths regarding medical cannabis use
Limited medical cannabis education
Absence of clinical guidelines (recommendations have been emerging)
Fear of repeating same mistakes (i.e. opioid crisis)
Perceived costs and limited insurance coverage
Main barriers for cannabinoid prescription

Fig. 20.1 Main barriers for medical cannabis prescription

the United States upon enactment of the Marihuana Tax Act in 1937 and is still classified federally as a Schedule 1 drug with a high potential of abuse under the Controlled Substances Act since 1970 [6, 7]. However, recent years have started to see some evolution, via various amendments since 1990, which allowed states to enact their own medical cannabis and cannabis laws and prohibit the Justice Department from interfering. The federal 2018 Farm Bill legalized the production of low-THC cannabis or *hemp* cultivars, coinciding with the FDA approval and effective de-scheduling of Epidiolex in the same year. Similar evolution of cannabis policy has progressed across the globe for the last 20 years, resulting in a patchwork of medical cannabis legalization and access in various countries.

Consequently, the prohibition of cannabis, or *marijuana*, and the lack of differentiation between medical and nonmedical uses of cannabis have encouraged the development of prejudice, myths, and social stigma. Such stigma persists among both healthcare professionals and patients despite the approval of several pharmaceutical cannabinoids and the improved characterization of the effects of cannabis in general. Patients may be uncomfortable or even afraid to try cannabinoid-based treatments and may be concerned about perception of their family and peers and may perceive a risk of psychoactive effects or addiction. For this reason, it is crucial to make a clear distinction between medical and recreational uses of cannabis. This exercise may elucidate the therapeutic objectives of incorporating cannabinoid-based medicines as an adjunct to chronic pain management.

Myths Versus Realities of Medical Cannabis Use

As medical use of cannabis has been reintroduced in several states and countries for specific clinical conditions, it is key to address misconceptions related to social stigma, lack of reliable information, and now commercial influence in the information age. Patient education or reeducation will support treatment adherence and allow for better acceptance and perception of medical cannabis among the general population. Table 20.1 summarizes the most frequent myths versus realities regarding the use of medical cannabis.

Research Gaps and Limitations to Justify Medical Cannabis Use

Over the last 40, years there has been emerging interest among researchers to investigate various properties of cannabis and cannabinoids. The

Table 20.1 Frequent myths versus reality of medical cannabis use

Myth	Reality
Smoking is the only way to administer medical cannabis	Drawing from historic use of cannabis, and inaccurately, cannabis has been administered as teas, tinctures, and butter or *bhang* in India since 1000 B.C. and in other Eastern cultures. In modern times, there are various routes of administration available for medical cannabis products such as oral (i.e., extracts), inhaled (i.e., vaporization), topical, etc. with specific pharmacokinetic characteristics that offer a diversity of treatment options for symptom control and patient accessibility [8]. The use of a particular method of administration will depend on the treatment objective. Due to its rapid onset, inhalation is recommended to control acute symptoms (i.e., breakthrough pain) [9]. The use of reliable and safe delivery system such as a vaporizer is highly recommended [10, 11]. For long-acting effects, consider oral route of administration [9, 12].
THC is for recreational use, whereas CBD is medicinal	A long-held stigma dating back to the origin of cannabis prohibition assumes that because THC is primarily responsible for the psychoactive effects of cannabis, it cannot be therapeutic. Conversely, THC has demonstrated potential therapeutic benefit for several indications. Clinically, many patients do not report psychoactivity or a feeling of "being high," indicating a potential pharmacological difference between medical and recreational users. For those patients who do experience negative psychoactive effects, dose titration and other strategies may be effective to mitigate effects.
Cannabis can cure cancer and/or other medical conditions ("the miracle drug")	A myth that is common among cancer patients or patients who may have sought information online where the effects and potential benefits of medical cannabis have been falsely and sometimes grossly overstated. No clinical evidence to support its use as a curative therapy in cancer patients or in other medical conditions [13]. However, cannabinoid-based treatments have shown benefit for cancer-related symptoms and may be considered as an adjunct clinical tool for symptom control. Cannabinoid therapy is not a first-line treatment, and while occasionally dose reduction of concomitant treatments is possible, it is unlikely to replace other medications. Healthcare professionals must be prepared to communicate accurate information, sometimes reeducating from misinformation found online, to patients, caregivers, and community in order to define realistic expectations [14].
Medical cannabis is natural and therefore must not produce any adverse effects or is inherently safer than pharmaceutical or "unnatural" products	The safety profile of THC and CBD has been characterized in several studies, and the expected adverse effects are well-documented for pharmaceutical cannabinoids [15]. Less is documented about the safety profile of cannabis; however, the risk of lethal overdose is almost negligible, with no known occurrence. Nevertheless, the risk of adverse effects still exists, and overdose may contribute to the severity of such effects. Cognitive, psychiatric, and cardiovascular such as tachycardia or hypotension adverse effects are mostly related to THC and its main active metabolite 11-OH-THC. Both THC and CBD may also produce adverse effects such as dry mouth, dizziness, somnolence, and fatigue. These effects are dose dependent and generally classified as mild to moderate. Slow titration of cannabinoid therapy is key to avoid severe adverse effects [12].
Any patient is eligible for cannabinoid therapy	Like any medication, cannabinoid-based treatment is not for everyone. There are specific indications and contraindications for cannabinoid prescription. A history of psychiatric illness such as schizophrenia or psychotic episodes and active, unstable cardiovascular illness such as unstable arrhythmia or uncontrolled hypertension are contraindications related primarily to THC [12]. A detailed and systematic medical history is required to decide who is a candidate for cannabinoid-based treatments [16].

(continued)

Table 20.1 (continued)

Myth	Reality
Medical cannabis will produce addiction	Previously termed cannabis dependence or cannabis abuse in *DSM-4* has been characterized in *DSM-5* as cannabis use disorder (CUD). Probability of becoming addicted to cannabis after lifetime exposure is 8.9% [17]. Lifetime probability of transition from cannabis use to CUD is around 27% [18]. Importantly, all this data comes from recreational use of cannabis, primarily of high-THC and unregulated products. Specific predictors for this risk of development of CUD include males, early-onset cannabis users, and childhood traumatic events. Cannabis withdrawal has been recognized in around 50% of heavy cannabis users upon cessation [19]. No clinical studies have yet been published related to the risk of development of CUD during medical cannabis use [20]. Undergoing CBD research for substance use disorder (i.e., opioid use disorder) is promising [21–23].

THC delta-9-tetrahydrocannabinol; *11-OH-THC* 11-hydroxy-tetrahydrocannabinol; *CBD* cannabidiol, *DSM-4* Diagnostic and Statistical Manual for Mental Disorders, fourth edition; *CUD* cannabis use disorder; *DSM-5* Diagnostic and Statistical Manual for Mental Disorders, fifth edition

characterization of the main components of the endocannabinoid system contributed significantly to this increase in interest [24]. Numerous systematic reviews and meta-analyses have supported the use of cannabinoid-based treatments in neuropathic pain and some other medical conditions [25, 26]. However, diverging conclusions and areas of debate have appeared as part of the discussion. Importantly, in several studies, the heterogeneity of study population, such as combination between different types of chronic pain, may have interfered with analysis and might have caused limitations to current evidence [27].

This lack of high-quality evidence for the use of medical cannabis in chronic pain patients is often out of step with observational studies, real-world evidence, and patient case reports that indicate significant potential benefit for cannabinoid-based treatments in chronic pain populations, including potential for opioid substitution [28]. To resolve these discrepancies, well-designed randomized controlled trials are required to validate efficacy and safety of medical cannabis. These study designs must consider population characteristics and adequate sample size calculation; must specify cannabinoid formulations and terpene profile, cannabinoid dosage, titration regimen, and route of administration, and must assess treatment changes and the use of concomitant medications in long-term follow-up. Perhaps most critically, investigators must dedicate attention to the classification of different types of pain within the study population. To bridge the gap between real-world evidence, evaluation of emotional, functional, and health-related quality-of-life impact and patient's satisfaction or perception of change is necessary. Finally, limitations related to placebo group blinding when delta-9-tetrahydrocannabinol (THC) is being used should be carefully addressed [29].

Lack of Knowledge Regarding Cannabis Regulatory Frameworks

With the existing and ever-evolving patchwork of cannabis legislation globally, it is understandably challenging to comprehend legal regulatory frameworks. By focusing on local status and regulatory requirements in local jurisdiction and on a developed understanding of available cannabinoid-based treatments, healthcare professionals play an important educational role [2].

In 2013, Uruguay was the first country to fully legalize cannabis, and in October of 2018, Canada became the largest country and the first G20 nation to legalize and regulate cannabis. Although the use of medical and recreational cannabis has not been federally legalized in the United States, several states have legalized its use. While still a Schedule 1 drug, the US Food and Drug Administration (FDA) has recognized the potential opportunities that cannabinoid-based therapies could offer [30]. So far, this regulatory agency has approved one purified, plant-derived cannabinoid-based treatment, a cannabidiol (CBD) oral solution for drug-resistant epilepsy [31, 32], and two synthetic cannabinoid formulations of THC and THC analogues, dronabinol and nabilone [15].

While more than 30 countries have now authorized the use of medical cannabis [33], access to cannabinoid-based treatments is still variable, and there remain barriers to access safe products with suitable quality control. Regardless of legal status, many patients are procuring "cannabis treatments" from illegal or unregulated sources and without appropriate clinical guidance and safe monitoring. Worryingly, some patients have been exposed to infectious risks associated with the administration of contaminated cannabis products [34, 35].

A robust regulatory framework, including consistent cannabis supply chain and complete testing for various pathogens, heavy metals, and contaminants, is essential. However, while regulations and the responsible healthcare agencies are still maturing in some jurisdictions, the application of the required quality standards may not be sufficiently regulated.

Finally, accurate testing of cannabinoid and terpene profile is essential to provide clinicians with the necessary information and confidence to give a medical cannabis prescription and accurate dosing. Unfortunately, when cannabis products are obtained from illegal or underregulated markets, the laboratory analyses are not reliable. Unsupported claims may be commonly found describing such illegal or underregulated products. In the United States, several manufacturers have been fined for claims that their THC and CBD products can treat and even cure some medical conditions, in violation of the Federal Food, Drug, and Cosmetic Act [30, 36].

Overall, regulatory frameworks and approval of cannabinoid-based treatments continue to evolve across many countries. Regulatory agencies in countries that have legalized medical cannabis continue to simplify access barriers and provide clear information under pressure from both patients and healthcare professionals.

Limited Medical Cannabis Education

Poor academic training is evident when healthcare practitioners are asked to rate their medical cannabis knowledge [3, 37]. Around 85% of health professionals would like more medical cannabis training and resources, mainly written summaries, and online learning programs [4].

Qualified educational curriculums in this field are scarce, and it is still uncommon to find recognized medical schools reviewing the endocannabinoid system, phytocannabinoids, terpenes, and their medical applications. Certified courses, symposiums, and prescribing training programs have emerged recently to bridge this important gap.

Development of Medical Cannabis Education Programs with High Scientific Content

Medical cannabis education should be designed to meet diverse learning objectives, including foundational, theoretical concepts and practical recommendations. As with the consideration of any new treatment option, responsible prescription in a collaborative, interdisciplinary setting should be encouraged. Some of the key elements to be considered in medical cannabis academic programs [38] are summarized in Table 20.2.

Table 20.2 Suggested content for medical cannabis continuing education programs

Level of knowledge	Content to be covered
Basic concepts	General aspects of the Cannabis plant
	Characteristics and components of the endocannabinoid system
	Pharmacology of phytocannabinoids, main differences between THC and CBD, terpene profile (potential therapeutic effects)
	Properties of pharmaceutical cannabinoids and natural cannabis products
	Routes of administration and pharmacokinetic differences
	Clinical evidence for the use of cannabinoids in various medical conditions, including results of systematic reviews and metanalyses
	Regulatory framework and legal access to medical cannabis according to specific jurisdictions
Advanced concepts	Critical aspects of patient's medical history to determine appropriateness of cannabinoid-based treatments: Indications and contraindications Precautions and warnings Screening for cannabis use disorder (CUD) Primary and secondary symptoms to be controlled History of cannabis use (recreational and medical)
	Considering potential drug-drug interactions
	Practical recommendations for the prescription of cannabinoid-based medicines as an adjunct to conventional treatments Design of the treatment plan: Chemovar selection Route of administration (i.e., inhaled, oral, combined) Initiation dose, titration regimen, frequency of administration Key components of effective patient education Follow-up, monitoring, and treatment changes: Monitoring adverse effects Treatment modification to improve efficacy and mitigate adverse effects
	Acute and long-term effects of cannabis use
	Clinical cases for a comprehensive review of the therapeutic use of medical cannabis (i.e., problem-based learning) in different settings
	Cannabinoid research development
	Development of clinical research program, including principles of controlled collection and analysis of real-world evidence

Conclusion

There remain many barriers to the understanding and possible acceptance of medical cannabis that affect healthcare professionals and patients across the globe. In the current context of limited training, reluctance and concern from healthcare professionals are valid but contrast with patient's interest. However, as clinical evidence and more reliable information of medical cannabis products develop, an increased patient awareness is expected, and healthcare professionals must also improve their knowledge and understanding of cannabinoid-based treatments. Medical cannabis regulation advancements have been crucial for improved access and the resulting societal understanding and acceptance of the therapeutic use of cannabis. There are still significant gaps in training opportunities and in high-quality clinical research that require commitment and cooperation between government, academic, and industry stakeholders.

References

1. Pergam SA, Woodfield MC, Lee CM, Cheng G-S, Baker KK, Marquis SR, et al. Cannabis use among patients at a comprehensive cancer center in a state

with legalized medicinal and recreational use. Cancer. 2017;123(22):4488–97.
2. Steele G, Arneson T, Zylla D. A comprehensive review of cannabis in patients with cancer: availability in the USA, general efficacy, and safety. Curr Oncol Rep. 2019;21(1):10.
3. Karanges EA, Suraev A, Elias N, Manocha R, McGregor IS. Knowledge and attitudes of Australian general practitioners towards medicinal cannabis: a cross-sectional survey. BMJ Open. 2018;8(7):e022101.
4. Zylla D, Steele G, Eklund J, Mettner J, Arneson T. Oncology clinicians and the Minnesota medical cannabis program: a survey on medical cannabis practice patterns, barriers to enrollment, and educational needs. Cannabis Cannabinoid Res. 2018;3(1):195–202.
5. Ko GD, Bober SL, Mindra S, Moreau JM. Medical cannabis — the Canadian perspective. J Pain Res. 2016;9:735–44.
6. Abrams DI, Guzman M. Cannabis in cancer care. Clin Pharmacol Ther. 2015;97(6):575–86.
7. Jensen B, Chen J, Furnish T, Wallace M. Medical marijuana and chronic pain: a review of basic science and clinical evidence. Curr Pain Headache Rep. 2015;19(10):50.
8. Borgelt LM, Franson KL, Nussbaum AM, Wang GS. The pharmacologic and clinical effects of medical cannabis. Pharmacotherapy. 2013;33(2):195–209.
9. Cyr C, Arboleda MF, Aggarwal SK, Balneaves LG, Daeninck P, Néron A, et al. Cannabis in palliative care: current challenges and practical recommendations. Ann Palliat Med. 2018;7(4):463–77.
10. Abrams DI, Vizoso HP, Shade SB, Jay C, Kelly ME, Benowitz NL. Vaporization as a smokeless cannabis delivery system: a pilot study. Clin Pharmacol Ther. 2007;82(5):572–8.
11. Tashkin DP. How beneficial is vaping cannabis to respiratory health compared to smoking? Addiction. 2015;110(11):1706–7.
12. MacCallum CA, Russo EB. Practical considerations in medical cannabis administration and dosing. Eur J Intern Med. 2018;49:12–9.
13. Abrams DI. Should oncologists recommend cannabis? Curr Treat Options in Oncol. 2019;20(7):59.
14. Shi S, Brant AR, Sabolch A, Pollom E. False news of a cannabis cancer cure. Cureus. 2019;11(1):e3918.
15. Schrot RJ, Hubbard JR. Cannabinoids: medical implications. Ann Med. 2016;48(3):128–41.
16. Arboleda MF, Prosk E, Cyr C, Gamaoun R, Vigano A. Medical cannabis in supportive cancer care: lessons from Canada. Support Care Cancer. 2020;28(7):2999–3001.
17. Lopez-Quintero C, Pérez de los Cobos J, Hasin DS, Okuda M, Wang S, Grant BF, et al. Probability and predictors of transition from first use to dependence on nicotine, alcohol, cannabis, and cocaine: results of the National Epidemiologic Survey on Alcohol and Related Conditions (NESARC). Drug Alcohol Depend. 2011;115(1–2):120–30.
18. Feingold D, Livne O, Rehm J, Lev-Ran S. Probability and correlates of transition from cannabis use to DSM-5 cannabis use disorder: results from a large-scale nationally representative study. Drug Alcohol Rev. 2020;39(2):142–51.
19. Budney AJ, Hughes JR, Moore BA, Vandrey R. Review of the validity and significance of cannabis withdrawal syndrome. Am J Psychiatry. 2004;161(11):1967–77.
20. Curran HV, Freeman TP, Mokrysz C, Lewis DA, Morgan CJA, Parsons LH. Keep off the grass? Cannabis, cognition and addiction. Nat Rev Neurosci. 2016;17(5):293–306.
21. Prud'homme M, Cata R, Jutras-Aswad D. Cannabidiol as an intervention for addictive behaviors: a systematic review of the evidence. Subst Abuse. 2015;9:33–8.
22. Hurd YL, Spriggs S, Alishayev J, Winkel G, Gurgov K, Kudrich C, et al. Cannabidiol for the reduction of cue-induced craving and anxiety in drug-abstinent individuals with heroin use disorder: a double-blind randomized placebo-controlled trial. Am J Psychiatry. 2019;176(11):911–22.
23. Chye Y, Christensen E, Solowij N, Yücel M. The endocannabinoid system and cannabidiol's promise for the treatment of substance use disorder. Front Psych. 2019;10:63.
24. Mechoulam R, Parker LA. The endocannabinoid system and the brain. Annu Rev Psychol. 2013;64:21–47.
25. National Academies of Sciences, Engineering, and Medicine, Health and Medicine Division, Board on Population Health and Public Health Practice, Committee on the Health Effects of Marijuana: An Evidence Review and Research Agenda. The health effects of cannabis and cannabinoids: the current state of evidence and recommendations for research. Washington (DC): National Academies Press (US); 2017. (The National Academies Collection: Reports funded by National Institutes of Health). Available from: http://www.ncbi.nlm.nih.gov/books/NBK423845/
26. Whiting PF, Wolff RF, Deshpande S, Di Nisio M, Duffy S, Hernandez AV, et al. Cannabinoids for medical use: a systematic review and meta-analysis. JAMA. 2015;313(24):2456–73.
27. Campbell G, Stockings E, Nielsen S. Understanding the evidence for medical cannabis and cannabis-based medicines for the treatment of chronic non-cancer pain. Eur Arch Psychiatry Clin Neurosci. 2019;269(1):135–44.
28. Ishida JH, Wong PO, Cohen BE, Vali M, Steigerwald S, Keyhani S. Substitution of marijuana for opioids in a national survey of US adults. PLoS One. 2019;14(10)
29. Wilsey B, Deutsch R, Marcotte TD. Maintenance of blinding in clinical trials and the implications for studying analgesia using cannabinoids. Cannabis Cannabinoid Res. 2016;1(1):139–48.
30. FDA Regulation of Cannabis and Cannabis-Derived Products, Including Cannabidiol (CBD). 2020.; Available from: https://www.fda.gov/news-events/

public-health-focus/fda-regulation-cannabis-and-cannabis-derived-products-including-cannabidiol-cbd
31. Thomas RH, Cunningham MO. Cannabis and epilepsy. Pract Neurol. 2018;18(6):465–71.
32. Yang YT, Szaflarski JP. The US Food and Drug Administration's authorization of the first cannabis-derived pharmaceutical: are we out of the haze? JAMA Neurol. 2019;76(2):135–6.
33. Maharajan MK, Yong YJ, Yip HY, Woon SS, Yeap KM, Yap KY, et al. Medical cannabis for chronic pain: can it make a difference in pain management? J Anesth. 2020;34(1):95–103.
34. Thompson GR, Tuscano JM, Dennis M, Singapuri A, Libertini S, Gaudino R, et al. A microbiome assessment of medical marijuana. Clin Microbiol Infect. 2017;23(4):269–70.
35. Stone T, Henkle J, Prakash V. Pulmonary mucormycosis associated with medical marijuana use. Respir Med Case Rep. 2019;26:176–9.
36. Rubin R. Cannabidiol products are everywhere, but should people be using them? JAMA. 2019;
37. Braun IM, Wright A, Peteet J, Meyer FL, Yuppa DP, Bolcic-Jankovic D, et al. Medical oncologists' beliefs, practices, and knowledge regarding marijuana used therapeutically: a nationally representative survey study. J Clin Oncol. 2018;36(19):1957–62. https://doi.org/10.1200/JCO.2017.76.1221.
38. Ware MA, Ziemianski D. Medical education on cannabis and cannabinoids: perspectives, challenges, and opportunities. Clin Pharmacol Ther. 2015;97(6):548–50.

Practical Recommendations for the Use of Medical Cannabis

21

Maria Fernanda Arboleda and Erin Prosk

Introduction

There has been a growing interest in the use of cannabinoid-based medicines among chronic pain patients worldwide [1–3]. While high-quality clinical research remains limited and regulatory frameworks slowly advance to approve the use of medical cannabis, healthcare providers of different specialties are now keen to acquire evidence-based information for best clinical practices. A significant difference between current and desired levels of medical cannabis knowledge among healthcare practitioners (HCPs) has limited the prescription of cannabinoid-based medicines and the provision of optimal medical guidance [4]. Worryingly, around 21% of patients are using cannabis therapeutically but without medical advice and safe monitoring [5], and more than 70% do so without legal authorization [6].

Existing clinical guidelines for cannabinoid use in chronic pain are scarce [7]. Currently, some literature supports the use of medical cannabis for neuropathic pain conditions as a third-line treatment [8]. However, such guidelines cite insufficient evidence to recommend medical cannabis for other types of chronic pain [9, 10]. To bridge the gap between recommendations and reality, some practical guidance for the safe and responsible prescription of medical cannabis have emerged [11–13]. Furthermore, some lessons learned have been shared from clinicians who practice in countries where cannabis has been fully legalized [14–15]. And finally, the use of cannabinoid-based medicines or medical cannabis has been proposed as an adjunct for several clinical settings [16].

While clinical evidence continues to evolve, there is a growing demand to implement medical cannabis training programs and educational resources to guide healthcare professionals in the often-unique prescription and regulatory process. As interest and access grows, experienced, multidisciplinary teams must be prepared to provide appropriate response to patient questions and to carefully identify patients who are potential candidates for cannabinoid-based medicines.

As a way to fulfill some current gaps, the aim of this chapter is to present a systematic approach to the prescription of cannabinoid-based medicines. Specific steps will guide HCPs to gain confidence and to be prepared to make informed recommendations. To accomplish this, best practices utilize common clinical tools and the collection of a detailed and focused medical history. Experience from a leading Canadian specialized medical cannabis clinic has been key to provide all these practical considerations.

M. F. Arboleda (✉) · E. Prosk
Research Department, Santé Cannabis Clinic, Montreal, QC, Canada
e-mail: mfarboleda@santecannabis.ca

S. N. Narouze (ed.), *Cannabinoids and Pain*, https://doi.org/10.1007/978-3-030-69186-8_21

Cannabinoid-Based Medicines: What Is Currently Available?

Before considering cannabinoid-based medicines as a complementary treatment, health professionals must identify which products are legally available in their countries [17].

In general, existing cannabinoid-based therapies are classified either as pharmaceutical cannabinoids or as natural cannabis. Figure 21.1 shows in detail the diverse cannabinoid-based medicines currently available.

Pharmaceutical cannabinoids may be synthetic or plant-derived and have been approved as pharmaceutical treatments or prescription drugs. Most randomized controlled trials (Phases I–III) have utilized pharmaceutical cannabinoids so more is known about their safety and efficacy in various clinical applications [18]. Consequently, regulatory agencies in specific countries have approved their use for certain medical conditions.

Products derived from natural cannabis are still considered unrecognized treatments. More clinical evidence is required to confirm their safety and efficacy [19]; however, it has been observed that patients may find their effects more tolerable [18].

Prescription or Pharmaceutical Cannabinoids

Learning about pharmaceutical cannabinoids is crucial because most clinical trials have been performed with these products. Nabilone, dronabinol, nabiximols, and Epidiolex® have met rigorous regulatory standards for specific medical approvals in diverse jurisdictions. Summarized practical information for each pharmaceutical cannabinoid is presented in Table 21.1 [18, 20–23]:

- *Nabilone* (Cesamet®) is a synthetic analogue of delta-9-tetrahydrocannabinol (THC) and was approved in 1986 by the US Food and Drug Administration (FDA) for the treatment of chemotherapy-induced nausea and vomiting which has failed conventional treatment. It is now quite widely available as a generic drug in several different countries [23]. In some cases, it has been used off label for acute and chronic pain management and has been evaluated for specific pain conditions [24–27]. It is approximately ten times more potent than natural THC and is administered in oral form [18, 28].

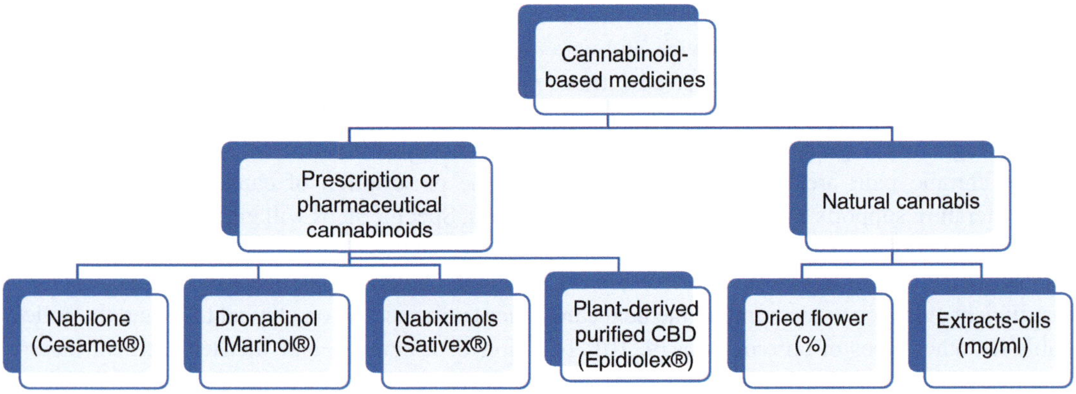

Fig. 21.1 Cannabinoid-based medicines: pharmaceutical versus natural cannabis

Table 21.1 Pharmaceutical cannabinoids: practical information

Pharmaceutical cannabinoid	Main characteristics and components	Pharmaceutical form and dosing	Approval (therapeutic indications)
Nabilone (Cesamet®)	Synthetic analogue of THC (10 times more potent than natural THC)	Capsules: 0.25 mg, 0.5 mg, 1 mg Oral administration Initiation dose: 0.25 mg HS Titrate dose according to symptoms Maximum dose: 2 mg 3 times a day (6 mg per day)	CINV which has failed conventional treatment
Dronabinol (Marinol®)	Synthetized THC	Capsules: 2.5 mg, 5 mg, 10 mg Oral administration Starting dosage *anorexia*: 2.5 mg, 1 hour before lunch and dinner. Maximum dose: 10 mg BID Starting dosage *CINV*: 5 mg/m^2, 1–3 hours prior to chemotherapy. Maximum dose: 15 mg/m^2 per dose, for four to six doses per day Titrate dose accordingly	1. Anorexia in HIV patients with weight loss 2. CINV which has failed conventional treatment
Nabiximols (Sativex®)	Natural extract of *Cannabis sativa* with THC and CBD in a balanced ratio (1:1) Each single 100 microliter spray contains 2.7 mg THC, 2.5 mg CBD Excipients: 0.04 ethanol and propylene glycol. Peppermint flavoring	Oromucosal spray, solution (10 mL), sublingual administration or inside of the cheeks. Site should be varied Starting dose: 1 spray HS Titration regimen: increase number of sprays according to symptoms and administer BID if needed Maximum dose: 12 sprays per day (~32 mg THC, 30 mg CBD)	1. Adjunct for spasticity in MS not responding to standard therapies
Epidiolex®	Plant-derived purified CBD Inactive ingredients: dehydrated alcohol, sesame seed oil, strawberry flavor, and sucralose	Oral solution: 100 mg/ml of CBD. Each bottle contains 100 mL Starting dose: 2.5 mg/kg BID (5 mg/kg/day) Titration regimen: after 1 week increase to 5 mg/kg BID (10 mg/kg/day) Weekly increments of 2.5 mg/kg BID as tolerated Maximum dose: 10 mg/kg BID (20 mg/kg/day) Measurement of liver function tests prior to starting treatment Adjust starting dose in *moderate* (1.25 mg/kg BID) and *severe* (0.5 mg/kg BID) hepatic impairment	1. Treatment of seizures associated with Lennox-Gastaut syndrome and Dravet syndrome (drug-resistant epilepsy) in patients 2 years of age or older[a]

BID twice daily, *CBD* cannabidiol, *CINV* chemotherapy-induced nausea and vomiting, *HIV* human immunodeficiency virus, *HS* at bedtime, *MS* multiple sclerosis, *THC* delta-9-tetrahydrocannabinol

[a]Precaution: concomitant use of valproate and high doses of Epidiolex® could increase AST and ALT [38]. If concomitant use of clobazam and Epidiolex®, measurement of clobazam and N-desmethylclobazam levels is necessary [39]

- *Dronabinol* (Marinol®) is a synthetized capsule of THC that is FDA-approved for anorexia in human immunodeficiency virus (HIV) patients with weight loss, since 1992. It is also approved for chemotherapy-associated nausea and vomiting that has failed traditional therapies [18].
- *Nabiximols* (Sativex®) was developed by GW Pharmaceuticals in the United Kingdom (UK). It is a natural extract blended from three cultivars of *Cannabis sativa* which comes in the form of an oromucosal spray. This balanced formulation of THC and cannabidiol (CBD) has been approved in more than 30 countries. However, it is not approved in the USA though it is recommended by the American Academy of Neurology mainly as an adjunct for spasticity in multiple sclerosis (MS), a common and disabling symptom affecting approximately 80% of this population [29–31]. A major limitation for its use relates to the high costs of the product and restricted insurance coverage.
- *Epidiolex®* is the first plant-derived cannabinoid treatment to be approved by the FDA. This authorization was released in 2018 for use in Lennox-Gastaut and Dravet syndrome for patients aged 2 years or older [32]. One year later, the European Drug Agency also approved its use for the same clinical conditions [33]. Epidiolex is an oral solution of purified CBD (98%) at a concentration of 100 mg/ml. Its safety and efficacy to treat drug-resistant epilepsy has be verified in multiple clinical trials [34–37].

Natural Cannabis

This class of cannabis-based medicines refers to herbal cannabis products or products derived from plant cannabis, mainly available as dried flower and oral products such as oils, extracts, capsules, and tinctures. Due to the complexity of these natural extracts and variable composition of active ingredients, including cannabinoids, terpenes, and flavonoids, it remains difficult to standardize and manufacture products to standards acceptable for use in clinical trials. Product diversity may be appreciated by some patients, but access to numerous strains and methods of administration are important limiting factors in a controlled clinical or research setting. Some authors have also questioned the validity of placebo group blinding to assess the effects of THC [40]. Given the abovementioned reasons, observational studies and real-world evidence have gained increasing attention in the cannabis field [41].

Inhalation

Dried cannabis is administered by inhalation, traditionally with a cigarette or a pipe, but now, much more commonly with an electronic vaporizer. Cannabinoid concentration in dried cannabis is expressed in percentage of dried weight (i.e., THC 10% w/w). Onset of effect occurs after 3–10 minutes of administration [42] and has a short duration of 2–4 hours [43]. Dose control may be limited as patients must implement a controlled inhalation technique in order to receive a consistent effect. Due to its rapid onset and short-acting effect, inhalation is recommended to control acute symptoms such as breakthrough pain, panic attacks, sleep induction, and appetite stimulation [12].

The use of a vaporizer could reduce the release of noxious chemicals due to temperature control (suggested between 180 and 220 °C) [44]. Some of these devices have been investigated to confirm safety and efficacy in chronic neuropathic pain [45–47].

Practical Recommendations [11, 12]

- Start with a single inhalation, pause for 10–15 minutes, and titrate according to symptoms.
- If a single inhalation is well tolerated and there is no therapeutic benefit, increase to two inhalations, and evaluate desired therapeutic effects.
- A slow dose escalation and waiting 10–15 minutes before increasing the number of inhalations is key to reduce the likelihood of developing adverse effects.

- Breath holding is not recommended due to increased exposure to harmful substances.
- Inhalation of cannabinoids should be avoided when a concomitant pulmonary condition such as chronic obstructive pulmonary disease (COPD) has been identified [48, 49].

Oral Administration

This method of administration has a unique pharmacokinetic profile from inhalation, and the cannabinoid concentration of oral products is expressed in mg/mL. Due to extensive first-pass effects among other factors, cannabinoid bioavailability is low and variable (5–20%). Onset of effect appears after 60–90 minutes of oral administration, and it has a long-lasting duration approximately 8–12 hours [43]. For this reason, when patients report persistent symptoms such as baseline chronic pain, sleep disturbance, and uncontrolled anxiety, this method of administration should be considered [12].

Practical Recommendations [11, 12]

- In most cases start with low doses of THC (1–2 mg) and CBD (2.5–5 mg). This is an individualized treatment; thus each patient will respond differently to cannabinoid therapy.
- Sublingual administration is generally recommended for a faster absorption.
- When initiating treatment or up-titrating the dose, always start at the evening or bedtime dose.
- Titrate slowly every 3–5 days until desired therapeutic benefits are achieved. If side effects are observed, return to previous dose.
- Consider administration twice daily (BID) or even three times per day (TID) if needed.
- In elderly patients always consider initiating with the lowest possible dose and titrate every 5–7 days.
- For previous occasional or regular consumers of cannabis: Consider the patient's experience to prescribe an appropriate starting dose. In many cases, patients may have taken unregulated products where no accurate cannabinoid concentration is provided.

In some cases, both inhalation and oral (combined) delivery methods are indicated such as when a patient presents with uncontrolled persistent pain and breakthrough or pain crisis.

When inhalation and oral administration are combined, practical recommendations for each may be followed; however it is recommended to stagger dose titration between the two methods.

Therapeutic Properties of Cannabinoids: THC Versus CBD

The complexity of the cannabis plant has been well characterized over the last few decades; it is known to contain more than 500 chemical compounds that might interact with the endocannabinoid system [28, 50]. In general, those compounds that are unique to the cannabis plant are known as cannabinoids or phytocannabinoids to differentiate from those that are synthetically derived. The primary phytocannabinoid is delta-9-tetrahydrocannabinol, or THC, a partial agonist to G-protein-coupled cannabinoid receptors CB1 and CB2. THC has been shown to be primarily responsible for the psychoactive effects of cannabis. Contrarily, cannabidiol, or CBD, is considered a nonintoxicating phytocannabinoid which is generally well tolerated. It does not appear to bind to CB1 or CB2 receptors at physiologically meaningful concentrations [51, 52]. When therapeutic doses of CBD are co-administered with THC, it might improve tolerability and safety versus THC alone. THC and CBD are the most studied cannabinoids in clinical trials [53–55].

The main therapeutic properties of THC and CBD as complementary treatments are summarized in Fig. 21.2 [16, 19]. The taxonomy of the cannabis plant is still widely debated, and it is estimated that more than 700 unique cultivars with unique chemical and morphological properties may exist [70]. Importantly, product selection may be greatly simplified by focusing on treatment objectives and determining (1) the preferred method of administration and (2) ratio of specific cannabinoid profile of THC versus CBD [71]. Generally, products may be classified as

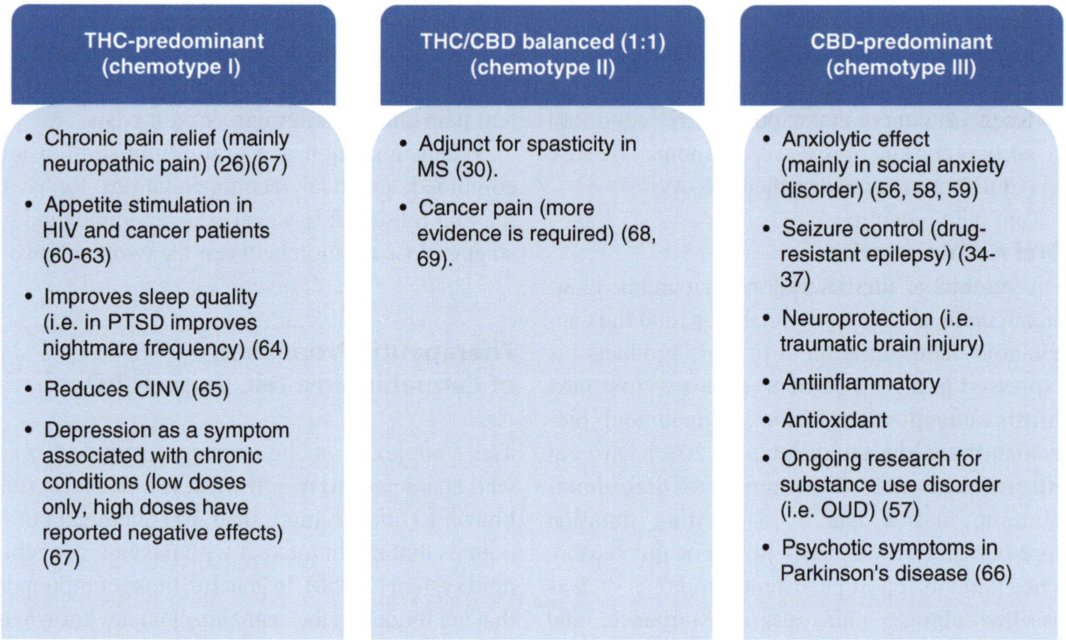

Fig. 21.2 Main therapeutic benefits of THC and CBD. CINV, chemotherapy-induced nausea and vomiting; HIV, human immunodeficiency virus; MS, multiple sclerosis; OUD, opioid use disorder; PTSD, posttraumatic stress disorder

THC-rich (chemotype I), THC and CBD balanced (chemotype II), or those considered CBD-rich (chemotype III) [72].

Practical Recommendations for the Prescription of Cannabinoid-Based Medicines

Key elements related to medical cannabis use are listed below [11]:

- Always define *clear therapeutic goals* with patients and/or family, and *manage* cannabinoid-based medicines *expectations* [12].
- A *comprehensive medical history* should always be recorded. *History of cannabis use* for medical and nonmedical purposes is also essential.
- *Screening for problematic cannabis use* with specific tools (i.e., CUDIT-r) might be useful [73]. However, there are still limitations to identify cannabis use disorder (CUD) among subjects using cannabis for medical purposes [74].
- Keep in mind that cannabinoids *are not a first-line treatment*. Conventional pharmacological and non-pharmacological treatments should be tried before considering cannabinoid-based therapy.
- *Medical cannabis is not for everyone.* There are specific indications and contraindications to be considered.
- Cannabinoid therapy is useful for *symptom control as an adjunct to conventional treatments*. In some cases, it might help to reduce concomitant medication dosage. This reduction should be carefully monitored by an HCP.
- There is some limited clinical evidence to support the *potential opioid-sparing effect* of cannabinoids [75]. Some literature supports opioid and cannabinoid synergistic effect for chronic pain management without significantly altering plasma opioid levels [76]. Opioid titration must be carefully monitored by an HCP.

- Some patients *might not feel any therapeutic benefit* even with significant cannabinoid doses. If possible, consider prescribing a different chemotype or changing the method of administration. As seen with other treatments, cannabinoids could also fail to show consistent pain reduction.
- If high doses of THC are utilized, do not stop cannabinoid therapy abruptly; consider tapering down to avoid withdrawal symptoms.

Clinical Evidence to Support Cannabinoid Use in Specific Medical Conditions

Although conclusions of systematic reviews and meta-analyses are inconsistent and generally limited by poor quality, the main conditions to consider cannabinoid-based medicines are [67, 77, 78]:

1. Chronic neuropathic pain. Most studies have been done with THC-rich inhaled products.
2. Spasticity in multiple sclerosis.
3. Chemotherapy-induced nausea and vomiting.
4. Drug-resistant epilepsy, specifically Lennox-Gastaut and Dravet syndromes.
5. Palliative care. For symptom control when conventional therapies have failed.

Is the Patient a Candidate for Cannabinoid Therapy? A Systematic Approach

After reviewing the regulatory status and availability of cannabis-based medicines in the country or state of practice, it is then important to develop a consistent, systematic approach to clinical assessments.

This systematic assessment to determine if a patient is potential candidate for cannabinoid-based medicines will guide the process and support physician's evaluation and treatment recommendations. The key steps are summarized in Table 21.2 and discussed in further detail below.

Table 21.2 Systematic assessment for potential cannabinoid therapy

Key steps	Description
1. Develop a complete clinical assessment and a thorough medical history	(a) Document a detailed medical history, and determine primary and secondary symptoms to be treated (application of validated measurement tools is recommended) (b) Record all pharmacological and non-pharmacological treatments previously tried (c) Document the patient's history of previous cannabis use and any adverse effects (for medical and nonmedical purposes) (d) Review any precautions and/or contraindications for cannabinoid treatment
2. Define treatment objectives and manage expectations	(a) Discuss the treatment objectives with patient and/or family, and ensure patient has reasonable expectations (b) Review the treatment agreement and required education about the treatment risks
3. Define a treatment plan: is the patient a candidate for cannabinoid therapy?	(a) Chemotype selection (THC versus CBD) according to the treatment objectives (b) Method of administration according to acute versus persistent symptoms and medical status (c) Starting dose and titration regimen
4. Elaborate a medical document or prescription, in line with specific regulatory requirements	(a) Explain process for safe access to cannabinoid-based medicines from authorized licensed producers (b) Keep in mind costs and product availability

(continued)

Table 21.2 (continued)

Key steps	Description
5. Monitor side effects and establish frequency of follow-up visits	(a) Always explain potential cannabinoid adverse effects (b) Recommend the use of a diary to record dose, frequency, symptom control, and side effects (c) Close monitoring is crucial. A phone follow-up during the titration phase is highly recommended (d) Determine frequency of follow-up visits according to patient's medical condition and treatment objectives

1. **Develop a Complete Clinical Assessment and a Thorough Medical History**
   (a) *Document a Detailed Medical History (Determine Primary and Secondary Symptoms)*

Once a complete medical history has been carefully developed, identification of primary and secondary symptoms is essential; this will guide treatment objectives. Application of validated and rapid assessment instruments such as the Brief Pain Inventory Short Form (BPI-SF) [79], the Edmonton Symptom Assessment System revised (ESAS-r) [80], and the EQ-5D [81] is highly recommended. This could be helpful to understand the intensity of various symptoms (i.e., pain, anxiety, insomnia, lack of appetite, nausea, etc.) and the consequent impact on health-related quality of life.

Additionally, the use of these tools could guide chemotype selection (i.e., if pain and important concomitant anxiety are the targeted symptoms, a THC/CBD-balanced or a CBD-predominant product might be considered). Finally, objective treatment response is possible when these tools are applied at each follow-up visit.

(b) *Record All Pharmacological and Non-pharmacological Treatments Previously Tried*

As previously mentioned, cannabinoids are not a first-line treatment. For this reason, identification of previous pharmacological and non-pharmacological treatments is extremely important.

(c) *Always Determine History of Previous Cannabis Use (Medical and Nonmedical)*

History of previous cannabis use will be an important factor to determine:

- The main interests and objectives for cannabinoid consumption (medical versus nonmedical purposes)
- What has the patient already tried and methods of administration
- Source of cannabinoid products (legal versus illegal markets)
- If there has been any previous therapeutic benefit
- If the patient has experienced any negative or adverse effects (i.e., paranoia, panic attacks, cognitive impairment, etc.)
- The risk for problematic cannabis use (screening tools could be helpful)
- Chemotype selection, starting and maintenance cannabinoid dosage (naïve versus regular users)

(d) *Any Precautions and/or Contraindications for Cannabinoid Treatment?*

Have in mind that cannabinoid therapy is not for everyone and selection of specific cannabinoid should be done carefully. Most contraindications are related to THC [19]:

- Unstable or uncontrolled cardiovascular conditions (i.e., ischemia, uncontrolled arrhythmia, and uncontrolled hypertension).
- Personal history of psychosis, schizophrenia, bipolar disorders.

- Patients under 18 years of age should not receive THC. However, CBD is not contraindicated and could be used for drug-resistant epilepsy in pediatric population.
- Patients under 25 years of age should be limited to CBD or CBD-rich chemotypes with limited quantities of THC.
- Avoid inhaled cannabinoids if concomitant severe pulmonary disease is present.
- Hypersensitivity to cannabinoids.
- Pregnancy or breastfeeding.

Some precautions to be considered when prescribing cannabinoid-based treatments are [11, 19]:

- Reduce starting dose if there is renal or liver function impairment. Dose escalation should be done carefully (i.e., every 5–7 days). Lowest effective dose should be used, and inhalation should be avoided. CBD may raise tacrolimus levels [82].
- History of substance use disorder and risk of CUD.
- Activities requiring coordination and concentration: driving should be avoided for at least 4 hours after inhaled cannabis use and 6–8 hours after oral administration [11] even when concomitant CBD has been used [83].
- Consider possible drug-drug interactions (i.e., clobazam, valproic acid, warfarin), and avoid using cannabinoids with alcohol.

2. **Define Treatment Objectives and Manage Expectations**

Always discuss with patients and/or family cannabinoid treatment objectives and manage their expectations. Clarify that cannabis-based medicines may help with symptom relief but there is no evidence of curative properties. Additionally, patient education is crucial to support a beneficial outcome and avoid adverse effects or other negative experiences. Take enough time to explain about cannabinoid treatments, address common misconceptions, and differentiate between medical and nonmedical cannabis use. Always confirm patient's commitment to follow the treatment plan, eliminate the use of illicit products, and continue contact with the healthcare team to report benefits or adverse effects.

3. **Define a Treatment Plan: Is the Patient a Candidate for Cannabinoid Therapy?**

Based on the patient's health status and past medical history, decide if that person is or not a candidate for cannabinoid-based medicines based on an analysis of the benefit-risk profile. Always keep in mind that cannabinoids are a personalized treatment and each patient may have an individualized response.

Identification of primary symptom and concomitant secondary symptoms will be key for chemotype selection. This could vary and will be done on a case-by-case basis.

Determining the appropriate method of administration will be defined according to acute versus persistent symptoms and the accessibility to the patient. Starting dose and titration regimen should always be fully and carefully explained to each patient.

4. **Elaborate a Medical Document or Prescription, in Line with Specific Regulatory Requirements**

Each country or state jurisdiction will have its own regulatory framework, and availability of cannabinoid-based medicines may differ. Therefore, make sure that you know which legal products are available and what documentation must be completed. Always recommend safe and consistent products with certified laboratory testing that ensures standardized quality control (i.e., from authorized licensed producers). To enable patients' access to medical cannabis products, keep in mind the costs to the patient, and try to recommend treatments that are sustainable and are consistently available.

5. **Monitor Side Effects and Establish Frequency of Follow-Up Visits**

Patients should be carefully monitored when cannabinoid therapy is initiated. The use of a diary is suggested to record product name and dose such as number of inhalations, or milliliters, the dose frequency, and resulting symptom control, side effects. A phone follow-up is generally a good strategy during the first few weeks of the titration phase to confirm treatment adherence and to identify potential side effects.

Establish a follow-up plan with your patient and/or family. At each visit evaluate if treatment objectives were achieved. If limited or no benefits are observed, consider a transition to a different chemotype or an increased cannabinoid dose or frequency.

Record adverse effects that may be related to cannabinoid treatment. Most adverse effects are related to THC and are dose dependent. Such adverse effects can often be avoided with careful titration and close follow-up [12]. The most frequent adverse effects related to both THC and CBD are somnolence, dizziness, sedation, and dry mouth. THC may also produce euphoria, anxiety, headache, blurred vision, cognitive effects, and not so common toxic psychosis and cardiovascular side effects such as tachycardia and orthostatic hypotension [11]. High doses of CBD in excess of 1000 mg per day may produce fatigue, diarrhea, and abnormal liver function tests [84]. Finally, cannabinoid hyperemesis syndrome is an unusual adverse effect that has been observed in chronic and heavy recreational cannabis users [85].

Conclusion

In the current climate and popularity of medical cannabis treatments, it is essential for HCPs to understand the main characteristics of cannabis and cannabinoid-based treatments. Before recommending cannabis-based medicines as an adjunct for specific conditions and symptoms, a foundational understanding of therapeutic potential, possible risks, and the regulatory framework must be developed. Existing clinical evidence has been primarily derived from the investigation of prescription or pharmaceutical cannabinoids. Well-designed studies are still required to identify the efficacy and safety of natural cannabis products in a controlled setting. Although conclusions of systematic reviews and meta-analyses are conflicting, cannabinoid recommendations have focused mostly on chronic neuropathic pain, spasticity in multiple sclerosis, and chemotherapy-induced nausea and vomiting. When considering a prescription for cannabis-based medicine, a systematic approach is essential to assess potential candidates. While clinical evidence of cannabinoid-based medicines develops slowly, anecdotal reports and patient interest grow at a steady pace, requiring healthcare teams to continue to keep pace with education and training opportunities.

References

1. Brady JP, Bruce D, Foster E, Shattell M. Self-efficacy in researching and obtaining medical cannabis by patients with chronic conditions. Health Educ Behav. 2020;1090198120914249
2. Baron EP, Lucas P, Eades J, Hogue O. Patterns of medicinal cannabis use, strain analysis, and substitution effect among patients with migraine, headache, arthritis, and chronic pain in a medicinal cannabis cohort. J Headache Pain. 2018;19(1):37.
3. Boehnke KF, Scott JR, Litinas E, Sisley S, Clauw DJ, Goesling J, et al. Cannabis use preferences and decision-making among a cross-sectional cohort of medical cannabis patients with chronic pain. J Pain. 2019;20(11):1362–72.
4. St Pierre M, Matthews L, Walsh Z. Cannabis education needs assessment among Canadian physicians-in-training. Complement Ther Med. 2020;49:102328.
5. Azcarate PM, Zhang AJ, Keyhani S, Steigerwald S, Ishida JH, Cohen BE. Medical Reasons for Marijuana Use, Forms of Use, and Patient Perception of Physician Attitudes Among the US Population. J Gen Intern Med. 2020;
6. Health Canada. Canadian cannabis survey 2019. Available from: https://www.canada.ca/en/health-canada/services/publications/drugs-health-products/canadian-cannabis-survey-2019-summary.html
7. Banerjee S, McCormack S. Medical cannabis for the treatment of chronic pain: a review of clinical effectiveness and guidelines. Canadian Agency for Drugs and Technologies in Health: Ottawa, ON; 2019.

Available from: http://www.ncbi.nlm.nih.gov/books/NBK546424/
8. Mu A, Weinberg E, Moulin DE, Clarke H. Pharmacologic management of chronic neuropathic pain: review of the Canadian Pain Society consensus statement. Can Fam Physician Med Fam Can. 2017;63(11):844–52.
9. Häuser W, Finn DP, Kalso E, Krcevski-Skvarc N, Kress H-G, Morlion B, et al. European Pain Federation (EFIC) position paper on appropriate use of cannabis-based medicines and medical cannabis for chronic pain management. Eur J Pain. 2018;22(9):1547–64.
10. Allan GM, Finley CR, Ton J, Perry D, Ramji J, Crawford K, et al. Systematic review of systematic reviews for medical cannabinoids: pain, nausea and vomiting, spasticity, and harms. Can Fam Physician Med Fam Can. 2018;64(2):e78–94.
11. MacCallum CA, Russo EB. Practical considerations in medical cannabis administration and dosing. Eur J Intern Med. 2018;
12. Cyr C, Arboleda MF, Aggarwal SK, Balneaves LG, Daeninck P, Néron A, et al. Cannabis in palliative care: current challenges and practical recommendations. Ann Palliat Med. 2018;7(4):463–77.
13. VanDolah HJ, Bauer BA, Mauck KF. Clinicians' guide to cannabidiol and hemp oils. Mayo Clin Proc. 2019;94(9):1840–51.
14. Arboleda MF, Prosk E, Cyr C, Gamaoun R, Vigano A. Medical cannabis in supportive cancer care: lessons from Canada. Support Care Cancer. 2020;28(7):2999–3001.
15. Ablin J, Ste-Marie PA, Schäfer M, Häuser W, Fitzcharles M-A. Medical use of cannabis products: lessons to be learned from Israel and Canada. Schmerz Berl Ger. 2016;30(1):3–13.
16. National Academies of Sciences, Engineering, and Medicine, Health and Medicine Division, Board on Population Health and Public Health Practice, Committee on the Health Effects of Marijuana: An Evidence Review and Research Agenda. The Health Effects of Cannabis and Cannabinoids: The Current State of Evidence and Recommendations for Research. Washington (DC): National Academies Press (US); 2017. (The National Academies Collection: Reports funded by National Institutes of Health). Available from: http://www.ncbi.nlm.nih.gov/books/NBK423845/
17. Steele G, Arneson T, Zylla D. A comprehensive review of cannabis in patients with cancer: availability in the USA, general efficacy, and safety. Curr Oncol Rep. 2019;21(1):10.
18. Schrot RJ, Hubbard JR. Cannabinoids: medical implications. Ann Med. 2016;48(3):128–41.
19. Health Canada. Information for Health Care Professionals: Cannabis (marihuana, marijuana) and the cannabinoids. 2013. Available from: https://www.canada.ca/en/health-canada/services/drugs-health-products/medical-use-marijuana/information-medical-practitioners/information-health-care-professiona ls-cannabis-marihuana-marijuana-cannabinoids.html.
20. GW Pharma Ltd. Sativex Oromucosal Spray – Summary of Product Characteristics (SmPC). 2018. Available from: https://www.medicines.org.uk/emc/product/602/smpc
21. Chen JW, Borgelt LM, Blackmer AB. Epidiolex (Cannabidiol): a new Hope for patients with Dravet or Lennox-Gastaut syndromes. Ann Pharmacother. 2019;1060028018822124
22. FDA. EPIDIOLEX (cannabidiol) oral solution. Available from: https://www.accessdata.fda.gov/drugsatfda_docs/label/2018/210365lbl.pdf
23. Fraguas-Sánchez AI, Torres-Suárez AI. Medical use of cannabinoids. Drugs. 2018;78(16):1665–703.
24. Walitt B, Klose P, Fitzcharles M-A, Phillips T, Häuser W. Cannabinoids for fibromyalgia. Cochrane Database Syst Rev. 2016;7:CD011694.
25. Skrabek RQ, Galimova L, Ethans K, Perry D. Nabilone for the treatment of pain in fibromyalgia. J Pain. 2008;9(2):164–73.
26. Mücke M, Phillips T, Radbruch L, Petzke F, Häuser W. Cannabis-based medicines for chronic neuropathic pain in adults. Cochrane Database Syst Rev. 2018;3:CD012182.
27. Beaulieu P. Effects of nabilone, a synthetic cannabinoid, on postoperative pain. Can J Anaesth. 2006;53(8):769–75.
28. Murnion B. Medicinal cannabis. Aust Prescr. 2015;38(6):212–5.
29. Yadav V, Bever C, Bowen J, Bowling A, Weinstock-Guttman B, Cameron M, et al. Summary of evidence-based guideline: complementary and alternative medicine in multiple sclerosis: report of the guideline development subcommittee of the American Academy of Neurology. Neurology. 2014;82(12):1083–92.
30. Patti F, Chisari CG, Solaro C, Benedetti MD, Berra E, Bianco A, et al. Effects of THC/CBD oromucosal spray on spasticity-related symptoms in people with multiple sclerosis: results from a retrospective multicenter study. Neurol Sci. 2020;
31. Oreja-Guevara C, González-Segura D, Vila C. Spasticity in multiple sclerosis: results of a patient survey. Int J Neurosci. 2013;123(6):400–8.
32. Thomas RH, Cunningham MO. Cannabis and epilepsy. Pract Neurol. 2018;18(6):465–71.
33. Wise J. European drug agency approves cannabis-based medicine for severe forms of epilepsy. BMJ. 2019;366:l5708.
34. Devinsky O, Marsh E, Friedman D, Thiele E, Laux L, Sullivan J, et al. Cannabidiol in patients with treatment-resistant epilepsy: an open-label interventional trial. Lancet Neurol. 2016;15(3):270–8.
35. Devinsky O, Cross JH, Wright S. Trial of cannabidiol for drug-resistant seizures in the Dravet Syndrome. N Engl J Med. 2017;377(7):699–700.
36. Szaflarski JP, Bebin EM, Comi AM, Patel AD, Joshi C, Checketts D, et al. Long-term safety and treatment effects of cannabidiol in children and adults with treatment-resistant epilepsies: expanded access program results. Epilepsia. 2018;59(8):1540–8.

37. Szaflarski JP, Bebin EM, Cutter G, DeWolfe J, Dure LS, Gaston TE, et al. Cannabidiol improves frequency and severity of seizures and reduces adverse events in an open-label add-on prospective study. Epilepsy Behav. 2018;87:131–6.
38. Gaston TE, Bebin EM, Cutter GR, Liu Y, Szaflarski JP. Interactions between cannabidiol and commonly used antiepileptic drugs. Epilepsia. 2017;58(9):1586–92.
39. Geffrey AL, Pollack SF, Bruno PL, Thiele EA. Drug–drug interaction between clobazam and cannabidiol in children with refractory epilepsy. Epilepsia. 2015;56(8):1246–51.
40. Wilsey B, Deutsch R, Marcotte TD. Maintenance of blinding in clinical trials and the implications for studying analgesia using cannabinoids. Cannabis Cannabinoid Res. 2016;1(1):139–48.
41. Ware MA. Medical Cannabis research: issues and priorities. Neuropsychopharmacol. 2018;43(1):214–5.
42. Huestis MA, Henningfield JE, Cone EJ. Blood cannabinoids. I. Absorption of THC and formation of 11-OH-THC and THCCOOH during and after smoking marijuana. J Anal Toxicol. 1992;16(5):276–82.
43. Borgelt LM, Franson KL, Nussbaum AM, Wang GS. The pharmacologic and clinical effects of medical cannabis. Pharmacotherapy. 2013;33(2):195–209.
44. Gieringer D, St. Laurent J, Goodrich S. Cannabis vaporizer combines efficient delivery of THC with effective suppression of pyrolytic compounds. J Cannabis Ther. 2004;4:7–27.
45. Abrams DI, Vizoso HP, Shade SB, Jay C, Kelly ME, Benowitz NL. Vaporization as a smokeless cannabis delivery system: a pilot study. Clin Pharmacol Ther. 2007;82(5):572–8.
46. Almog S, Aharon-Peretz J, Vulfsons S, Ogintz M, Abalia H, Lupo T, et al. The pharmacokinetics, efficacy, and safety of a novel selective-dose cannabis inhaler in patients with chronic pain: a randomized, double-blinded, placebo-controlled trial. Eur J Pain. 2020;
47. Eisenberg E, Ogintz M, Almog S. The pharmacokinetics, efficacy, safety, and ease of use of a novel portable metered-dose cannabis inhaler in patients with chronic neuropathic pain: a phase 1a study. J Pain Palliat Care Pharmacother. 2014;28(3):216–25.
48. Tashkin DP, Roth MD. Pulmonary effects of inhaled cannabis smoke. Am J Drug Alcohol Abuse. 2019;0(0):1–14.
49. Owen KP, Sutter ME, Albertson TE. Marijuana: respiratory tract effects. Clin Rev Allergy Immunol. 2014;46(1):65–81.
50. Abrams DI, Guzman M. Cannabis in cancer care. Clin Pharmacol Ther. 2015;97(6):575–86.
51. Jensen B, Chen J, Furnish T, Wallace M. Medical marijuana and chronic pain: a review of basic science and clinical evidence. Curr Pain Headache Rep. 2015;19(10):50.
52. Russo EB. Cannabidiol claims and misconceptions. Trends Pharmacol Sci. 2017;38(3):198–201.
53. Bridgeman MB, Abazia DT. Medicinal Cannabis: history, pharmacology, and implications for the acute care setting. P T Peer-Rev J Formul Manag. 2017;42(3):180–8.
54. Abrams DI. Integrating cannabis into clinical cancer care. Curr Oncol Tor Ont. 2016;23(2):S8–14.
55. Russo EB. Taming THC: potential cannabis synergy and phytocannabinoid-terpenoid entourage effects. Br J Pharmacol. 2011;163(7):1344–64.
56. Crippa JA, Derenusson GN, Ferrari TB, Wichert-Ana L, Duran FL, Martin-Santos R, et al. Neural basis of anxiolytic effects of cannabidiol (CBD) in generalized social anxiety disorder- a preliminary report. J Psychopharmacol. 2011. Available from: https://www.theroc.us/researchlibrary/Neural%20basis%20of%20anxiolytic%20effects%20of%20cannabidiol%20(CBD)%20in%20generalized%20social%20anxiety%20disorder-%20a%20preliminary%20report.pdf
57. Chye Y, Christensen E, Solowij N, Yücel M. The endocannabinoid system and cannabidiol's promise for the treatment of substance use disorder. Front Psych. 2019;10:63.
58. Zuardi AW, Rodrigues NP, Silva AL, Bernardo SA, Hallak JE, Guimarães FS, et al. Inverted U-shaped dose-response curve of the anxiolytic effect of cannabidiol during public speaking in real life. Front Pharmacol. 2017;8:259.
59. Black N, Stockings E, Campbell G, Tran LT, Zagic D, Hall WD, et al. Cannabinoids for the treatment of mental disorders and symptoms of mental disorders: a systematic review and meta-analysis. Lancet Psychiatry. 2019;6(12):995–1010.
60. Jatoi A. Dronabinol versus megestrol acetate versus combination therapy for cancer-associated anorexia: a north central cancer treatment group study. J Clin Oncol. 2002;20(2):567–73.
61. Cannabis-In-Cachexia-Study-Group, Strasser F, Luftner D, Possinger K, Ernst G, Ruhstaller T, et al. Comparison of orally administered cannabis extract and delta-9-tetrahydrocannabinol in treating patients with cancer-related anorexia-cachexia syndrome: a multicenter, phase III, randomized, double-blind, placebo-controlled clinical trial from the Cannabis-In-Cachexia-Study-Group. J Clin Oncol Off J Am Soc Clin Oncol. 2006;24(21):3394–400.
62. Badowski ME, Yanful PK. Dronabinol oral solution in the management of anorexia and weight loss in AIDS and cancer. Ther Clin Risk Manag. 2018;14:643–51.
63. Bar-Sela G, Zalman D, Semenysty V, Ballan E. The effects of dosage-controlled cannabis capsules on cancer-related cachexia and anorexia syndrome in advanced cancer patients: pilot study. Integr Cancer Ther. 2019;18:1–8.
64. Jetly R, Heber A, Fraser G, Boisvert D. The efficacy of nabilone, a synthetic cannabinoid, in the treatment of PTSD-associated nightmares: a preliminary randomized, double-blind, placebo-controlled cross-over design study. Psychoneuroendocrinology. 2015;51:585–8.

65. Badowski ME. A review of oral cannabinoids and medical marijuana for the treatment of chemotherapy-induced nausea and vomiting: a focus on pharmacokinetic variability and pharmacodynamics. Cancer Chemother Pharmacol. 2017;80(3):441–9.
66. Zuardi AW, JAS C, JEC H, Pinto JP, MHN C, GGR R, et al. Cannabidiol for the treatment of psychosis in Parkinson's disease. J Psychopharmacol. 2009;23(8):979–83.
67. Whiting PF, Wolff RF, Deshpande S, Di Nisio M, Duffy S, Hernandez AV, et al. Cannabinoids for medical use: a systematic review and meta-analysis. JAMA. 2015;313(24):2456–73.
68. Johnson JR, Burnell-Nugent M, Lossignol D, Ganae-Motan ED, Potts R, Fallon MT. Multicenter, double-blind, randomized, placebo-controlled, parallel-group study of the efficacy, safety, and tolerability of THC:CBD extract and THC extract in patients with intractable cancer-related pain. J Pain Symptom Manag. 2010;39(2):167–79.
69. Boland EG, Bennett MI, Allgar V, Boland JW. Cannabinoids for adult cancer-related pain: systematic review and meta-analysis. BMJ Support Palliat Care. 2020;10(1):14–24.
70. Hazekamp A, Tejkalová K, Papadimitriou S. Cannabis: from cultivar to chemovar II—A metabolomics approach to cannabis classification. Cannabis Cannabinoid Res. 2016;1(1):202–15.
71. Russo EB. Current therapeutic cannabis controversies and clinical trial design issues. Front Pharmacol. 2016;7:309.
72. Lewis MA, Russo EB, Smith KM. Pharmacological foundations of cannabis chemovars. Planta Med. 2018;84(4):225–33.
73. Adamson SJ, Kay-Lambkin FJ, Baker AL, Lewin TJ, Thornton L, Kelly BJ, et al. An improved brief measure of cannabis misuse: the cannabis use disorders identification test-revised (CUDIT-R). Drug Alcohol Depend. 2010;110(1–2):137–43.
74. Loflin M, Babson K, Browne K, Bonn-Miller M. Assessment of the validity of the CUDIT-R in a subpopulation of cannabis users. Am J Drug Alcohol Abuse. 2018;44(1):19–23.
75. Nielsen S, Sabioni P, Trigo JM, Ware MA, Betz-Stablein BD, Murnion B, et al. Opioid-sparing effect of cannabinoids: a systematic review and meta-analysis. Neuropsychopharmacol. 2017;42(9):1752–65.
76. Abrams DI, Couey P, Shade SB, Kelly ME, Benowitz NL. Cannabinoid-opioid interaction in chronic pain. Clin Pharmacol Ther. 2011;90(6):844–51.
77. Inglet S, Winter B, Yost SE, Entringer S, Lian A, Biksacky M, et al. Clinical data for the use of cannabis-based treatments: a comprehensive review of the literature. Ann Pharmacother. 2020;1060028020930189
78. Allan GM, Ramji J, Perry D, Ton J, Beahm NP, Crisp N, et al. Simplified guideline for prescribing medical cannabinoids in primary care. Can Fam Physician Med Fam Can. 2018;64(2):111–20.
79. Atkinson TM, Rosenfeld BD, Sit L, Mendoza TR, Fruscione M, Lavene D, et al. Using confirmatory factor analysis to evaluate construct validity of the Brief Pain Inventory (BPI). J Pain Symptom Manag. 2011;41(3):558–65.
80. Hui D, Bruera E. The Edmonton symptom assessment system 25 years later: past, present, and future developments. J Pain Symptom Manag. 2017;53(3):630–43.
81. Matter-Walstra K, Klingbiel D, Szucs T, Pestalozzi BC, Schwenkglenks M. Using the EuroQol EQ-5D in Swiss cancer patients, which value set should be applied? PharmacoEconomics. 2014;32(6):591–9.
82. Leino AD, Emoto C, Fukuda T, Privitera M, Vinks AA, Alloway RR. Evidence of a clinically significant drug-drug interaction between cannabidiol and tacrolimus. Am J Transplant. 2019;19(10):2944–8.
83. Arkell TR, Lintzeris N, Kevin RC, Ramaekers JG, Vandrey R, Irwin C, et al. Cannabidiol (CBD) content in vaporized cannabis does not prevent tetrahydrocannabinol (THC)-induced impairment of driving and cognition. Psychopharmacology. 2019;236(9):2713–24.
84. Chesney E, Oliver D, Green A, Sovi S, Wilson J, Englund A, et al. Adverse effects of cannabidiol: a systematic review and meta-analysis of randomized clinical trials. Neuropsychopharmacology. 2020:1–8.
85. Sorensen CJ, DeSanto K, Borgelt L, Phillips KT, Monte AA. Cannabinoid hyperemesis syndrome: diagnosis, pathophysiology, and treatment—a systematic review. J Med Toxicol. 2017;13(1):71–87.

Cannabinoid-Based Medicines: Dosing, Titration & Monitoring

22

Caroline A. MacCallum, Lauren de Freitas, Lindsay A. Lo, and Michael Boivin

Introduction

Cannabis formulation and administration methods play an important role in onset, duration, and effects experienced by patients. Since impairment and adverse events are THC dependent, the use of oral ingested oils is often recommended for medical cannabis, as it allows for precise dosing of THC vs. inhaling vaporized flower. In order for patients to experience minimal/no side effects, while also achieving pain/treatment goals, a safe cannabis dosing strategy is to "start low and go slow". Patients using cannabis flower may benefit from using a "mindful vaping technique". Using THC and CBD products concurrently, or a CBD-dominant product can help balance THC-mediated adverse effects, and may allow for higher tolerance of THC than THC-predominant products. Once cannabis treatment has been initiated, ongoing monitoring by a healthcare professional is essential to achieve optimal dose and reduce unwanted adverse events.

Methods of Administration

Inhalation: Smoking and Vaporizing

Inhaled cannabis products can be either smoked (i.e., via a "joint," bong, pipe) or vaporized (i.e., via a vaporizer); however, vaporization is preferred since it releases fewer harmful by-products and is associated with decreased adverse pulmonary symptoms [3]. Smoking heats cannabis to 600–900 °C, releasing harmful carcinogens (e.g., tar, ammonia, polyaromatic hydrocarbons) and carbon monoxide [4]. Smoking can also reduce THC delivery, as 30–60% of cannabinoids are lost in "sidestream smoke", resulting in only 10–60% absorption of the administered dose [2, 3, 5, 9]. In contrast, vaporization requires 160–220 °C of heat, releasing little, if any, carbon monoxide, although more longitudinal research is needed as hydrocarbons may still potentially be produced [4]. Due to reduced combustion and more efficient decarboxylation than smoking, vaporization allows for greater precision of dosing with minimal side-

C. A. MacCallum (✉)
Department of Medicine, Faculty of Medicine, University of British Columbia, Vancouver, BC, Canada
e-mail: info@drcarolinemaccallum.com

L. de Freitas
Centre for Addiction and Mental Health, Toronto, ON, Canada

L. A. Lo
Department of Psychology, Queen's University, Kingston, ON, Canada

M. Boivin
CommPharm Consulting, Barrie, ON, Canada

S. N. Narouze (ed.), *Cannabinoids and Pain*, https://doi.org/10.1007/978-3-030-69186-8_22

stream smoke loss, requiring 30–50% less dried cannabis with reduced adverse events [5]. Some vaporizers are considered medical devices by regulatory bodies in different countries.

The rapid onset and duration of action of inhaling cannabis products provides an advantage in managing intermittent or acute symptoms such as breakthrough pain, nausea, panic attacks, appetite, and sleep initiation. Vaporization should be considered as an "as-needed" option for the daytime to supplement a background of oral cannabis when not operating heavy machinery, including driving.

When considering inhalation as a route of administration, it is important to consider sight and fine motor abilities in using an inhalation device. Patient education and counseling regarding proper inhalation techniques, including how to dose cannabis flower consistently, are essential. Other considerations for inhalation include the cost, frequency of dosing, and odor (vaporization produces less odor than smoking but more than oral route). Dosing specific factors to be aware of include the size of the chamber, depth of the inhalation taken, how long the inhalation is held, temperature that the cannabis is heated to, and more [6].

Recent advances have led to "metered dose" inhaler devices, which contain decarboxylated THC and/or CBD in a powdered form that is inhaled without heat, similar to asthma inhalers. The Syqe® Inhaler device has shown a promise in a recent clinical trial among medical cannabis patients [7]. Other vaporizers can be tethered to an individual's personal smartphone or device, which can set the desired temperature for the vaporizer among other factors. Some vaporizer pen devices have vibration features to notify an individual when a specific amount of THC and/or CBD has been inhaled.

Oral

Oral cannabis preparations (i.e., oils and capsules) have the longest onset and duration of action of all the delivery methods (Table 22.1), and are therefore advantageous in managing chronic conditions, namely, chronic pain and associated symptom clusters (see Chap. 25 on Cannabinoids and Pain: Clinical Evidence). Ingested oils allow for precise dosing by using a graduated syringe or medicine dropper. Using a 1.0-milliliter (mL) syringe with 0.1 graduations is preferred, as it will accurately dose the oil to 0.01 ml (vs. medicine droppers which may be 0.25 ml graduations), therefore making oral dosing easier and a more accurate method of titrating than other routes [2]. When using a new bottle of product, consider decreasing the dose slightly, as cannabinoid content can vary between batches.

Oral cannabis preparations have an absorption rate of 20–30% [9]. As such, they should be swallowed directly and not mixed in a food where the dose can be lost, especially if doses are small. However, if a patient must put it in food prior to ingestion, it is recommended to place it directly on a spoon with the food (ie yogurt, applesauce) to ensure that the full dose is ingested. Cannabis should never be mixed in a liquid where it will adhere to the side of the glass (cannabis is very hydrophobic). Some patients report a faster onset of action when ingesting cannabis with food containing fat, and even delayed absorption until food with fat has been ingested [8]. Although some patients report a faster absorption sublingually, pharmacokinetic studies demonstrate minimal absorption of THC oil directly into the bloodstream via the oral mucosa [9, 10]. Conversion of THC to THC-COOH, the main long-acting molecule, occurs through first-pass metabolism by the liver upon swallowing [11].

Edibles are unlike pharmaceutical preparations in the sense that they are prepared in the form of mints, gummies, brownies, energy shots, teas, dissolvable powders, breath strips, and more. Edible routes are usually harder to dose, and have the potential to overconsume them as a snack [12]. Refer to Chap. 36 on Cannabinoid-Related Adverse Events and Impairment for information about recreational vs. medical populations, paying attention to the differences in their intent and choice of product route and potency. Edibles are not designed as a means of standardized dosing for medical patients, but more for recreational use. However, some medical patients on stable dosing may prefer edibles instead of an unpalatable oil.

Table 22.1 Cannabis methods of administration

Routes	Smoking/vaporization	Oral	Oromucosal	Topical
Onset (min)	5–10	60–180	15–45	Variable
Duration (h)	2–4	6–8	6–8	Variable
Form(s) and Uses	Dried flower and concentrates[a] Smoking can involve using a cannabis "cigarette" (joint, spliff), pipe or water pipe (bong), dabs, shatter[a] Vaporization requires the use of an electronic device that heats the cannabis loaded into the vape chamber and releases the resulting vapor	Oils/extracts, capsules (dronabinol, nabilone), edibles (cannabis-infused food and beverages)	Sprays (nabiximols), tinctures Oromucosal preparations are applied either sublingually, buccally, or through the nose to the nasopharyngeal tract via a pump-action spray	Creams, balms, salves, ointments, patches, oils Topicals are directly applied to the skin externally
Pros	Rapid onset of action Doses can be quickly titrated to desired effect Commonly used for acute/episodic symptoms (e.g., breakthrough pain). Vaporization requires lower heat and produces less exposure to toxicants compared to smoked cannabis	Longer duration of action to provide relief for chronic conditions/symptoms Wide range of products No inhalation required No respiratory risks involved No odor and are more convenient, discrete, and accurate dosing when using oils	Intermediate onset and duration of action Nabiximols are pharmaceutically developed with evidence of its efficacy in specific patient populations (i.e., multiple sclerosis)	Act locally, recommended for smaller areas No respiratory risk. Minimal systemic effects (when applied to intact skin) and therefore minimal risk of intoxication
Cons	Smoking and vaporizing require dexterity to prepare and administer cannabis Vaporizers can be expensive and some are not portable Smoking should not be recommended due to the harmful carcinogens and by-products released Vaporizers produce less CO and pulmonary symptoms than smoking but can still release some harmful polyaromatic hydrocarbons and tar Potential respiratory consequences (bronchial irritation, cough, sputum). Long-term lung safety is still unknown with both smoking and vaporization	Slower titration due to delayed onset, delayed peak of action, and interindividual variability in dosing requirements Unintended effects can last for several hours	Expensive and availability can vary based on country/region	Limited data on topical preparations; including the extent of systemic absorption Local effects may not be strong enough/penetrate to depth to produce desired symptom relief

 Information gathered from [1, 2]

[a]See Chap. 31 on Product Safety and Quality Control, Table 31.2, for more information on concentrates

Oromucosal

Oromucosal preparations are available as buccal sprays, tinctures, and lozenges, and generally contain an alcohol base to enhance absorption from the oral cavity. The best evidence for oromucosal cannabis preparations is for nabiximols (such as Sativex©) which are pharmaceutically developed, plant-derived cannabis products that deliver a standardized 1:1 ratio of THC and CBD with each spray (see Chap. 17 on Nabiximols (Sativex®)) [13].

The onset of action of oromucosal products is between that of the inhalation and oral routes, where it is slower than inhalation, but faster than oral cannabis onset [9]. However, the duration of action of oromucosal products are comparable to oral cannabis preparations, (Table 22.1) since some of the spray is swallowed [2]. Oromucosal sprays (i.e., nabiximols) may be particularly helpful among those experiencing difficulty in measuring daily doses with other cannabis products (e.g., cannabis oils, vaporizing). However, they may be limited in use due to a lack of availability and affordability for some individuals and populations. There is limited evidence for products such as lozenges and other tinctures; however, this is certainly a very desired route for patients who are not interested in inhaling cannabis and want a faster onset of action.

Topical

A summary of the differences and similarities of the varying routes of administration can be found in Table 22.1. Due to first-pass metabolism and digestion, oral consumption of cannabis has a reduced bioavailability compared to inhaling cannabis, translating into a greater onset of action and increased duration of effects. In comparison, smoking and vaporization provide a more rapid, delivery of THC via alveoli in the lungs, allowing for rapid absorption into the bloodstream [14]. However, smoking requires full combustion of dried flower, which also releases harmful by-products such as tar, carbon monoxide, ammonia, and polycyclic aromatic hydrocarbons [3], thus increasing the risk for acute and/or chronic pulmonary-bronchial harms [15]. Vaporization requires less heat application than smoking and therefore has been increasingly popular as a "safer" method to consume cannabis, as it produces fewer toxic by-products, including significantly decreased CO concentrations when used appropriately [3, 4]. It is important to consider the varying onset of effects between routes of administration and the cannabinoid composition (i.e., CBD vs. THC) when titrating doses and making recommendations to patients in avoiding adverse events, discussed below.

There is limited evidence for topical formulations, which demonstrate variable kinetic profiles [16]. Patients report that some preparations may have a fast onset of action, similar to inhalation, however, with a slightly longer duration of action (still less than oral). Topicals may contain cannabis that is either CBD-dominant, THC-dominant, or combinations of both THC and CBD. This route is generally not effective in managing systemic symptoms, such as sleep initiation, generalized pain, and nausea, as topical preparations do not penetrate intact skin deep enough to enter the bloodstream, or contain large enough cannabinoid quantities. This factor may be advantageous in patients with localized symptoms who want to minimize daytime exposure to THC while also decreasing potential risks such as impairment during work/driving hours.

It is generally recommended to use topicals on small-to-medium areas. Variables to consider which affect topical skin penetration (and hence efficacy) include the carrier base, covering the site after application, skin integrity, and essential oils/terpenes from the cannabis plant (which may disrupt the skin barrier). Topicals may be more effective in areas with minimal adipose tissue. Patients have reported that topicals help with joint pain including small joints in the hands, wrists, knees, feet, and elbows. This may be due to CB1 receptors found in the synovial membrane, as demostrated in some animal models [17]. It has also been reported by patients that topicals can be especially helpful for musculoskeletal pain including inflammatory, non-inflammatory, and connective tissue injuries including sprains and strains [14]. Another common use of topicals is to treat headaches (scalp, temporal, and jaw area), myalgias – especially paraspinal/cervical area, and musculoskeletal injuries [14]. There has been an increasing demand for topicals in skin conditions including psoriasis, eczema, and challenging ulcers (i.e., pyoderma gangrenosum and sickle cell), as well as more common household conditions such as burns and wound pain [18].

Dosing

Concentration and Potency

Cannabis dosing is dependent on the THC and/or CBD content of each plant chemovar, which is labeled as a percentage of CBD or THC in the total weight of the dried cannabis flower (%/g), or by concentration in cannabis oils (mg/ml). The cannabinoid concentration in the cannabis flower can typically range from 0.1% to 30% of CBD and/or THC. In unregulated markets, THC concentrations have large variability, as do the ratios of other cannabinoids in these products, including CBD and other cannabinoids, as well as terpenes.

In order to dose cannabis products accurately, given that impairment and adverse events are THC dose-dependent, recommendations should be based on the mg of THC, not on the concentration (%) [2]. The exact mg of THC consumed in each dose can be calculated (approximately) if the potency (%) and mg of the product consumed are both known [19]. This tends to be easier when working with oils than with dried flower. For example, assuming 100% absorption, a chemovar containing 24% THC would theoretically deliver 240 mg of THC to a patient if they inhaled 1 gram of that dried product. However, if the chemovar contained 12% THC, it would instead provide 120 mg of THC per 1 gram of dried flower, meaning that the patient would need to consume 2 grams of the 12% THC to receive the same mg of THC as the chemovar containing 24% THC. Generally, consider recommending a higher concentration chemovar for patients with limited income, as it may be more cost-efficient given that less product is needed to deliver the desired dose (see Chap. 31 on Product Safety and Quality Control, Table 31.2, for more information on concentrates).

Cannabis Flower Dosing

Dosing strategy for cannabis flower is described in Fig. 22.1. First, the chemovar is selected, and then "mindful vaping" technique is used. The vast majority of patients vaporize for acute symptomatic relief. As a result, THC:CBD in a

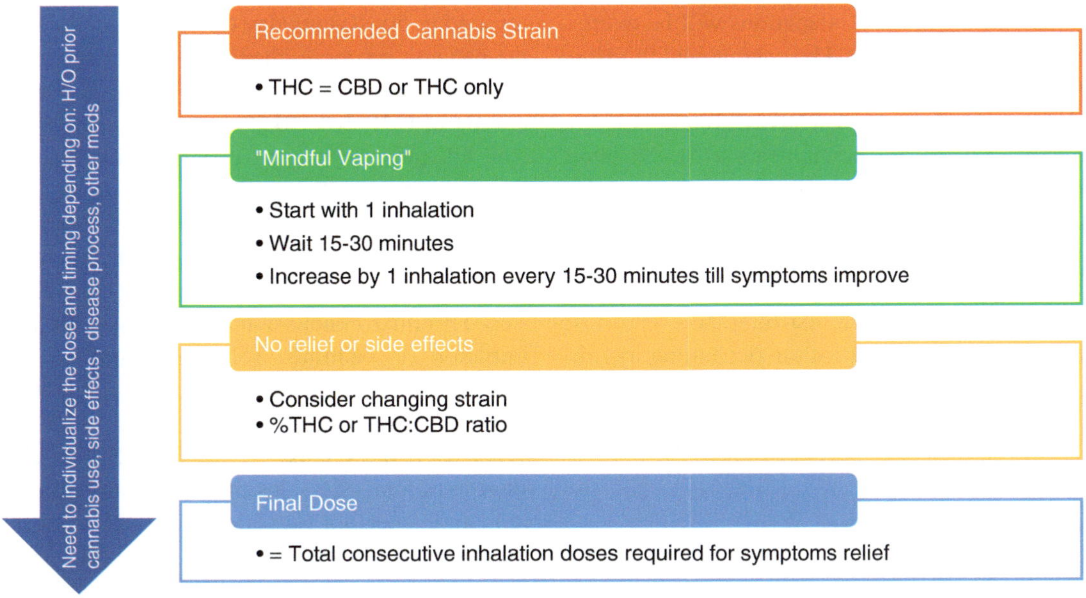

Fig. 22.1 Suggested algorithm for initiating and titrating cannabis flowers (© Caroline MacCallum, MD, and Samer Narouze, MD, PhD, used with permission)

1:1 ratio, or THC dominant chemovars are most commonly used by patients (CBD does not have the "breakthrough" effect). This is a way to encourage patients to take an one inhalation, then wait 15–30 minutes, and then check in and see how they feel. The lowest effective dose ("less is more") is especially important for new patients. Since the onset of action for inhalation is 5–10 minutes (Table 22.1); as long as a patient waits atleast 15 minutes between inhalations that should be acceptable. Subsequently, they can continue increasing by one inhalation each time they take another dose, again waiting set time between doses. Their total dose is the sum of all the inhalations required to achieve symptom control in one "sitting". So, for example, if a patient took one inhalation, waited 15–30 minutes; then two inhalations, waited 15–30 minutes; and then three inhalations and then had relief of symptoms, their optimal dose would be six inhalations for that specific flower. The next time they dose, they can take six inhalations consecutively, without waiting 15–30 minutes between inhalations. Take caution in summing up the number of inhalations if there are gaps longer than 30 minutes between inhalations, as the concentration of cannabinoids will be reduced and the total inhalations will be overestimated. Patients should be encouraged to restart this process for each new type of cannabis flower they use. Each flower can have different potency, and even if the potency appears to be the same, the cannabinoid profile will likely vary and that can increase or decrease the efficacy for that flower. If a patient stops using cannabis for more than 5 days, they should restart this whole process as they will have lost tolerance. The dose can vary with vaporization depending on the severity of symptoms, and it is common for patients to adjust the dose based on symptoms.

Cannabis Oil Dosing

Although THC-mediated adverse events are often early and transient, improving the safety profile of medicinal cannabis can be achieved through low dosing and slow titration. The safest dosing strategy for cannabis is to "start low, go slow", and to stay at the lowest dose that allows the patient to reach their treatment goals with minimal/no side effects. With safe appropriate dosing, side effects (such as euphoria) can be avoided/minimized while achieving symptom management [2]. Adverse events are also mitigated when patients develop a tolerance to these effects over a number of days, without developing a tolerance to the benefit.

Patients do not need to experience euphoria in order to achieve symptom improvement. Incorporating CBD into a THC-dominant regimen can be helpful in balancing THC-mediated adverse events, especially for cannabis-naïve patients. Patients can better tolerate higher doses of THC when CBD is present with THC vs. THC (or synthetic THC) "monotherapy" [2, 20, 21].

Another alternative to minimize THC adverse events is to start patients on a CBD-dominant regimen, as many patients may not need to use THC to manage their daytime symptoms. Figure 22.2 demonstrates a safe initiation and titration for cannabis oil. Consider starting patients on 5 mg of CBD-dominant oil twice daily (Fig. 22.2, step 1), and titrate by 5 mg CBD twice daily (Fig. 22.2, step 2), every 2–3 days. The majority of patients respond to 50–100 mg/day (2, 28). Depending on the patient's response, the titration increase could be drawn out to increase every 2–7 days. However, a 5 mg of CBD twice daily increment increase is well tolerated, and most patients can increase by this amount every 2–3 days.

Daytime CBD oil can continue to be titrated alone, or if there are issues with sleep, 1–2.5 mg of THC can also be initiated at bedtime (Fig. 22.2, step 1); either concurrently with daytime CBD initiation or bedtime. THC initiation can be delayed until daytime CBD is optimized. Continue increasing bedtime THC by 1–2.5 mg every 2–7 days (Fig. 22.2, step 2) [2, 22]. Beginning oral THC dosing at bedtime is common and beneficial for patients who do not want to experience the effects of THC during the day. Consider dosing cannabis oil 1–2 hours prior to bed for those with difficulty initiating sleep or administering it at bedtime for those with sleep maintenance issues.

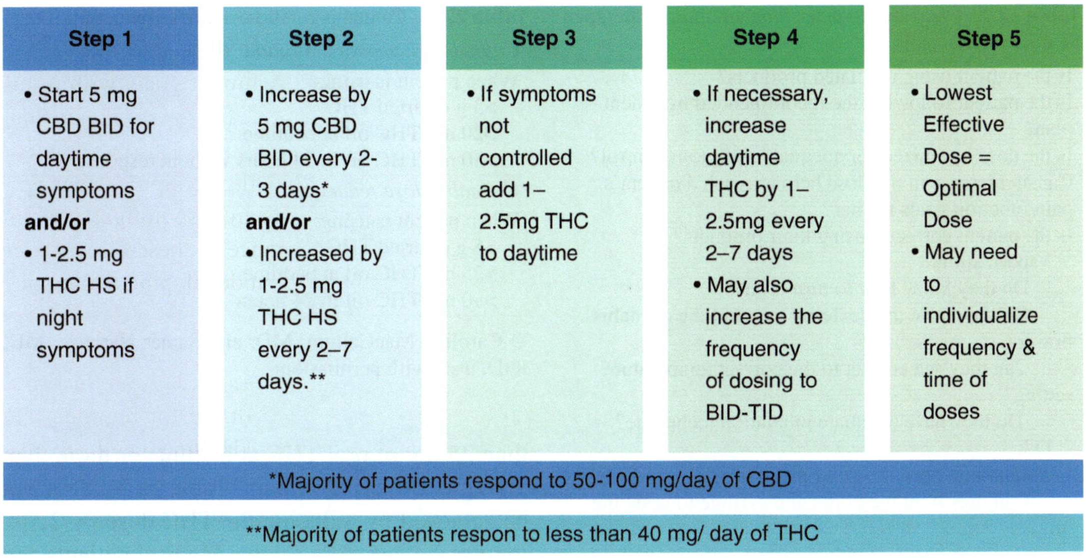

Fig. 22.2 Suggested algorithm for initiating and titrating cannabis oils (© Caroline MacCallum, MD, and Julia JA Clark used with permission)

If daytime symptom alleviation is not achieved after titrating daytime CBD dose to target as well as nighttime THC to target (Fig. 22.2, step 2), consider initiating 1–2.5 mg of THC during daytime and titrating by 1–2.5 mg every 2–7 days (Fig. 22.2, step 3). The majority of patients respond to less than 40 mg THC/day while maintaining the patient's CBD dose from this point on (28). If this is well-tolerated, continue to increase the dose of THC in 1–2.5 mg increments and increase the frequency to two to three times per day (Fig. 22.2, step 4). Titrate the dose to the optimal dose or the lowest effective dose (Fig. 22.2, step 5) until adequate symptom management is achieved, aiming for less than 40 mg of THC total dose daily [2]. If considering going above 40 mg/day of THC, expert consultation is recommended. Since adverse events of cannabis are due to THC, it is important to modify the dose of cannabis based on the milligrams of THC.

For patients suffering from severe pain and/or functional impairment, those in palliative care, or patients who have experience with cannabis use (either medically or recreationally), a "rapid treatment" protocol is suggested [28]. Patients could start on a balanced THC/CBD product at a slightly higher dose of 2.5–5 mg (THC/CBD) once day increasing to twice daily and titrating by 2.5–5 mg (THC/CBD) every 2–3 days until the patient's goals are met or until 40 mg of THC has been reached [22].

Patients should be informed that if they experience any THC adverse events (see Chap. 36 on Cannabinoid-Related Adverse Events and Impairment), they should transition back to the previous, most well-tolerated dose. If the patient is an older adult and/or has complex comorbidities or extensive polypharmacy, a lower starting dose of 1 mg of THC should be considered which can be increased by the same dose every 2–7 evenings.

Achieving Optimal Therapeutic Dose and Cannabis Rotation

The optimal therapeutic dose is the dose which allows the patient to reach their pain/function treatment goals with minimal or no side effects. Slow dose increase over time helps tolerance to build slowly (i.e., to minimize potential euphoria

Table 22.2 Questions to determine an optimal therapeutic dose for cannabis

Is the patient using regulated products?
Is the patient following the recommended treatment plan?
Is the dose optimized for adequate symptom control?
Can an increase in the dose help to reach a patient's pain/function goals further?
Is the patient correctly using their products?
Vaporization:
Do they know how to turn it on?
Do they have the dexterity to grind the cannabis flower?
Can they see and set to the correct temperature setting?
Do they have adequate inhalation technique?
Oil:
Can they open the child-proof top?
Can they hold the bottle and syringe to draw the oil?
Can they see the graduations on the syringe?
Are there any adverse events experienced?
Does the product type or route of administration or chemovar need to be changed?
Does the chemovar cannabinoid composition need to be changed?
Is the patient adherent to treatment? Are there cost barriers to optimizing cannabis dose (especially for CBD)? If they have a drug plan, would a prescription for nabilone help affordability?

and side effects) as dose is titrated to manage symptoms. Please see Table 22.2 for questions to ask patients in determining their therapeutic dose.

Cannabis Chemovar Rotation and Reduction

Changing the type of cannabis plant, route of administration, and dose may be helpful for some individuals to achieve better control of their symptoms. Additionally, adherence can be another important consideration if treatment goals are not being met, and this should be regularly assessed (Tables 22.2 and 22.3).

Based on clinical experience, consider reducing cannabis if a patient is using more than 5 g of THC predominant dried cannabis or dose of more than 25 mg of oral THC at bedtime or more than 50 mg oral oil in 24 hours (Table 22.3). This can be achieved by reducing the THC dose by 2.5–5 mg per day every 2–7 days. Medical patients can frequently reduce quickly depending on their starting dose. If consuming higher doses of THC or concerns of cannabis use disorder, a longer and slower taper may be required. CBD could be incorporated if the patient is not tolerating the reduction in THC or symptoms are bothersome.

Table 22.3 Cannabis rotation and dose reduction

Cannabis chemovar "rotation"
When patient is using:
>3 g of dried THC
>20 mg THC oil at bedtime
>30 mg THC oil in 24 hours without response
Cannabis dose reduction
When patient is using:
>5 g of dried THC
>25 mg THC oil at bedtime
>50 mg THC oil in 24 hours

Patients will normally have a reduced THC tolerance ('washout') after 5 days of stopping THC-containing cannabis. However, in some patients this can take up to two weeks or more. It has been observed that after this washout, patients respond to cannabis as if they were previously naive to THC. If reinnitiating THC containing cannabis, it is suggested to restart THC at a dose of 2.5 mg.

There are many situations where a patient may need to stop or reduce cannabis use (e.g., travelling, hospitalization, incarceration). Practically, if the patient is using less than 2 g of THC-predominant dried cannabis, or less than 20 mg of THC oil per day, they are unlikely to have any signs of withdrawal and, therefore, there is no need to slowly taper the THC dose. Even above these doses, withdrawal symptoms are infrequently seen in medical cannabis patients. The primary concern with stopping medical cannabis is a decrease in control of their health condition for which this medication is being used to manage.

Monitoring

Monitoring is an essential component of the cannabis treatment plan as it aids in establishing the patient's effective cannabis dose, and in reaching their desired pain/function goals, while also ensuring safety. When determining the monitoring strategy for cannabis with an individual patient, prior experience with cannabis, comorbid medical conditions, and the ability to adhere to a treatment plan, should be taken into consideration. Special populations (see Chaps. 23, 33 and 34) in particular may need more regular follow-up visits than others. Initially, consider follow-up within 1–3 months of starting the treatment plan to review the dose and corresponding symptom outcomes, concurrent medications, and potential drug interactions, with the possibility of tapering other medications, if appropriate. After the patient is stabilized on a particular dose, consider follow-up appointments every 3–6 months, depending on the patient's medical history, prior cannabis experience, and their ability to adhere to the treatment plan [2] (Table 22.4).

Patients should be encouraged to track their cannabis use, including the products they use, route of administration, dose, and a record of individual symptoms and/or condition outcomes and adverse events (see Chap. 36 on Cannabinoid-Related Adverse Events and Impairment). The use of a mobile cannabis tracking app may be helpful for patients, as well as for clinicians, in attaining an optimal cannabis dose for their patients. Alternatively, this can be done in the form of a journal (see Fig. 22.3). Finally, healthcare providers can also implement validated questionnaires such as GAD-7 (General Anxiety Disorder-7) [23], depression PHQ-9 (Patient Health Questionnaire) [24], and the BPI (Brief Pain Inventory) pain scale [25], which may provide some objective measures. These results can be tracked in subsequent follow-up visits to help inform future cannabis dosing and direction as well as for research and pharmacovigilance purposes.

Table 22.4 Proposed management of cannabis adverse events

Mild/moderate	Severe	Possible cannabis adjustments to address adverse events
Encourage patient to reach out for support Use breathing (i.e. "box breathing") and mindfulness techniques Use distraction techniques	Recommend patient to safely proceed to ER (i.e., someone else to drive) Stop cannabis use	Return to previously tolerated dose Add or increase CBD Reduce THC dose Change chemovar Change route of administration Stop cannabis use if risk outweighs benefit

Summary

Patients should be educated on proper vaporization and/or cannabis oil dosing and titration regimens (Fig. 22.1). The optimal therapeutic dose is the dose that allows the patient to reach his/her pain/function treatment goals with minimal or no side effects. Euphoria or impairment (i.e., feeling "high") does not have to occur in order to experience symptom improvement.

It is preferred to start low and go slow when titrating to the optimal dose. The most accurate dosing uses mg of THC and CBD via oils. This is more challenging with cannabis flower due to many variables. Starting with CBD primarily for daytime symptom control as a standalone (without THC) is preferential, with THC for night time symptoms. If daytime symptoms are not well controlled, THC can be added to daytime regimen. Inhaled THC is short-acting over oils and may be preferred as a "PRN" depending on lifestyle factors. If using THC flower for daytime, consider recommending a chemovar that also contains CBD to reduce adverse events. Patients require ongoing monitoring by a healthcare provider to achieve optimal therapeutic dose, as they may require adjustments to their products and regimen (Fig. 22.4).

Date: ______________________

Licensed Producer: ____________ Product/Strain: ____________________

Route of Administration: ☐ Inhalation ☐ Oral Oil ☐ Topical

Dose Consumed: ________________________________

if you are consuming oral oil use the ilustralid below and fill in the dose you consumed.

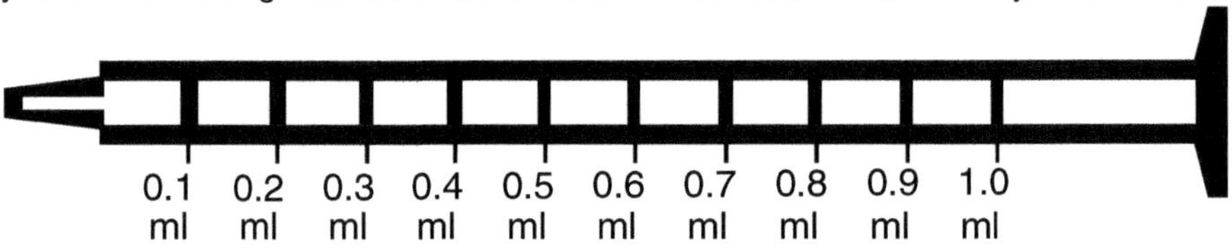

Time Taken: ___________ am pm Onset Time: _____ Duration of Effects= ________

Positive Effects On Symptoms

☐ Pain Relief
☐ Muscle Relaxation
☐ Energizing
☐ Motivating
☐ Inflamation Reduct.
☐ Improved Sleep
☐ Tremor Reduction
☐ Seizure Reduction
☐ Intestinal Ease
☐ Appetite Stimulated
☐ Mental Focus
☐ Mood lilted
☐ Other ______________________

Negatives

☐ Anxiety
☐ Dizziness
☐ Drowsiness
☐ Sleepiness
☐ Nausea
☐ Diarrhea
☐ Headache
☐ Impaired
☐ Memory Issues
☐ Brain Fog
☐ Fatique
☐ Dry Mouth
☐ Other: ____________________

How effective was your medication?

Mark an X or circle your overall feeling after taking your medication. Your optimal dose is the dose what gives you the most amount of symptom relief with the least amolun of side effects.

–4	–3	–2	–1	0	1	2	3	4

Much Worse **No Change** **Optimal**

Notes

____

____

____

Fig. 22.3 Patient journal to monitor cannabis efficacy and adverse events (© Caroline MacCallum, MD, and Fonda Betts, use with permission)

1. Does symptom occur during day or night?

- **Night** - sleep is a great place to start THC.

  –**High myrcene/ "sedating" THC** may be more helpful than CBD for sleep. It helps with pain, anxiety, insomnia. If sleep improves, so will ability to cope with daytime symptoms

- **Daytime - try CBD alone, or CBD with THC, or low close THC** to minimize impairment.

2. Type of symptom?

- Acute/Intermittent symptom = **vaporize**
- Chronic/persistent symptom = **oil**

3. Pathophysiology of Condition

- Inflammatory = CBD
- Neurological =THC (+/- CBD)
- Exceptions: seizures, psychosis/bipolar = CBD

4. Special populations consideraions

- Geriatric, severe cardiac disease, frail = may start even lower than low for THC (ie 1mg)
- Children= avoid THC

5. Add cannabis on to other prescription, then consider slow reduce opioids/other medications one at a time if appropriate.

Fig. 22.4 Cannabis treatment algorithm (© Caroline MacCallum, MD, used with permission)

References

1. Kansagara D, Becker WC, Ayers C, Tetrault JM. Priming primary care providers to engage in evidence-based discussions about cannabis with patients. Addict Sci Clin Pract. 2019;14(1):42.
2. MacCallum CA, Russo EB. Practical considerations in medical cannabis administration and dosing. Eur J Intern Med. 2018;49:12–9.
3. Russell C, Rueda S, Room R, Tyndall M, Fischer B. Routes of administration for cannabis use–basic prevalence and related health outcomes: a scoping review and synthesis. Int J Drug Policy. 2018;52:87–96.
4. Abrams DI, Vizoso HP, Shade SB, Jay C, Kelly ME, Benowitz NL. Vaporization as a smokeless cannabis delivery system: a pilot study. Clin Pharm Therap. 2007;82(5):572–8.
5. Ko GD, Bober SL, Mindra S, Moreau JM. Medical cannabis–the Canadian perspective. J Pain Res. 2016;9:735.
6. Repka MA, Munjal M, ElSohly MA, Ross SA. Temperature stability and bioadhesive properties of Δ9-tetrahydrocannabinol incorporated hydroxypropylcellulose polymer matrix systems. Drug Dev Ind Pharm. 2006;32(1):21–32.
7. Vulfsons S, Ognitz M, Bar-Sela G, Raz-Pasteur A, Eisenberg E. Cannabis treatment in hospitalized patients using the SYQE inhaler: results of a pilot open-label study. Palliat Support Care. 2020;18(1):12–7.
8. Zgair A, Wong JC, Lee JB, Mistry J, Sivak O, Wasan KM, et al. Dietary fats and pharmaceutical lipid excipients increase systemic exposure to orally administered cannabis and cannabis-based medicines. Am J Transl Res. 2016;8(8):3448.
9. Huestis MA. Human cannabinoid pharmacokinetics. Chem Biodivers. 2007;4(8):1770.
10. Karschner EL, Darwin WD, Goodwin RS, Wright S, Huestis MA. Plasma cannabinoid pharmacokinetics following controlled oral Δ9-tetrahydrocannabinol and oromucosal cannabis extract administration. Clin Chem. 2011;57(1):66–75.
11. Huestis M. Pharmacokinetics of THC in inhaled and oral preparations. In: Marihuana and medicine. Totowa, NJ: Humana Press; 1999. p. 105–16.
12. Hammond D. Communicating THC levels and 'dose' to consumers: implications for product labelling and packaging of cannabis products in regulated markets. Int J Drug Policy. 2019:102509.
13. Guy GW, Stott CG. The development of Sativex®—a natural cannabis-based medicine. In: Cannabinoids as therapeutics. Birkhäuser Basel; 2005. p. 231–63.

14. Li X, Vigil JM, Stith SS, Brockelman F, Keeling K, Hall B. The effectiveness of self-directed medical cannabis treatment for pain. Complement Ther Med. 2019;46:123–30.
15. Jett J, Stone E, Warren G, Cummings KM. Cannabis use, lung cancer, and related issues. J Thorac Oncol. 2018;13(4):480–7.
16. Bartner LR, McGrath S, Rao S, Hyatt LK, Wittenburg LA. Pharmacokinetics of cannabidiol administered by 3 delivery methods at 2 different dosages to healthy dogs. Can J Vet Res. 2018;82(3):178–83.
17. McDougall JJ. Cannabinoids and pain control in the periphery. In: Peripheral receptor targets for analgesia. Hoboken, NJ: Wiley; 2009. p. 325–46.
18. Maida V, Corban J. Topical medical cannabis: a new treatment for wound pain—three cases of Pyoderma Gangrenosum. J Pain Symptom Manag. 2017;54(5):732–6.
19. Freeman TP, Lorenzetti V. Moving forwards with the standard THC unit. Addiction. 2020;
20. Sellers EM, Schoedel K, Bartlett C, Romach M, Russo EB, Stott CG, et al. A multiple-dose, randomized, double-blind, placebo-controlled, parallel-group QT/QTc study to evaluate the electrophysiologic effects of THC/CBD spray. Clin Pharm Drug Dev. 2013;2(3):285–94.
21. Favrat B, Ménétrey A, Augsburger M, Rothuizen LE, Appenzeller M, Buclin T, et al. Two cases of "cannabis acute psychosis" following the administration of oral cannabis. BMC Psychiatry. 2005;5(1):1–6.
22. Bhaskar A, Bell A, Boivin M, Briques W, Brown M, Clarke H, Cyr C, Eisenberg E, Silva RFDO, Frohlich E, Georgius P, Hogg M, Horsted TI, MacCallum CA, Müller-Vahl KR, O'Connell C, Sealey R, Seibolt M, Sihota A, Smith B, Sulak D, Vigano A, Moulin DE. Global Task Force on Dosing and Administration of Medical Cannabis for Treatment of Chronic Pain; 2020. (submitted).
23. Spitzer RL, Kroenke K, Williams JB, Löwe B. A brief measure for assessing generalized anxiety disorder: the GAD-7. Arch Intern Med. 2006;166(10):1092–7.
24. Kroenke K, Spitzer RL, Williams JB. The PHQ-9: validity of a brief depression severity measure. J Gen Intern Med. 2001;16(9):606–13. https://doi.org/10.1046/j.1525-1497.2001.016009606.x.
25. Tan G, Jensen MP, Thornby JI, Shanti BF. Validation of the Brief Pain Inventory for chronic nonmalignant pain. J Pain. 2004;5(2):133–7.

Cannabinoid-Based Medicines: Patient Safety Considerations

23

Caroline A. MacCallum, Lindsay A. Lo, and Michael Boivin

Introduction

Cannabis education can mitigate risks and promote patient safety. There are considerations, precautions, relative contraindications, and contraindications for cannabinoids use. It is important for clinicians recommending cannabis (CRC) to assess the benefits and risks of medical cannabis use for each patient individually. General contraindications for cannabis use include those who have severe and unstable cardiac and pulmonary conditions, psychosis, those who are pregnant/breastfeeding, and adolescents (Table 23.1).

Patients need to be evaluated on a case-by-case basis, as there may still be options available, and contraindications may not necessarily be "absolute." Further research is needed to assert definitive conclusions around contraindications for cannabis use, as data pertaining to this topic remains varied.

Practical Considerations for Cannabis Use

It is important to understand some of the generalization and assumptions implied in Table 23.1:

1. Contraindications typically pertain to the use of THC and are dose-dependent.
2. CBD may be an option even where THC may be a contraindication. CBD does not have the same adverse event profile as THC.
3. CBD and THC can be used as a means for harm reduction for substances with greater risk of morbidity and mortality (i.e., opioids).
4. CBD could be an appropriate harm reduction in patients who have a contraindication to THC and/or are currently using high doses of THC (i.e., psychosis or pregnancy).
5. Finally, some contraindications are specific to the route of administration (smoking) especially in those with respiratory conditions. Ingestible cannabis oils and even vaporization would be safer options in these patients where smoking would be contraindicated.

C. A. MacCallum (✉)
Department of Medicine, Faculty of Medicine, University of British Columbia, Vancouver, BC, Canada
e-mail: info@drcarolinemaccallum.com

L. A. Lo
Department of Psychology, Queen's University, Kingston, ON, Canada

M. Boivin
CommPharm Consulting, Barrie, ON, Canada

S. N. Narouze (ed.), *Cannabinoids and Pain*, https://doi.org/10.1007/978-3-030-69186-8_23

Table 23.1 Considerations and potential contraindication for cannabinoid

Considerations	Precautions	Relative contraindications	Contraindications
Immunocompromised Chronic kidney disease Older adults Patients with concurrent medical conditions Polypharmacy Potential drug interactions	Concurrent mood or anxiety disorder Have risk factors for cardiovascular disease Tobacco use E-cigarette use Severe liver dysfunction /disease Medications associated with sedation or cognitive impairment Driving or safety sensitive occupations	Under 25 years of age Current or past cannabis use disorder Current or past substance use disorder	Unstable cardiovascular disease Respiratory disease (if smoking cannabis) Personal or strong family history of psychosis/ bipolar Pregnant, planning on becoming pregnant, or breastfeeding

© Caroline MacCallum, MD, used with permission. Information gathered from Refs. [1–3]

Considerations

Immunocompromised Patients

When recommending cannabis to immunocompromised patients, clinicians should ensure high-quality products that are free of contaminants and toxins. Due to cannabis being a plant, there is a possibility that it can become infected with microorganisms. Immunocompromised users are at a higher risk of developing infections from contaminated cannabis, especially when using inhaled cannabis. As such, a regulated source that is compliant with mandatory contaminant testing should always be used for immunocompromised populations. Best practice is to select producers using gamma radiation on dried flower and carbon dioxide extraction when extracting CBD and THC for oils to ensure microorganisms such as fungus and bacteria are killed.

Calcineurin Inhibitors, Protein Disulfide Isomerase (PD1) Inhibitors, and Biologics

The immunosuppressive calcineurin inhibitors such as cyclosporine and tacrolimus are metabolized by CYP 3A4 (see Table 23.2 cannabinoid-drug interactions below). The use of these agents with CBD can increase the level of calcineurin inhibitor toxicity. Therefore, it may be best to avoid cannabis in this patient population, unless the risk benefit ratio for other symptoms favors otherwise as that point considering lower dose of cannabis should be done under the direction of a cannabis expert.

Caution should be used with PD1 inhibitors, also known as immune checkpoint inhibitors. In a retrospective analysis, cannabis (CBD) may worsen the efficacy of nivolumab in those with advanced melanoma, non-small cell lung cancer, and renal clear cell carcinoma [4]. Cannabis can help relieve many symptoms associated with cancer and chemotherapy and allow for full completion of immunotherapy, as well as reduce the need for glucocorticosteroids. It is recommended to hold cannabis a few days pre- and post-immunotherapy infusion [5], although more research is required to determine the significance of this interaction on treatment outcomes.

Biologic therapies are commonly used for autoimmune inflammatory conditions, multiple sclerosis, asthma, and some malignancies. These medications do not have the same mechanism of action as PD1 inhibitors and are not metabolized by CYP 3A4. They may safely be used concurrently with cannabinoids.

Chronic Kidney Disease

It is important for patients with chronic kidney disease (CKD) to avoid smoking and to abstain from illicit sources of cannabis that may contain contaminants such as heavy metals, pesticides,

Table 23.2 Potential cannabinoid drug interactions[a]

Enzyme	Interaction and effect	Drugs
CYP 3A4	*Inducers:* may decrease THC and/or CBD *Inhibitors:* may increase THC and/or CBD *Substrates:* CBD is potential inhibitor of CYP3A4 and could increase 3A4 substrates. Caution with medications with smaller therapeutic index (e.g., tacrolimus). Unlikely to have effect on THC	Carbamazepine, phenobarbital, phenytoin, rifampin, St. John's wort Azole antifungals, clarithromycin, diltiazem, erythromycin, grapefruit, HIV protease inhibitors, macrolides, mifepristone, verapamil Alprazolam, atorvastatin, carbamazepine, clobazam, cyclosporine, diltiazem, HIV protease inhibitors, buprenorphine, tacrolimus, cyclosporine, phenytoin, sildenafil, simvastatin, sirolimus, verapamil, zopiclone
CYP 2C9	*Inducers:* may decrease THC concentration. Unlikely to have effect on CBD *Inhibitors:* may increase THC concentration. Unlikely to have effect on CBD *Substrates:* THC and/or CBD may increase drug levels, should monitor for toxicity	Amiodarone, fluconazole, fluoxetine, metronidazole, valproic acid, sulfamethoxazole Carbamazepine, rifampin Warfarin, rosuvastatin, phenytoin
CYP 2C19	*Inducers:* may decrease CBD and THC *Inhibitors*: may increase CBD and THC *Substrates:* CBD may increase the level of medications metabolized by 2C19 such as norclobazam (active metabolite in clobazam). CBD may also prevent clopidogrel from being activated. Unlikely to have effect on THC	Carbamazepine, rifampin, St. John's wort Cimetidine, omeprazole, esomeprazole, ticlopidine, fluconazole, fluoxetine, isoniazid Aripiprazole, citalopram, clopidogrel, diazepam, escitalopram, moclobemide, norclobazam, omeprazole, pantoprazole, sertraline
CYP 1A1 and 1A2	*Substrates:* smoking cannabis can stimulate these isoenzymes and increase the metabolism of these medications	Amitriptyline, caffeine, clozapine, duloxetine, estrogens, fluvoxamine, imipramine, melatonin, mirtazapine, olanzapine, theophylline
p-glycoprotein	*Substrates:* CBD may inhibit p-glycoprotein drug transport. Should monitor for toxicity. No effect from use of THC	Dabigatran, digoxin, loperamide

© Caroline MacCallum, MD, used with permission. Information gathered from Refs. [11, 15–21, 49]

[a]Formal drug interaction studies with cannabinoids have not been conducted. Other drug interactions are possible as more individuals use cannabinoids with other medications

and solvents [6]. However, cannabinoids are generally safe among patients with CKD. For instance, when administered orally, cannabinoids are primarily metabolized by the liver, and then excreted in feces, with only 20% of metabolites being excreted in urine. There is no evidence to suggest that CBD adversely affects kidney function, although there may be a concern with CBD-drug interactions involving kidney transplantation [6]. Cannabis has a potential role in improving many symptoms associated with end-stage renal disease (ESRD) and CKD [7]. Two-thirds of individuals with stage 3–5 CKD experience pain, with many using opioids. Nausea and vomiting are common for those on hemodialysis (1 in 5 patients). Anorexia, insomnia, and uremic pruritus are also common in ESRD. These symptoms may be responsive to cannabis therapy and may be an option for some of these individuals.

Older Adults and Patients with Concurrent Medical Conditions

Cannabis can be a useful tool in elderly populations. It may be an appropriate choice in elderly patients exhibiting a poor response or inability to take traditional treatments. Elderly patients are more likely to use cannabis for medical purposes compared to other age cohorts, and have been reported to experience associated improvements in quality of life, sleep, appetite, and pain [8]. There has been no preclinical or clinical evidence to suggest that higher CBD levels may be toxic among older subjects. To make this statement, strong, high-quality evidence is required. It may be that risks due to cannabis use among the elderly are related to chronic histories of recreational use rather than acute impairments and toxicities [9].

Importantly, there is increasing evidence in the potential role of cannabis to reduce polypharmacy. Data from a large elderly sample population ($N = 901$) supports medical cannabis as a safe and efficacious treatment option for elderly people [8]. The most common indications for medical use of cannabis were cancer-associated pain (36.6%), nonspecific pain (30%), and symptoms related to chemotherapy treatment (24.2%). After 6 months of cannabis use, 93.7% showed slight to significant improvement with 41.9% showing a significant improvement. The median in pain intensity reduction on a 10-point pain scale was from 8/10 to 4/10. Interestingly, the number of falls actually decreased from 53.4% to 21.9%. There was also a reduction in opioid analgesic use or complete cessation in 18.1% of patients. Quality of life also significantly improved 6 months post-cannabis treatment among this sample ($p < 0.001$, n = 861). Only 3.6% of participants reported a severe adverse event. The authors reported that 31.7% of participants experienced an adverse event with the most common being dizziness (9.7%) and dry mouth (7.1%) [8]. Overall, the authors concluded cannabis to be safe and efficacious in elderly populations. They noted improvements in all conditions and pain levels and that cannabis treatment may reduce the use of other medications [8]. Though evidence supports the benefits of medical cannabis for some elderly patients, it should still be used with caution. Specifically, lower starting dose, slower titration, and later THC introduction are recommended in order to avoid adverse events such as falls and orthostatic hypotension, which are more common among this population.

Polypharmacy and Drug Interactions [10]

Cannabis is generally safe to use concomitantly with other medications, as significant drug interactions are uncommon [10]. To date, there are no known drugs that cannot be used with cannabis if necessary [11]. Most of the concern for drug interactions involves the use of cannabis with CNS depressants. While it should be stressed no drug-drug interactions with cannabis pose a risk for cardiac or respiratory arrest, there is potential for additive side effects at the pharmacodynamic level. For instance, when clobazam is taken with a high dose of CBD (>200–300mg), higher levels of N-desmethylclobazam, a sedating metabolite, may be produced. This could result in increased sedation, and therefore caregivers should be counselled on such. A slow CBD titration is recommended in these patients so that if sedation was to increase, it would be gradual in onset. At that point, clobazam could be reduced, providing treatment goals are being met (ie reduction in seizures) [12]. Blood testing for metabolites could be considered, however, typically the increase sedation is evident clinically (and gradually) before lab tests result. Worsened sedation and cognitive impairment can occur with the concomitant use of cannabis and alcohol, opioids, antipsychotics, benzodiazepines, tricyclic antidepressants, or antiepileptics [13]. Recent evidence has suggested CBD may cause elevated liver enzymes in some individuals [14]. The influence of CBD dose and co-morbidities has not yet been established. Baseline and repeat liver enzymes during the initiation period of CBD may be warranted in some cases.

THC is oxidized predominantly by CYP family enzymes 2C9, 2C19, and 3A4, while CBD is metabolized predominantly by CYP2C19 and CYP3A4. Therefore, CYP inhibitors may increase serum levels, while CYP enzyme inducers may decrease serum levels. Potential pharmacokinetic drug interactions involving CYP enzymes are outlined in Table 23.2. It is important to note that, although theoretically drugs metabolized by the CYP enzyme family may interact with cannabis, many of these findings have not been established in humans. The most robust data regarding drug interactions comes from clinical trials with Nabiximols, which found most data to not be clinically significant. If a patient is deemed at risk for an actual or potential drug interaction, increased monitoring should be implemented.

Precautions

Concurrent Active Mood or Anxiety Disorder

Cannabis does not appear to increase the likelihood of developing depression, anxiety, and post-traumatic stress disorder [1]. In bipolar disorder, a near-daily use may be linked to increased symptoms compared to nonusers [1]. Evidence suggests either a bidirectional relationship between cannabis use and anxiety disorders or no association between cannabis use and anxiety [22]. While there is not enough evidence to infer causality, there is a risk associated with increased levels of cannabis use and increased risk of developing psychosis [1]. The risk increased further with genetic vulnerabilities, experiences of childhood trauma/maltreatment or early stressors in life, early age of initiation, and regular use, therefore making some individuals more vulnerable to the effects of cannabis than others (see Chap.33 on Cannabinoids and Mental Health Risks) [1, 23].

Patients with Risk Factors for Cardiovascular Disease (CVD)

To date, the evidence is inconclusive if cannabis use is associated with cardiovascular disease [1]. In populations that are more likely to experience CVD, cannabis use is fairly low [1]. However, CVD is a relative contraindication for cannabis, and precaution should be exercised in patients with risk factor for CVD.

Tobacco Use

Smoking tobacco is a known risk factor for cardiovascular disease, respiratory disorders, and strokes [1]. As such, patients who are smoking tobacco in addition to cannabis may be at an elevated risk. In terms of cannabis use patterns, nicotine dependence alone is not a risk factor for the development of problematic cannabis use [1]. However, the behavior of smoking may also make those who smoke tobacco more likely to smoke cannabis.

E-Cigarette Use

There has been an increase in the incidence of e-cigarette or vaping product use-associated lung injury (EVALI) over the last several years. E-cigarettes are battery-operated devices that heat a liquid to deliver an aerosolized product [24]. E-cigarette use has been linked to severe respiratory illness, marked by bilateral infiltrates on chest imaging [24]. As of January 2020, the United States had reported 2558 hospitalizations with nonfatal cases and 60 fatal cases [25]. In a 98 patient report, 89% of patients reported using THC products in e-cigarette devices [24]. THC e-cigarette or vaping products were commonly reported to be obtained from illicit sources. As such, the CDC recommends to not use e-cigarette or vaping products obtained from unregulated sources [26]. It should be noted that EVALI has not been associated with dried product cannabis vaporization. Dried product vaporization has been legal for medical use in Canada since 2001 with no reported cases of EVALI. Cautions should be taken when recommending vaporization pens; This is especially true for those with respiratory conditions (see Chap. 37 on Cannabis Vaping Hazards).

Severe Liver Dysfunction or Disease

There is no strong evidence of an association between cannabis use and the progression of existing liver disease [1]. In individuals with viral hepatitis C, there is limited evidence of no association between the progression of liver fibrosis or hepatic disease with daily cannabis use [1]. A recent systematic review and meta-analysis supports that cannabis does not increase the prevalenc or progression of liver fibrosis in individuals with viral hepatitic C [27].

Additionally, as cannabis is metabolized by CYP enzymes, patients with any progressive liver disease, or those on multiple concomitant medications metabolized by the CYP enzymes outlined in Table 23.2 may lead to drug interaction with CBD/THC, and therefore require a dose adjustment for CBD/THC or their prescription medication.

Medications Associated with Sedation or Cognitive Impairment

There is moderate evidence for association between cannabis use and the development of substance dependence or a substance use disorder (e.g., alcohol, tobacco) [1]. However, alcohol dependence alone was not found to increase the risk of developing problematic cannabis use [1]. Additionally, there is limited evidence for the association between cannabis use and changes in patterns of use of licit and illicit substances such as opioids, alcohol, and tobacco/nicotine [1]. There should be precautions taken with the additive effect of sedating or cognitive impairing medications. Cannabis, specifically THC, can cause sedation and cognitive impairment. In patients taking these medications, caution should be exercised when starting a patient on THC.

Driving and Safety Sensitive Occupations

CRCs should be aware if patients will be engaging in safety sensitive activities (e.g. driving) or occupations. Safety sensitive occupations are those in which impairment may lead to significant risk of injury or death to oneself or others. Cannabis may cause impairment in a variety of neurocognitive and psychomotor domains [28]. Evidence supports that daily use of THC, as is seen with medical patients, may build tolerance to to the impairing effects of THC, particularly at lower doses [28–31]. Risk of impairment increases as THC dose increases [28, 30]. While evidence supports a THC-dose dependent risk, there is debate around the risk, if any, for CBD consumption. However, recent studies show that there is no neurocognitive or psychomotor impairment, including for driving tasks, associated with CBD doses of up to 100 mg [32, 33]. Although CBD is believed to be non-impairing, other terpenes and cannabinoids may impact impairment, particularly in naive users. Individuals using THC should not drive or partake in safety-sensitive activities for at least 4 hours post inhalation, 6 hours post oral ingestion, or for 8 hours if euphoria is experienced [11, 28]. For individuals using CBD, a careful risk vs benefit ratio should be considered. If CBD use causes improved function (e.g. less impairment compared to untreated condition or other medications) and there are no alternative options, the same guidelines should be employed until absence of impairment is established.

Relative Contraindications

Individuals Under the Age of 25

The use of cannabis in children and teens is controversial. There are several risks that should be known by healthcare providers involving the use of cannabis under 25 years of age. Youth may have an increased chance of cannabis use disorder. Regular cannabis use by youth may also be associated with increased risk of persistent cognitive effect, increased social dysfunction, anxiety, and depression [34–36]. In those at risk, younger initiation of cannabis use is associated with earlier onset of schizophrenia and bipolar disorder, as well as worse outcomes [37]. There are some cases where cannabis may be useful and appropriate if conventional treatments have failed, such as in epilepsy and autism. However, these chemovars typically contain predominantly CBD. Careful evaluation by the healthcare provider and caution over problematic use and addiction must be taken, especially if using chemovars containing higher ratios of THC/CBD or no CBD (see Chap. 32 on Cannabinoids and Brain Development).

Cannabis Use Disorder (CUD)

Cannabis is generally contraindicated in patients with a current or past cannabis use disorder (CUD). CUD is primarily a concern with recreational use and is reported in the literature to have an approximately 9% occurrence [38]. Self-reported problematic cannabis use in Canadian cannabis users was 6.8% [39]. While it is usually less of an issue in medical cannabis use, it remains important to assess potential risk factors for CUD. Risk factors include depression, male gender, current tobacco use, use of other illicit drugs, poor school performance, oppositional behaviors, younger age of first alcohol use, parental substance abuse, antisocial behaviors, and childhood sexual abuse (see Chap. 38 on Cannabis Use Disorder).

Substance Use Disorder (SUD) and Consideration for Harm Reduction

Medical cannabis should be used with caution in patients with a current or past substance use disorder. Precautions should always be taken to assess abuse potential, and history with substance use disorder may increase the risk of abuse. However, some clinicians have used cannabis as a harm reduction strategy in select patient populations with frequent monitoring and follow-up. The use of nabiximols (a 1:1 ratio of THC/CBD) has also showed promise in the treatment of substance use disorders including CUD. The lack of overdose death risk with cannabis generally makes it a safer option compared to other medications such as opioids or benzodiazepines.

Contraindications

Cardiovascular Disease

Cannabis should be used with caution in cardiovascular conditions. Cannabis, more specifically THC, may cause acute cardiovascular effects, such as increased heart rate and postural hypotension [1]. While cannabis produces no QTc issues [40], it should be used with caution in unstable cardiac conditions, such as acute congestive heart failure, critical aortic stenosis, poorly controlled atrial fibrillation or hypertensive heart disease, and angina, due to possible tachycardia and hypertension. To date, there is limited evidence of statistical significant association between THC use and myocardial infarction, stroke, and increased risk of diabetes [1].

Respiratory Disease

Smoking cannabis is heated to 600–900 °C, leading to the production of carbon monoxide and carcinogens through combustion. In contrast, vaporization of cannabis is approximately 160–220 °C causing little, if any, release of carbon monoxide [41]. Smoking cannabis releases the same harmful chemicals also found in tobacco smoking such as polyaromatic hydrocarbons, carbon monoxide, and tar. Smoked cannabis has been shown to have an approximately threefold increase in the amount of tar inhaled compared to smoked tobacco, with up to 30% more tar retained in the respiratory tract than tobacco [42].

Vaporization is a more efficient method for decarboxylation (i.e., conversion of raw acids in the plant THCA and CBDA to THC and CBD, respectively). There is also a reduction in the loss of cannabinoids and terpenes. Sidestream smoke leads to a 30% to 50% loss of cannabinoids, thus increasing the overall cost of cannabinoid-based medicine.

There is substantial evidence associating cannabis smoking and worsening of respiratory symptoms, as well as more frequent chronic bronchitis episodes [1]. However, it remains unclear if cannabis use is associated with the development of COPD, asthma, or a worsening of lung function. When considering the evidence, there is limited data to support an association between cannabis smoking and increased risk of developing chronic obstructive pulmonary disease (COPD), when controlling for tobacco use [1]. Further, there is no or insufficient evidence to evaluate if there is association between cannabis smoking and hospital admission for COPD, asthma development, or asthma exacerbation [1]. It is always best to recommend alternative routes of consumption to smoking; this is particularly important for patients with preexisting respiratory conditions.

Despite smoked cannabis having a lower incidence of COPD and lung cancer than tobacco [43], smoking cannabis is not recommended. Moderate evidence supports the lack of association between cannabis use (smoked) and incidence of lung, head, and neck cancers [1]. Alternatives to smoking, such as using ingestibles (i.e., oils/capsules) or oromucosal products may be preferred over vaporizing dried flower in those with lung disease.

Psychosis and Bipolar Disorders

Cannabis is contraindicated in psychosis, unless CBD-predominant preparations are being used, as a risk is related to THC content of cannabis. CBD has been shown to help alleviate psychotic symptoms of schizophrenia [44]. Caution should be used when patients have a personal or family history of psychosis, schizophrenia, or bipolar disorder (for more information, See Chap. 33 on Cannabinoids and Mental Health Risks). If deemed appropriate for cannabis use, careful guidance from the treating healthcare provider must be taken to ensure symptoms are being well managed and not exacerbated. In addition, monitoring for problematic use and cannabis use disorder is also important in these patients. For more information on the risks of cannabis use among individuals with personal or familial histories of mental health disorders, see Chap. 33 on Cannabinoids and Mental Health Risks.

Pregnancy and Breastfeeding

The use of cannabis during pregnancy may increase adverse outcomes for women and the fetus [42]. While there is a lack of evidence for an increased risk of major malformations related to in utero cannabis exposure, continuous cannabis exposure may produce negative effects on fetal growth and development. However, evidence supporting this is largely varied. Maternal cannabis use in pregnancy has been associated with increased odds of maternal anemia, decreased birth weight, and infants needing placement in neonatal intensive care [45]. Conversely, a large meta-analysis ($N = 32{,}483$) found inadequate evidence associating infant exposure to cannabis in utero with low birth weight [46]. Additionally, another large retrospective cohort study ($N = 12{,}069$) also found that cannabis alone was not associated with significant adverse outcomes [47]. However, concurrent cannabis and tobacco smoking was found to increase the risk of adverse perinatal outcomes such as maternal asthma, preterm birth, decreased head circumference, and decreased birth weight [47]. As such, the possibility cannot be ignored that neonatal morbidity may exist when cannabis is used during pregnancy. For breastfeeding mothers, it is important to note that THC can be detectable in breast milk for up to 6 days after last use [48].

In summary, current evidence does not support an increased risk of major malformations. There is a possible negative effect on fetal growth with continuous exposure to cannabis in utero and possible increased transient neonatal morbidity. There is concern regarding the negative effect on neurodevelopment, especially with frequent and continuous maternal cannabis use during pregnancy.

Summary

Healthcare providers should be aware of considerations including special populations, preexisting or past history of medical conditions, substance use history, and other medications before initiating a cannabinoid-based medicine. CRCs are encouraged to engage patients in a shared decision process to weigh the risks and benefits of cannabis, allowing for an individualized cannabis treatment plan for each patient.

As with any psychoactive medication, strategies to mitigate adverse events include “starting low and going slow," shorter trial period, more frequent monitoring and reassessment for efficacy, adverse events, and drug interactions. The majority of adverse events are THC dose-dependent. As such, CBD-dominant products may be a useful alternative to THC or in addition to mitigate risk (see Chap. 22 on Cannabinoid-Based Medicines: Dosing, Titration and Monitoring). With proper education, a treatment plan, patient engagement, and appropriate product selection, many of these adverse events can be avoided. Alternatively, these complex patients could also be referred to a physician with additional experience in cannabinoid medicine as these patients can require additional support and expertise.

References

1. National Academies of Sciences, Engineering, and Medicine. The health effects of Cannabis and cannabinoids: the current state of evidence and recommendations for research. Washington, DC: The National Academies Press; 2017.
2. College of Family Physicians of Canada. Authorization Dried Cannabis For Chronic Pain or Anxiety: Preliminary Guidance from the College of Family Physicians of Canada: College of Family Physicians of Canada; 2014.
3. Health Canada. Information for health care professionals: cannabis (marihuana, marijuana) and the cannabinoids. 2019. Available at: https://www.canada.ca/content/dam/hc-sc/documents/services/drugs-medication/cannabis/information-medical-practitioners/information-health-care-professionals-cannabis-cannabinoids-eng.pdf
4. Taha T, et al. Cannabis impacts tumor response rate to nivolumab in patients with advanced malignancies. Oncol. 24, 2019;(4):549–54.
5. Sulak D. Handbook of cannabis for clinicians: principles and practice. New York: Norton Professional Books. Forthcoming,; 2020.
6. Rein JL, Wyatt CM. Marijuana and cannabinoids in ESRD and earlier stages of CKD. Am J Kidney Dis. 2018;71:267–74.
7. Ho C, Martinusen D, Lo C. A review of cannabis in chronic kidney disease symptom management. Can J Kidney Health Dis. 2019;6:1–14.
8. Abuhasira R, Schleider LB, Mechoulam R, Novack V. Epidemiological characteristics, safety and efficacy of medical cannabis in the elderly. Eur J Intern Med. 2018;49:44–50.
9. Scott EP, Brennan E, Benitez A. A systematic review of the neurocognitive effects of cannabis use in older adults. Curr Addict Rep. 2019;6(4):443–55.
10. Russo EB. Current therapeutic cannabis controversies and clinical trial design issues. Front Pharmacol. 2016;7
11. MacCallum CA, Russo EB. Practical considerations in medical cannabis administration and dosing. Eur J Intern Med. 2018;49:12–9.
12. Devinsky O, Cross JH, Laux L, March E, Miller I, Nabbout R, et al. Trial of cannabidiol for drug-resistant seizures in the Dravet syndrome. N Engl J Med. 2017;376(21):2011–20.
13. Lucas CJ, Galettis P, Schneider J. The pharmacokinetics and the pharmacodynamics of cannabinoids. Br J Clin Pharmacol. 2018;84(11):2477–82.
14. Watkins PB, Church RJ, Li J, Knappertz V. Cannabidiol and Abnormal Liver Chemistries in Healthy Adults: Results of a Phase I Clinical Trial. Clin Pharmacol Ther. 2021;109(5):1224–31. https://doi.org/10.1002/cpt.2071. Epub 2020 Nov 21. PMID: 33022751.
15. Antoniou T, Bodkin J, Ho JM-W. Drug interactions with cannabinoids. Can Med Assoc J. 2020;192(9):E206.
16. Health Canada. (2018). For health care professionals: cannabis and cannabinoids. Government of Canada.
17. Alsherbiny MA, Li CG. Medicinal cannabis-potential drug interactions. Medicines (Basel). 2018;6(1)
18. Rong C, Carmona NE, Lee YL, Ragguett RM, Pan Z, Rosenblat JD, et al. Drug-drug interactions as a result of co-administering Δ9-THC and CBD with other psychotropic agents. Expert Opinion Drug Safety. 2018;17(1):51–4.
19. Cascorbi I. Drug interactions—principles, examples and clinical consequences. Dtsch Arztebl Int. 2012;109(33–34):546–56.
20. Foster BC, Abramovici H, Harris CS. Cannabis and cannabinoids: kinetics and interactions. Am J Med. 2019;132(11):1266–70.
21. Brown JD, Winterstein AG. Potential adverse drug events and drug–drug interactions with medical and consumer cannabidiol (CBD) use. J Clin Med. 2019;8(7):989.
22. Walsh Z, Gonzalez R, Crosby K, Thiessen MS, Carroll C, Bonn-Miller MO. Medical cannabis and mental health: a guided systematic review. Clin Psychol Rev. 2017;51:15–29.
23. Ragazzi TCC, Shuhama R, Menezes PR, Del-Ben CM. Cannabis use as a risk factor for psychotic-like experiences: a systematic review of non-clinical populations evaluated with the Community Assessment of Psychic Experiences. Early Interv Psychiatry.
24. Layden J, Ghinai I, Pray I, Kimball A, Layer M, Tenforde MW, et al. Pulmonary illness related to E-cigarette use in Illinois and Wisconsin – final report. N Engl J Med. 2020;382:903–16.
25. Werner AK, Koumans EH, Chatham-Stephens K, Salvatore PP, Armatas C, Byers P, et al. Hospitalizations and deaths associated with EVALI. N Engl J Med. 2020;382(17):1589–98.
26. Centers for Disease Control and Prevention (CDC). (2020). Outbreak of lung injury associated with the

use of E-cigarette, or vaping, products. Centers for Disease Control and Prevention.
27. Farooqui MT, Khan MA, Cholankeril G, Khan Z, Mohammed Abdul MK, Li AA, Shah N, Wu L, Haq K, Solanki S, Kim D, Ahmed A. Marijuana is not associated with progression of hepatic fibrosis in liver disease: a systematic review and meta-analysis. Eur J Gastroenterol Hepatol. 2019 Feb;31(2):149-156. doi: 10.1097/MEG.0000000000001263.
28. Eadie L, Lo LA, Christiansen A, Brubacher JR, Barr A, Panenka WJ, MacCallum CA. Duration of neurocognitive impairment with medical cannabis use: a scoping review. Front Psychiatry. 2021. https://doi.org/10.3389/fpsyt.2021.638962
29. Nordstrom BR, Hart CL. Assessing cognitive functioning in cannabis users: cannabis use history an important consideration. Neuropsychopharmacology. 2006 Dec;31(12):2798-9; author reply 2800-1. doi: 10.1038/sj.npp.1301210
30. Ramaekers JG, Kauert G, Theunissen EL, Toennes SW, Moeller MR. Neurocognitive performance during acute THC intoxication in heavy and occasional cannabis users. J Psychopharmacol. 2009 May;23(3):266-77. doi: 10.1177/0269881108092393.
31. Ramaekers JG, Theunissen EL, de Brouwer M, Toennes SW, Moeller MR, Kauert G. Tolerance and cross-tolerance to neurocognitive effects of THC and alcohol in heavy cannabis users. Psychopharmacology (Berl). 2011 Mar;214(2):391-401. doi: 10.1007/s00213-010-2042-1.
32. Spindle TR, Cone EJ, Goffi E, Weerts EM, Mitchell JM, Winecker RE, Bigelow GE, Flegel RR, Vandrey R. Pharmacodynamic effects of vaporized and oral cannabidiol (CBD) and vaporized CBD-dominant cannabis in infrequent cannabis users. Drug Alcohol Depend. 2020 Jun 1;211:107937. doi: 10.1016/j.drugalcdep.2020.107937.
33. Arkell TR, Vinckenbosch F, Kevin RC, Theunissen EL, McGregor IS, Ramaekers JG. Effect of Cannabidiol and Δ9-Tetrahydrocannabinol on Driving Performance: A Randomized Clinical Trial. JAMA. 2020 Dec 1;324(21):2177-2186. doi: 10.1001/jama.2020.21218.
34. Urbanoski KA, Strike CJ, Rush BR. Individuals seeking treatment for cannabis-related problems in Ontario: demographic and treatment profile. Eur Addict Res. 2005;11(3):115–23.
35. Crean RD, Crane NA, Mason BJ. An evidence based review of acute and long-term effects of cannabis use on executive cognitive functions. J Addict Med. 2011;5(1):1–8.
36. Fergusson DM, Horwood LJ, Swain-Campbell N. Cannabis use and psychosocial adjustment in adolescence and young adulthood. Addiction. 2002;97: 1123–35.
37. Hanna RC, Perez JM, Ghose S. Cannabis and development of dual diagnoses: a literature review. Am J Drug Alcohol Abuse. 2017;43(4):442–55.
38. Anthony JC, Warner LA, Kessler RC. Comparative epidemiology of dependence on tobacco, alcohol, controlled substances, and inhalants: basic findings from the National Comorbidity Survey. Exp Clin Psychopharmacol. 1994;3:244–68.
39. Statistics Canada. Cannabis Stats Hub, Canadian Community Health Survey: Cannabis use disorder. 2020. Retrieved from: https://www150.statcan.gc.ca/n1/pub/13-610-x/cannabis-eng.htm. Accessed on 8 July 2020.
40. Sellers EM, Schoedel K, Bartlett C, Romach M, Russo EB, Stott CG, et al. A multiple- dose, randomized, double-blind, placebo-controlled, parallel-group QT/QTc study to evaluate the electrophysiologic effects of THC/CBD spray. Clin Pharm Drug Dev. 2013;2:285–94.
41. Abrams DI, Vizoso HP, Shade SB, Jay C, Kelly ME, Benowitz NL. Vaporization as a smokeless cannabis delivery system: a pilot study. Clin Pharm Therap. 2007;82(5):572–8.
42. Wu TC, Tashkin DP, Djahed B, Rose JE. Pulmonary hazards of smoking marijuana as compared with tobacco. N Engl J Med. 1988;318(6):347–51.
43. Tashkin DP. Does smoking marijuana increase the risk of chronic obstructive pulmonary disease? CMAJ. 2009;180(8):797–8.
44. Leweke FM, Piomelli D, Pahlisch F, Muhl D, Gerth CW, Hoyer C, et al. Cannabidiol enhances anandamide signaling and alleviates psychotic symptoms of schizophrenia. Transl Psychiatry. 2012;2(3):e94.
45. Gunn JKL, Rosales CB, Center KE, Nuñez A, Gibson SJ, Christ C, Ehiri E. Prenatal exposure to cannabis and maternal and child health outcomes: a systematic review and meta-analysis. Br Med J Open. 2016;6(4):e009986.
46. English DR, Hulse GK, Milne E, Holman CD, Bower CI. Maternal cannabis use and birth weight: a meta-analysis. Addiction. 1997;92(11):1553–60.
47. Chabarria KC, Racusin DA, Antony KM, Kahr M, Suter MA, Mastrobattista JM, Aagaard KM. Marijuana use and its effects in pregnancy. Am J Obstet Gynecol. 2016;215(4):506.e1–7.
48. Bertrand KA, Hanan NJ, Honerkamp-Smith G, Best BM, Chambers CD. Marijuana use by breastfeeding mothers and cannabinoid concentrations in breast milk. Pediatrics. 2018;142(3)
49. Greger J, Bates V, Mechtler L, Gengo F. A Review of Cannabis and Interactions With Anticoagulant and Antiplatelet Agents. J Clin Pharmacol. 2020 Apr;60(4):432-438. doi: 10.1002/jcph.1557.

Part V

Cannabinoids and Pain

Cannabinoids and Pain: Mechanisms of Action

24

Samer N. Narouze

Introduction

Cannabinoids act simultaneously or synergistically on multiple pain targets within the peripheral and CNS [1–3]. Alongside acting on cannabinoid receptors (CB1 and CB2), cannabinoids may modulate pain through interaction with the putative non-CB1/non-CB2 cannabinoid G protein-coupled receptor 55 (GPR55) and GPR18 which is also known as the N-arachidonoyl glycine (NAGly) receptor [4, 5], as well as other well-known G protein-coupled receptors (GPCRs) such as serotonin (5-HT) and opioid receptors [6, 7].

Moreover, cannabinoids can interact with different transient receptor potential ion channel subfamilies (TRPV, TRPA, and TRPM) [2, 3]. TRPV1 is involved with temperature control, pain transmission, and modulation, as well as the integration of diverse painful stimuli [8–10].

Cannabinoids have various effects on the cys-loop ligand-gated ion channel superfamily (e.g., nicotinic acetylcholine, glycine, $GABA_A$, $GABA_A$-ρ, $5\text{-}HT_3$ receptors) [11–19]. Anandamide, THC, and cannabidiol directly activate glycine receptors, contributing to cannabinoid-induced analgesia in inflammatory and neuropathic pain [12–15], while 2-arachidonoylglycerol (2-AG) and cannabidiol (CBD) are positive allosteric modulators mainly at the α2-containing $GABA_A$ receptor subtypes [16, 17]. On the other hand, cannabinoids (THC) negatively allosterically modulate and inhibit nicotinic and 5-HT3 receptors [11, 18, 19].

The anti-inflammatory action of cannabinoids may contribute to their analgesic effects [20, 21]. Cannabinoid (CBD) action as a CB2 inverse agonist may explain its anti-inflammatory properties [22]. Some cannabinoids modulate and activate different isoforms of the nuclear receptor peroxisome proliferator-activated receptors (PPARα, β, and γ) [23].

Additionally, non-cannabinoid constituents of the cannabis plant (e.g., terpenoids and flavonoids) may contribute to the analgesic and anti-inflammatory effects of cannabis [24, 25].

Endocannabinoids' Mechanism of Action

Anandamide (AEA)

Anandamide is a partial agonist at both CB_1 and CB_2 receptors, but a full agonist at the transient receptor potential vanilloid 1 (TRPV1) receptor. Although anandamide is a partial agonist, it has a selectivity and higher affinity to the CB_1 receptor than 2-AG [26]. Once actions are carried out at the receptor, anandamide is thought to possibly be taken up by transport proteins on both neurons

S. N. Narouze (✉)
Western Reserve Hospital, Center For Pain Medicine, Cuyahoga Falls, OH, USA
e-mail: narouzs@hotmail.com
Twitter: @NarouzeMD

S. N. Narouze (ed.), *Cannabinoids and Pain*, https://doi.org/10.1007/978-3-030-69186-8_24

and glia that mediate endocannabinoid uptake [27]. Anandamide can play a dual role in nociception: antinociceptive at cannabinoid receptors and pronociceptive at the TRPV1 receptor [28]. Anandamide has a noted "tetrad effect" when injected into mice. The tetrad is a combination of inhibition of motor activity, catalepsy, hypothermia, and hypoalgesia [29, 30].

Anandamide also interacts with other neurotransmitter systems that may play a role in nociception. Cannabinoids might directly inhibit 5-HT_3 receptors, leading to analgesia and neuroprotection effects [29]. Anandamide exerts part of its CNS effects through the 5-HT_3 receptors [29]. In addition, it was shown that micromolar concentrations of anandamide bind to 5-HT_1 and 5-HT_2 receptors, thus further describing the role of anandamide in other neurotransmitter systems [31].

2-Arachidonoylglycerol (2-AG)

2-AG is a full agonist at CB_1 and CB_2 receptors. 2-AG may be secreted from the postsynaptic neuron by simple diffusion or through a passive carrier protein [27]. Once bound to CB_1, activation leads to inhibition of neurotransmitter release in the presynaptic cell via inhibition of voltage-activated calcium channels and enhancement of inwardly rectifying K^+ channels in the cell [27, 32].

Subsequent to neuronal depolarization, the Ca2+-dependent release of glutamate from presynaptic vesicles activates NMDA receptors at the postsynaptic neurons leading to excitatory postsynaptic currents (EPSCs). This variation of membrane excitability quickly triggers the synthesis of 2-AG. Then, 2-AG travels retrograde to stimulate CB1 receptors on presynaptic terminals, which in turn activate K+ channels and inversely inhibit Ca2+ channels, thus inhibiting excitatory neurotransmitter release [32] (Fig. 24.1).

Endocannabinoids and Pain Modulation

Endocannabinoids are sensitized on demand. When noxious stimuli occur, there is an increase in endocannabinoid release, thus leading to pain modulation effects [30]. Animal studies show endocannabinoids to have analgesic actions in the periphery, spinal, and supraspinal pain pathways [30] (Table 24.1).

Peripheral Mechanisms

Models of inflammatory pain show elevated concentrations of anandamide and 2-AG in peripheral tissues [28]. The cannabinoid receptor, CB2, in the periphery plays a vital role in analgesia. 2-AG has been studied to show multiple mechanisms leading to pain modulation which include inhibiting production and release of reactive oxygen species and cytokines, and in addition 2-AG will release peripheral endogenous opioids [28]. There is more research describing the anti-inflammatory and antinociceptive mediated actions of 2-AG compared to anandamide. There are also CB1 receptors in the periphery that localize on sensory afferent terminals where endocannabinoids act to gate the transduction of pain from noxious stimuli [28].

Spinal Mechanisms

Endocannabinoids have antinociceptive effects at the dorsal horn in the spinal cord due to high expression of CB_1 receptors. At this level, 2-AG inhibits the release of pronociceptive neurotransmitters from primary afferent terminals mediated by CB_1 receptors [28]. In contrast, anandamide was shown to have effects on acute and chronic pain via mediation of CB_2 receptors expressed on inhibitory interneurons and glial cells [28]. In a surgical incision model, it was shown that hours

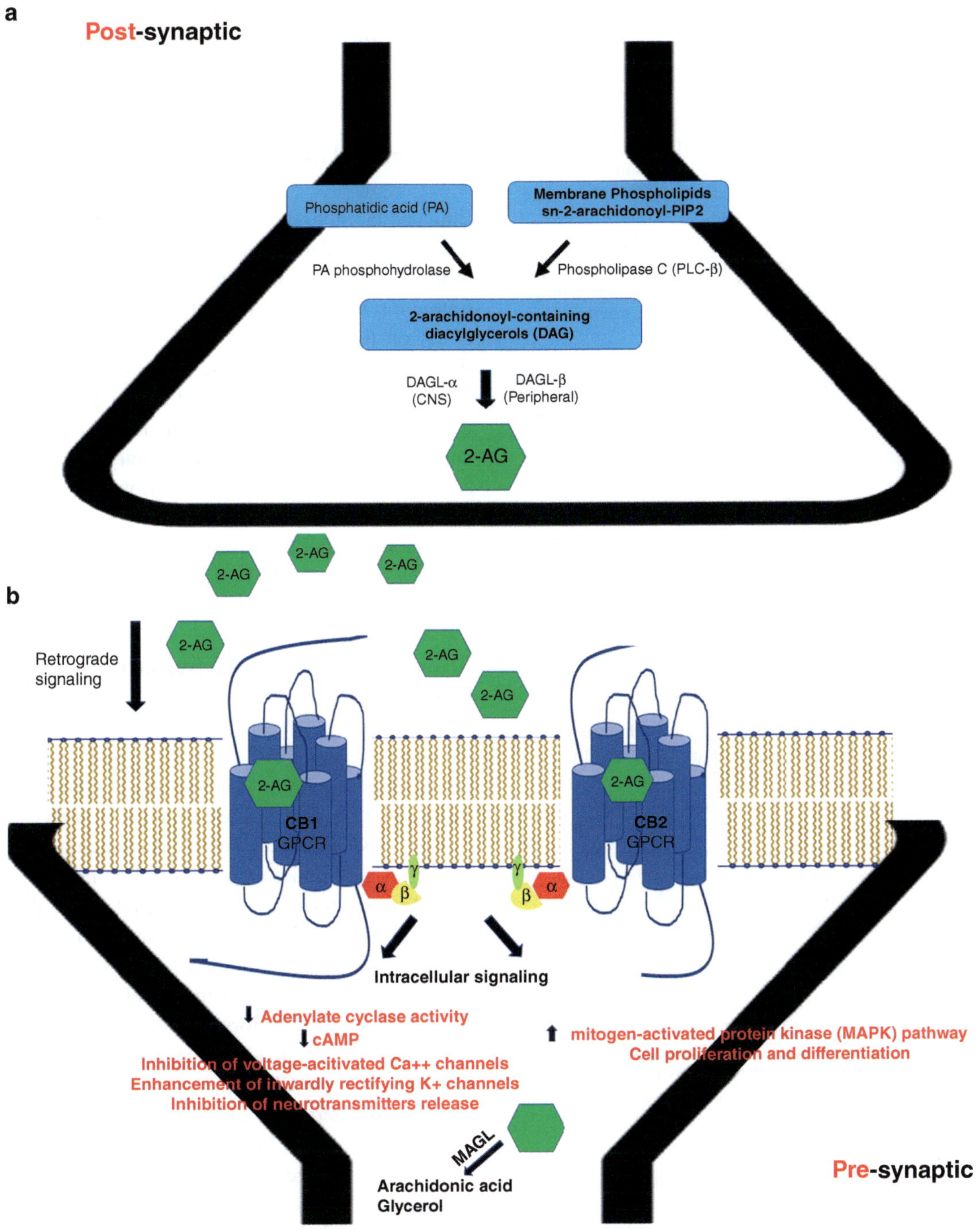

Fig. 24.1 Synthesis of 2-AG and the retrograde signaling. (**a**) The variation of postsynaptic membrane excitability triggers the synthesis of 2-AG. (**b**) 2-AG travels retrograde to stimulate CB1 receptors on presynaptic terminals, which in turn activate K+ channels and inversely inhibit Ca2+ channels, thus inhibiting excitatory neurotransmitter release. 2-AG is metabolized in the presynaptic neuron with MAGL into arachidonic acid and glycerol. 2-AG, 2-arachidonoylglycerol; CB1, cannabinoid receptor 1; CB2, cannabinoid receptor 2; COX2, cyclooxygenase 2; DAG, diacylglycerol; DAGL-α and DAGL-β, diacylglycerol lipase-α or diacylglycerol lipase-β; MAGL, monoacylglycerol lipase; PA, phosphatidic acid; PLCβ, phospholipase Cβ; PLD, phospholipase D; PIP2, sn-2-arachidonoyl-phosphatidylinositol-4,5-bisphosphate. (Used with permission from ©Samer Narouze, MD, PhD)

Table 24.1 Cannabinoid multimodal analgesic mechanisms of action

Cannabinoid antinociception pathways	
Peripheral	
	Peripheral CB2 receptor activation can lead to pain modulation by inhibiting production and release of inflammatory mediators (reactive oxygen species and cytokines) Endocannabinoids can release peripheral endogenous opioids Peripheral CB1 receptors act to gate the transduction of pain from noxious stimuli
Spinal	
	CB1 receptors are highly expressed on dorsal horn and DRG. CB1 activation leads to inhibition of pronociceptive neurotransmitter release from primary afferent terminals CB2 receptors expressed on spinal inhibitory interneurons and glial cells Anandamide exerts its actions at the onset of pain, whereas 2-AG plays a role in the resolution of pain
Supraspinal	
	Cannabinoids modulate: Ascending pain signals in the thalamus Descending signals in the brain stem Pain sensation in the frontal-limbic circuits (THC targets preferentially the affective qualities of pain) Anandamide has a "biphasic effect." On-demand release during acute pain causes antinociceptive effects. High concentration of anandamide due to prolonged stimulation leads to pronociceptive responses via TRPV1 binding

CB1 cannabinoid receptor type 1, *CB2* cannabinoid receptor type 2, *DRG* dorsal root ganglion, *THC* Δ^9-tetrahydrocannabinol, *CBD* cannabidiol, *AEA* anandamide, *2-AG* 2-arachidonoylglycerol, *TRPV1* transient receptor potential vanilloid type 1. (By ©Samer Narouze, MD, PhD, used with permission)

after a peripheral surgical incision, there was a marked decrease in anandamide concentrations, whereas there were no changes in 2-AG concentration [28]. Anandamide concentrations returned to baseline as nociceptive behavior subsides. 2-AG concentrations increased later in conjunction with glial cell activation, CB_2 receptor upregulation, and resolution of the pain state [28]. Endocannabinoids have different effects on pain modulation. Anandamide exerts its action at the onset of pain, whereas 2-AG plays a role in the resolution of pain.

Supraspinal Mechanisms

Endocannabinoids modulate ascending pain signals in the thalamus, descending signals in the brain stem, and pain sensation in the frontal-limbic circuits [28]. Anandamide has a biphasic effect on the supraspinal level of pain modulation. Anandamide is released due to stimulation of the periaqueductal gray (PAG) or peripheral inflammatory insult [27]. In acute pain, anandamide that is released causes antinociceptive actions. When high concentrations of anandamide occur due to prolonged stimulation, anandamide modulates pronociceptive responses via TRPV1 binding [27].

Anandamide and 2-AG Synergistic Effect

Anandamide and 2-AG have synergistic yet different roles in pain modulation at the spinal and supraspinal levels. Stress-induced analgesia exhibits a synergistic effect of anandamide and 2-AG through induction of descending inhibitory GABAergic signaling to the spinal cord, thus mediating stress-induced analgesia [27]. In a prolonged foot shock modulation study, both endocannabinoids were found to be released in the ipsilateral lumbar V dorsal root ganglion upon stimulation [33]. The CB_1 receptors at the dorsal root ganglion and CB_2 receptors at the periphery involve a synergistic interplay between anandamide and 2-AG [33]. Both endocannabinoids levels were enhanced after 3 and 7 days of chronic constriction injury at the sciatic nerve of a rat [33]. After the 3-day mark, endocannabinoid levels were increased only at the spinal cord and PAG. However, after 7 days, elevated concentrations were detected in the rostral ventral medulla as well [33]. This study provides evidence of endocannabinoid cooperation regarding synergistic involvement in the regulation of pain.

Chronic pain enhances the endocannabinoid signaling effects of both anandamide and 2-AG. An upregulation of CB_2 receptors found in such pain states would benefit from endocannabinoid agonism [27]. 2-AG signaling cascades from microglial cells mediate effects in persistent pain [27].

Endocannabinoid Receptors

CB1 Receptors

Central CB1 Receptors

CB1 receptor is the most abundant GPCR in the mammalian brain; thus it is referred to as the "brain cannabinoid receptor" [34]. CB1 receptors are expressed centrally in all brain structures and in decreasing density from the olfactory bulb, cerebellum, hippocampus, basal ganglia, cortex, and amygdala to the hypothalamus, thalamus, and brain stem [35].

They are expressed in most brain areas on presynaptic terminals of both glutamatergic and gamma aminobutyric acid (GABA)-ergic neurons [36]. Moreover, CB1 receptors can also be expressed postsynaptically where it can form heterodimers in association with other GPCRs including the dopamine D2, adenosine A2, or orexin type-1 receptors [37–39].

The intracellular region of CB1 is most regularly coupled to Gi/o proteins. Consequently, the activation of CB1 receptors inhibits adenylate cyclase activity with subsequent reduction of intracellular cyclic adenosine monophosphate (cAMP) level or promotes mitogen-activated protein kinase (MAPK) activity [34] (Fig. 24.2). Decreased cAMP level leads to activation of voltage-gated K+ and inhibition of Ca2+ channels, thus inhibiting neurotransmitter release [40–42]. In neurons, CB1 activation of Gi/o can also directly inhibit voltage-activated Ca2+ channels [32].

Neuronal depolarization rapidly triggers the synthesis of endocannabinoids, particularly 2-AG, at postsynaptic neurons. Subsequently, 2-AG travel backward to stimulate CB1 receptors on presynaptic terminals, and then after it is inactivated by hydrolytic enzymes. This "on-demand"

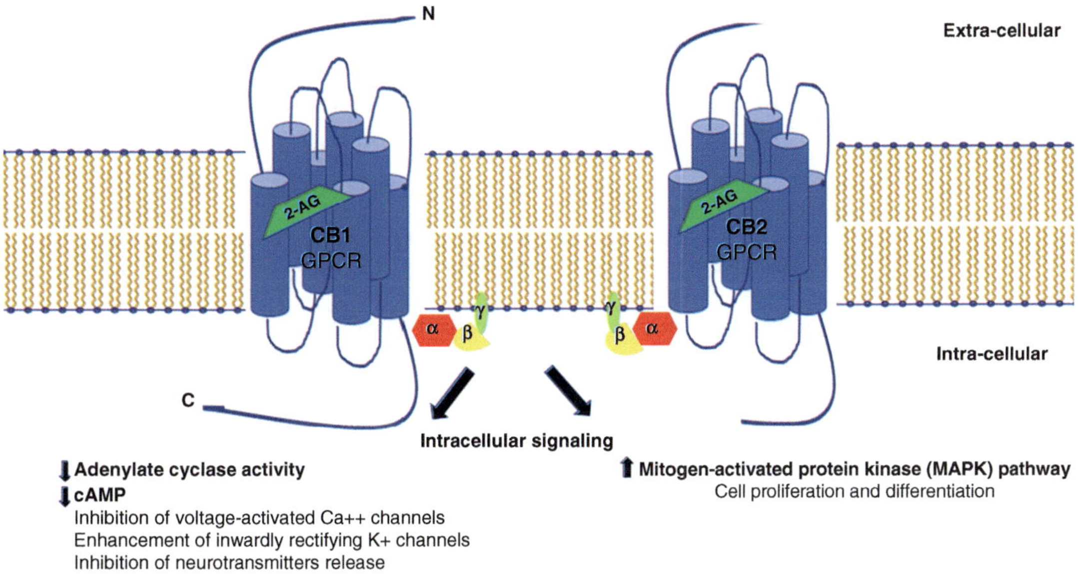

Fig. 24.2 CB1 receptor activation. The intracellular region of CB1 is most regularly coupled to Gi/o proteins. The activation of CB1 receptors by binding to a ligand (2-AG) inhibits adenylate cyclase activity with subsequent reduction of intracellular cyclic adenosine monophosphate (cAMP) level or enhances mitogen-activated protein kinase (MAPK) activity. Decreased cAMP level leads to activation of voltage-gated K+ and inhibition of Ca2+ channels, thus inhibiting neurotransmitter release. (Used with permission from ©Samer Narouze, MD, PhD)

synthesis of endocannabinoids leads to CB1-mediated activation of K+ and inhibition of Ca2+ channels, thus controlling both excitatory and inhibitory neurotransmitter releases, which eventually tunes the duration of synaptic activity and synaptic plasticity [43, 44].

CB1 is also found in non-neuronal cells of the brain, predominately in astrocytes, where its activation stimulates the release of neurotransmitters. Unexpectedly, astroglial CB1 receptor activation seems to induce intracellular Ca2+ levels, triggering the release of glutamate and the subsequent activation of presynaptic metabotropic glutamate receptors [45–47] (Table 24.2).

Peripheral CB1 Receptors

CB1 receptors are also expressed in the peripheral nervous system and in almost all mammal tissues and organs including the adrenal glands, smooth and skeletal muscle, heart, lung, gastrointestinal tract, liver, male and female reproductive systems, bone, adipose tissue, and skin [32]. The CB1 receptors play a vital role in the maintenance of homeostasis and regulating adrenal, cardiovascular, lung, gastrointestinal, and reproduction functions, among others.

Peripheral CB1 receptors are mainly localized on sensory afferent terminals where endocannabinoids act to gate the transduction of pain

Table 24.2 Cannabinoids mechanism of action in chronic pain

Cannabinoids' mechanism of action in chronic pain	
CB1 receptors	
Central	Expressed abundantly centrally (CNS and spinal) On presynaptic terminals of both glutamatergic and gamma aminobutyric acid (GABA) neurons GPCR receptors, coupled to Gi/Go α proteins CB1 receptor activation inhibits adenylate cyclase activity and reduces intracellular cAMP Activation of voltage-gated K+ and inhibition of Ca2+ channels, inhibiting neurotransmitter release
Peripheral	Peripheral CB1 receptors are mainly localized on sensory afferent terminals, modulating the transduction of pain from noxious stimuli, an important role in peripheral pain sensitization
CB2 receptors	
Central	The role of CB2 in the brain is still controversial Expressed in activated spinal microglia and astrocytes Like CB1, CB2 receptor is a GPCR and is coupled to Gi/Go α proteins. Thus, its stimulation inhibits adenylate cyclase activity
Peripheral	CB2 receptors are abundantly expressed in the immune system cells CB2 receptor activation reduces the release of pro-inflammatory cytokines and lymphoangiogenic factors CB2 receptors represent key regulators of inflammatory and nociceptive responses CB2 receptors can control the activation and migration of immune cells
TRPV1	
	TRPV1 channels are largely expressed in dorsal root ganglia and sensory nerve fibers (Aδ and C-type) TRPV1 has paradoxical effect on pain TRPV1 activation contributes to pain transmission and neurogenic inflammation TRPV1 "desensitization" occurs following TRPV1 stimulation due to increase of intracellular Ca2+ (see text) This fast process of TRPV1 desensitization and inactivation leads to the paradoxical analgesic and anti-inflammatory effects of TRPV1 agonists There is intracellular cross talk between TRPV1 and CB1 or CB2 as they are colocalized in peripheral and central neurons
GPR55	
	GPR55 is activated by THC while antagonized by CBD There are heteromers between GPR55 and CB1 receptors GPR55 activation may play an opposite role to CB1 by enhancing neurotransmitter release GPR55 also involved in mechanical hyperalgesia resulted from neuropathic and inflammatory pain

Table 24.2 (continued)

Cannabinoids' mechanism of action in chronic pain	
Other receptors	
	THC activates 5-HT7, 5-HT2A, and alpha-2 adrenoceptors (descending inhibitory pathway) THC, CBD, and anandamide directly activate glycine receptors, contributing to cannabinoid-induced analgesia in inflammatory and neuropathic pain 2-AG and CBD are positive allosteric modulators at the α2-containing GABAA receptor subtypes Cannabinoids (THC) inhibit nicotinic, 5-HT3, andNMDA receptors contributing to analgesia THC, CBD, and endocannabinoids activate PPARα and PPARγ receptors contributing to the analgesic, anti-inflammatory, and neuroprotective effects
Opioid receptors	
	Cross talk and heteromers between cannabinoids and opioids receptors (see text) Synergistic interactions between cannabinoid and opioid analgesia CB2 activation triggers the release of beta-endorphin
Transport proteins and metabolizing enzymes	
	CBD augments anandamide effects by inhibiting its uptake and metabolizing enzyme, FAAH This is an area of ongoing research

CB1 cannabinoid receptor type 1, *CB2* cannabinoid receptor type 2, *cAMP* cyclic adenosine monophosphate, *THC* Δ^9-tetrahydrocannabinol, *CBD* cannabidiol, *AEA* anandamide, *2-AG* 2-arachidonoylglycerol, *GPCR* G protein-coupled receptor, *GPR55* G protein-coupled receptor 55, *TRPV1* transient receptor potential vanilloid type 1, *NMDA* N-methyl-D-aspartate, *FAAH* fatty acid amide hydrolase. (By ©Samer Narouze, MD, PhD, used with permission)

from noxious stimuli [3], thus playing an important role in peripheral pain sensitization.

Central CB2 Receptors

The role of CB2 in the brain is still controversial. In contrast to CB1, CB2 receptors in the brain are limited, and its expression is restricted to specific neuronal cells and becomes abundant in activated microglia and astrocytes [45, 48].

Like CB1, CB2 receptor is a GPCR and is coupled to Gi/Go α proteins. Thus, its stimulation inhibits adenylate cyclase activity and activates MAPK [32].

Peripheral CB2 Receptors

In contrast, CB2 receptors are abundantly expressed in the immune system cells such as monocytes, macrophages, B and T cells, and mast cells. CB2 receptor activation reduces the release of pro-inflammatory cytokines and lymphoangiogenic factors [49–51]. Moreover, CB2 receptors are also present in other peripheral organs playing a role in the immune response, including the spleen, tonsils, thymus gland, and keratinocytes, as well as in the gastrointestinal system [32].

Accordingly, CB2 receptors represent key regulators of inflammatory and nociceptive responses and can control the activation and migration of immune cells [52, 53].

Other Putative Endocannabinoid Receptors: TRPV1 and GPR55

TRPV1

The transient receptor potential vanilloid type 1 (TRPV1) channel, also known as the capsaicin receptor, was the first member of the TRPV channel subfamily to be discovered and cloned [54]. TRPV1 channels are activated by capsaicin, endocannabinoids, and phytocannabinoids [55–57].

TRPV1 function is heavily dependent on the binding of key regulatory proteins that induce changes in its phosphorylation state. The phosphorylation induced by adenosine triphosphate (ATP), protein kinase A (PKA), PKC, phosphoinositide-binding protein (PIRT), and phosphatidylinositol 4,5-bisphosphate (PIP2) is required for TRPV1 activation and cation gating. TRPV1 activation contributes to pain transmission, neurogenic inflammation, synaptic plasticity, neuronal overexcitability, and neurotoxicity [57–60].

TRPV1 "desensitization" occurs as the rise of intracellular Ca2+ following TRPV1 stimulation activates proteins (i.e., calmodulin) that stabilize the channel in a closed conformational state or Ca2+-dependent phosphatases (i.e., calcineurin), which dephosphorylate and inactivate TRPV1 [59–63]. This fast process of TRPV1 desensitization and inactivation is thought to underlie the paradoxical analgesic, anti-inflammatory, and anti-convulsant effects of TRPV1 agonists [57, 64, 65].

TRPV1 channels are largely expressed in dorsal root ganglia and sensory nerve fibers (Aδ and C-type) [66]. In sensory neurons, TRPV1 channels work as molecular integrators for multiple types of sensory inputs that contribute to generate and transmit pain. In central neurons, lower amounts of TRPV1 channels are expressed both pre- and postsynaptically, where they act to regulate synaptic strength [66–68]. They usually affect pain, anxiety, and depression by inducing effects opposite to those exerted by CB1 receptors in the same context [32].

Moreover, there is intracellular cross talk between TRPV1 and CB1 or CB2 as they are colocalized in peripheral and central neurons (sensory neurons, dorsal root ganglia, spinal cord, brain neurons) [67, 69]. Recently, a multiplicity of interactions between cannabinoid, opioid, and TRPV1 receptors in pain modulation was discovered [70]. This provides a great opportunity for the development of new multiple target ligands for pain control with improved efficacy and side effects profile [71].

GPR55

GPR55 is considered by some experts as the third cannabinoid receptor, CB3. GPR55 belongs to the large family of GPCRs, and its endogenous ligand is lysophosphatidylinositol (LPI) [72, 73].

GPR55 is activated by Δψ-THC while antagonized by cannabidiol (CBD). Conflicting data exist regarding the likelihood that low concentrations of endocannabinoids may activate GPR55 [74, 75]. These controversies might be explained by biased signaling depending on the cell type and condition or the formation of heteromers between GPR55 and CB1 receptors [76, 77]. Activation of GPR55 might play an opposite role to CB1 by enhancing neurotransmitter release [32]. GPR55 may play a role in mechanical hyperalgesia associated with inflammatory and neuropathic pain [78].

Phytocannabinoids (THC and CBD)

THC

Δ^9-tetrahydrocannabinol (THC) is an analog to the endocannabinoid, anandamide (AEA). It is responsible for most of the pharmacological actions of cannabis, including the psychoactive, memory, analgesic, anti-inflammatory, antioxidant, antipruritic, bronchodilator, antispasmodic, and muscle relaxant activities [79, 80]. THC acts as a partial agonist at CB1 and CB2 receptors [22]. THC has a very high binding affinity to CB1 receptor which mediates its psychoactive properties. Interestingly, most of the negative effects of THC, psychogenic effects, impaired memory, anxiety, and immunosuppression, can be reversed by other constituents of the cannabis plant (other cannabinoids, CBD, terpenoids, and flavonoids) [24, 80].

CBD

Cannabidiol (CBD) is the other important cannabinoid in the cannabis plant. It is the non-psychoactive analog of THC. CBD have significant analgesic, anti-inflammatory, anticonvulsant, and anxiolytic activities without the psychoactive effect of THC [81]. CBD has little binding affinity for either CB1 or CB2 receptors, but it can antagonize them in the presence of THC. CBD behaves as a non-competitive negative allosteric modulator of CB1 receptor, and it reduces the efficacy of THC and AEA [82]. This may explain the "entourage effect" that CBD displays, as it improves the tolerability and safety of THC by reducing the likelihood of psychoactive effects and other adverse effects such as tachycardia, sedation, and anxiety [80, 83].

Mechanisms of Action in Pain Modulation

The phytocannabinoids THC and CBD are lipophilic substances that readily cross the blood-brain barrier and interact with receptors in both the central and peripheral nervous systems, exerting analgesic effects especially in hyperalgesia and inflammatory states [84, 85] (Table 24.3).

THC

THC exhibits CB1 receptor-mediated antinociception through activation of supraspinal sites and descending serotonergic and noradrenergic pain modulatory pathways to produce antinociceptive effects via spinal 5-HT7, 5-HT2A, and alpha-2 adrenoceptor activation [86, 87].

The frontal-limbic distribution of cannabinoid receptors explains the central mechanism of THC analgesia as it targets preferentially the affective qualities of pain. Functional magnetic resonance imaging revealed that amygdala activity contributes to the dissociative effect of THC on pain perception related to cutaneous ongoing pain and hyperalgesia that were temporarily induced by capsaicin [88]. THC reduced the reported unpleasantness, but not the intensity of ongoing pain and hyperalgesia. THC also reduced func-

Table 24.3 THC and CBD mechanisms of action in pain modulation

THC and CBD mechanisms of action in pain modulation	
THC	
	Partial agonist at CB1 and CB2 receptors (see Table 24.2) High binding affinity to CB1 receptor The frontal-limbic distribution of CB1 receptors explains the central mechanism of THC analgesia as it targets preferentially the affective qualities of pain Activation of supraspinal descending serotonergic and noradrenergic pain modulatory pathways Spinal 5-HT7, 5-HT2A, and alpha-2 adrenoceptor activation CB2 receptor activation reduces cytokine-mediated neuro-inflammation Non-CB1/non-CB2 receptor-mediated antinociception by inhibiting nicotinic, 5HT3, and NMDA receptors Activation of glycine receptors, contributing to analgesia in inflammatory and neuropathic pain
CBD	
	Weak binding affinity for either CB1 or CB2 receptors. However, antagonist of CB1 and CB2, in the presence of THC Non-competitive negative allosteric modulator of the CB1 Act synergistically with THC and contribute to its analgesic effect while providing an "entourage effect" Regulates the perception of pain through non-CB1/non-CB2 mechanisms Modulation of non-cannabinoid GPCRs (5-HT1A), ion channels (TRPV1, TRPA1, TPRM8, NAGlyR), and PPARs Activation of glycine receptors, contributing to analgesia in inflammatory and neuropathic pain Augments anandamide (AEA) effects by inhibiting its uptake as well as its metabolizing enzyme, FAAH

CB1 cannabinoid receptor type 1, *CB2* cannabinoid receptor type 2, *THC*, Δ^9-tetrahydrocannabinol, *CBD* cannabidiol, *AEA* anandamide, *2-AG* 2-arachidonoylglycerol, *GPCR* G protein-coupled receptor, *GPR55* G protein-coupled receptor 55, *TRPV1* transient receptor potential vanilloid type 1, *NMDA* N-methyl-D-aspartate, *PPAR* peroxisome proliferator-activated receptors, *NAGlyR* N-arachidonoyl glycine receptor, *FAAH* fatty acid amide hydrolase. (By ©Samer Narouze, MD, PhD, used with permission)

tional connectivity between the amygdala and primary sensorimotor areas during the ongoing pain state. The authors concluded that peripheral mechanisms alone cannot account for the dissociative effects of THC on the pain that was observed and amygdala activity contributes to inter-individual response to cannabinoid analgesia [88].

The analgesic effects of THC are mediated through mechanisms distinct from those responsible for the psychoactive effects. THC has additive analgesic effect with kappa opioid receptor agonists. This effect is blocked by kappa antagonism, but opioid receptor antagonism does not alter the psychoactive effects of THC [89].

Cannabinoids may exert other non-CB1/non-CB2 receptor-mediated antinociceptive effects by interacting with 5HT3 and N-methyl-d-aspartate receptors [89, 90].

CB2 receptors serve an important role in immune function, inflammation, and pain modulation specially in allodynia and hyperalgesia states [91, 92]. The presence of CB2 receptors on microglia within the nervous system may explain the cannabinoids' role in neuropathic pain modulation by reducing cytokine-mediated neuroinflammation [91, 92].

CB2 receptor expression has been demonstrated in areas of the peripheral and central nervous system relevant to pain perception and modulation, including the dorsal root ganglion, spinal cord, and microglia. This explains the analgesic effects produced by CB2 agonists [93–97].

CB2-selective agonists suppress neuronal activity in the dorsal horn via reduction in C-fiber activity and wind-up involving wide dynamic range (WDR) neurons [98, 99]. There is increase in peripheral CB2 receptor protein or mRNA expression in inflamed tissues and in the dorsal root ganglion in neuropathic states [100–102].

CBD

CBD regulates the perception of pain mainly through non-CB1/non-CB2 mechanisms. CBD interacts with a significant number of other targets, including non-cannabinoid GPCRs (e.g., 5-HT1A), ion channels (TRPV1, TRPA1, TPRM8, GlyR), and PPARs. Moreover, CBD augments anandamide (AEA) effects by inhibiting its uptake as well as its hydrolysis by the enzyme fatty acid amide hydrolase (FAAH) [3, 78, 103].

CBD can act synergistically with THC and contribute to its analgesic effect while providing an "entourage effect," minimizing the negative psychoactive effects of THC [80]. This depends on the differences in concentration of THC/CBD in the cannabis chemovar. Although CBD as a monotherapy has not been evaluated clinically in the management of pain, its anti-inflammatory and anti-spasmodic effects and good safety profile suggest that it could be a safe and effective analgesic [104, 105].

References

1. Vučković S, Srebro D, Vujović KS, Vučetić Č, Prostran M. Cannabinoids and pain: new insights from old molecules. Front Pharmacol. 2018;9:1259.
2. Pertwee RG, Howlett AC, Abood ME, Alexander SP, Di Marzo V, Elphick MR, et al. International union of basic and clinical pharmacology. LXXIX. Cannabinoid receptors and their ligands: beyond CB1 and CB2. Pharmacol Rev. 2010;62:588–631. https://doi.org/10.1124/pr.110.003004.
3. Morales P, Hurst DP, Reggio PH. Molecular targets of the phytocannabinoids-a complex picture. Prog Chem Org Nat Prod. 2017;103:103–31.
4. Staton PC, Hatcher JP, Walker DJ, Morrison AD, Shapland EM, Hughes JP, et al. The putative cannabinoid receptor GPR55 plays a role in mechanical hyperalgesia associated with inflammatory and neuropathic pain. Pain. 2008;139:225–36.
5. Huang SM, Bisogno T, Petros TJ, Chang SY, Zavitsanos PA, Zipkin RE, et al. Identification of a new class of molecules, the arachidonyl amino acids, and characterization of one member that inhibits pain. J Biol Chem. 2001;276:42639–44.
6. Russo EB, Burnett A, Hall B, Parker KK. Agonistic properties of cannabidiol at 5-HT1a receptors. Neurochem Res. 2005;30:1037–43.
7. Scavone JL, Sterling RC, Van Bockstaele EJ. Cannabinoid and opioid interactions: implications for opiate dependence and withdrawal. Neuroscience. 2013;248:637–54. https://doi.org/10.1016/j.neuroscience.2013.04.034.
8. Horvath G, Kekesi G, Nagy E, Benedek G. The role of TRPV1 receptors in the antinociceptive effect of

anandamide at spinal level. Pain. 2008;134:277–84. https://doi.org/10.1016/j.pain.2007.04.032.
9. Cui M, Honore P, Zhong C, Gauvin D, Mikusa J, Hernandez G, et al. TRPV1 receptors in the CNS play a key role in broad-spectrum analgesia of TRPV1 antagonists. J Neurosci. 2006;26(37):9385–93.
10. Huang SM, Bisogno T, Trevisani M, Al-Hayani A, De Petrocellis L, Fezza F, et al. An endogenous capsaicin-like substance with high potency at recombinant and native vanilloid VR1 receptors. Proc Natl Acad Sci U S A. 2002;99(12):8400–5.
11. Oz M, Al Kury L, Keun-Hang SY, Mahgoub M, Galadari S. Cellular approaches to the interaction between cannabinoid receptor ligands and nicotinic acetylcholine receptors. Eur J Pharmacol. 2014;731:100–5.
12. Hejazi N, Zhou C, Oz M, Sun H, Ye JH, Zhang L. Delta9-tetrahydrocannabinol and endogenous cannabinoid anandamide directly potentiate the function of glycine receptors. Mol Pharmacol. 2006;69:991–7.
13. Ahrens J, Demir R, Leuwer M, de la Roche J, Krampfl K, Foadi N, et al. The nonpsychotropic cannabinoid cannabidiol modulates and directly activates alpha-1 and alpha-1-Beta glycine receptor function. Pharmacology. 2009;83:217–22.
14. Xiong W, Cheng K, Cui T, Godlewski G, Rice KC, Xu Y. Cannabinoid potentiation of glycine receptors contributes to cannabis-induced analgesia. Nat Chem Biol. 2011;7:296–303.
15. Xiong W, Cui T, Cheng K, Yang F, Chen SR, Willenbring D, et al. Cannabinoids suppress inflammatory and neuropathic pain by targeting a3 glycine receptors. J Exp Med. 2012;209:1121–34. https://doi.org/10.1084/jem.20120242.
16. Sigel E, Baur R, Rácz I, Marazzi J, Smart TG, Zimmer A, et al. The major central endocannabinoid directly acts at GABA(A) receptors. Proc Natl Acad Sci U S A. 2011;108:18150–5.
17. Bakas T, van Nieuwenhuijzen PS, Devenish SO, McGregor IS, Arnold JC, Chebib M. The direct actions of cannabidiol and 2-arachidonoylglycerol at GABA(A) receptors. Pharmacol Res. 2017;119:358–70.
18. Shi B, Yang R, Wang X, Liu H, Zou L, Hu X. Inhibition of 5-HT(3) receptors-activated currents by cannabinoids in rat trigeminal ganglion neurons. J Huazhong Univ Sci Technolog Med Sci. 2012;32:265–71.
19. Barann M, Molderings G, Brüss M, Bönisch H, Urban BW, Göthert M. Direct inhibition by cannabinoids of human 5-HT3A receptors: probable involvement of an allosteric modulatory site. Br J Pharmacol. 2002;137:589–96.
20. Klein TW. Cannabinoid-based drugs as anti-inflammatory therapeutics. Nat Rev Immunol. 2005;5:400–11.
21. Jesse Lo V, Fu J, Astarita G, La Rana G, Russo R, Calignano A, et al. The nuclear receptor peroxisome proliferator-activated receptor-alpha mediates the anti-inflammatory actions of palmitoylethanolamide. Mol Pharmacol. 2005;67:15–9.
22. Pertwee RG. The diverse CB1 and CB2 receptor pharmacology of three plant cannabinoids: Δ9-tetrahydrocannabinol, cannabidiol and Δ9-tetrahydrocannabivarin. Br J Pharmacol. 2008;153(2):199–215.
23. O'Sullivan SE. An update on PPAR activation by cannabinoids. Br J Pharmacol. 2016;173:1899–910.
24. Andre CM, Hausman JF, Guerriero G. Cannabis sativa: the plant of the thousand and one molecules. Front Plant Sci. 2016;7:19.
25. ElSohly MA, Radwan MM, Gul W, Chandra S, Galal A. Phytochemistry of Cannabis sativa L. Prog Chem Org Nat Prod. 2017;103:1–36.
26. Hillard CJ. Biochemistry and pharmacology of the endocannabinoids arachidonylethanolamide and 2-arachidonylglycerol. Prostaglandins Other Lipid Mediat. 2000;61(1–2):3–18.
27. Reggio PH. Endocannabinoid binding to the cannabinoid receptors: what is known and what remains unknown. Curr Med Chem. 2010;17(14):1468–86.
28. Woodhams SG, Sagar DR, Burston JJ, Chapman V. The role of the endocannabinoid system in pain. Handb Exp Pharmacol. 2015;227:119–43.
29. Mechoulam R, Fride E, Marzo VD. Endocannabinoids. Eur J Pharmacol. 1998;359(1):1–18.
30. Manzanares J, Julian MD, Carrascosa A. Role of the cannabinoid system in pain control and therapeutic implications for the management of acute and chronic pain episodes. Curr Neuropharmacol. 2006;4(3):239–57.
31. Kimura T, Ohta T, Watanabe K, Yoshimura H, Yamamoto I. Anandamide, an endogenous cannabinoid receptor ligand, also interacts with 5-hydroxytryptamine (5-HT) receptor. Biol Pharm Bull. 1998;21(3):224–6.
32. Iannotti FA, Di Marzo V, Petrosino S. Endocannabinoids and endocannabinoid-related mediators: targets, metabolism and role in neurological disorders. Prog Lipid Res. 2016;62:107–28. https://doi.org/10.1016/j.plipres.2016.02.002.
33. Luchicch A, Pistis M. Anandamide and 2-arachidonoylglycerol: pharmacological properties, functional features, and emerging specificities of the two major endocannabinoids. Mol Neurobiol. 2012;46:374–92.
34. Turu G, Hunyady L. Signal transduction of the CB1 cannabinoid receptor. J Mol Endocrinol. 2010;44:75–85.
35. Herkenham M, Lynn AB, Little MD, Johnson MR, Melvin LS, de Costa BR, et al. Cannabinoid receptor localization in brain. Proc Natl Acad Sci U S A. 1990;87:1932–6.
36. Elphick MR, Egertová M. The neurobiology and evolution of cannabinoid signaling. Philos Trans R Soc Lond Ser B Biol Sci. 2001;356:381–408.
37. Przybyla JA, Watts VJ. Ligand-induced regulation and localization of cannabinoid CB1 and dopamine

D2L receptor heterodimers. J Pharmacol Exp Ther. 2010;332:710–9.
38. Ferré S, Lluís C, Justinova Z, Quiroz C, Orru M, Navarro G, et al. Adenosine-cannabinoid receptor interactions implications for striatal function. Br J Pharmacol. 2010;160:443–53.
39. Ward RJ, Pediani JD, Milligan G. Heteromultimerization of cannabinoid CB(1) receptor and orexin OX(1) receptor generates a unique complex in which both protomers are regulated by orexin a. J Biol Chem. 2011;286:37414–28.
40. Pertwee RG. Pharmacology of cannabinoid CB1 and CB2 receptors. Pharmacol Ther. 1997;74:129–80.
41. Howlett AC, Mukhopadhyay S. Cellular signal transduction by anandamide and 2-arachidonoylglycerol. Chem Phys Lipids. 2000;108:53–70.
42. Witkowski G, Rola R, Szulczyk P. Effect of cyclic adenosine monophosphate on the G protein-dependent inward rectifier K(+)-like channel current in medial prefrontal cortex pyramidal neurons. J Physiol Pharmacol. 2012;63:457–62.
43. Mu J, Zhuang SY, Kirby MT, Hampson RE, Deadwyler SA. Cannabinoid receptors differentially modulate potassium A and D currents in hippocampal neurons in culture. J Pharmacol Exp Ther. 1999;291:893–902.
44. Wilson RI, Nicoll RA. Endogenous cannabinoids mediate retrograde signaling at hippocampal synapses. Nature. 2001;410:588–92.
45. Stella N. Cannabinoid and cannabinoid-like receptors in microglia, astrocytes, and astrocytomas. Glia. 2010;58:1017–30.
46. Oliveira da Cruz JF, Robin LM, Drago F, Marsicano G, Metna-Laurent M. Astroglial type-1 cannabinoid receptor (CB1): a new player in the tripartite synapse. Neuroscience. 2015;S0306-4522(15):00434.
47. Navarrete M, Araque A. Endocannabinoids potentiate synaptic transmission through stimulation of astrocytes. Neuron. 2010;68(1):113–26.
48. Demuth DG, Molleman A. Cannabinoid signalling. Life Sci. 2006;78:549–63.
49. Matias I, Di Marzo V. Endocannabinoids and the control of energy balance. Trends Endocrinol Metab. 2007;18:27–37.
50. Staiano RI, Loffredo S, Borriello F, Iannotti FA, Piscitelli F, Orlando P, Secondo A, Pertwee RG. The pharmacology of cannabinoid receptors and their ligands: an overview. Int J Obes. 2006;30:S13–8.
51. Granata F, Lepore MT, Fiorelli A, Varricchi G, Santini M, Triggiani M, Di Marzo V, Marone G. Human lung-resident macrophages express CB1 and CB2 receptors whose activation inhibits the release of angiogenic and lymphangiogenic factors. J Leukoc Biol. 2016;99(4):531–40.
52. Malan TP Jr, Ibrahim MM, Lai J, Vanderah TW, Makriyannis A, Porreca F. CB2 cannabinoid receptor agonists: pain relief without psychoactive effects? Curr Opin Pharmacol. 2003;3:62–7.
53. Whiteside GT, Lee GP, Valenzano KJ. The role of the cannabinoid CB2 receptor in pain transmission and therapeutic potential of small molecule CB2 receptor agonists. Curr Med Chem. 2007;14:917–36.
54. Caterina MJ, Schumacher MA, Tominaga M, Rosen TA, Levine JD, Julius D. The capsaicin receptor: a heat-activated ion channel in the pain pathway. Nature. 1997;389:816–24.
55. De Petrocellis L, DiMarzo V. Lipids as regulators of the activity of transient receptor potential type V1 (TRPV1) channels. Life Sci. 2005;77:1651–66.
56. Di Marzo V, De Petrocellis L. Endocannabinoids as regulators of transient receptor potential (TRP) channels: a further opportunity to develop new endocannabinoid-based therapeutic drugs. Curr Med Chem. 2010;17:1430–49.
57. Iannotti FA, Hill CL, Leo A, Alhusaini A, Soubrane C, Mazzarella E, et al. Nonpsychotropic plant cannabinoids, cannabidivarin (CBDV) and cannabidiol (CBD), activate and desensitize transient receptor potential vanilloid 1 (TRPV1) channels in vitro: potential for the treatment of neuronal hyperexcitability. ACS Chem Neurosci. 2014;5:1131–41.
58. Nagy I, Friston D, Valente JS, Torres Perez JV, Andreou AP. Pharmacology of the capsaicin receptor, transient receptor potential vanilloid type-1 ion channel. Prog Drug Res. 2014;68:39–76.
59. Julius D. TRP channels and pain. Annu Rev Cell Dev Biol. 2013;29:355–84.
60. Nilius B, Mahieu F, Karashima Y, Voets T. Regulation of TRP channels: a voltage–lipid connection. Biochem Soc Trans. 2007;35:105–8.
61. Cortright DN, Szallasi A. Biochemical pharmacology of the vanilloid receptor TRPV1. An update. Eur J Biochem. 2004;271:1814–9.
62. Planells-Cases R, Garcìa-Sanz N, Morenilla-Palao C, Ferrer-Montiel A. Functional aspects and mechanisms of TRPV1 involvement in neurogenic inflammation that leads to thermal hyperalgesia. Pflugers Arch. 2005;451:151–9.
63. Mandadi S, Tominaga T, Numazaki M, Murayama N, Saito N, Armati PJ, et al. Increased sensitivity of desensitized TRPV1 by PMA occurs through PKCepsilon-mediated phosphorylation at S800. Pain. 2006;123:106–16.
64. Brederson JD, Kym PR, Szallasi A. Targeting TRP channels for pain relief. Eur J Pharmacol. 2013;716:61–76.
65. Iwaoka E, Wang S, Matsuyoshi N, Kogure Y, Aoki S, Yamamoto S, et al. Evodiamine suppresses capsaicin-induced thermal hyperalgesia through activation and subsequent desensitization of the transient receptor potential V1 channels. J Nat Med. 2016;70(1):1–7.
66. Edwards JG. TRPV1 in the central nervous system: synaptic plasticity, function, and pharmacological implications. Prog Drug Res. 2014;68:77–104.
67. Cristino L, de Petrocellis L, Pryce G, Baker D, Guglielmotti V, Di Marzo V. Immunohistochemical localization of cannabinoid type 1 and vanilloid transient receptor potential vanilloid type 1 receptors in the mouse brain. Neuroscience. 2006;139:1405–15.

68. Mori F, Ribolsi M, Kusayanagi H, Monteleone F, Mantovani V, Buttari F, et al. TRPV1 channels regulate cortical excitability in humans. J Neurosci. 2012;32:873–9.
69. Anand P, Whiteside G, Fowler CJ, Hohmann AG. Targeting CB2 receptors and the endocannabinoid system for the treatment of pain. Brain Res Rev. 2009;60:255–66. https://doi.org/10.1016/j.brainresrev.2008.12.003.
70. Zádor F, Wollemann M. Receptome: interactions between three pain-related receptors or the "triumvirate" of cannabinoid, opioid and TRPV1 receptors. Pharmacol Res. 2015;102:254–63. https://doi.org/10.1016/j.phrs.2015.10.015.
71. Reddy AS, Zhang S. Polypharmacology: drug discovery for the future. Expert Rev Clin Pharmacol. 2013;6:41–7. https://doi.org/10.1586/ecp.12.74.
72. Oka S, Nakajima K, Yamashita A, Kishimoto S, Sugiura T. Identification of GPR55 as a lysophosphatidylinositol receptor. Biochem Biophys Res Commun. 2007;362:928–34.
73. Henstridge CM, Balenga NA, Ford LA, Ross RA, Waldhoer M, Irving AJ. The GPR55 ligand L-alpha-lysophosphatidylinositol promotes RhoA-dependent Ca2+ signaling and NFAT activation. FASEB J. 2009;23:183–93.
74. Sharir H, Console-Bram L, Mundy C, Popoff SN, Kapur A, Abood ME. The endocannabinoids anandamide and virodhamine modulate the activity of the candidate cannabinoid receptor GPR55. J Neuroimmune Pharmacol. 2012;7:856–65.
75. Pertwee RG. GPR55: a new member of the cannabinoid receptor clan? Br J Pharmacol. 2007;152:984–6.
76. Kargl J, Balenga N, Parzmair GP, Brown AJ, Heinemann A, Waldhoer M. The cannabinoid receptor CB1 modulates the signaling properties of the lysophosphatidylinositol receptor GPR55. J Biol Chem. 2012;287:44234–48.
77. Martínez-Pinilla E, Reyes-Resina I, Oñatibia-Astibia A, Zamarbide M, et al. CB1 and GPR55 receptors are co-expressed and form heteromers in rat and monkey striatum. Exp Neurol. 2014;261:44–52.
78. Staton PC, Hatcher JP, Walker DJ, Morrison AD, et al. The putative cannabinoid receptor GPR55 plays a role in mechanical hyperalgesia associated with inflammatory and neuropathic pain. Pain. 2008;139(1):225–36.
79. Rahn EJ, Hohmann AG. Cannabinoids as pharmacotherapies for neuropathic pain: from the bench to the bedside. Neurotherapeutics. 2009;6:713–37.
80. Russo EB. Taming THC: potential cannabis synergy and phytocannabinoid-terpenoid entourage effects. Br J Pharmacol. 2011;163:1344–64. https://doi.org/10.1111/j.1476-5381.2011.01238.x.
81. Costa B, Trovato AE, Comelli F, Giagnoni G, Colleoni M. The non-psychoactive cannabis constituent cannabidiol is an orally effective therapeutic agent in rat chronic inflammatory and neuropathic pain. Eur J Pharmacol. 2007;556:75–83. https://doi.org/10.1016/j.ejphar.2006.11.006.
82. Laprairie RB, Bagher AM, Kelly ME, Denovan-Wright EM. Cannabidiol is a negative allosteric modulator of the cannabinoid CB1 receptor. Br J Pharmacol. 2015;172:4790–805. https://doi.org/10.1111/bph.13250.
83. Abrams DI, Guzman M. Cannabis in cancer care. Clin Pharmacol Ther. 2015;97:575–86. https://doi.org/10.1002/cpt.108.
84. Chin CL, Tovcimak AE, Hradil VP. Differential effects of cannabinoid receptor agonists on regional brain activity using pharmacological MRI. Br J Pharmacol. 2008;153:367–79.
85. versen L, Chapman V. Cannabinoids: a real prospect for pain relief? Curr Opin Pharmacol. 2002;2:50–5.
86. Dogrul A, Seyrek M, Yalcin B, Ulugol A. Involvement of descending serotonergic and noradrenergic pathways in CB1 receptor-mediated antinociception. Prog Neuro-Psychopharmacol Biol Psychiatry. 2012;38:97–105.
87. Seyrek M, Kahraman S, Deveci MS, Yesilyurt O, Dogrul A. Systemic cannabinoids produce CB_1-mediated antinociception by activation of descending serotonergic pathways that act upon spinal 5-HT(7) and 5-HT(2A) receptors. Eur J Pharmacol. 2010;649(1–3):183–94.
88. Lee MC, Ploner M, Wiech K, et al. Amygdala activity contributes to the dissociative effect of cannabis on pain perception. Pain. 2013;154(1):124–34. https://doi.org/10.1016/j.pain.2012.09.017.
89. Welch SP. Blockade of cannabinoid-induced antinociception by norbinaltorphimine, but not N,N-diallyl-tyrosine-Aib-phenylalanine-leucine, ICI 174,864 or naloxone in mice. J Pharmacol Exp Ther. 1993;265:633–40.
90. Pertwee RG, Howlett AC, Abood ME, et al. International Union of Basic and Clinical Pharmacology. LXXIX. Cannabinoid receptors and their ligands: beyond CB1 and CB2. Pharmacol Rev. 2010;62:588–631.
91. Hulsebosch CE. Special issue on microglia and chronic pain. Exp Neurol. 2012;234:253–4.
92. Beltramo M. Cannabinoid type 2 receptor as a target for chronic pain. Mini Rev Med Chem. 2009;9:11–25.
93. Beltramo M, Bernardini N, Bertorelli R, et al. CB2 receptor-mediated antihyperalgesia: possible direct involvement of neural mechanisms. Eur J Neurosci. 2006;23:1530–8.
94. Van Sickle MD, Duncan M, Kingsley PJ, et al. Identification and functional characterization of brainstem cannabinoid CB2 receptors. Science. 2005;310:329–32.
95. Jhaveri MD, Elmes SJ, Richardson D, et al. Evidence for a novel functional role of cannabinoid CB(2) receptors in the thalamus of neuropathic rats. Eur J Neurosci. 2008;27:1722–30.
96. Anand U, Otto WR, Sanchez-Herrera D, et al. Cannabinoid receptor CB2 localisation and agonist mediated inhibition of capsaicin responses in human sensory neurons. Pain. 2008;138:667–80.

97. Jhaveri MD, Sagar DR, Elmes SJ, Kendall DA, Chapman V. Cannabinoid CB2 receptor-mediated anti-nociception in models of acute and chronic pain. Mol Neurobiol. 2007;36:26–35.
98. Nackley AG, Zvonok AM, Makriyannis A, Hohmann AG. Activation of cannabinoid CB2 receptors suppresses C-fiber responses and windup in spinal wide dynamic range neurons in the absence and presence of inflammation. J Neurophysiol. 2004;92:3562–74.
99. Quartilho A, Mata HP, Ibrahim MM, et al. Inhibition of inflammatory hyperalgesia by activation of peripheral CB2 cannabinoid receptors. Anesthesiology. 2003;99:955–60.
100. Richardson D, Pearson RG, Kurian N, et al. Characterisation of the cannabinoid receptor system in synovial tissue and fluid in patients with osteoarthritis and rheumatoid arthritis. Arthritis Res Ther. 2008;10:R43.
101. Walczak JS, Pichette V, Leblond F, Desbiens K, Beaulieu P. Behavioral, pharmacological and molecular characterization of the saphenous nerve partial ligation: a new model of neuropathic pain. Neuroscience. 2005;132:1093–102.
102. Wotherspoon G, Fox A, McIntyre P, Colley S, Bevan S, Winter J. Peripheral nerve injury induces cannabinoid receptor 2 protein expression in rat sensory neurons. Neuroscience. 2005;135:235–45.
103. Burstein S. Cannabidiol (CBD) and its analogs: a review of their effects on inflammation. Bioorg Med Chem. 2015;23:1377–85. https://doi.org/10.1016/j.bmc.2015.01.059.
104. Ko GD, Bober SL, Mindra S, Moreau JM. Medical cannabis – the Canadian perspective. J Pain Res. 2016;9:735–44. https://doi.org/10.2147/JPR.S98182.
105. Wade DT, Robson P, House H, Makela P, Aram J. A preliminary controlled study to determine whether whole-plant cannabis extracts can improve intractable neurogenic symptoms. Clin Rehabil. 2003;17:21–9. https://doi.org/10.1191/0269215503cr581oa.

Cannabinoids and Pain: Clinical Evidence

25

Caroline A. MacCallum, Lauren Eadie, and Samer N. Narouze

Introduction

In this chapter, we have summarized systematic reviews of randomized controlled trials using cannabis-based medicine for pain, including, but not limited to, chronic pain (non-cancer pain, neuropathic pain, centralized pain disorders such as fibromyalgia, rheumatic inflammatory pain, cancer pain) and acute pain.

There have been many cannabis-based medicine studies in patients with chronic non-cancer pain; only the most recent studies were included.

Chronic Non-cancer Pain

There are a series of systematic reviews completed on the chronic non-cancer pain population that demonstrate a significant analgesic effect of cannabis-based medicines. In 2020, a thorough systematic review and meta-analysis (N = 36 RCTs; n = 4006 patients) was conducted investigating the effects of cannabinoids on chronic non-cancer pain [1]. Various cannabinoid products and methods of administration (smoked cannabis, oromucosal cannabis sprays, and oral cannabinoids) were compared to placebo for analgesia. The authors concluded that there was moderate evidence to support cannabinoids for the use of chronic non-cancer pain. The best results were seen with study durations of 2–8 weeks (weighted mean difference, −0.68; [95% CI, −0.96, −0.40]; I^2 = 8%; $p < 0.00001$) with longer studies showing only a mild benefit. Another meta-analysis and meta-regression by the American Psychological Association found that cannabis therapy has a medium-to-large analgesic effect across the chronic non-cancer pain studies they investigated (Cohen's d = −0.58; 95% CI: −0.74, −0.43) [2].

A large systematic review and meta-analysis of systematic reviews (containing two or more RCTs) examined medical cannabinoids for the management of chronic pain, spasticity, or nausea and vomiting [3]. The authors completed a responder rate analysis (an analysis of benefit determined by the proportion of patients who attained at least a 30% improvement in VAS (visual analog scale) pain scores or reached a defined minimal clinically important difference).

C. A. MacCallum (✉) · L. Eadie
Department of Medicine, Faculty of Medicine, University of British Columbia, Vancouver, BC, Canada
e-mail: info@drcarolinemaccallum.com

S. N. Narouze
Western Reserve Hospital, Center For Pain Medicine, Cuyahoga Falls, OH, USA

S. N. Narouze (ed.), *Cannabinoids and Pain*, https://doi.org/10.1007/978-3-030-69186-8_25

The meta-analysis ($N = 15$ RCTs) revealed that a greater proportion of patients (39%) taking cannabinoids for chronic pain had at least a 30% reduction in pain compared to the proportion taking placebo (30%) (RR = 1.37; 95% CI, 1.14 to 1.64; NNT = 11). Among seven of the included systematic reviews with meta-analyses examining pain and cannabis [4–10], three studies found significant improvement in pain ratings by 0.4–0.8 points compared to placebo [1, 4, 7, 9]. Five reviews reported a 30% or greater reduction in pain [5–7, 10], with only two of the five reviews producing statistically significant findings [6–10]. One of the meta-analyses mentioned above compared inhaled cannabis to placebo in 178 patients with chronic neuropathic pain [6].This study noted an NNT of 5.6 to produce a > 30% reduction in VAS neuropathic pain score across chronic painful neuropathies of different etiologies [6].

Neuropathic pain was examined among 13 of the 15 RCTs [11–23], and cancer pain was assessed in the remaining two [24, 25]. These findings should be interpreted with caution due to high attrition, exclusion of patients with variable pain scores, and lack of clarity on blinding and randomization. Sensitivity analysis found study size and duration affected findings (subgroup differences, $p \leq 0.03$), with larger and longer RCTs finding no benefit. Specifically, inhaled cannabinoids had an RR of 1.52 (95% CI 1.17 to 1.99) and an NNT of six, while oromucosal cannabinoids had an RR of 1.28 (95% CI 1.02 to 1.61) and an NNT of 16, with no significant differences among subgroups ($p = 0.34$). Small studies (≤150 patients) had an RR of 1.56 (95% CI 1.26 to 1.92) and an NNT of six, while large studies (>150 patients) had a nonsignificant RR of 1.09 (95% CI 0.86 to 1.39), with a statistically significant difference in subgroups ($p = 0.03$). RCTs lasting less than one week had an RR of 1.58 (95% CI 1.13 to 2.20) and an NNT of five; RCTs of 2–5 weeks had an RR of 1.79 (95% CI 1.31 to 2.43) and an NNT of seven; and RCTs of 9–15 weeks had a nonsignificant RR of 1.07 (95% CI 0.87 to 1.32). Subgroup comparisons were statistically significant ($p = 0.01$) [3]. Evidence for benefit was classified as low or very low as per GRADE (Grading of Recommendations, Assessment, Development and Evaluation), with the highest risk of bias among RCTs of inhaled medical cannabinoids [3].

Interestingly, low-dose THC (1.29% THC) seems to be as effective as an analgesic as moderate dose THC (3.53% THC) compared to placebo on neuropathic pain patients. A double-blinded, placebo-controlled, randomized controlled trial, included in the systematic review mentioned above, compared the effect of low-dose vaporized THC compared to medium-dose vaporized THC and to placebo on 39 patients with neuropathic pain [16]. There was a significant reduction in neuropathic pain using the VAS ($P < 0.0001$ at 3 hours, $p = 0.0018$ at 5 hours) with minimal psychoactive effects [16].

In addition to analgesia, some studies showed improvement in factors negatively associated with chronic pain, such as sleep, anxiety, and depression. Numerous phase 1–3 studies in over 2000 patients with 1000 patient years of exposure utilizing nabiximols 1:1 THC/CBD oromucosal spray demonstrated marked improvement in sleep parameters in patients with a wide variety of pain conditions including multiple sclerosis, peripheral neuropathic pain, intractable cancer pain, and RA [26]. 40–50% of patients in these studies attained good or very good sleep quality, and showed no tolerance to the benefit of nabiximols with no need for dosage increase over four years [27]. This added benefit on the symptom clusters associated with chronic non-cancer pain is somewhat novel to cannabis-based medicines compared to the alternative pharmaceuticals currently used.

Health Canada concludes on neuropathic pain and chronic non-cancer pain, "A few studies that have used experimental methods having predictive validity for pharmacotherapies used to alleviate chronic pain, have reported an analgesic effect of smoked cannabis. Furthermore, there is more consistent evidence of the efficacy of cannabinoids (smoked/vaporized cannabis, nabiximols, dronabinol) in treating chronic pain of various etiologies, especially in cases where conventional treatments have been tried and have failed" [28].

Chronic Neuropathic Pain

The Cochrane Database of Systematic Reviews in 2018 published its review on cannabis-based medicines for chronic neuropathic pain in adults, which included 16 studies with 1750 participants [26]. Studies ranged from two to 26 weeks in duration, and compared placebo (15 studies) or dihydrocodeine (one study) to a plant-derived combination of THC and CBD oromucosal spray (10 studies), synthetic oral THC (nabilone, two studies), inhaled herbal cannabis (two studies), or oral plant-derived THC (dronabinol, two studies). Findings among eight of the studies examined ($n = 1001$) showed that cannabis-based medicines may increase the number of people achieving 50% or greater pain relief compared with placebo [21% versus 17%; RD, 0.05 (95% CI 0.00 to 0.09); NNTB 20 (95% CI 11 to 100); low-quality evidence] [26].

The results were uncertain regarding whether herbal cannabis reduced mean pain intensity (very low-quality evidence), which may be a reflection of the exclusion of participants with a history of substance abuse and other significant comorbidities from the studies, together with their small sample sizes [23]. The authors concluded that "the potential benefits of cannabis-based medicine (herbal cannabis, plant-derived or synthetic THC, THC/CBD oromucosal spray) in chronic neuropathic pain might be outweighed by their potential harms" [25] .

Fibromyalgia

Systematic reviews focusing on pain reduction, in particular pain populations, yielded inconsistent results. Registry data on patients initiating medical cannabis for treatment of fibromyalgia showed that after commencing medical cannabis treatment, all patients reported significant improvement in every parameter on the questionnaire [29]. Additionally, 50% of patients stopped taking other medications for fibromyalgia [29]. A randomized controlled trial (RCT) on the use of nabilone, an oral synthetic cannabinoid, on sleep in patients with fibromyalgia showed that it was superior to amitriptyline, a drug currently used for chronic non-cancer pain [30]. Another randomized double-blind trial in 40 patients with fibromyalgia utilizing nabilone showed a significant decrease in VAS for both pain and anxiety to placebo [31]. A recent larger scale study (n = 878) reported promising results for the utility of CBD for fibromyalgia [32]. Within this sample, 72% of participants substituted CBD for pain medications, including opioids (53.3%) and benzodiazapines (23.1%). Fewer side effects and better symptom control were the most commonly reported reasons for substituition. As such, CBD may be a useful in not only improving symptom control, but also decreasing risk of harm associated with common pain medications such as opioids.

Rheumatoid Arthritis

A double-blind, randomized, parallel group trial compared nabiximols, to placebo in 58 patients with pain due to rheumatoid arthritis (RA) [33]. There were statistically significant improvements in pain on movement and at rest, quality of sleep, 28-joint Disease Activity Score (DAS28), and short-form McGill Pain Questionnaire "pain at present" component [33, 34, 35]. Notably, there were no adverse event-related withdrawals or serious adverse events in the nabiximol group [33].

Despite these promising results, the above studies on patients with fibromyalgia and rheumatoid arthritis have small sample sizes, and two systematic reviews have reported that there is currently still insufficient evidence for analgesic benefit with cannabis-based medicines in patients with fibromyalgia, back pain, osteoarthritis, and rheumatoid arthritis [36, 37].

Cancer Pain

Regarding cancer pain, the results of two systematic reviews are unclear and inconsistent, [8, 38] with meta-analytic findings not reaching statistical significance for the therapeutic potential of cannabis on cancer pain [8].

A systematic review (n = 6 RCTs; n = 1460 participants) and a meta-analysis (n = 5 RCTs) investigating the effects of cannabis/cannabinoids on cancer-related pain compared with placebo or another alternative active agent showed that for adults with advanced cancer, cannabinoid adjunctive therapy did not reduce cancer-associated pain.

Health Canada concluded that "the limited available clinical evidence with certain cannabinoids (dronabinol, nabiximols) suggests a modest analgesic effect of dronabinol and a modest and mixed analgesic effect of nabiximols on cancer pain" [28].

For more detailed review on cannabinoids and cancer pain, please refer to Chap. 26.

Acute Nociceptive Pain

A systematic review and meta-analysis of 18 RCTs (n = 422) compare cannabis to placebo on several acute pain measures including acute pain threshold, pain intensity, pain unpleasantness, pain tolerance, and mechanical hyperalgesia [39]. There was a small increase in pain threshold, a small-to-medium increase in pain tolerance, and a small-to-medium reduction in unpleasantness with cannabis compared to placebo, but no change in pain intensity or mechanical hyperalgesia. This study concluded that cannabis may improve the negative effect associated with pain, rather than decrease the acute pain signal itself [39].

A review of seven RCTs for acute pain found a reduction in pain among one of the included studies, no effect among five of the studies, and worse pain in the remaining study. They concluded that cannabinoids have no role in acute pain [40].

More recently, a systematic review and meta-analysis suggests that the analgesic role of perioperative cannabinoid compounds is limited, with no clinically important benefits detected when cannabinoids are added to traditional systemic analgesics. Particularly, there seems to be an increased incidence of postoperative pain and hypotension associated with the addition of perioperative cannabinoids to traditional systemic analgesics. These results do not support the routine use of cannabinoids to manage acute postoperative pain at the present time [41].

Summary

The National Academies of Sciences, Engineering and Medicine [42] conducted an exhaustive review of the medical literature on the health effects of cannabis and cannabinoids. Findings from the report state "there is conclusive or substantial evidence that cannabis or cannabinoids are effective for the treatment of chronic pain in adults." The report noted that only a handful of studies specifically evaluated outcomes related to dispensary cannabis in the United States and that little is known about dosing or side effects. It appears that more consistent methodology is needed among future research designs with regard to cannabis product, dosing, method of intake, timing of administration, pain scale measurements, and how pain is subjectively measured and reported. Without this, it is challenging to compare the breadth of data that now exists on cannabis and its effect on pain. Expert physicians and researchers in cannabis-based medicines are working on a systematic review that will provide a detailed, up-to-date tool for healthcare providers and patients to assist them with decisions about CBP derived from the cannabis plant as a treatment option for chronic pain and co-occurring conditions [43].

References

1. Johal H, Devji T, Chang Y, Simone J, Vannabouathong C, Bhandari M. Cannabinoids in chronic non-cancer pain: a systematic review and meta-analysis. Clin Med Insights Arthritis Musculoskelet Disord. 2020;13:1179544120906461. https://doi.org/10.1177/1179544120906461.
2. Yanes JA, McKinnell ZE, Reid MA, Busler JN, Michel JS, Pangelinan MM, et al. Effects of can-

nabinoid administration for pain: a meta-analysis and meta-regression. Exp Clin Psychopharmacol. 2019;27(4):370–82.

3. Allan GM, Finley CR, Ton J, Perry D, Ramji J, Crawford K, Lindblad AJ, Korownyk C, Kolber MR. Systematic review of systematic reviews for medical cannabinoids: pain, nausea and vomiting, spasticity, and harms. Can Fam Physician. 2018 Feb;64(2):e78–94.
4. Martin-Sanchez E, Furukawa TA, Taylor J, Martin JL. Systematic review and meta-analysis of cannabis treatment for chronic pain. Pain Med. 2009;10(8):1353–68.
5. Whiting PF, Wolff RF, Deshpande S, Di Nisio M, Duffy S, Hernandez AV, et al. Cannabinoids for medical use: a systematic review and meta-analysis. JAMA. 2015;313(24):2456–73. Errata in: JAMA 2016;315(14):1522, JAMA 2015;314(21):2308, JAMA 2015;314(5):520, JAMA 2015;314(8):837.
6. Andreae MH, Carter GM, Shaparin N, Suslov K, Ellis RJ, Ware MA, et al. Inhaled cannabis for chronic neuropathic pain: a meta-analysis of individual patient data. J Pain. 2015;16(12):1221–32. Epub 2015 Sep 9.
7. Petzke F, Enax-Krumova EK, Häuser W. Efficacy, tolerability and safety of cannabinoids in neuropathic pain syndromes [article in German]. Schmerz. 2016;30(1):62–88.
8. Lobos Urbina D, Peña DJ. Are cannabinoids effective for treatment of pain in patients with active cancer? Medwave. 2016;16(Suppl 3):e6539.
9. Iskedjian M, Bereza B, Gordon A, Piwko C, Einarson TR. Meta-analysis of cannabis based treatments for neuropathic and multiple sclerosis-related pain. Curr Med Res Opin. 2007;23(1):17–24.
10. Mücke M, Carter C, Cuhls H, Prüß M, Radbruch L, Häuser W. Cannabinoids in palliative care: systematic review and meta-analysis of efficacy, tolerability and safety [article in German]. Schmerz. 2016;30(1):25–36.
11. Langford RM, Mares J, Novotna A, Vachova M, Novakova I, Notcutt W, et al. A double-blind, randomized, placebo-controlled, parallel-group study of THC/CBD oromucosal spray in combination with the existing treatment regimen, in the relief of central neuropathic pain in patients with multiple sclerosis. J Neurol 2012. 2013;260(4):984–97.
12. Wilsey B, Marcotte T, Deutsch R, Gouaux B, Sakai S, Donaghe H. Low-dose vaporized cannabis significantly improves neuropathic pain. J Pain. 2013;14(2):136–48.
13. Ware MA, Wang T, Shapiro S, Robinson A, Ducruet T, Huynh T, et al. Smoked cannabis for chronic neuropathic pain: a randomized controlled trial. CMAJ. 2010;182(14):E694–701.
14. Selvarajah D, Gandhi R, Emery CJ, Tesfaye S. Randomized placebo-controlled double-blind clinical trial of cannabis-based medicinal product (Sativex) in painful diabetic neuropathy: depression is a major confounding factor. Diabetes Care. 2010;33(1):128–30.
15. Ellis RJ, Toperoff W, Vaida F, van den Brande G, Gonzales J, Gouaux B, et al. Smoked medicinal cannabis for neuropathic pain in HIV: a randomized, crossover clinical trial. Neuropsychopharmacology (New York, N.Y.) 2008. 2009;34(3):672–80.
16. Wilsey B, Marcotte T, Tsodikov A, Millman J, Bentley H, Gouaux B, et al. A randomized, placebo-controlled, crossover trial of cannabis cigarettes in neuropathic pain. J Pain. 2008;9(6):506–21.
17. Nurmikko TJ, Serpell MG, Hoggart B, Toomey PJ, Morlion BJ, Haines D. Sativex successfully treats neuropathic pain characterised by allodynia: a randomised, double-blind, placebo-controlled clinical trial. Pain. 2007;133(1–3):210–20.
18. Abrams DI, Jay CA, Shade SB, Vizoso H, Reda H, Press S, et al. Cannabis in painful HIV-associated sensory neuropathy: a randomized placebo-controlled trial. Neurology. 2007;68(7):515–21.
19. Rog DJ, Nurmikko TJ, Friede T, Young CA. Randomized, controlled trial of cannabis-based medicine in central pain in multiple sclerosis. Neurology. 2005;65(6):812–9.
20. Berman JS, Symonds C, Birch R. Efficacy of two cannabis based medicinal extracts for relief of central neuropathic pain from brachial plexus avulsion: results of a randomised controlled trial. Pain. 2004;112(3):299–306.
21. Lynch ME, Cesar-Rittenberg P, Hohmann AG. A double-blind, placebo-controlled, crossover pilot trial with extension using an oral mucosal cannabinoid extract for treatment of chemotherapy-induced neuropathic pain. J Pain Symptom Manag. 2014;47(1):166–73.
22. Serpell M, Ratcliffe S, Hovorka J, Schofield M, Taylor L, Lauder H, et al. A double-blind, randomized, placebo-controlled, parallel group study of THC/CBD spray in peripheral neuropathic pain treatment. Eur J Pain. 2014;18(7):999–1012.
23. GW Pharmaceuticals Ltd. A study of Sativex® for pain relief due to diabetic neuropathy. ClinicalTrials.gov. http://ClinicalTrials.gov/show/NCT00710424. Accessed 4 June 2019.
24. Portenoy RK, Ganae-Motan ED, Allende S, Yanagihara R, Shaiova L, Weinstein S, et al. Nabiximols for opioid-treated cancer patients with poorly-controlled chronic pain: a randomized, placebo-controlled, graded-dose trial. J Pain. 2012;13(5):438–49.
25. Johnson JR, Burnell-Nugent M, Lossignol D, Ganae-Motan ED, Potts R, Fallon MT. Multicenter, double-blind, randomized, placebo-controlled, parallel-group study of the efficacy, safety, and tolerability of THC:CBD extract and THC extract in patients with intractable cancer-related pain. J Pain Symptom Manag. 2010;39(2):167–79.
26. Mücke M, Phillips T, Radbruch L, Petzke F, Häuser W. Cannabis-based medicines for chronic neuropathic pain in adults. Cochrane Database Syst Rev. 2018;3 https://doi.org/10.1002/14651858.CD012182.pub2.
27. Russo E, Guy G, Robson P. Cannabis, pain, and sleep: lessons from therapeutic clinical trials of Sativex®,

a cannabis-based medicine. Chem Biodivers. 2007;4(8):1729–43.
28. Health Canada. Information for healthcare professionals: cannabis (marihuana, marijuana) and the cannabinoids. 2019. Retrieved from: https://www.canada.ca/content/dam/hc-sc/documents/services/drugs-medication/cannabis/information-medical-practitioners/information-health-care-professionals-cannabis-cannabinoids-eng.pdf
29. Habib G, Artul S. Medical Cannabis for the Treatment of Fibromyalgia. J Clin Rheumatol. 2018;24(5):255-258. https://doi.org//10.1097/RHU.0000000000000702. PMID: 29461346.
30. Ware MA, Fitzcharles M, Joseph L, Shir Y. The effects of nabilone on sleep in fibromyalgia: results of a randomized controlled trial. Anesth Analg. 2010;110(2):604–10.
31. Skrabek RQ, Galimova L, Ethans K, Perry D. Nabilone for the treatment of pain in fibromyalgia. J Pain. 2008;9(2):164–73.
32. Boehnke KF, Gagnier JJ, Matallana L, Williams DA. Substituting Cannabidiol for Opioids and Pain Medications Among Individuals with Fibromyalgia: a Large Online Survey. J Pain. 2021:S1526-5900(21)00220-0. https://doi.org/10.1016/j.jpain.2021.04.011.
33. Blake DR, Robson P, Ho M, Jubb RW, McCabe CS. Preliminary assessment of the efficacy, tolerability and safety of a cannabis-based medicine (Sativex) in the treatment of pain caused by rheumatoid arthritis. Rheumatology (Oxford). 2006;45(1):50–2.
34. Wells G, Becker J, Teng J, Dougados M, Schiff M, Smolen J, et al. Validation of the 28-joint Disease Activity Score (DAS28) and European League Against Rheumatism response criteria based on C-reactive protein against disease progression in patients with rheumatoid arthritis, and comparison with the DAS28 based on erythrocyte sedimentation rate. Ann Rheum Dis. 2009;68(6):954–60.
35. Strand LI, Ljunggren AE, Bogen B, Ask T, Johnsen TB. The Short-Form McGill Pain Questionnaire as an outcome measure: test–retest reliability and responsiveness to change. Eur J Pain. 2008;12(7):917–25.
36. Fitzcharles MA, Ste-Marie PA, Häuser W, Clauw DJ, Jamal S, Karsh J, et al. Efficacy, tolerability, and safety of cannabinoid treatments in the rheumatic diseases: a systematic review of randomized controlled trials. Arthrit Care Res. 2016;68(5):681–8.
37. Walitt B, Klose P, Fitzcharles MA, Phillips T, Häuser W. Cannabinoids for fibromyalgia. Cochrane Database Syst Rev. 2016;7:CD011694.
38. Tateo S. State of the evidence: cannabinoids and cancer pain-a systematic review. J Am Assoc Nurse Pract. 2017;29(2):94–103. Epub 2016 Nov 10.
39. De Vita MJ, Moskal D, Maisto SA, Ansell EB. Association of Cannabinoid administration with experimental pain in healthy adults: a systematic review and meta-analysis. JAMA Psychiat. 2018;75(11):1118–27. https://doi.org/10.1001/jamapsychiatry.2018.2503.
40. Stevens AJ, Higgins MD. A systematic review of the analgesic efficacy of cannabinoid medications in the management of acute pain. Acta Anaseth Scand. 2017;61(3):268–80.
41. Abdallah FW, Hussain N, Weaver T, Brull R. Analgesic efficacy of cannabinoids for acute pain management after surgery: a systematic review and meta-analysis. Reg Anesth Pain Med. 2020;45(7):509–19. https://doi.org/10.1136/rapm-2020-101340.
42. National Academies of Sciences, Engineering, and Medicine. 2017. The Health Effects of Cannabis and Cannabinoids: The Current State of Evidence and Recommendations for Research. Washington, DC: The National Academies Press.
43. Wright P, Walsh Z, Margolese S, Sanchez T, Arlt S, Belle-Isle L, et al. Canadian clinical practice guidelines for the use of plant-based cannabis and cannabinoid-based products in the management of chronic non-cancer pain and co-occurring conditions: protocol for a systematic literature review. BMJ Open. 2020;10:e036114. https://doi.org/10.1136/bmjopen-2019-036114.

Cannabinoids and Cancer Pain

26

Matthew Chung, Barlas Benkli, Salman Hirani,
and Christina Le-Short

Introduction

Pain is one of the most distressing and debilitating symptoms that cancer patients can experience and is often a cause for severe impairment of quality of life [1, 2]. A systematic review and meta-analysis reported that 51% of patients with cancer experienced pain regardless of staging [2]. Elevated rates of pain were reported by patients with advanced, metastatic, or terminal disease at a rate of 52% [2]. In addition, 28% of patients continued to report pain following curative and anti-cancer therapies [2]. Patients with a cancer diagnosis may also have pain prior to their diagnosis, which may be further compounded by cancer-related treatment (i.e., surgery) [3]. Patients are often reluctant to mention their pain or raise concerns related to their discomfort, restricting function. It is imperative to adequately address the topic of pain during cancer treatment, as insufficiently controlled pain during this period can predispose patients toward the development of chronic pain following treatment cessation [4].

M. Chung (✉) · S. Hirani · C. Le-Short
Department of Pain Medicine, Division of Anesthesiology, Critical Care and Pain Medicine, The University of Texas MD Anderson Cancer Center, Houston, TX, USA
e-mail: mchung1@mdanderson.org

B. Benkli
Department of Neurology, The University of Texas McGovern Medical School, Houston, TX, USA

Early detection and improved cancer treatment have led to an increasing number of cancer survivors along with an increased life expectancy following diagnosis. With increasing prevalence of cancer patients and cancer survivors, pain control has become a cornerstone for cancer management, as it supports the ideals of quality of life, compliance with therapy, physical function, and overall outlook on life [3]. This population has potential for multiple medical and psychosocial complications that can have a direct effect on adequately controlling their pain [5]. As pain shifts from the short-term effects of treatment to a long-term issue, providers rely on chronic pain management strategies to optimize pain relief [6]. Chronic pain syndromes that cancer survivors often experience include neuropathy, lymphedema, myalgia, arthralgia, post-surgical pain, and genital pain to name a few [7]. This population is far different from those with chronic pain without a history of cancer as they have localizable tissue damage while also being at risk for recurrence of disease [6]. Yet the source of chronic pain in cancer survivors without active disease is often secondary to cancer treatment rather than the cancer itself [6]. Cancer treatment in the form of surgery, radiation, chemotherapy, hormonal therapy, steroids, hematopoietic stem-cell transplantation, and bisphosphonates is all known to have associated pain in cancer survivors [6, 8, 9]. The mechanisms underlying cancer treatments and chronic pain are largely unknown, with neural injury as a possible consequence of

S. N. Narouze (ed.), *Cannabinoids and Pain*, https://doi.org/10.1007/978-3-030-69186-8_26

surgery and radiation. Sources of chemotherapy-related pain include associated neuronal damage, mitochondrial damage, and heightened oxidative stress resulting in further inflammation and alteration of neurotransmission [10].

With an ever-growing survivorship population, cancer survivors with chronic pain may benefit from similar treatment strategies employed in chronic pain of non-cancer origin [4, 6]. Among cancer survivors, chronic nociceptive, neuropathic, and postoperative pain is largely managed with systemic pain medications including opiates as first-line therapy [11]. Growing concerns regarding long-term use of systemic opiates, including adverse events, lack of effectiveness, abuse, dependence, and tolerance, are similar for patients with cancer- and non-cancer-related chronic pain and have resulted in consideration of non-opioid as well as noninvasive modalities to control chronic cancer pain.

Cannabis is the most commonly used controlled substance in the United States and is more commonly used in an inhalational format for its psychoactive properties [7]. Use of cannabis in the cancer population has been studied with variable levels of evidence in the treatment of nausea, anorexia, pain, cancer itself, anxiety, and sleep disorders [12–19]. Among various symptoms encountered among cancer patients, pain has been commonly cited as one of the most common indications for use [20]. Although a significant portion of cancer patients use cannabinoids, the ratio of those who receive medical guidance on this topic is relatively low and has been reported by Pergam et al. as low as 15% [21].

Cannabinoids (CB) have previously been identified as potential adjuvant analgesics in the setting of cancer pain [22, 23]. CBs are developed within trichomes or glands that are found on flowers and fan leaves of cannabis plants [20]. The term cannabinoids encompasses endocannabinoids, phytocannabinoids, and synthetic cannabinoid analogues [24]. This alternative form of analgesia has been used by cancer patients both with and without medical guidance in various formulations. More medically relevant preparations of CB and CB analogues include cannabis extracts with varying THC/CBD ratios, nabiximols (an extract with a 1:1 THC/CBD ratio), and THC analogues such as nabilone and dronabinol [24]. The cannabis plant itself is consumed by patients through smoking, vaping, and oral ingestion. Other studied forms of cannabinoids include THC oils, THC oromucosal spray, and nabiximols (THC/CBD) oromucosal spray [25].

At the time of publication of this chapter, cannabinoids have had no approved indication in the United States for cancer pain. Canada, Israel, and several European countries currently use cannabinoids in symptomatic treatment of cancer, although there is no EU-wide framework for medical use of cannabinoids [26]. As of 2019, nabiximols, nabilone, and dronabinol were used for varying indications including multiple sclerosis-related spasticity, neuropathic pain, loss of appetite, and nausea in several European countries. In this chapter we aim to explore relevant mechanisms of cancer pain that are addressed by cannabis and cannabinoids, current understanding with a summary of pre-clinical and clinical studies to date, clinical considerations, as well as commentary on the future of cannabinoids in cancer pain.

Relevant Mechanisms of Cancer Pain

Nociception in cancer pain can take on various forms of visceral, somatic, and neuropathic pain. Cancer pain can be encountered as a consequence of a combination of changes within the body at various cellular, tissue, and systemic levels during any phase of cancer including proliferation, invasion, and metastasis. Notably, the type of cancer can also impose variable types and severity of pain. Added, the corresponding immune system and its response to cancer are a well-known contributor of cancer pain. During inception and progression of a tumor mass, several immune mediators (including prostaglandins, endothelins, protons, bradykinin, proteases, nerve growth factor, and tumor necrosis factor) are released and interact with receptors found on peripheral nociceptive nerve terminals that engage abnormal discharge and increased excitability. Tumor growth in the area of peripheral nerves can further degenerate neural integrity and consequentially impose neuropathic complaints including hyperalgesia and/or allodynia. The impact of tumor growth on the peripheral nervous system in this fashion can perpetuate the development of central sensitization, further enhancing neurotransmission of nociceptive input via the dorsal horn and perception of spontaneous and breakthrough pain.

Although the medicinal properties of cannabis have been known for quite some time, it was not until the discovery of THC and subsequent revelations surrounding the components of the endocannabinoid system that led to further understanding of cannabinoid-induced analgesia [27, 28]. Following tissue injury, neural and non-neural cells produce arachidonic acid derivatives called endocannabinoids. Specifically, anandamide and 2-arachidonoylglycerol (2-AG) are two endocannabinoids that modify sensitization and inflammation following injury through its targeted interaction with cannabinoid receptors [29]. CB type 1 (CB_1) and CB type 2 (CB_2) are two G protein cannabinoid receptor subtypes that are coupled to potassium and calcium channels that are involved in postsynaptic membrane hyperpolarization as well as presynaptic reduction in neurotransmitter release. CB_1 receptors can be found in the central and peripheral nervous system, with predominance in the former. CB_2 can be found predominantly in the peripheral nervous system, with its specific expression on immune cells and keratinocytes [30]. Direct action on the CB_1 and CB2 receptors in the peripheral nervous system contributes toward attenuated release of inflammatory agents and enhanced release of analgesic opioids in various inflammatory and neuropathic pain models [31]. CB_1 receptor activation in the periphery of afferent nociceptive nerve endings reduces hyperalgesia by opening G protein-coupled potassium channels, inhibiting voltage-dependent calcium channels, as well as inhibiting release of substance P and calcitonin gene-related peptide (CGRP). CB_2 receptor activation leads to secretion of beta-endorphins that subsequently activate mu opioid receptors in the adjacent peripheral nociceptive afferent nerve endings which open similar G protein-coupled potassium channels for anti-nociception through hyperpolarization of transmitting action potentials. Although many studies and pain models predicate involvement of the CB_1 and CB_2 receptors in the periphery, more recent studies also reveal CB_1 in the central nervous system which can be a promising target in pain management [32, 33]. CB_1 receptors in the central nervous system (CNS) are shown to be modulated by THC, with promising results in mice pain models. There are also studies on how CBD modulates CB_1 receptors in CNS; however further studies are needed to assess utility in pain management [32].

Apart from direct effects of CB effector mechanisms, cannabinoids attempt to quell concerns pertaining to opiate use. CB receptor activation is suggested to potentiate response to mu opioid receptors when concomitantly used with opiates [34–36]. Additionally CB receptor activation may prevent opioid tolerance [37]. This assumption is based on previously demonstrated parallels in agonism of CB_2 and endothelin B receptors (the latter of which is commonly involved in cancer pain) and its downstream effect on mu opioid receptors [14]. The endocannabinoid system and its discovery have brought increasing focus and attention toward targeting the activation of CB receptors with exogenous cannabinoids in pain.

Current Understanding of Clinical Studies

As mentioned previously, cancer pain can arise from one or more various mechanisms, inflammatory, visceral, or neuropathic. Patients may also have an underlying history of non-cancer-related pain coexisting with their cancer pain.

Additionally, pain may be further enhanced by or manifested from psychiatric disease or psychological disturbance in the form of pain catastrophizing. Thus, it is imperative to keep all facets of pain or pain contributors in mind during the management of a cancer patient rather than treating the cancer pain itself. Since the breadth of evidence of cannabinoids and overall pain may supersede the extent of this chapter, we aim to address the evidence specifically pertaining to cannabinoids in cancer pain.

The first study examining cannabinoids (specifically oral THC) with advanced cancer pain included ten patients that were double blinded and placebo controlled. This study by Noyes et al. examined pain relief, pain intensity, as well as other symptoms using a range of doses from 5 to 20 mg and found that higher doses demonstrated improved analgesia [9, 38]. In a follow-up study, the authors compared various doses of THC and codeine for similar analgesic effects and demonstrated higher doses of THC to be more sedating than codeine [9].

In a multicenter, double-blind, placebo-controlled study, nabiximols and THC were compared among advanced cancer patients who had insufficient analgesia from their opiate regimen. The nabiximols arm demonstrated significant relief of cancer pain [16]. In a follow-up, open lab study from Johnson et al., the same group of nabiximols patients continued to have sustained relief in their pain from chronic use without need for titration or any other medication meant for pain control [39]. To further study potential levels of cannabinoid components, Portenoy et al. further investigated nabiximols in a graded-dose trial in a randomized study that included similarly opiate-treated advanced cancer patients. Noyes et al. found that lower doses (fewer sprays) had significant pain control while higher doses (greater sprays daily) had higher associated adverse effects [38, 40].

In a prospective observational study, 112 advanced cancer patients, who had pain and a variety of other cancer-related symptoms (i.e., anorexia), were given nabilone, a synthetic cannabinoid. Maida et al. demonstrated that nabilone use had associated improvement of cancer-related symptoms including pain [41]. Furthermore, these patients tapered their existing analgesic regimens (including nonsteroidal anti-inflammatory drugs, tricyclic antidepressants, gabapentin, etc.) and required lower starting doses for analgesic relief [35, 41].

In a randomized, placebo-controlled study involving 360 cancer patients with opioid refractory cancer pain patients, nabiximols in various dosages were administered and compared to placebo. Low-dose (2.7–10.8 mg THC/2.5–10.0 mg CBD) and medium-dose nabiximols (10.8–16.2 mg THC/10.0–15.0 mg CBD) were shown to have more effectiveness in reduction of pain from baseline to end of study (low $p = 0.008$, medium $p = 0.038$). High-dose nabiximols (29.7–43.2 mg THC/27.5–40.0 mg CBD) had insignificant effects on pain and were also shown to have higher frequency of adverse events [40].

In a randomized, placebo-controlled pilot study of nabiximols, Lynch et al. investigated chronic induced neuropathic pain (CIPN) in cancer patients. No significant difference was seen for pain control given the small sample size, yet it demonstrated some associated improvement for CIPN [42].

Among clinical studies investigating cannabinoids and cancer pain, side effects and adverse events were consistent with other symptoms encountered in other studies exploring cannabinoid use for other indications [43]. THC was commonly associated with euphoria, mental clouding, and drowsiness [9, 17]. Nabiximols in several studies had commonly reported somnolence, dizziness, confusion, nausea, hypotension, fatigue, and dry mouth. It was also reported that most side effects were often mild, temporary, and curtailed with adjustment of treatment doses [9, 38, 40–42].

In historical human studies, cannabinoids at tolerable doses were shown to have efficacy comparable to low-dose opioid treatment [9, 38]. More recently, THC/CBD combination medications have been studied as an adjunctive treatment for pain relief with mixed results [16, 39, 40, 44]. Nabiximols, a THC/CBD combination, is approved for use in multiple sclerosis to treat spasticity in Canada, New Zealand, and some European countries, while in Canada it is also indicated for cancer pain. In a randomized placebo-controlled study, an oral formulation of nabiximols was shown to be associated with increased pain relief at stable, tolerable doses [39, 40]. In another large randomized placebo-controlled study, Lichtman showed nabiximols was not superior to placebo [44]. An additional study investigating pain along with other cancer-related symptoms (i.e., chemotherapy induced nausea) showed nabilone was associated with improvement in multiple cancer-related symptoms along with pain in addition to decreased analgesic use [41]. A phase 3 study by Fallon et al. investigating nabiximols' efficiency in chronic pain failed to show superiority to placebo; however in a subset of patients that included 30% of patients from the United States, all under the age of 65 years demonstrated significant improvement [23].

There are multiple challenges in conducting trials and the subsequent development of guidelines in management of cancer pain including but not limited to heterogeneity of this patient population, patient safety, and variable methods of administration. Future studies on cannabis and cannabinoids with these challenges addressed are needed to establish efficacy, side effect profile, and pharmacokinetics to explore any semblance of a guideline for clinical practice. With its current federal classification as a Schedule 1 substance, cannabis and cannabinoids are limited to investigation as a medical product [45].

Clinical Considerations

The management of pain and suffering is uniquely tailored to each individual regardless of a diagnosis of cancer. Therein, it is of utmost importance to continue to explore novel classes of analgesics and noninvasive therapies. The growth and popularity in the use of cannabis and cannabinoids have led to significant crossover of medical and recreational use among consumers inclusive of cancer patients. Most experienced clinicians will have encountered anecdotal benefits among their patients; however the danger lies in the largely unregulated and inconsistent product which is of grave concern even among those involved in research of these drugs. It is imperative to caution use among cancer patients due to dynamic factors of immunocompetence, physiology, and chemotoxic medication regimen, alongside potential disease recurrence or regression.

Cannabinoid use incites concerns due to the impact and potential side effects throughout the body, including nervous, cardiac, gastrointestinal, and pulmonary systems. The neuropsychiatric effects of cannabinoids largely stem from the THC components given its anxiety and psychoactive properties. This may explain why most formulations of synthetic cannabinoids that include THC also have CBD components [46, 47]. Untoward effects of cannabinoids have been demonstrated to cause tachycardia and high blood pressure among patients with existing cardiac disease and can subsequently cause complications [47]. In an inhalational form, cannabis has demonstrated impaired immunological response and consequent infections [48].

It is also important to keep in mind growing concern of potential cross-reactivity of chemotherapy, regular opiate use, and psychotropic agents among cancer patients using cannabinoids. To date, there are both in vitro and in vivo studies suggesting THC and CBD effect induction and inhibition of liver enzymes; however further studies are needed. At this time, there is simply insufficient evidence to guide clinical decision-making [49–52]. Providers should keep an open dialogue with cancer patients regarding cannabinoid use for education and treatment-related clinical decision-making.

The topic of cannabinoid and concurrent opiate use is a question commonly brought up by cancer patients, caregivers, and physicians as regular opiate use has been a part of standard of care in cancer pain management. Current practice based on federal regulations has inevitably led patients to choose one treatment over the other or with the physician turning a blind eye to dual therapy. In chronic pain, cannabinoids are thought to have both primary pain-relieving effects in addition to synergistic analgesia, decreasing tolerance and minimizing side effects with concomitant opiate use. Studies have shown that cannabinoids decrease the risk of opioid addiction by amplifying analgesic effects of opioids at mu receptors while dampening positive reinforcing effects [53, 54]. Reassuringly, many cancer-related studies have suggested the inclusion of cannabinoids and opiate therapy as part of future randomized control studies. The question of how cannabinoids can potentially address our growing concerns of opiate overuse, tolerance, and dependence in cancer pain largely remains unanswered with an inability to provide any guidance for clinical decisions at this time.

It is important as clinicians and scientists dedicated toward the health and well-being of patients that we continue to educate and promote the refinement of current knowledge.

Commentary on the Future of Cannabinoids in Cancer Pain

Current environment regarding cannabis and cannabinoid use in the United States is consumer driven with the oncologist and pain provider often taking the stance of turning a blind eye or running the risk of guiding patients into unknown and potentially deleterious territory. Due to state-level approval, the marketplace for under-regulated cannabis-based products will continue to escalate as patients seek out an alternative route for pain control. According to the National Conference of State Legislature (NCSL), a vast majority of states (all except 4) permit medical cannabis/cannabinoid use in some form; among them 12 also have legislature to allow recreational use approved or in progress [17]. Although an increasing number of US states have legalized medical cannabinoids in the last decade, lack of federal regulations, regulatory bodies, and paucity of guidelines limits use by healthcare professionals and patients while also making it difficult to have large-scale studies to determine its efficiency in treatment of cancer pain. Without further study, patients who exercise cannabis/cannabinoid use may be subject to suboptimal therapy (from factors of poor medication selection and improper dosing) and be at risk of becoming ostracized by their opiate-prescribing physicians (given their risk of liability).

Following the review of updated clinical and pre-clinical data available, the authors agree that while treatment of cancer pain with cannabis and cannabinoid appears promising, tolerability remains questionable, and efficacy is lacking requiring further study. Added, the authors suggest that cannabinoids (dronabinol, nabilone, nabiximols, medical cannabis) should not be considered as part of regular management in cancer pain given their lack of evidence thus far. Alternatively, CB agents can be considered for other cancer-related symptoms (such as nausea and vomiting), but only in situations of standard treatment failure or as an adjunct to certain agents when appropriate. Lastly, we recognize that increased awareness and advocacy for change by policymakers are paramount for successful study of this form of analgesia.

Cannabinoids in cancer pain – clinical trial summary

Authors, year of publication	Study type	Cannabis or cannabinoid formulation	Study population	Patients enrolled; treatment arm(s); placebo or no control	Adjuvant therapies	Degree of benefit documented
Lynch et al. 2014 [42]	Randomized placebo-controlled crossover pilot study	Nabiximols spray (mean treatment of 8 sprays; range of 3–12 sprays)	Cancer patients with chemotherapy-induced neuropathic pain	16;16;0	Unknown	No significant difference between nabiximols and placebo; however, 5 participants reported two-point or greater reduction in pain. An extension study (10 patients) carried out 6 additional months demonstrated modest improvement beyond initial pain reduction
Portenoy et al. 2012 [40]	Randomized placebo controlled	Nabiximols spray (low dose, 4 sprays; medium dose, 10 sprays; and high dose, 16 sprays) and placebo	Advanced cancer and opioid-refractory pain	360; 268; 91	Opiates	1.Primary end point involving comparison of proportion of patients in each study group obtaining 30% reduction in baseline pain was not significant 2. Improved pain in low-dose group (100 microL to 600 mL involving concentrations of 2.7 mg THC/2.5 mg CBD with each 100 microL spray)
Johnson et al. 2010 [16]	Randomized placebo-controlled parallel group study	Nabiximols spray (2.7 mg THC and 2.5 mg CBD in 100 microL pump) vs. THC spray (2.7 mg per 100 microL)	Advanced cancer with inadequate analgesia despite chronic opioid dosing	177; THC/ CBD 60; THC 58; placebo 59	Opiates	Nabiximols arm demonstrated improved pain compared to placebo ($p = 0.024$); nabiximols arm participants took fewer doses of breakthrough pain medication compared to placebo ($p = 0.004$); THC arm without any significant pain changes

Authors, year of publication	Study type	Cannabis or cannabinoid formulation	Study population	Patients enrolled; treatment arm(s); placebo or no control	Adjuvant therapies	Degree of benefit documented
Maida et al. 2008 [41]	Prospective observational	Nabilone (Cesamet)	Advanced cancer patients	112; 47; 65	Opiates, nonsteroidal anti-inflammatory drugs, tricyclic antidepressants, gabapentin	Improved pain score and decreased total morphine equivalent doses compared to baseline were demonstrated in the treatment arm. Additionally lower rate of starting adjuvant therapies of and greater tendency to discontinue active adjuvant therapies of NSAID, TCA, and gabapentin
Noyes et al. 1975 [38]	Randomized control study	THC oil capsules	Advanced cancer	10; 10; 0	Opiates (methadone specifically)	Increased pain relief correlation with higher doses of THC ($p < 0.001$); doses studied included placebo, 5 mg, 10 mg, 15 mg, or 20 mg
Noyes et al. 1975 [9]	Randomized control study	THC oil capsules	Advanced cancer	36;36;0	Opiates	Pain reduction demonstrated in 20 mg of THC over placebo ($p < 0.05$); no significant difference in analgesia between THC and codeine. A rotation of placebo, THC, and codeine was given to all participants)

Disclosures No financial disclosures to report.

Conflict of Interest No conflicts of interest to report.

References

1. Carr D, Goudas L, Lawrence D, et al. Management of cancer symptoms: pain, depression, and fatigue. Evid Rep Technol Assess. 2002;61:1–5.
2. Van den Beuken-van Everdingen MH, de Rijke JM, Kessels AG, et al. Update on prevalence of pain in patients with cancer: a systematic review and meta-analysis. J Pain Symptom Manag. 2016;51(6):1070–190.
3. Jacobs M, Macefield RC, Elbers RG, et al. Meta-analysis shows clinically relevant and long-lasting deterioration in health-related quality of life after esophageal cancer surgery. Qual Life Res. 2014;23:1097–115.
4. Burton AW, Fanciullo GJ, Beasley RD, Fisch MJ. Chronic pain in the cancer survivor: a new frontier. Pain Med. 2007;8:189–98.

5. Moryl N, Coyle N, Essandoh S, Glare P. Chronic pain management in cancer survivor. J Natl Compr Canc Netw. 2010;8(9):1104–10.
6. Glare PA, Davies PS, Finlay E, Gulati A, Lemanne D, Moryl N, Oeffinger KC, Paice JA, Stubblefield MD, Syrjala KL. Pain in cancer survivors. J Clin Oncol. 2014;32(16):1739–47.
7. Syrjala KL, Jensen MP, Mendoza E, Yi JC, Fisher HM, Keefe FJ. Psychological and behavioral approaches to cancer pain management. J Clin Oncol. 2014;32(16):1703–11.
8. Levy MH, Chwistek M, Mehta RS. Management of chronic pain in cancer survivors. Cancer J. 2008;14(6):401–9.
9. Noyes R, Brunk SF, Avery DA, et al. The analgesic properties of delta-9-tetrahydrocannabinol and codeine. Clin Pharmacol Ther. 1975;18(1):84–9. [PUBMED Abstract]
10. Boyette-Davis JA, Hou S, Abdi S, Dougherty PM. An updated understanding of the mechanisms involved in chemotherapy-induced neuropathy. Pain Manag. 2018;8(5):363–75.
11. Denlinger CS, Ligibel JA, Are M, et al. Survivorship: pain version 1.2014, clinical practice guidelines in oncology. J Natl Compr Canc Netw. 2014;12(4):488–500.
12. Ananth P, Reed-Weston A, Wolfe J. Medical marijuana in pediatric oncology: a review of the evidence and implications for practice. Pediatr Blood Cancer. 2018;65(2).
13. Bertrand A, Boyle H, Moreaux J. Does consumption of tobacco, alcohol, and cannabis in adolescents and young adults with cancer affect the use of analgesics during hospitalizations? Arch Pediatr. 2016;23:353–9.
14. Cathcart P, de Giorgio A, Stebbing J. Cannabis and cancer: reality or pipe dream? Lancet Oncol. 2015;16:1291–2.
15. Jatoi A, Windschitl HE, Loprinzi CL, et al. Dronabinol versus megestrol acetate versus combination therapy for cancer-associated anorexia: a North Central Cancer Treatment Group study. J Clin Oncol. 2002;20:567–73.
16. Johnson JR, Burnell-Nugent M, Lossignol D, et al. Double-blind, randomized, placebo-controlled, parallel-group study of the efficacy, safety, and tolerability of THC: CBD extract and THC extract in patients with intractable cancer-related pain. J Pain Symptom Manag. 2010;39:167–79.
17. National Academies of Sciences, Engineering and Medicine. The health effects of cannabis and cannabinoids: the current state of evidence and recommendations for research. Washington, DC: National Academies Press; 2017. https://www.ncsl.org/research/civil-and-criminal-justice/marijuana-overview.aspx
18. Schleider LB, Mechoulam R, Lederman V, et al. Prospective analysis of safety and efficacy of medical cannabis in a large unselected population of patients with cancer. Eur J Intern Med. 2018;1:37–43.
19. Todaro B. Cannabinoids in the treatment of chemotherapy-induced nausea and vomiting. J Natl Compr Canc Netw. 2012;10:487–92.
20. Pertwee RG. Pharmacological actions of cannabinoids. In: Pertwee RG, editor. Cannabinoids. Berlin: Springer; 2005. p. 1–51.
21. Pergam SA, Woodfield MC, Lee CM, et al. Cannabis use among patients at a comprehensive cancer center in a state with legalized medicinal and recreational use. Cancer. 2017;123(22):4488–97.
22. Campbell FA, Tramer MR, Carroll D, et al. Are cannabinoids an effective and safe treatment option in the management of pain? A qualitative systematic review. BMJ. 2001;323(7303):13–6.
23. Fallon MT, Lux EA, Sanchez R, Sun W, Wright S, Lichtman AH, Kornyeyeva E. Sativex oromucosal spray as adjunctive therapy in advanced cancer patients with chronic pain unalleviated by optimized opioid therapy: two double-blind, randomized, placebo-controlled phase 3 studies. Br J Pain. 2017;11:119–33.
24. Fraguas-Sánchez AI, Torres-Suárez AI. Medical use of cannabinoids. Drugs 2018;78(16):1665–1703. https://doi.org/10.1007/s40265-018-0996-1. Review. PubMed PMID: 30374797.
25. Blake A, Wan BA, Malek L, DeAngelis C, Diaz P, Lao N, Chow E, O'Hearn S. A selective review of medical cannabis in cancer pain management. Ann Palliat Med. 2017;6(Suppl 2):S215-S222. https://doi.org/10.21037/apm.2017.08.05. Epub 2017 Aug 23. Review. PubMed PMID: 28866904.
26. European Monitoring Centre for Drugs and Drug Addiction. Medical use of cannabis and cannabinoids: questions and answers for policymaking. Luxembourg: Publications Office of the European Union; 2018.
27. Matsuda LA, Lolait SJ, Brownstein MJ, Young CA, Bonner TI. Structure of a cannabinoid receptor and functional expression of the cloned cDNA. Nature. 1990;346:561–4.
28. Munro S, Thomas KL, Abu-Shaar M. Molecular characterization of a peripheral receptor for cannabinoids. Nature. 1993;365:61–5.
29. Maccarrone M, Guzman M, Mackie K, Doherty P, Harkany T. Programming of neural cells by (endo) cannabinoids: from physiological rules to emerging therapies. Nat Rev Neurosci. 2014;15:786–801. https://doi.org/10.1038/nrn3846.
30. Rahn EJ, Makriyannis A, Hohmann AG. Activation of cannabinoid Cb1 and Cb2 receptors suppresses neuropathic nociception evoked by the chemotherapeutic agent vincristine in rats. Br J Pharmacol. 2007;152(5):765–77.
31. Ibrahim MM, Porreca F, Lai J, et al. CB2 cannabinoid receptor activation produces antinociception by stimulating peripheral release of endogenous opioids. Proc Natl Acad Sci. 2005;102(8):3093–8.
32. Al-Zoubi R, Morales P, Reggio PH. Structural insights into CB1 receptor biased signaling. Int J Mol Sci. 2019;20:E1837.

33. Baker D, Pryce G, Giovannoni G, Thompson AJ. The therapeutic potential of cannabis. Lancet Neurol. 2003;2(5):291–8.
34. Cichewicz DL, Welch SP. Modulation of oral morphine anti Nociceptive tolerance and naloxone-precipitated withdrawal signs by oral Delta 9-tetrahydrocannabinol. J Pharmacol Exp Ther. 2003;305:812–7.
35. Maida V, Daeninck PJ. A user's guide to cannabinoid therapies in oncology. Curr Oncol. 2016;23(6):398–406. https://doi.org/10.3747/co.23.3487. Epub 2016 Dec 21. Review. PubMed PMID: 28050136; PubMed Central PMCID: PMC5176373
36. Yuill MB, Hale DE, Guindon J, Morgan DJ. Anti-nociceptive interactions between opioids and a cannabinoid receptor 2 agonist in inflammatory pain. Mol Pain. 2017;13:1744806917728227. https://doi.org/10.1177/1744806917728227. PubMed PMID: 28879802; PubMed Central PMCID: PMC5593227
37. Cichewicz DL, McCarthy EA. Antinociceptive synergy between delta(9)-tetrahydrocannabinol and opioids after oral administration. J Pharmacol Exp Ther. 2003;304:1010–5.
38. Noyes R, Brunk SF, Baram DA, et al. Analgesic effect of delta-9-tetrahydrocannabinol. J Clin Pharmacol. 1975;15(2–3):139–43. [PUBMED Abstract]
39. Johnson JR, Lossignol D, Burnell-Nugent M, Fallon MT. An open-label extension study to investigate the long-term safety and tolerability of THC/CBD oromucosal spray and oromucosal THC spray in patients with terminal cancer-related pain refractory to strong opioid analgesics. J Pain Symptom Manag. 2013;46(2):207–18. https://doi.org/10.1016/j.jpainsymman.2012.07.014. Epub 2012 Nov 8. PubMed PMID: 23141881
40. Portenoy RK, Ganae-Motan ED, Allende S, Yanagihara R, Shaiova L, Weinstein S, McQuade R, Wright S, Fallon MT. Nabiximols for opioid-treated cancer patients with poorly-controlled chronic pain: a randomized, placebo-controlled, graded-dose trial. J Pain. 2012;13(5):438–49. https://doi.org/10.1016/j.jpain.2012.01.003. Epub 2012 Apr 5. PubMed PMID: 22483680
41. Maida V, Ennis M, Irani S, Corbo M, Dolzhykov. Adjunctive Nabilone in cancer pain and symptom management: a prospective observational study using propensity scoring. J Support Oncol. 2008;6:119–24.
42. Lynch ME, Cesar-Rittenberg P, Hohmann AG. A double-blind, placebo-controlled, crossover pilot trial with extension using an oral mucosal cannabinoid extract for treatment of chemotherapy-induced neuropathic pain. J Pain Symptom Manag. 2014;47(1):166–73. https://doi.org/10.1016/j.jpainsymman.2013.02.018. Epub 2013 Jun 4. PubMed PMID: 23742737
43. Grotenhermen F, Muller-Vahl K. The therapeutic potential of cannabis and cannabinoids. Dtsch Arztebl Int. 2012;109:495–501.
44. Lichtman AH, Lux EA, McQuade R, Rossetti S, Sanchez R, Sun W, Wright S, Kornyeyeva E, Fallon MT. Results of a double-blind, randomized, placebo-controlled study of Nabiximols Oromucosal spray as an adjunctive therapy in advanced cancer patients with chronic uncontrolled pain. J Pain Symptom Manag. 2018;55(2):179–188.e1. https://doi.org/10.1016/j.jpainsymman.2017.09.001. Epub 2017 Sep 18. PubMed PMID: 28923526
45. Borgelt LM, Franson K, Nussbaum AM, et al. The pharmacologic and clinical effects of medical cannabis. Pharmacotherapy. 2013;33:195–209.
46. Cooper ZD. Adverse effects of synthetic cannabinoids: management of acute toxicity and withdrawal. Curr Psychiatry Rep. 2016;18(5):52. https://doi.org/10.1007/s11920-016-0694-1. Review. PubMed PMID: 27074934; PubMed Central PMCID:PMC4923337
47. Schrot RJ, Hubbard JR. Cannabinoids: medical implications. Ann Med. 2016;48(3):128–41. https://doi.org/10.3109/07853890.2016.1145794. Epub 2016 Feb 25. Review. PubMed PMID: 26912385
48. Taskin D, Baldwin G, Sarafian T, Dubinett M, Roth M. Respiratory and immunologic consequences of marijuana smoking. J Clin Pharmacol. 2002;42:71Supplement–81Supplement.
49. Rong C, Carmona NE, Lee YL, Ragguett RM, Pan Z, Rosenblat JD, Subramaniapillai M, Shekotikhina M, Almatham F, Alageel A, Mansur R, Ho RC, McIntyre RS. Drug-drug interactions as a result of co-administering Δ(9)-THC and CBD with other psychotropic agents. Expert Opin Drug Saf. 2018;17(1):51–4. https://doi.org/10.1080/14740338.2017.1397128. Epub 2017 Oct 31. Review. PubMed PMID: 29082802
50. Stout SM, Cimino NM. Exogenous cannabinoids as substrates, inhibitors, and inducers of human drug metabolizing enzymes: a systematic review. Drug Metab Rev. 2014;46(1):86–95. https://doi.org/10.3109/03602532.2013.849268. Epub 2013 Oct 25. Review. PubMed PMID: 24160757
51. Yamaori S, Okamoto Y, Yamamoto I. Cannabidiol, a major phytocannabinoid, as a potent atypical inhibitor for CYP2D6. Drug Metab Dispos. 2011;39(11):2049–56.
52. Zendulka O, Dovrtělová G, Nosková K, Turjap M, Šulcová A, Hanuš L, Juřica J. Cannabinoids and Cytochrome P450 interactions. Curr Drug Metab. 2016;17(3):206–26. Review
53. Grenald SA, Young MA, Wang Y, Ossipov MH, Ibrahim MM, Largent-Milnes TM, Vanderah TW. Synergistic attenuation of chronic pain using mu opioid and cannabinoid receptor 2 agonists. Neuropharmacology. 2017;116:59–70.
54. Maguire DR, France CP. Interactions between cannabinoid receptor agonists and mu opioid receptor agonists in rhesus monkeys discriminating fentanyl. Eur J Pharmacol. 2016;784:199–206. https://doi.org/10.1016/j.ejphar.2016.05.018. Epub 2016 May 13. PubMed PMID: 27184925; PubMed Central PMCID: PMC4939121

Part VI

Cannabinoids as a Substitute for Opioids

Cannabinoids as a Substitute for Opioids: Basic Science and Clinical Evidence

27

Caroline A. MacCallum, Lauren de Freitas, Lauren Eadie, and Samer N. Narouze

Introduction

Opioid (illicit, prescription, nonmedical prescription) overdose mortality is the leading cause of accidental death in the United States. In 2016, opioid overdose was responsible for 42,249 deaths in the United States, the equivalent of 115 people/day [1]. There is a strong dose-dependent risk of harm related to opioids, especially with regard to fatal overdose [2]. The CDC reports that a dose of 50 mg morphine equivalent dose (MED) doubles the risk of fatal overdose compared to 20 mg MED, and when the dose is greater than 90 mg MED, the risk increases tenfold [3].

Alternative analgesics are necessary to address this crisis since chronic non-cancer pain (CNCP) is estimated to affect 20% of the adult population. Current CNCP guidelines recommend reassessing risk-benefit ratios for opioid doses exceeding a 90 mg MED due to accompanied increases in morbidity and mortality and a lack of evidence for associated improvements in pain and function. Opioids are considered second-line therapy for CNCP and are used frequently after unsuccessful attempts with first-line agents [4]. Despite the frequent use of opioids for CNCP conditions, opioids were unable to produce superior analgesia compared to non-opioid treatments among a 12-month RCT of neuropathic pain patients [5].

Physicians face an increasing number of CNCP patients not achieving their pain management goals and a lack of options to safely address their patients' pain. Given the complexity of chronic pain, most agents used for the management of neuropathic pain are off-label [6]. There is a growing public and professional interest in the possibility that cannabis might help curb the opioid epidemic. The major distinct differences that might give cannabinoids an edge over opioids are:

1. Cannabis has a superior safety profile in comparison to opioids, with no reported deaths directly due to overdose.
2. Patients develop selective tolerance to the psychoactive effects of cannabis quickly over a period of days, without concomitant tolerance to the benefits, and therefore maintain the same daily dose for many years.

C. A. MacCallum (✉) · L. Eadie
Department of Medicine, Faculty of Medicine, University of British Columbia, Vancouver, BC, Canada
e-mail: info@drcarolinemaccallum.com

L. de Freitas
Centre for Addiction and Mental Health, Toronto, ON, Canada

S. N. Narouze
Western Reserve Hospital, Center For Pain Medicine, Cuyahoga Falls, OH, USA

S. N. Narouze (ed.), *Cannabinoids and Pain*, https://doi.org/10.1007/978-3-030-69186-8_27

Pharmacology

Anatomical, biochemical, and molecular studies support the existence of reciprocal interactions between the endocannabinoid and opioid systems. The mesolimbic DA pathway represents the main common link allowing for crosstalk between these two systems, although the glutamatergic and GABAergic systems are also important targets for this interaction [7]. There are synergistic interactions between cannabinoid and opioid analgesics [8].

Cannabinoids have multimodal mechanisms of action to produce analgesia, including the inhibition of nociceptive processing through modulation of neuronal circuits in the CNS, pro-inflammatory molecule release, mast cell activation (via indirect activation of CB1 and CB2 receptors), as well as modulating endogenous opioid receptors in primary afferent pathways [9–11]. Several lines of evidence support the interconnection between cannabinoid and opioid signally. Specifically, THC has additive analgesic efficacy with kappa opioid receptor agonists. THC may also displace opiates from the μ-opioid receptor, as well as allosterically modulate the μ- and δ-opioid receptor to inhibit their activity [12, 13]. Preclinical evidence demonstrates that CB1 receptor antagonists can potentially reverse morphine-induced peripheral antinociception among inflammatory pain models, indicating the endocannabinoid system's role in opioid-related actions [14, 15]. CB2 receptor agonists have also been shown to can evoke peripheral analgesia by triggering the release of beta-endorphin in response to stimulation of CB2 receptors expressed in human keratinocytes [16]. As such, there is a strong evidence that cannabinoid and opioid effects share receptor interactivity as well as downstream second messenger effects. From a clinical standpoint, this may provide an opportunity for therapeutic synergy [16]. In intractable or difficult-to-control pain, using low-dose cannabis as an adjunctive therapy may be an approach to decrease opioid dosed, and thus risk of opioid related harm, while improving control of pain [17, 18].

When combined with THC, the effective dose 50 (ED50) for morphine is 3.6 times lower than that of morphine alone [19]. Similarly, the combination of THC with codeine reduces the ED50 by 9.5 times [19]. It was shown that vaporized cannabis augments the analgesic effects of opioids without significantly altering plasma opioid levels [20]. Specifically, adjunctive vaporized cannabis (3.56% THC, three times a day) significantly decreased pain by 27% among chronic pain patients without significantly altering the opioid pharmacokinetics or plasma opioid levels [20, 21]. With a therapeutic index of 1:>1000, cannabis is considered one of the least physiologically toxic analgesics, compared to codeine (1:20), alcohol (1:10), and heroin (1:5) [22]. A paucity of cannabinoid (CB) receptors in the brainstem, and therefore a lack of respiratory depression, may account for the lower toxicity. In comparison, there is significant risk of sleep-disordered breathing associated with opioids, especially if combined with other CNS depressants such as benzodiazepines [23]. cannabinoids

Observational and Epidemiological Evidence

There is preliminary evidence to suggest that medical cannabis initiation may either reduce the opioid dose required for pain relief or it may replace the use of opioids altogether, decreasing the risk of opioid-related fatalities due to overdose [21, 24]. Specifically, 97% of medical cannabis patients "strongly agreed/agreed" that they are able to decrease the amount of opiates they consume when they also use cannabis, and 81% "strongly agreed/agreed" that taking cannabis by itself was more effective at treating their condition than taking cannabis with opioids [21]. Another survey revealed high self-reported use of cannabis as a substitute for prescription drugs (63%), particularly pharmaceutical opioids (30%), benzodiazepines (16%), and antidepressants (12%). Interestingly, 42% of patients reported accessing cannabis from illegal/unregulated sources [24].

Other cross-sectional survey evidence suggests that medical cannabis use is associated with a 64% reduction in opioid use, in addition to improved quality of life and decreased medication-related side effects [25]. Cannabis may alleviate symptom clusters that can accompany CNCP, including nausea, anxiety, insomnia, and depression [11, 26]: thereby potentially reducing the psychological distress associated with chronic pain [27, 28]. The COMPASS study (n = 431) determined that the medical use of cannabis, even after adjusting for confounders, produced a greater reduction in pain among the cannabis group compared to controls (Difference = 1.10; 95% CI = 0.72–1.56) and, moreover, that physical components of quality of life and mood also significantly improved compared to the control group [29].

However, there are conflicting reports showing that cannabis use may increase risk for opioid abuse. Investigators analyzed data from wave one (2001–2002) and wave two (2004–2005) of the National Epidemiologic Survey on Alcohol and Related Condition to assess the associations between cannabis use and change in risk for incident nonmedical prescription opioid use and opioid use disorder at 3 years. Results indicated that cannabis use at wave one was associated with an increased incidence of nonmedical prescription opioid use (OR = 5.78; 95% CI, 4.23–7.9) and opioid use disorder (OR = 7.76; 95% CI, 4.95–12.16) at wave two. Adjustment for background characteristics did not impact the statistical significance of these associations. The authors concluded that "cannabis use, even among adults with moderate to severe pain, was associated with a substantially increased risk of nonmedical prescription opioid use at 3-year follow-up" [30].

Campbell et al. reported the effect of cannabis use in people with chronic non-cancer pain prescribed opioids. At 4-year follow-up, cannabis users had a greater pain severity score (risk ratio 1·14, 95% CI 1·01–1·29, for less frequent cannabis use; and 1·17, 1·03–1·32, for daily or near-daily cannabis use) and greater generalized anxiety disorder severity scores (1·07, 1·03–1·12; and 1·10, 1·06–1·15). The authors concluded there was no evidence that cannabis use reduced pain severity or exerted an opioid-sparing effect [31].

Medical marijuana laws (MCLs) reduce prescription medication use in Medicare part D and Medicaid populations [32, 33]. States with medical cannabis laws between 1999 and 2010 had a 24.8% lower mean annual opioid overdose mortality rate (95% CI, −37.5% to −9.5%; P = 0.003) compared to states without medical cannabis laws [34]. However, extending the analysis through 2017, the association between state medical cannabis laws and opioid overdose mortality reversed direction from negative 21% to positive 23%, and remained positive after accounting for recreational cannabis laws [35] (Fig. 27.1). However, authors concluded that they found it was unlikely medical cannabis exerted a

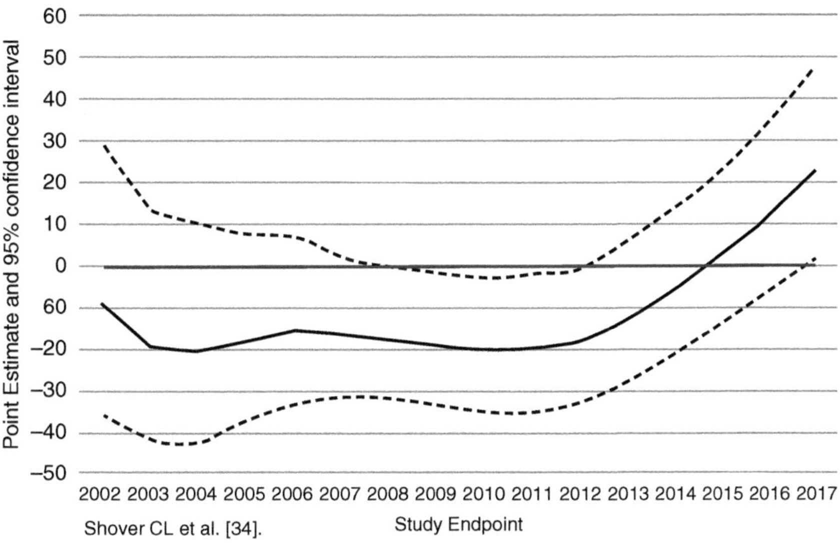

Fig. 27.1 The association between MCLs and opioids overdose mortality

true effect on opioid outcomes, and the association was most likely spurious [36].

Other recent evidence from the United States using Medicaid data between 2011 and 2016 supports lower opioid prescribing rates among legalized cannabis states [37, 36]. Specifically, opioid prescribing decreased by 5.88% (95% CI −11.5% to −0.21%) in states with medical cannabis laws and by 6.38% (95% CI, −12.20% to −0.56%) in states with both recreational and medical laws [36].

Clinical and Meta-Analytic Evidence

As per the 2014 treatment algorithm for the pharmacological management of neuropathic pain (Fig. 27.2) by the Canadian Pain Society Consensus Statement for Chronic Neuropathic Pain, cannabinoids are considered as a third-line treatment, with a number needed to treat (NNT) of 3.4 in comparison to TCAs (2.1), pregabalin (4.5), and gabapentin (6.5) [4]. For the majority of patients with neuropathic pain, opioid risk may exceed the benefits; As such, many physicians would consider cannabinoids as a second line treatment. More recently, data from clinical trials, systematic reviews, and meta-analyses have demonstrated moderate level of evidence for the use of medical cannabis in chronic pain and neuropathic pain populations [29, 38–42]. Specifically, when pooling all cannabis-based medicines together, cannabis was superior to placebo in producing substantial and moderate pain relief, decreasing pain intensity, while also improving sleep, psychological distress, and overall global improvement [42–45]. Other meta-analytic evidence (n = 33 RCTs) found that cannabinoids reduced mean pain scores by −0.70 compared to placebo ($p < 0.001$), and that all routes of administration (inhaled, oral and oromucosal) equally significantly reduced mean pain scores compared to placebo (all $p < 0.001$) [44]. Meta-regression revealed similar analgesic effects for neuropathic and non-neuropathic pain (p = 0.262) [44]. The Canadian Pain Society Consensus Statement for Chronic Neuropathic Pain, designated opioids as a second-line treatment, while cannabinoids were considered third-line (Fig 27.2). For most patients with neuropathic pain, opioid risk may exceed the benefits; As such, many physicians would consider cannabinoids as a second line treatment. This has led to the investigation of using cannabis as a substitution or adjunctive therapy option for opioids.

An RCT investigating if cannabis enhanced the analgesic effects of low dose oxycodone, found that while neither low-dose cannabis (5.6% THC, 560 mg cannabis cigarette) or low-dose oxycodone

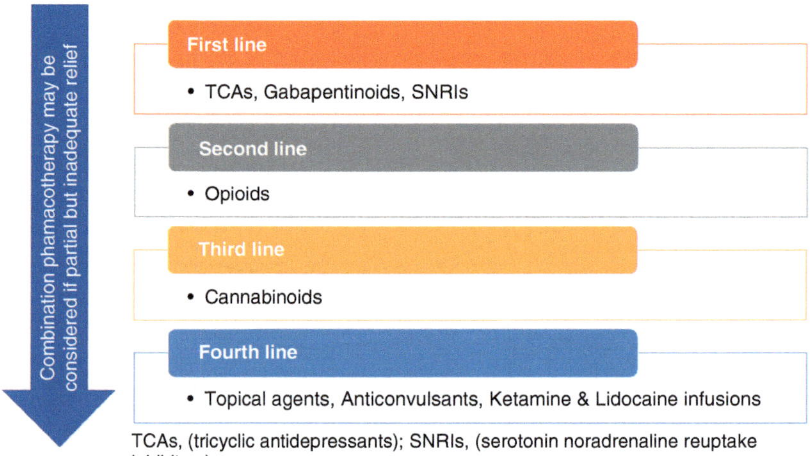

TCAs, (tricyclic antidepressants); SNRIs, (serotonin noradrenaline reuptake inhibitors).

Data gathered from references [4, 47, 48]

Fig. 27.2 Algorithm for the pharmacological management of neuropathic pain

(2.5 mg) elicited analgesia alone, when used concomitantly participants had increased pain threshold and tolerance [46]. Interestingly, the higher dose of oxycodone (5 mg) did not show improved analgesia when used concomitantly with cannabis [46]. A recent Phase II study also reported improved analgesia with the concomitant use of 4 mg hydromorphone and 2.5 mg dronabinol [47]. This time, no benefit was seen at the higher doses dronabinol (5 mg and 10 mg), in addition to there being an increased risk for abuse and adverse events [47]. As such, the optimal range for therapeutic synergy appears to be within the lower dosing ranges of THC and opioids. It should be noted that there is some conflicting evidence with respect to how efficacious concomitant use of low dose THC and opioids is for improving analgesia [48].

In a recent study with 600 chronic pain patients, some of whom were using more than 90 MED/day, opioid doses were individually tapered (~10% reduction every 1–2 weeks) while adjunctive medical cannabis was provided (maximum rate of 0.5 g/day per 10% decrease in opioid dose) [49]. After six months, 26% stopped taking opioids, 55% decreased opioid use by ~30%, and 19% had no response. In line with this, a recent systematic review (n = 9 studies; 7222 participants) found a 64–75% reduction in opioid dose when used concomitantly with cannabis, with 32–59.3% of the CNCP patient sample using cannabis for opioid substitution [49].

Proposed Cannabis Adjunct Initiation Trial with Opioid Therapy

Utilizing adjunctive agents for pain relief is a well-recognized treatment approach, such as the concomitant use of TCAs and gabapentinoids in neuropathic pain syndromes. Table 27.1 describes a proposed cannabis adjunct initiation trial with opioid therapy. This approach would allow for cautious initiation of cannabis with a focus on efficacy, safety, titration, and monitoring. Cannabis should be considered especially for patients who are taking ≥90 MED and not achieving pain management goals, or when further escalations in opioid dose would produce harms that exceed the benefits [50].

It is important to reassess patients at two to four week intervals during the initial titration phase in order to monitor for adverse events and response, and to provide education and support. A greater than 30% decrease in pain intensity and/or improvement in overall function are indicative of a successful trial and optimal dose. Once the optimal dose is achieved, follow-up may be less frequent (every three months). Cannabis adjunct therapy may allow clinicians to use lower opioid doses and reach better pain management outcomes, without an exposure to the equivalent level of risk and harm. An opioid taper could be considered two to four weeks post-cannabis initiation. This may be appropriate if symptoms are improving, or if there is an increase in opioid-related adverse events. It is important for patients to be educated on symptoms of opioid withdrawal as they may mistake withdrawal symptoms as indication of increased baseline chronic pain. Proper education and counseling are paramount to a successful opioid taper. It is advisable to consider a slow taper, 5–10% reduction in opioid every 2–4 weeks (or even longer) as tolerated. The tapering process should be individualized, and the progress is re-evaluated frequently and adjusted as needed. Cannabis, namely THC more so than CBD, may be helpful in ameliorating the symptoms of opioid withdrawal such as pain,

Table 27.1 Proposed steps for cannabis adjunct trial with opioid therapy

Step 1 – Assessment
Step 2 – Starting cannabis at a low dose
Step 3 – Slow titration until optimal dose
Step 4 – Frequent monitoring
Step 5 – Optimizing the titration
Step 6 – Consider stopping the trial and discontinuing cannabis if no response

MacCallum et al. [39]

anxiety, tremor, insomnia, irritability, nausea, diarrhea, and malaise.

Sihota et al. proposed a similar titration and taper regime as above [51]. They reported that chronic pain patients not reaching treatment goals should start with CBD-dominant oral extracts and add THC if needed. They proposed starting at 0.5–3 mg THC, increasing 1–2 mg once or twice a week, with a maximum of 30-40 mg/day. When improvement to daily functioning, desire for less medication to control pain, or optimized cannabis dose was reported begin opioid tapering. A very similar taper schedule of 5–10% MED every 1–4 weeks was suggested. Finally, they recommened defining clinical successs as improvement to quality of life or function, ≥30% reduction in pain intensity, ≥25% reduction in opioid dose, a reduction in opioid dose <90 mg MED and/or reduced opioid related adverse events. Approaches such as the ones defined above may be beneficial to chronic pain patients not reaching treatment goals with their current opioid treatment regime.

We acknowledge that comprehensive assessments for psychological dependency and addiction risk are essential components for long-term opioids or cannabinoids use in the management of chronic pain. The goal of the above suggested algorithms is to mitigate harms associated with long term opioid use and reduce the overall opioid burden, especially in those taking high MED. Additionally, these strategies are intended to be used with biopsychosocial tools for best results. Those with substance use disorder, are at a higher risk of cannabis use disorder and as such need to be considered with additional caution if these strategies are to be applied to this population. We recommend all patients, even without history of substance use disorder, have ongoing monitoring for risk of addiction using appropriate validated questionnaires.

Summary

Opioid overdose (prescription and illicit) is the leading cause of accidental deaths in the United States. Investigations into alternate analgesics such as cannabis are warranted. Cannabinoids not only have a superior adverse event profile compared to opioids, with no reported deaths directly related to overdose, but they also allow patients to be maintained on a stable dose over a number of years, unlike opioids.

Preclinical evidence supports the existence of reciprocal interactions between the endocannabinoid and opioid systems, and illustrates that the antinociceptive effects of cannabinoids are mediated through mechanisms distinct from those responsible for the psychoactive effects. Observational studies point to a reduction of opioid use with concomitant cannabis use, which is typically associated with reduced side effects, symptom clusters, and improved quality of life. Further evidence has shown a reduction in opioid prescribing among states with medical cannabis laws, and those with both medical and recreational cannabis laws.

Improved pain-related outcomes and reduced opioid-related harm are observed when low-dose THC is introduced as an adjunctive therapy with lower doses of opioids. Long-term administration of opioids can lead to tolerance and opioid-induced hyperalgesia, so co-administration of low doses of THC in conjunction with low doses of opioids seems to be an attractive regimen reducing the need to escalate opioid dose while increasing opioid potency and reducing side effects. It is imperative to use addiciton risk and psychological dependency assessments as well as other biopsychosocial tools for best outcomes.

In short, small doses of opioids in combination with cannabinoids may provide an alternate method of treating refractory or complex pain, while overcoming the undesirable effects of opioids and psychotropic effects of cannabinoids. Further research is warranted to clarify this relationship further.

References

1. National Institute on Drug Abuse (NIDA). Overdose Death Rates. 2019. Retrieved from: https://www.drugabuse.gov/related-topics/trends-statistics/overdose-death-rates.
2. Busse J, Guyatt G, Carrasco A, Akl E, Agoritsas T. The 2017 Canadian guideline for opioids for chronic non-cancer pain. Hamilton: McMaster University; 2017.

3. Centers for Disease Control and Prevention (CDC). Protect patients from opioid overdose. 2017. Retrieved from: https://www.cdc.gov/vitalsigns/opioids/index.html.
4. Moulin DE, Boulanger A, Clark AJ, Clarke H, Dao T, Finley GA, Sessle BJ. Pharmacological management of chronic neuropathic pain: revised consensus statement from the Canadian Pain Society. Pain Res Manag. 2014;19(6):328–35.
5. Krebs EE, Gravely A, Nugent S, Jensen AC, DeRonne B, Goldsmith ES, et al. Effect of opioid vs nonopioid medications on pain-related function in patients with chronic back pain or hip or knee osteoarthritis pain: the SPACE randomized clinical trial. JAMA. 2018;319(9):872–82.
6. Goodman CW, Brett AS. A clinical overview of off-label use of gabapentinoid drugs. JAMA Intern Med. 2019;179(5):695–701.
7. Robledo P, Berrendero F, Ozaita A, Maldonado R. Advances in the field of cannabinoid–opioid cross-talk. Addict Biol. 2008;13(2):213–24. https://doi.org/10.1111/j.1369-1600.2008.00107.x.
8. Cichewicz DL. Synergistic interactions between cannabinoid and opioid analgesics. Life Sci. 2004;74(11):1317–24.
9. Meng ID, Manning BH, Martin WJ, Fields HL. An analgesia circuit activated by cannabinoids. Nature. 1998;395(6700):381–3. https://doi.org/10.1038/26481.
10. Finn DP, Jhaveri MD, Beckett SRG, Roe CH, Kendall DA, Marsden CA, Chapman V. Effects of direct periaqueductal grey administration of a cannabinoid receptor agonist on nociceptive and aversive responses in rats. Neuropharmacology. 2003;45(5):594–604.
11. Manzanares J, Julian MD, Carrascosa A. Role of the cannabinoid system in pain control and therapeutic implications for the management of acute and chronic pain episodes. Curr Neuropharmacol. 2006;4(3):239–57.
12. Lichtman AH, Sheikh SM, Loh HH, Martin BR. Opioid and cannabinoid modulation of precipitated withdrawal in Δ9-tetrahydrocannabinol and morphine-dependent mice. J Pharmacol Exp Ther. 2001;298(3):1007–14.
13. Pertwee RG, Howlett AC, Abood ME, Alexander SPH, Di Marzo V, Elphick MR, et al. International Union of Basic and Clinical Pharmacology. LXXIX. Cannabinoid receptors and their ligands: beyond CB1 and CB2. Pharmacol Rev. 2010;62(4):588–631.
14. da Fonseca Pacheco D, Klein A, de Castro Perez A, da Fonseca Pacheco CM, De Francischi JN, Duarte IDG. The μ-opioid receptor agonist morphine, but not agonists at δ-or κ-opioid receptors, induces peripheral antinociception mediated by cannabinoid receptors. Br J Pharmacol. 2008;154(5):1143–9.
15. da Fonseca Pacheco D, Klein A, Perez AC, da Fonseca Pacheco CM, de Francischi JN, Lopes Reis GM, Duarte IDG. Central antinociception induced by μ-opioid receptor agonist morphine, but not δ-or κ-, is mediated by cannabinoid CB1 receptor. Br J Pharmacol. 2009;158(1):225–31.
16. Ibrahim MM, Porreca F, Lai J, Albrecht PJ, Rice FL, Khodorova A, et al. CB2 cannabinoid receptor activation produces antinociception by stimulating peripheral release of endogenous opioids. Proc Natl Acad Sci. 2005;102(8):3093–8.
17. Bushlin I, Rozenfeld R, Devi LA. Cannabinoid–opioid interactions during neuropathic pain and analgesia. Curr Opin Pharmacol. 2010;10(1):80–6.
18. Cichewicz DL, McCarthy EA. Antinociceptive synergy between Δ9-tetrahydrocannabinol and opioids after oral administration. J Pharmacol Exp Ther. 2003;304(3):1010–5.
19. Nielsen S, Sabioni P, Trigo JM, Ware MA, Betz-Stablein BD, Murnion B, et al. Opioid-sparing effect of cannabinoids: a systematic review and meta-analysis. Neuropsychopharmacology. 2017;42(9):1752–65.
20. Abrams DI, Couey P, Shade SB, Kelly ME, Benowitz NL. Cannabinoid–opioid interaction in chronic pain. Clin Pharmacol Therap. 2011;90(6):844–51.
21. Reiman A, Welty M, Solomon P. Cannabis as a substitute for opioid-based pain medication: patient self-report. Cannabis Cannabinoid Res. 2017;2(1):160–6.
22. Gable RS. Macroscope: the toxicity of recreational drugs. Am Sci. 2006;94(3):206–8.
23. Zutler M, C Holty JE. Opioids, sleep, and sleep-disordered breathing. Curr Pharm Des. 2011;17(15):1443–9.
24. Lucas P, Walsh Z. Medical cannabis access, use, and substitution for prescription opioids and other substances: a survey of authorized medical cannabis patients. Int J Drug Policy. 2017;42:30–5.
25. Boehnke KF, Litinas E, Clauw DJ. Medical cannabis use is associated with decreased opiate medication use in a retrospective cross-sectional survey of patients with chronic pain. J Pain. 2016;17(6):739–44.
26. Giorgi V, Bongiovanni S, Atzeni F, Marotto D, Salaffi F, Sarzi-Puttini P. Adding medical cannabis to standard analgesic treatment for fibromyalgia: a prospective observational study. Clin Exp Rheumatol. 2020;38(123):S53–9.
27. Feingold D, Brill S, Goor-Aryeh I, Delayahu Y, Lev-Ran S. Depression and anxiety among chronic pain patients receiving prescription opioids and medical marijuana. J Affect Disord. 2017;218:1–7.
28. Lavie-Ajayi M, Shvartzman P. Restored self: a phenomenological study of pain relief by cannabis. Pain Med. 2019;20(11):2086–93.
29. Ware MA, Wang T, Shapiro S, Collet JP, Boulanger A, Esdaile JM, et al. Cannabis for the management of pain: assessment of safety study (COMPASS). J Pain. 2015;16(12):1233–42.
30. Olfson M, Wall MM, Liu SM, Blanco C. Cannabis use and risk of prescription opioid use disorder in the United States. Am J Psychiatr. 2018;175(1):47–53.
31. Campbell G, Hall WD, Peacock A, Lintzeris N, Bruno R, Larance B, et al. Effect of cannabis use in people with chronic non-cancer pain prescribed opioids: findings from a 4-year prospective cohort study. Lancet Public Health. 2018;3(7):e341–50.

32. Bradford AC, Bradford WD. Medical marijuana laws reduce prescription medication use in Medicare Part D. Health Aff. 2016;35(7):1230–6.
33. Bradford AC, Bradford WD. Medical marijuana laws may be associated with a decline in the number of prescriptions for Medicaid enrollees. Health Aff. 2017;36(5):945–51.
34. Bachhuber MA, Saloner B, Cunningham CO, Barry CL. Medical cannabis laws and opioid analgesic overdose mortality in the United States, 1999–2010. JAMA Intern Med. 2014;174(10):1668–73.
35. Shover CL, Davis CS, Gordon SC, Humphreys K. Association between medical cannabis laws and opioid overdose mortality has reversed over time. Proc Natl Acad Sci. 2019;116(26):12624–6.
36. Wen H, Hockenberry JM. Association of medical and adult-use marijuana laws with opioid prescribing for Medicaid enrollees. JAMA Intern Med. 2018;178(5):673–9.
37. Bradford AC, Bradford WD, Abraham A, Adams GB. Association between US state medical cannabis laws and opioid prescribing in the Medicare Part D population. JAMA Intern Med. 2018;178(5):667–72.
38. National Academies of Sciences, Engineering, and Medicine; Health and Medicine Division; Board on Population Health and Public Health Practice; Committee on the Health Effects of Marijuana: An Evidence Review and Research Agenda. The Health Effects of Cannabis and Cannabinoids: The Current State of Evidence and Recommendations for Research. Washington (DC): National Academies Press (US); 2017 Jan 12. Available from: https://www.ncbi.nlm.nih.gov/books/NBK423845/doi:10.17226/24625.
39. MacCallum CA, Eadie L, Barr AM, Boivin M, Lu S. Practical Strategies Using Medical Cannabis to Reduce Harms A ssociated With Long Term Opioid Use in Chronic Pain. Front. Pharmacol. 2021;12:633168. https://doi.org/10.3389/fphar.2021.633168.
40. Andreae MH, Carter GM, Shaparin N, Suslov K, Ellis RJ, Ware MA, et al. Inhaled cannabis for chronic neuropathic pain: a meta-analysis of individual patient data. J Pain. 2015;16(12):1221–32.
41. Yanes JA, McKinnell ZE, Reid MA, Busler JN, Michel JS, Pangelinan MM, et al. Effects of cannabinoid administration for pain: a meta-analysis and meta-regression. Exp Clin Psychopharmacol. 2019;27(4):370.
42. Mücke M, Phillips T, Radbruch L, Petzke F, Häuser W. Cannabis-based medicines for chronic neuropathic pain in adults. Cochrane Database Syst Rev. 2018;3:CD012182.
43. Johal H, Devji T, Chang Y, Simone J, Vannabouathong C, Bhandari M. Cannabinoids in chronic non-cancer pain: a systematic review and meta-analysis. Clin Med Insights Arthritis Musculoskelet Disord. 2020;13:1179544120906461.
44. Wong SSC, Chan WS, Cheung CW. Analgesic effects of cannabinoids for chronic non-cancer pain: a systematic review and meta-analysis with meta-regression. J Neuroimmune Pharmacol. 2020;15(4):801–29.
45. Vulfsons S, Minerbi A, Sahar T. Cannabis and pain treatment—a review of the clinical utility and a practical approach in light of uncertainty. Rambam Maimonides Med J. 2020;11(1):e0002.
46. Cooper ZD, Bedi G, Ramesh D, Balter R, Comer SD, Haney M. Impact of co-administration of oxycodone and smoked cannabis on analgesia and abuse liability. Neuropsychopharmacology. 2018;43(10):2046–55.
47. Dunn KE, Bergeria CL, Huhn AS, Speed TJ, Mun CJ, Vandrey R, Campbell CM. Within-subject, double-blinded, randomized, and placebo-controlled evaluation of the combined effects of the cannabinoid dronabinol and the opioid hydromorphone in a human laboratory pain model. Neuropsychopharmacology. 2021;0:1–9.
48. Babalonis S, Lofwall MR, Sloan PA, Nuzzo PA, Fanucchi LC, Walsh SL. Cannabinoid modulation of opioid analgesia and subjective drug effects in healthy humans. Psychopharmacology (Berl). 2019 Nov;236(11):3341–352.
49. Rod K. A pilot study of a medical cannabis-opioid reduction program. Am J Psychiatr Neurosci. 2019;7(3):74–7.
50. Busse JW, Craigie S, Juurlink DN, Buckley DN, Wang L, Couban RJ, et al. Guideline for opioid therapy and chronic noncancer pain. CMAJ. 2017;189(18):E659–66.
51. Sihota A, Smith BK, Ahmed SA, Bell A, Blain A, Clarke H, Cooper ZD, Cyr C, Daeninck P, Deshpande A, Ethans K, Flusk D, Le Foll B, Milloy MJ, Moulin DE, Naidoo V, Ong M, Perez J, Rod K, Sealey R, Sulak D, Walsh Z, O'Connell C. Consensus-based recommendations for titrating cannabinoids and tapering opioids for chronic pain control. Int J Clin Pract. 2020 Nov 28:e13871.
52. Cohen SP, Bhatia A, Buvanendran A, Schwenk ES, Wasan AD, Hurley RW, Viscusi ER, Narouze S, Davis FN, Ritchie EC, Lubenow TR, Hooten WM. Consensus guidelines on the use of intravenous ketamine infusions for chronic pain from the American Society of Regional Anesthesia and Pain Medicine, the American Academy of Pain Medicine, and the American Society of Anesthesiologists. Reg Anesth Pain Med. 2018;43(5):521–46.
53. Kim YC, Castañeda AM, Lee CS, Jin HS, Park KS, Moon JY. Efficacy and safety of lidocaine infusion treatment for neuropathic pain: a randomized, double-blind, and placebo-controlled study. Reg Anesth Pain Med. 2018;43(4):415–24.
54. Cooper ZD, Comer SD, Haney M. Opioid modulation of cannabis-induced analgesia and subjective effects in cannabis smokers. Drug Alcohol Depend. 2017;100(171):e44–5.
55. Portenoy RK, Ganae-Motan ED, Allende S, Yanagihara R, Shaiova L, Weinstein S, et al. Nabiximols for opioid-treated cancer patients with poorly-controlled chronic pain: a randomized, placebo-controlled, graded-dose trial. J Pain. 2012;13(5):438–49.
56. Liu Y, Williamson V, Setlow B, Cottler LB, Knackstedt LA. The Importance of Considering Polysubstance Use: Lessons from Cocaine Research. Drug Alcohol Depend. 2018;192:16–28.

28 Cannabinoids as a Substitute for Opioids: Suggested Algorithm

Tolulope Oso, Salman Hirani, Matthew Chung, Barlas Benkli, and Christina Le-Short

Introduction

Physicians and clinics are inundated on a daily basis with questions by patients regarding cannabis use. The rate of acceptance and availability of cannabis products has outpaced physician knowledge to adequately answer these questions [1]. Patient interest in cannabis use to treat various ailments has increased drastically over the past several years. Internet searches for the phrases "cannabidiol" or "CBD" rose 126% from 2016 to 2017 and another 160% from 2017 to 2018 [2]. In April 2019 alone, the terms were searched 6.4 million times [2]. As it stands, some form of medicinal marijuana has been legalized in 33 states and the District of Columbia. These states are attempting to legislate which conditions qualify for treatment with cannabis, with little scientific basis for those decisions [3]. With over 22 million Americans consuming cannabis, and that number rising on an annual basis, there has never been a more critical time for doctors to be armed with appropriate guidelines and algorithms [4]. If physicians fail to appropriately and adequately address questions regarding cannabis use, patients will turn to the Internet and to budtenders in search of answers in lieu of medical guidance [1, 5, 6].

Current data is not enough to establish the benefit of cannabinoids in the management of pain; however there are many studies providing insight to potential benefits of cannabinoids in pain management. In particular, there is evidence of potential benefits of cannabis-based medicine in the treatment of chronic neuropathic pain [7] and spasticity due to multiple sclerosis [8].

Building a widely accepted algorithm for cannabis is difficult given how the drug is classified and still controversial. Given that cannabis is still considered illegal at the federal level, the research needed to assess for a safety profile has yet to be done at the scale needed to definitively provide one algorithm for all patients.

Multiple guidelines and algorithms have recently been published for opiate use for numerous medical conditions through various specialties and societies. The goal of such an algorithm for the use of cannabinoids would be to standardize care for patients across providers so that all patients are treated equally. As further

T. Oso
Department of Anesthesia, The University of Texas McGovern Medical School, Houston, TX, USA

S. Hirani (✉)
Department of Anesthesiology and Perioperative Medicine, Oregon Health and Science University, Portland, OR, USA
e-mail: hirani@ohsu.edu

M. Chung · C. Le-Short
Department of Pain Medicine, Division of Anesthesiology, Critical Care and Pain Medicine, The University of Texas MD Anderson Cancer Center, Houston, TX, USA

B. Benkli
Department of Neurology, The University of Texas McGovern Medical School, Houston, TX, USA

S. N. Narouze (ed.), *Cannabinoids and Pain*, https://doi.org/10.1007/978-3-030-69186-8_28

research, understanding, and acceptance across the political and medical spectrum is gained, the algorithm and guidelines should be continuously updated.

Suggested Algorithm for Use of Cannabinoids in Pain Management

Upon evaluation of the patient's history and a thorough physical exam, certain questions must be answered before initiation of a cannabinoid as an adjuvant for pain management. First, the patient should be a minimum of 18 years of age. Cannabis has been associated with developmental delay in children and adolescents [9–11]. Ehrenreich and colleagues' behavioral study showed an association between attentional deficits in adults after cannabis abuse in early-onset users (younger than age 16 when cannabis use started) compared to those who were older [9]. In a study of 122 lifetime cannabis users, Pope et al. found that early-onset users, those who initiated cannabis use at an age less than 17, were associated with overall poorer cognitive performance in neuropsychological tests [10]. Lastly, Schneider and Koch's findings showed that chronic synthetic cannabinoid receptor stimulation in peri-pubertal rats, in comparison to adults, exhibited long-lasting deficits in sensorimotor gating, object recognition memory, and the performance of instrumental tasks [11]. Therefore, ensuring that the patient is at least 18 years old can help circumvent some of these concerns.

Obtaining a thorough history of prior drug abuse is an imperative next step. If there is a current or former abuse of alcohol or drugs, cannabis therapy is not recommended. There is a scarcity of human trials pertaining to cannabinoid pain therapy and drug abuse; however, there are several rodent studies that can be referenced. The CB1 receptor antagonist, SR-141716A, was found to attenuate the reward system for many substances including heroin and ethanol, therefore decreasing the addictive potential of these substances [12]. Cannabinoid agonists also elicited relapse and heroin-seeking behavior in animals with a history of addiction [13]. These findings suggest that the CB1 receptor may play a role in addictive behavior and the activation of it may promote relapse in patients with a history of drug abuse.

If the patient is greater than 18 years of age with no history of drug or alcohol abuse, methods of categorizing the chronicity of pain will help in determining whether cannabis therapy will be beneficial. The efficacy of cannabinoid receptor agonists on acute postoperative pain has been inconclusive with some studies claiming less than or no analgesic effect compared to placebo/other medications, while others have shown significant analgesic effect in postoperative or trauma-induced pain [14–17]. Given these findings, we cannot recommend the initiation of cannabinoids in the acute setting. However, these studies did not compare the use of THC agonists in patients with a prior history of THC use, which is a patient population that could benefit in the acute postoperative setting.

CB1 agonists have been found to have an analgesic effect in patients with chronic pain, especially in the management of neuropathic, cancer pain, and spasticity management. As referenced above, studies have shown great efficacy in relief of those types of pain. Consroe et al. found that within their study population of 112 multiple sclerosis (MS) patients, 95% found cannabis improved not only spasticity but also chronic pain in their extremities [18]. Some also found symptomatic relief of stress, sleep, mood, stiffness, and spasm with the use of cannabis [19]. In a study by Wade et al., pathologies including MS, spinal cord injury (SCI), brachial plexus injury, and limb amputation all showed increased pain relief with both TCH and CBD compared to placebo [20]. CB receptor agonist, WIN 55, 212–2, has been shown to be more efficacious than morphine in the inhibition of the "wind up phenomenon" (a phenomenon that contributes to the development of hyperalgesia and allodynia) [21]. These findings are especially important because they target neuropathic pain, which has proven to be difficult to treat. Endogenous and exogenous cannabinoids continue to be studied for their role in cancer pain management. Guerrero and colleagues' mice study resulted in cannabinoids aiding in increasing the pain threshold for tumor-afflicted mice [22]. For chemotherapy-induced nausea and vomiting, cannabinoids have been found to be a useful antiemetic as well as an appetite stimulant [23, 24].

Once establishing the type of pain, the next step is to determine prior methods of pain control. Cannabinoids are usually not the first line of pain control, likely due to the controversy surrounding them and a small number of human trials pertaining to their efficacy. Per the Canadian Pain Society, cannabinoids are a third-line agent for the management of neuropathic pain following SSRIs, methadone, and topical lidocaine [25]. For cancer pain, studies including nabiximols as add-on therapy to opioids vs placebo showed increased efficacy in intractable cancer pain [26]. Both opioids and cannabinoids attenuate nociception via G protein-coupled mechanisms and thus have a synergistic interaction [24]. Engagement of the cannabinoid receptor, HU-210, was also shown to help with the antinociceptive effects of morphine and prevent the development of tolerance. This could aid in prolonging the use of opioids without incremental dose increases, thus aiding to prevent the unwanted side effects of opioid ingestion [27]. Naef et al. showed that THC alone had enhanced hyperalgesia compared to antinociception when combined with morphine [28]. Therefore, cannabinoids should likely not be used solely or as the first agent in the management of chronic pain conditions.

For neuropathic pain, synthetic cannabinoids such as nabilone or nabiximols, can be added as a third-line treatment. For chronic cancer and non-cancer-related pain, it may be beneficial to tailor the addition of the cannabinoid to the patient's opioid tolerance threshold. Adding a synthetic cannabinoid when the patient develops tolerance to their opioid regimen or when adverse effects of opioids become limiting may aid in the efficacy of the opioid without worsening the side effect profile (Fig. 28.1).

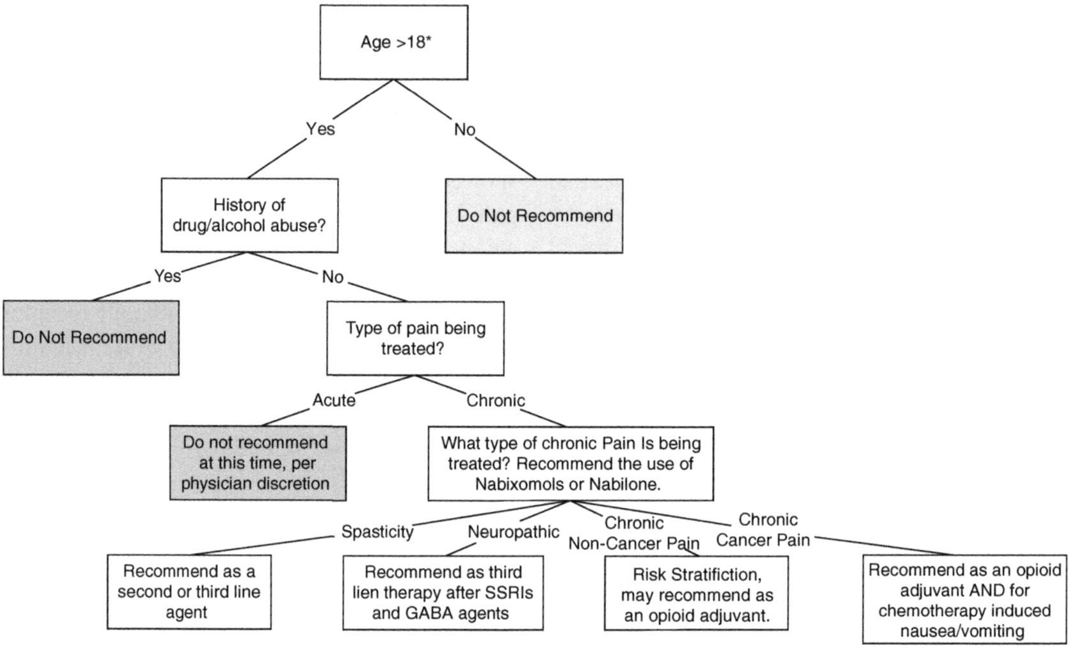

Fig. 28.1 Medical Cannabinoids Analgesic Algorithm. *Some experts prefer age > 25

Disclosures No financial disclosures to report.

Conflict of Interest No conflicts of interest to report.

References

1. Narouze S, Hakim S, Kohan L, Adams D, Souza D. Medical Cannabis attitudes and beliefs among pain physicians. Medical cannabis attitudes and beliefs among pain physicians. Reg Anesth Pain Med. 2020:rapm-2020-101658. https://doi.org/10.1136/rapm-2020-101658. Online ahead of print
2. Leas EC, Nobles AL, Caputi TL, Dredze M, Smith DM, Ayers JW. Trends in internet searches for Cannabidiol (CBD) in the United States. JAMA Netw Open. 2019;2(10):e1913853. https://doi.org/10.1001/jamanetworkopen.2019.13853.
3. Boehnke KF, Gangopadhyay S, Clauw DJ, Haffajee RL. Qualifying conditions of medical Cannabis license holders in the United States. Health Affairs (Project Hope). 2019;38(2):295–302. https://doi.org/10.1377/hlthaff.2018.05266.
4. NIDA. 2020, April 8. What is the scope of marijuana use in the United States?. Retrieved from https://www.drugabuse.gov/publications/research-reports/marijuana/what-scope-marijuana-use-in-united-states on 2020, June 14.
5. Greiner C, Chatton A, Khazaal Y. Online self-help forums on cannabis: a content assessment. Patient Educ Couns. 2017;100(10):1943–50. https://doi.org/10.1016/j.pec.2017.06.001.
6. Mitchell JT, Sweitzer MM, Tunno AM, Kollins SH, McClernon FJ. "I use weed for my ADHD": a qualitative analysis of online forum discussions on Cannabis use and ADHD. PLoS One. 2016;11(5):e0156614. https://doi.org/10.1371/journal.pone.0156614. Published 2016 May 26
7. Mücke M, Phillips T, Radbruch L, Petzke F, Häuser W. Cannabis-based medicines for chronic neuropathic pain in adults. Cochrane Database Syst Rev. 2018;3(3):CD012182. https://doi.org/10.1002/14651858.CD012182.pub2.
8. Rice J, Cameron M. Cannabinoids for treatment of MS symptoms: state of the evidence. Curr Neurol Neurosci Rep. 2018;18:50. https://doi.org/10.1007/s11910-018-0859-x.
9. Ehrenreich H, Kunert HJ, Moeller MR, Poser W, Schilling L, Gigerenzer G, Hoehe MR, Rinn T. Specific attentional dysfunction in adults following early start of cannabis use. Psychopharmacology. 1999;142:295–301.
10. Pope HG, Gruber AJ, Hudson JI, Cohane G, Huestis MA, Yurgelun-Todd D. Early-onset cannabis use and

cognitive deficits: what is the nature of the association? Drug Alcohol Depend. 2003;69:303–10.
11. Schneider M, Koch M. Chronic pubertal, but not adult chronic cannabinoid treatment impairs sensorimotor gating, recognition memory, and the performance in a progressive ratio task in adult rats. Neuropsychopharmacology. 2003;28:1760–9.
12. Parolaro D, Rubino T. Cannabinoids and drugs of abuse. Cannabinoids as Therapeutics Milestones in Drug Therapy MDT 207–218.
13. Fattore L, Spano MS, Cossu G, Deiana S, Fratta W. Cannabinoid mechanism in reinstatement of heroin-seeking after a long period of abstinence in rats. Eur J Neurosci. 2003;17:1723–6.
14. Raft D, Gregg J, Ghia J, Harris L. Effects of intravenous tetrahydrocannabinol on experimental and surgical pain; psychological correlates of the analgesic response. Clin Pharmacol Therap. 1977;21:26–33.
15. Buggy DJ, Toogood L, Maric S, Sharpe P, Lambert DG, Rowbotham DJ. Lack of analgesic efficacy of oral δ-9-tetrahydrocannabinol in postoperative pain. Pain. 2003;106:169–72.
16. Beaulieu P. Effects of nabilone, a synthetic cannabinoid, on postoperative pain. Can J Anaesth. 2006;53:769–75.
17. Jain AK, Ryan JR, Mcmahon FG, Smith G. Evaluation of intramuscular Levonantradol and placebo in acute postoperative pain. J Clin Pharmacol. 1981; https://doi.org/10.1002/j.1552-4604.1981.tb02610.x.
18. Consroe P, Musty R, Rein J, Tillery W, Pertwee R. The perceived effects of smoked Cannabis on patients with multiple sclerosis. Eur Neurol. 1997;38:44–8.
19. Clark AJ, Ware MA, Yazer E, Murray TJ, Lynch ME. Patterns of cannabis use among patients with multiple sclerosis. Neurology. 2004;62:2098–100.
20. Wade DT, Robson P, House H, Makela P, Aram J. A preliminary controlled study to determine whether whole-plant cannabis extracts can improve intractable neurogenic symptoms. Clin Rehabil. 2003;17:21–9.
21. Strangman NM, Walker JM. Cannabinoid WIN 55,212-2 inhibits the activity-dependent facilitation of spinal nociceptive responses. J Neurophysiol. 1999;82:472–7.
22. Guerrero AV, Quang P, Dekker N, Jordan RC, Schmidt BL. Peripheral cannabinoids attenuate carcinoma-induced nociception in mice. Neurosci Lett. 2008;433:77–81.
23. Slatkin NE. Cannabinoids in the treatment of chemotherapy-induced nausea and vomiting: beyond prevention of acute emesis. J Support Oncol. 2007;5(5 Suppl 3):1–9.
24. Elikottil MJ, Gupta MP, Gupta PK. The analgesic potential of cannabinoids. J Opioid Manag. 2018;5:341–57.
25. Moulin D, Boulanger A, Clark A, et al. Pharmacological management of chronic neuropathic pain: revised consensus statement from the Canadian Pain Society. Pain Res Manag. 2014;19:328–35.
26. Portenoy RK, Ganae-Motan ED, Allende S, Yanagihara R, Shaiova L, Weinstein S, Mcquade R, Wright S, Fallon MT. Nabiximols for opioid-treated cancer patients with poorly-controlled chronic pain: a randomized, placebo-controlled, graded-dose trial. J Pain. 2012;13:438–49.
27. Johnson JR, Burnell-Nugent M, Lossignol D, Ganae-Motan ED, Potts R, Fallon MT. Multicenter, double-blind, randomized, placebo-controlled, parallel-group study of the efficacy, safety, and tolerability of THC:CBD extract and THC extract in patients with intractable cancer-related pain. J Pain Symptom Manag. 2010;39:167–79.
28. Naef M, Curatolo M, Petersen-Felix S, Arendt-Nielsen L, Zbinden A, Brenneisen R. The analgesic effect of oral delta-9-tetrahydrocannabinol (THC), morphine, and a THC-morphine combination in healthy subjects under experimental pain conditions. Pain. 2003;105:79–88.

Perioperative Management of Patients on Cannabis/Cannabinoids

29

Amita Kundra

Introduction

Cannabis plants produce chemicals known as cannabinoids, which induces a wide range of effects on its consumers. At least 100 of these cannabinoids have been identified within the plant, of which the two popular ones are cannabidiol (CBD) and tetrahydrocannabinol (THC). THC is psychoactive (mind-altering), whereas CBD is not.

Cannabis remains the most widely used illicit drug in the USA. An estimated 22 million people over the age of 12 consume cannabis products per year. With the widespread legalization of cannabis for medicinal and recreational purposes, this chapter will evaluate marijuana's effects and potential complications that may occur in the surgical setting.

Perioperative Effects

Pulmonary Effects

The consumption of cannabis can lead to a higher risk of various types of pulmonary complications. When cannabis is consumed in the hand-rolled and unfiltered cigarette form, it can lead to inhalation of carcinogenic chemicals and irritants such as benzopyrene and benzanthracene into the lungs. The cannabis oil that is used in e-cigarettes also contains chemical irritants such as propylene glycol. When propylene glycol is heated, it can lead to the inhalation of several chemical irritants and respiratory carcinogens such as formaldehyde. When these chemicals are inspired, it can lead to opacification of the centrilobular airspaces that resembles pneumonia. The inhalation of cannabis in the cigarette form can also lead to higher carboxyhemoglobin levels and tar retention in the airways [1].

The inhalation of marijuana results in a peak effect of cannabinoids in just 15 minutes, which can last up to 4 hours. Smoking cannabis can have similar effects on the lungs as cigarettes [2].

It can cause cough, increased mucous production, and inflammation of the lungs. This inflammation can cause an asthmatic effect, which may lead to bronchospasm. Cannabis consumption can also cause adverse breathing patterns in patients called hypoventilation and increase their risk for aspiration [3].

Cardiovascular Effects

Cardiovascular effects of cannabis can range from increasing heart rate, increasing risk for arrhythmias, and increased risk of myocardial infarctions. The mechanism is believed to be secondary to beta-adrenergic stimulation of CB1-R

A. Kundra (✉)
South Shore Hospital Department of Anesthesiology, Northwell Health, Bay Shore, NY, USA

S. N. Narouze (ed.), *Cannabinoids and Pain*, https://doi.org/10.1007/978-3-030-69186-8_29

receptors. Stimulation of these receptors leads to sympathetic stimulation and inhibition of parasympathetic system [1].

One of the most common sequalae of cannabis consumption is tachycardia. One study showed that an elevated heart rate (tachycardia) could last for 90 minutes after the onset of marijuana inhalation [2].

Young patients who received higher doses were at risk for developing premature ventricular contractions, atrial fibrillation, and atrial flutter [4, 5]. Patients were also observed to have hypertension. These affects were observed to be dose dependent. When the plasma concentration of cannabis increased, it can lead to an increase in systolic pressure compared to baseline lasting for up to 60 min after smoking.

Most importantly, marijuana use has been shown to be an independent risk factor (fivefold risk in the first hour of marijuana use) for myocardial infarction [6, 7].

Hemostatic Effects

Cannabis has been shown to affect bleeding patterns in patients, which can be a significant consideration during surgery. Several studies have evaluated marijuana's anticoagulation effects [8, 9]. Cannabinoids and their metabolites are believed to inhibit platelet aggregation, a crucial step in the process of clot formation. Furthermore, this has been shown to be a dose-dependent, implying that high-dose marijuana consumers have a higher risk of bleeding diathesis during surgery [10].

Another recent study shed more light on the anticoagulant effects of cannabis. Cannabis was found to inhibit platelet activation, the step that precedes platelet aggregation [11].

On the contrary, others documented an increased platelets' aggregation in the presence of THC [12].The increased clot formation could be why patients who use cannabis have a higher risk of developing heart attacks and strokes [13].

THC stimulates the sympathetic system, inhibits the parasympathetic system, and induces arterial wall inflammatory response through oxidative stress, platelets activation, deformation of oxidize LDL, and over-reactivation of factor VII which may lead to endothelial erosion and thrombus formation in normal coronary arteries [13].

Recent studies have shown that ischemic stroke is one of the most common vascular side effects in cannabis consumers [14]. In fact, young patients (25–35 years old) who consume cannabis have a 2.3- to 2.9-fold risk of stroke compared to tobacco smokers [15, 16]. However, preexisting conditions may also play a role in these sequelae. The mechanism is believed to occur secondary to action of the CB1-R receptors. Typically CB1-R receptors will increase blood flow secondary to vasodilation [16]. However in situations of hypoxia and hypercapnia, the activation of these receptors leads to decreased cerebral blood flow [17].

Temperature Regulation

Cannabis exposure has been associated with temperature dysregulation. Cannabinoid-induced hypothermia seems to be mediated by CB1-R activation. It can be reversed with administering a CB1-R antagonist such as rimonabant [18].

Cannabis exposure was shown to be associated with hypothermia and shivering in the perioperative period. Shivering can be a concerning phenomenon in the postanesthetic period. It can lead to increased heart rate, blood pressure, myocardial oxygen consumption, and myocardial ischemia.

Drug Interactions

Cannabis can interact with many drugs used in anesthesia practice.

Patients who consume cannabis regularly can have significantly increased anesthetic requirements. A small randomized, single-blinded study showed that routine marijuana users required significantly higher doses of propofol (almost twice the normal dose) for appropriate sedation [19].

THC is primarily metabolized in the liver, by the CYP 450 system of enzymes; furthermore,

THC and CBD concentrations are high in the liver after oral ingestion, which results in an even greater hepatic load for metabolism. This underpins the reason why patients who consume cannabis may have an increased tolerance for opioids, chlorpromazine, and barbiturates, which are routinely used in sedation and are also metabolized by the liver.

In terms of inhaled anesthetics, studies have shown that cannabis consumers have a higher tolerance of inhaled anesthetics such as isoflurane and sevoflurane [20].

Therefore, most practitioners recommend that patients hold off on consuming cannabis before their surgery. As states prepare for the legalization of recreational marijuana, more research is being performed to study the effects of cannabis on those who are undergoing anesthesia and surgery.

Preoperative Evaluation

During the preoperative interview, it is important to determine the patient's level of exposure to cannabinoids. It is important to ask about the duration of the consumption, the frequency of consumption, and how the cannabis is consumed. It is also important to determine the time elapsed since last use. If the patient has had surgery in the past, it is important to inquire whether the patient has had any complications such as any history of hyperreactive airway or severe shivering with the previous anesthetic.

It is important to distinguish the patients who are chronic cannabis users from those who are new users. Patients who are new users tend to have different perioperative findings than those who are chronic users. New users are more likely to develop tachycardia and systolic hypertension within 2 hours of consumption. They are predisposed to develop malignant arrhythmias such as atrial fibrillation, ventricular fibrillation, ventricular tachycardia, and Brugada pattern. If they have a previous history of coronary artery disease, they are at risk of developing coronary spasm. From a pulmonary standpoint, they are at risk of developing airway hyperreactivity or uvulitis [20].

Patients who are chronic users are more likely to have different perioperative findings that occur due to inhibition of the sympathetic system. Their heart rate may range from a bradycardia to a tachycardia. They have a tendency to develop orthostatic hypotension, sinus arrest, and intraoperative hypothermia. They are also at risk of developing coronary vasospasm and/or myocardial infarction [20].

Conclusion

As states continue to legalize the use of recreational marijuana, there will continue to be more patients seen who consume cannabis. In the perioperative setting, there is more to learn about the safety and efficacy of cannabis and cannabinoids. As more information is obtained, hopefully the anesthesiology community will come together to establish protocols to reduce perioperative complications and improve outcomes.

References

1. Echeverria-Villalobos M, Todeschini AB, Stoicea N, Fiorda-Diaz J, Weaver T, Bergese SD. Perioperative care of cannabis users: a comprehensive review of pharmacological and anesthetic considerations. J Clin Anesth (Elsevier Inc). 2019;59:41–9.
2. Johnson S, Domino EF. Some cardiovascular effects of marihuana smoking in normal volunteers. Clin Pharmacol Ther. 1971;12(5):762–8.
3. Schwilk B, Bothner U, Schraag S, et al. Perioperative respiratory events in smokers and nonsmokers undergoing general anaesthesia. Acta Anaesthesiol Scand. 1997;41(3):348–55.
4. Fisher BAC, et al. Cardiovascular complications induced by cannabis smoking: a case report and review of the literature. Emerg Med J [Internet]. 2005 Sep [cited 2020 Feb 17];22(9):679–80. Available from: https://www.ncbi.nlm.nih.gov/pmc/articles/PMC1726916/.
5. Akins D, Awdeh MR. Marijuana and second-degree AV block. Journal. 1981;74(3):371–2.
6. Hodcroft C, Rossiter MC, Buch AN. Cannabis-associated myocardial infarction in a young man with normal coronary arteries. J Emerg Med [Internet]. 2014 Sep [cited 2020 Feb 17];47(3):277–81.

Available from: https://www.jem-journal.com/article/S0736-4679(13)01403-0/abstract.
7. Mittleman MA, Lewis RA, et al. Triggering Myocardial Infarction by Marijuana. Circulation [Internet]. 2001 Jun [cited 2020 Feb 17];103(23):2805–9. Available from: https://www.ahajournals.org/doi/10.1161/01.CIR.103.23.2805.
8. Zakrzeska A, Gredzinski T, KIsel W, Chabielska E. Cannabinoids and haemostasis. Postepy Hig Med Dosw (Online). 2016;70(0):760–74.
9. Schaefer C, Brackett DGC, et al. Decreased platelet aggregation following marihuana smoking in man. J Okla State Med Assoc. 1979;72(12):435–6.
10. Formukong EA, Evans AT, Evans FJ. The inhibitory effects of cannabinoids, the active constituents of Cannabis sativa L. on human and rabbit platelet aggregation. J Pharm Pharmacol [Internet]. 1989 [cited 2020 Feb 18];41(10):705–9. Available from: https://onlinelibrary.wiley.com/doi/abs/10.1111/j.2042-7158.1989.tb06345.x.
11. De Angelis V, Koekman AC, Weeterings C, Roest M, De Groot PG, Herczenik E, et al. Endocannabinoids control platelet activation and limit aggregate formation under flow. PLoS One. 2014;9(9):e108282.
12. Levy, R, Schurr, A, Nathan I, Dvilanksi A. Impairment of ADP-induced platelet aggregation by Hashish components [Internet]. Thromb Haemost. 1976 [cited 2020 Jun 19]. p. 634–40. Available from: https://pubmed.ncbi.nlm.nih.gov/1037158/.
13. Dahdouh Z, Roule V, Lognoné T, Sabatier R, Grollier G. Cannabis and coronary thrombosis: what is the role of platelets? 2011 [cited 2020 Jun 25.]; Available from: https://www.tandfonline.com/action/journalInformation?journalCode=iplt20.
14. Jouanjus E, Raymond V, Lapeyre-Mestre M, Wolff V. What is the current knowledge about the cardiovascular risk for users of cannabis-based products? A systematic review [Internet]. Curr Atheroscler Rep. Current Medicine Group LLC 1; 2017 [cited 2020 Jun 30]. 19. Available from: https://pubmed.ncbi.nlm.nih.gov/28432636/.
15. Hemachandra D, McKetin R, Cherbuin N, Anstey KJ. Heavy cannabis users at elevated risk of stroke: evidence from a general population survey. Aust N Z J Public Health [Internet]. 2016 Jun 1 [cited 2020 Jun 30];40(3):226–30. Available from: https://pubmed.ncbi.nlm.nih.gov/26558539/
16. Rumalla K, Reddy AY, Mittal MK. Recreational marijuana use and acute ischemic stroke: A population-based analysis of hospitalized patients in the United States. J Neurol Sci [Internet]. 2016 May 15 [cited 2020 Jun 30];364:191–6. Available from: http://www.jns-journal.com/article/S0022510X16300661/fulltext.
17. Szekeres M, Nádasy GL, Turu G, Soltész-Katona E, Tóth ZE, Balla A, et al. Angiotensin II induces vascular endocannabinoid release, which attenuates its vasoconstrictor effect via CB1 cannabinoid receptors. J Biol Chem. 2012;287(37):31540–50.
18. Pryce G, Baker D. Antidote to cannabinoid intoxication: the CB1 receptor inverse agonist, AM251, reverses hypothermic effects of the CB1 receptor agonist, CB-13, in mice. Br J Pharmacol. 2017;174(21):3790–4.
19. Flisberg P, Paech MJ, Shah T, Ledowski T, Kurowski I, Parsons R. Induction dose of propofol in patients using cannabis. Eur J Anaesthesiol [Internet]. 2009 Mar [cited 2020 Jun 25];26(3):192–5. Available from: https://pubmed.ncbi.nlm.nih.gov/19237981/.
20. Echeverria-Villalobos M, Todeschini AB, Stoicea N, Fiorda-Diaz J, Weaver T, Bergese SD. Perioperative care of cannabis users: a comprehensive review of pharmacological and anesthetic considerations. J Clin Anesth. 2019;57:41–9. https://doi.org/10.1016/j.jclinane.2019.03.011. Epub 2019 Mar 7

Part VII

The Challenges with Medical Cannabis

The Colorado Experience

30

Alexander Shustorovich

The Colorado Experience

Colorado has been a pioneer state in the forefront of marijuana legislature reform. Following medical cannabis legalization in California in 1996 [1], Colorado legalized limited amounts of cannabis for medicinal use in November 2000. Patients with debilitating disease (e.g., cancer, HIV/AIDS) and associated signs and symptoms, such as cachexia, severe pain, severe nausea, seizures related to epilepsy, and spasticity in setting of neuromuscular disorders (e.g., multiple sclerosis), qualified for medicinal cannabis use [2]. Upon recommendation by their physicians, patients were issued registry identification cards by the Colorado Department of Public Health and Environment (CDPHE) [3] for possession of up to 2 ounce of usable cannabis and up to 6 marijuana plants (with 3 or fewer being mature, flowering plants) [2]. There was no form of regulated market available, and most of the medical supply came from individual grow operations or caregiver grow operations arbitrarily limited to five patients [2]. Caregiver grow operations also had to be registered with CDPHE. For the next decade, the medical cannabis market in Colorado functioned in a rather "wild west" fashion, based upon the integrity of the growers to produce high-quality medicine. Quality caregivers mostly operated delivery services or used discreet retail locations in fear of federal persecution, demonstrated by multiple raids and seizures of California dispensaries during this period [4].

The Ogden Memorandum of 2009 issued an official "hands-off" policy by the Justice Department, which instructed US Attorneys not to "focus federal resources in your States on individuals whose actions are in clear and unambiguous compliance with existing state laws providing for the medical use of marijuana" [2]. This federal memo provided a sense of security to facilitate medicinal cannabis commercialization across the states. It was regarded as the "green light" from the federal government to open a medical cannabis business. Meanwhile, a non-profit organization in Colorado, Sensible Colorado, sued the state over the arbitrary limitation of five patients per caregiver and eventually triumphed in 2007, lifting the patient restriction and paving the way for storefront dispensaries [4]. In 2009, Colorado legislature passed HB 10-1284 and SB 10-109, enacting the Colorado Medical Marijuana Code, which established a medical marijuana distribution system and commercialized distribution of cannabis. This not only provided licensure to businesses for production and distribution but also imposed regulations on patients, caregivers, and doctors [4]. Various state revisions followed to "clean up" the Colorado Medical Marijuana Code and required joint efforts from the CDPHE and the Colorado Medical Marijuana Enforcement

A. Shustorovich (✉)
Department of Physical Medicine & Rehabilitation, Johns Hopkins University School of Medicine, Baltimore, MD, USA

S. N. Narouze (ed.), *Cannabinoids and Pain*, https://doi.org/10.1007/978-3-030-69186-8_30

Table 30.1 Amendment 64 provisions

Amendment 64
Regulate the growth, manufacture, and sale of marijuana in a system of licensed establishments overseen by state and local governments
Allow individuals who are 21 years old or older to possess, use, display, purchase, transport, and transfer—to individuals who are 21 years old or older—one ounce or less of marijuana
Allow individuals who are 21 years old or order to possess, grow, process, and transport up to 6 marijuana plants, with certain restrictions
Require the state legislature to enact an excise tax on marijuana sales, of which the first $40 million in revenue raised annually must be credited to a state fund used for constructing public schools. The excise tax must be approved by a separate statewide vote
Require the state legislature to enact legislation concerning the growth, processing, and sale of industrial hemp

Source: https://www.colorado.gov/pacific/sites/default/files/13%20Amendment%2064%20LEGIS.pdf

Division (CMED) to implement regulations. The number of registered patients with the CDPHE dramatically increased from about 5000 in 2009 to almost 119,000 in 2011 [3].

Near the end of 2012, Colorado became the first state in the world to legalize recreational cannabis use with the passage of Amendment 64 [5]. Although medical cannabis continued to be regulated in a commercial market, recreational cannabis had specific personal possession and grow limitations [3]. See Table 30.1 for details of Amendment 64 provisions.

Nonetheless, as intended by Amendment 64, full regulation and commercialization were achieved by 2014. The established infrastructure allowed for growth, manufacture, processing, and sale of cannabis products recreationally to adults over the age of 21. The implemented taxes were meant to support public health initiatives and fund the public school capital construction assistance fund [6]. Many entrepreneurs viewed the legalization of marijuana as a lucrative business opportunity. Recreational sales boomed after legalization, increasing yearly, while medical marijuana sales only saw a modest increase initially, with relative leveling off and decline over the most recent years [7] (Fig. 30.1). The sales of retail marijuana products more than tripled, from $303 million in 2014 to $1.09 billion in 2017 [7] (Table 30.2). An average of $90 million in retail marijuana products were sold in 2017 up from $25 million in 2014 (Table 30.2). "Since 2014 sales of retail flower have gone up 516%, infused edibles up 226%, and infused non-edibles up 135%" [7]. With the growing sales of recreational marijuana, the state government appreciated a significant rise in tax and license revenue over the next 4 years (data only available through June 2018), although it is important to note that marijuana taxes only made up about 1.52% of the tax revenue collected by the state [7] (Fig. 30.2).

And yet, the seemingly glamorous sales and tax revenue did not come without public health and social concerns. Colorado has set the stage for the country and the rest of the world by becoming the innovator of marijuana reform. To some it is considered the big social experiment demonstrating a plausible model for cannabis legalization, while to others, it has posed even more questions. What would the end of cannabis prohibition truly look like? What is the long-term safety of daily use of recreational marijuana? How do I talk to my kids about this? Anecdotally, it was anticipated that there would be large increases in recreational marijuana use (both adults and minors), reduced marijuana-related crime, and increased motor vehicle accidents (MVA). Short-term effects of cannabis intoxication include deficits in attention, memory, learning, and decision-making [8], but due to decades of prohibition, proper research on the effects of chronic cannabis use has been limited. What has been gathered thus far and what is reliably known are that marijuana use in developing minds (e.g., the youth) causes both structural brain abnormalities and altered neural activity in the user [8]. More importantly, we must further our understanding of how these neurological changes translate to psychological and functional outcomes.

Dr. Roberts conducted a thorough cautionary review in 2019 evaluating health and safety effects of marijuana in Colorado [3]. At the time of publication, the state had legal recreational marijuana use for about 5 years. He noted that

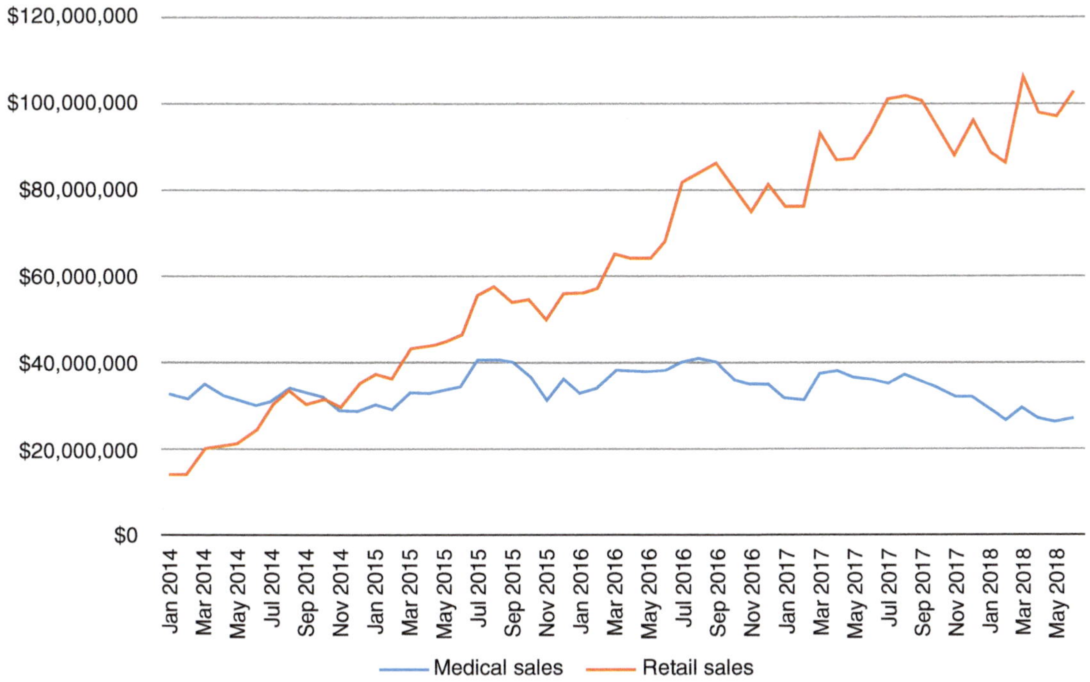

Fig. 30.1 Monthly marijuana sales, by type, 2014 to June 2018. Note: Medical marijuana sales (gross sales minus wholesale) and sales of accessories/other products that do not contain medical marijuana. Retail marijuana sales (gross sales minus wholesale) and does not include sales of accessories/other products that do not contain retail marijuana. (Source: Colorado Department of Revenue, Marijuana Enforcement Division [11])

Table 30.2 Annual and average monthly sales of marijuana products, 2014 to June 2018

Calendar year	Annual total sales			Average monthly sales		
	Medical	Retail	Total	Medical	Retail	Total
2014	$380,284,040	$303,239,699	$683,523,739	$31,690,337	$25,269,975	$56,960,312
2015	$418,054,912	$577,536,343	$995,591,255	$34,837,909	$48,128,029	$82,965,938
2016	$445,616,062	$861,587,411	$1,307,203,473	$37,134,672	$71,798,951	$108,933,623
2017	$416,516,782	$1,091,185,437	$1,507,702,219	$34,709,732	$90,932,120	$125,641,852
2018	$138,387,136	$474,477,654	$612,864,790	$27,677,427	$94,895,531	$122,572,958

Source: Colorado Department of Revenue, Marijuana Enforcement Division [11]
Notes: Medical marijuana sales (gross sales minus wholesale) and sales of accessories/other products that do not contain medical marijuana. Retail marijuana sales (gross sales minus wholesale) and does not include sales of accessories/other products that do not contain retail marijuana

cannabis potency had increased over the last several decades, and the "weed our parents smoked in the 60s and 70s" was far less potent compared to the presently cultured breeds. Current commercialized cannabis is near 20% tetrahydrocannabinol (THC), while in the 1980s the concentration was <2%. This increase only considers cannabis flower, yet other formulations such as waxes and oils can reach 80–90% THC [3]. The review demonstrated an increase in cannabis-related presentations to the emergency departments (ED) and hospitalizations across the state. Most prevalent were admissions for acute psychosis related to intolerance to the cannabis potency [3, 9]. This was consistent with large reviews conducted by the World Health Organization (WHO) and the National Academies of Sciences, Engineering, and Medicine (NASEM) that identified statistically significant association between cannabis use and develop-

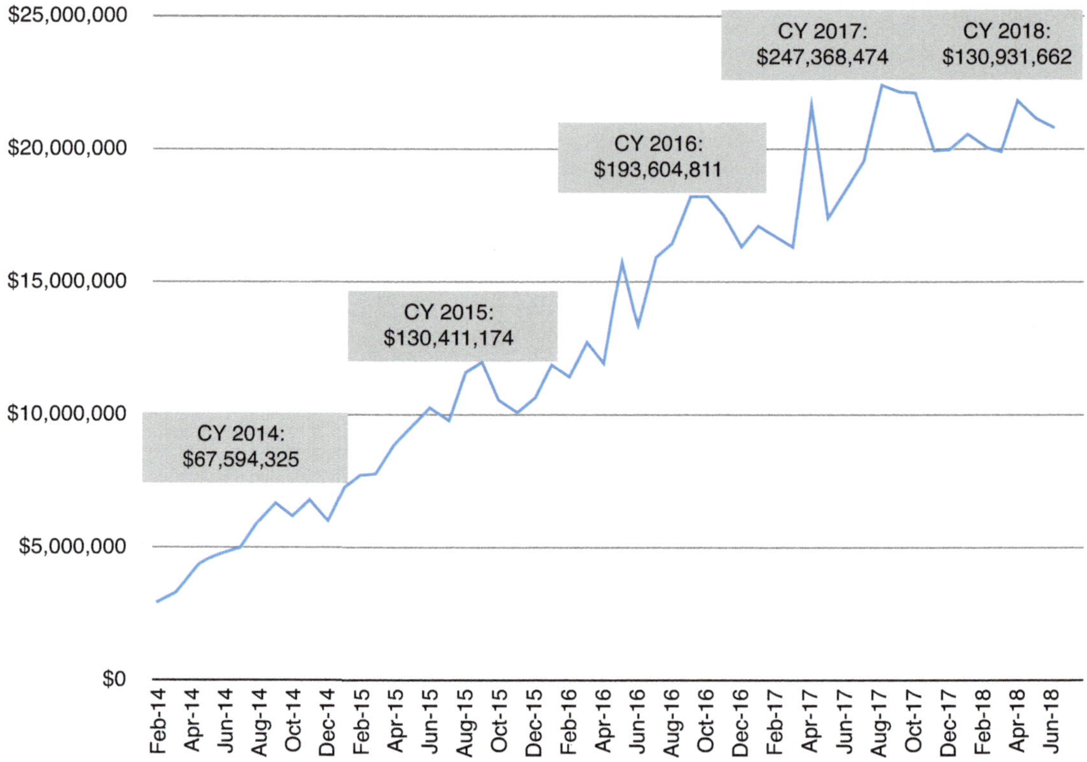

Fig. 30.2 Total taxes, licenses, and fees, 2014 to June 2018. Note: Calendar year 2018 taxes reported through June 2018. (Source: Marijuana Enforcement Division [12])

ment of schizophrenia and psychoses in genetically predisposed, frequent users [3, 8, 9]. Nonetheless, thousands of other users have continued to partake in ingesting and inhaling cannabis products without these negative effects [10].

Surprisingly, the youth marijuana use has not dramatically increased since legalization of recreation marijuana in Colorado [3, 7, 9, 10]. Both Dr. Roberts and Dr. Leyton demonstrated that although many high schoolers had tried marijuana, there was no significant overall increase in sustained marijuana use [3, 9]. There has been an objective increase in marijuana use among adults (age 21 and over), but this was likely to be expected, as adults were the targeted demographic group. However, most significant was the overall decrease in marijuana-related arrests. There was a total of 302 marijuana-related arrests in Denver, CO, in 2017, which is considerably reduced from the 1605 arrests in 2012 [7]. But unfortunately, a statistical racial divide has persisted, which likely pokes holes at our society's cultural construct and not necessarily cannabis reform [7, 10]. Contradictory to common belief, cannabis-related MVAs only initially increased within the first year of recreational legalization but then leveled off to rates similar in states without legalization [9].

The Colorado experience over the last 6 years has been a trying time filled with legislative, social, and economic reform. Being the first to legalize recreational marijuana use pushed the state government into uncharted territory. As expected, it was not smooth sailing, and many concerned citizens and families have left the state to find refuge from the "reefer" movement [10]. There is still much to learn about the long-term psychological and physiological effects on daily users. The data we have now suggests we should tread with caution, but further research with large cohorts is required to truly understand the risks, benefits, and safety of cannabis use. Economically, it has proven to be a sound business venture, but at a relatively high risk. Previously protected by the Ogden and Cole memorandums, US Attorney General Jeff Sessions rescinded these provisions in January 2018 reminding everyone cannabis is still considered a Schedule I substance by the Drug Enforcement Agency (DEA) and business owners remain at risk of being persecuted at the federal level [3]. It is difficult to not compare marijuana prohibition to prohibition of alcohol in the early twentieth century. Nonetheless, objectively speaking, Colorado has shown us what a leap in marijuana reform looks like. Time will only tell when social norms, cultures, and political values adjust accordingly. It seems we have a potential working model (although not perfect) for cannabis reform, but the rate of progression will depend on the ever-changing social climate.

References

1. PBS Frontline Marijuana Timeline. https://www.pbs.org/wgbh/pages/frontline/shows/dope/etc/cron.html.
2. Amendment 20 to Colorado's state constitution. Americans for Safe Access. https://www.safeaccessnow.org/amendment_20_to_colorado_s_state_constitutionnew. Accessed 12 Apr 2020.
3. Roberts BA. Legalized Cannabis in Colorado Emergency Departments: a cautionary review of negative health and safety effects. West J Emerg Med. 2019;20(4):557–72. https://doi.org/10.5811/westjem.2019.4.39935.
4. History of Colorado's marijuana laws. Sensible Colorado. http://sensiblecolorado.org/history-of-co-medical-marijuana-laws/. Accessed 12 Apr 2020.
5. Coffman K, Neroulias N. Colorado, Washington first states to legalize recreational pot. Reuters. 6 Nov 2012. Accessed 12 Apr 2020.
6. Amendment 64 implementation. https://www.colorado.gov/pacific/sites/default/files/13%20Amendment%2064%20LEGIS.pdf. Accessed 5 Apr 2020.
7. Impacts of marijuana in Colorado: a report pursuant to Senate Bill 13-283. Oct 2018. http://cdpsdocs.state.co.us/ors/docs/reports/2018-SB13-283_Rpt.pdf. Accessed 5 Apr 2020.
8. Weir K. Marijuana and the developing brain. Monitor on Psychology. Published Nov 2015. https://www.apa.org/monitor/2015/11/marijuana-brain. Accessed 16 Apr 2020.
9. Leyton M. Cannabis legalization: did we make a mistake? Update 2019. J Psychiatry Neurosci. 2019;44(5):291–3. https://doi.org/10.1503/jpn.190136.
10. Healy J. Reefer madness or pot paradise? The surprising legacy of the place where legal weed began. The New York Times. Published 30 June 2019. https://www.nytimes.com/2019/06/30/us/marijuana-colorado-legalization.html. Accessed 16 Apr 2020.
11. Colorado Department of Revenue, Marijuana Enforcement Division. Marijuana sales report. 2018. https://cdor.colorado.gov/data-and-reports/marijuana-data/marijuana-sales-reports.
12. Colorado Department of Revenue, Marijuana Enforcement Division. Marijuana tax data. 2018. https://cdor.colorado.gov/data-and-reports/marijuana-data/marijuana-tax-reports.

Product Safety and Quality Control 31

Caroline A. MacCallum, Lindsay A. Lo,
Fonda Betts, and Michael Koehn

Introduction

There are a number of quality control variables to consider when choosing medical cannabis products including the presence of contaminants, microorganisms, and pesticides. Patients may unknowingly assume that cannabis from any source is equally safe to use. Clinicians and patients must be aware of the potential differences between regulated cannabis products and those from unregulated sources in order to make informed decisions that best fit the medical needs of the patient.

Cannabis as a "Natural" Medicine

Many patients assume that cannabis, being a plant and thereby a "natural" medicine, implies inherent safety with no side effects. Subsequently, patients may have a false sense of security that CBD is "safe", and that THC is "harmful." While CBD may have less serious adverse events when compared to THC, potential health concerns relating to product standardization, labelling, and integrity including contaminants, microorganisms, and pesticides are discussed in the next section.

Standardization and Quality Control

Where medical cannabis is still illegal, and even in countries where cannabis is only legal at the state level, there are frequent gaps in quality control processes, which may be overcome with federal legaliztion and implementation of standards of practice for growing and testing cannabis. Many cannabis products lack mandatory standardized laboratory testing to ensure a safe final product, which are free of or contain acceptable range for human consumption of contaminants, pesticides, microorganisms, and even diluents/

C. A. MacCallum (✉)
Department of Medicine, Faculty of Medicine, University of British Columbia, Vancouver, BC, Canada
e-mail: info@drcarolinemaccallum.com

L. A. Lo
Department of Psychology, Queen's University, Kingston, ON, Canada

F. Betts
Greenleaf Medical Clinic, Langley, BC, Canada

M. Koehn, MACP
CannSolve Medical Clinic, Mental Health Agency and Cannabis Education Centre, Kamloops, BC, Canada

S. N. Narouze (ed.), *Cannabinoids and Pain*, https://doi.org/10.1007/978-3-030-69186-8_31

fillers (see Chap. 37 on Cannabis Vaping Hazards).

There is much confusion surrounding cannabis product labelling, terminology, and marketing. Companies may use terms such as "organic," "sustainably grown," "pesticide-free," or "grown in living soil" to differentiate themselves in the marketplace. Without regulation, these terms may or may not reflect the efficacy or purity of the final product sold to consumers. The integrity of cannabis products depends on the standard of practice of the grow facility and the company's own inherent quality assurance processes, policies, and procedures.

While some cannabis companies may claim to produce a cleaner and safer product, to date there is no substantial evidence that any one of these growing methods is inherently safer than another. Even with good manufacturing processes (GMP) compliant cannabis, there are still many contributing factors and potential for contaminants from the environment to be present in the final product [1–3]. For example, cannabis grown outdoors could contain pesticides released from the air or water from a neighboring contaminated crop [2, 3]. This affirms the need for mandatory regulated testing and standardized labelling to provide reassurance that patients' health and safety are preserved. It is best practice to ask the seller to provide the "Certification of Analysis" (COA) for each product to ensure that the product labelling meets the labelling requirements by state.

Contaminants

Product contaminant exposure may vary from region to region depending on regulatory protocols and where patients choose to purchase their cannabis. Products obtained from legal cannabis producers, such as in Canada, have passed mandatory government regulations that are enforceable through licensing. Cannabis products that are legally sold in Canada through retail and online stores must pass standardized testing for contaminants.

In unregulated markets, there are several issues healthcare providers and patients should be aware of. Cannabinoids can be extracted from the plant to form concentrates in a process involving polar solvents, such as naphtha, butane, or petroleum ether, which may leave toxic residues that the patient will consume. This process of extraction results in highly concentrated contaminants and THC content (up to 80% THC). These highly potent concentrates or "dabs" are commonly used by recreational users who acknowledge greater tolerance and withdrawal in accordance with their use [4]. In contrast, in a regulated medical cannabis market where butane, propane, ethanol, and CO2 are used as solvents, high-quality products can be produced and tested for residual contamination. Solvent quality and manufacturing processes both play an important role in the creation of high-quality extracts. Medical professionals, in collaboration with their patients, should assess both the medical effects and product safety of concentrated cannabis products used in treatment.

Although the hazards of vaping are mentioned in Chap. 37, particular factors regarding contaminants are important to reiterate. E-cigarettes may use propylene glycol (1,2 propanediol) and glycerol as propellants, which when heated can produce formaldehyde, a Group 1 carcinogen (International Agency for Research on Cancer - IARC) [5]. 1,3 Propanediol is a new propellant being studied and tested as a replacement for these, but more research on the long-term safety profile is needed [6]. Vitamin E acetate has been associated with e-cigarette and vaping-associated lung illness (EVALI) related to vaping devices, liquids, refill pods, and cartridges [7]. Evidence from the CDC among 49 states in the United States suggests that illicit products with THC were associated with a higher risk of EVALI, likely resulting from the vitamin E concentration within the devices and products.

An additional preliminary report on pulmonary illness related to e-cigarette use found that in 53 cases, 84% of patients were using THC in their e-cigarette device [8]. Patients most commonly presented with respiratory (98%) and gastrointestinal (81%) symptoms, and bilateral infiltrates were seen on CT chest scans [8]. While 94% of cases were hospitalized and 32% were intubated/

ventilated, only one death was reported [8]. A variety of products and devices were reported however the most common THC-containing device (67%) was under the "dank vape" label, a black-market product [8]. An additional study revealed up to 91% of patients reported obtaining their THC-containing e-cigarette device from an informal, illegal source [7].

In summary, the majority of pulmonary illnesses related to vaporization have been associated with illicit product use [7–9]. Further, they tend to be seen in younger people using THC and nicotine containing e-cigarettes recreationally. Currently, there are no safety or long-term studies on pen ingredients. Ideally, ingestible oil products should be encouraged for medical use. If a patient wishes to use a vaporization pen, it is best practice to advise on potential risks, check the ingredients being reported on the label, and recommend regulated products. If any respiratory symptoms occur, stop and report them to your governing agency.

While no vaporizer to date has demonstrated a complete absence of polyaromatic hydrocarbon production [10], it appears that there may be a reduction of toxic high molecular weight compounds (including tar) with vaporization of dried flower. There may still be exposure to low weight compounds such as ammonia [10]. However, it has been suggested that ammonia levels in vaporized dried cannabis may be due to synthetic fertilizers. More research on flower contaminants as well as by-products of vaporization of dried cannabis is required [10].

Microorganisms

Cannabis may become contaminated with a variety of microorganisms such as pathogenic bacteria, yeast, and mold. This may occur during cultivation, harvesting, drying, storage, and distribution [3]. Humid conditions can make cannabis more vulnerable to microbial contamination. Common microbial contaminants include powdery mildew, *Salmonella* species, *Escherichia coli*, *Penicillium* species, *Aspergillum* species, and other bile-tolerant Gram-negative bacteria [3]. While care should always be taken when sourcing products for any patient, there is an elevated need when dealing with at-risk populations, such as those who are immunocompromised. Patients with immunocompromising conditions are at a higher risk for microbial infection, especially for inhaled cannabis. A more serious contaminant, the *Aspergillus* species, can cause serious effects when inhaled [3]. Additionally, cannabis may also become contaminated with mycotoxins, a harmful metabolite produced by fungi. The main mycotoxins of concern are aflatoxins, ochratoxins, and vomitoxins [3]. While several factors, such as growing/handling practices and humidity, influence the risk of cannabis becoming contaminated, it is best practice to source products from producers who adhere to rigorous contaminant testing and quality assurance protocols.

Pesticides

Lack of federal regulation in the United States does pose some risk for pesticide use in certain cannabis products. Out of 26 samples from legal dispensaries in Washington state, 22/26 (86%) tested positive for pesticides. Many had multiple contaminants and had levels of 10,000–100,000 parts per billion (ppb), exceeding the upper limit of quantification. There were 24 distinct pesticide agents including insecticides, miticides, fungicides, and insecticidal synergist and growth regulators [11]. Several factors contribute to this issue including unregulated pesticide use, lack of regulatory and industry oversight, lack of available organic certification, and lack of federal/state laboratory standardization. Pesticide-contaminated products are dangerous, particularly to young patients with epilepsy or other neurological conditions. Further, this could also result in exposure to known carcinogens. In order to safeguard cannabis consumers, proper standards must be applied as with any product intended for human consumption. Health standards may improve under federal legalization and regulation of cannabis where ongoing laboratory testing is required for the issuance of a sales license. Additional measures may include mandating integrated pest management that effectively restricts the use of many synthetic pesticides while testing, and tracking to ensure that all products sold in dispensaries can be traced from seed to sale. An example of such regulation can be seen in Canada.

Prior to a 2017 mandate, Health Canada testing found roughly 5% of tested samples came back positive for restricted pesticides such as fungicides. Currently, license holders are permitted to only use pesticides or pest control products that are approved for use on cannabis in accordance with the pest control products act (PCPA) [12]. Adequate controls at the site of production must be in place to ensure unauthorized pest control products are not used. Health Canada requires mandatory testing for pesticide active ingredients for all cannabis products before being sold. Testing for microbes and heavy metals is also done. Due to mandatory testing, a sample of medical cannabis in 2018 was found to contain the banned pesticide myclobutanil, a known carcinogen. Regulation drastically improves the quality, safety, and consistency of cannabis products, although healthcare providers should be aware that even regulated cannabis can occasionally be contaminated. This is especially the case when recommending products for at-risk patient population such as those that are immunocompromised.

Gamma Irradiation

Gamma irradiation is commonly used in agriculture to sterilize food products through exposure to ionizing radiation. The FDA, WHO, CDC, Health Canada, and USDA have all found irradiation to be safe for food products. While there are limited safety studies regarding cannabis and gamma radiation, currently available evidence suggests cannabis is also safe following irradiation; there are no "mutations" or alterations to the product or any "residual" radiation observed on cannabis as a result of using gamma radiation [13, 14]. However, monoterpene content may be slightly reduced as is seen in other agricultural products [13]. Some researchers feel that this reduction in monoterpenes could reduce the efficacy of the cannabis plant, however, the impact has not been well characterized in clinical studies.

Gamma irradiation will kill pathogenic fungi; however it will not neutralize mycotoxins that are already present. There have been no studies to date that have proven the safety of an irradiated product that is smoked, but many licensed producers in Canada irradiate their cannabis in order to meet the strict limit of 1000 colony forming units (CFU) per gram of finished product. There are cannabis producers globally who irradiate cannabis in order to consistently meet government-mandated testing limits of microbial contamination throughout the production process. Consistent irradiation may help better manage product supply to meet the needs of patient, rather than waiting for a failed test to identify a product that will need further treatment or disposal after months of growing and processing. Much of the popularity of irradiation among licensed producers is directly tied to strict standards set out by the government in the legalized and regulated market. In order to maintain consistently low microbial counts from production to consumption, gamma irradiation may be seen as a necessity. Alternatively, the extraction process for making cannabis oils (including CO2 and ethanol extraction) seems to result in the most "sterile" product possible, suggesting this to be the best route for immunocompromised individuals over inhaled gamma-radiated products where possible (see Chap. 23 on Cannabinoid-Based Medicines: Patient Safety Considerations for more information).

Labelling

While understanding labelling is an essential component of promoting product safety, it can be challenging to ascertain how the labelling of a product relates to dose and expected effect. There is little guidance on "dose expression" or how a specific dose of THC that is labelled on a particular product translates into the amount to consume for desired effects [13]. This has left both novice and more frequent users of cannabis unsure of the appropriate dose to take, especially among edible and oral products [15].

Evidence has shown that available cannabis products frequently fail to meet basic label accuracy standards for pharmaceuticals. Edible cannabis products ($N = 75$) from three major metropolitan areas (San Francisco, Los Angeles, and Seattle) were analyzed in one study. With respect to THC content, 17% were accurately labelled, 23% were under-labelled, and 60% were over-labelled [16]. The median THC:CBD ratio of products with detectable CBD was 36:1. Products containing significantly more THC than labelled place patients at risk of experiencing significant adverse events. On the other hand, under-labelled products might not achieve the desired therapeutic benefits [16]. Another report analyzed 84 cannabidiol extracts purchased online and found that 69% had mislabelled cannabinoid content [17]. Recently, a class action lawsuit was launched against several large Canadian cannabis companies for incorrect labelling claims on medical and recreational cannabis packaging [18]. This incident demonstrates the variation in analytical results and difficulties with cannabis labelling, even in a highly regulated market like Canada.

In a medical context, cannabis is "recommended" or "certified" by a physician. This is based on policy rather than science indications. Therefore, practicioners may have little influence over the dose or frequency of cannabis; this may be left to the dispensary and patient. This is in contrast to recreational use, which may lead to greater acute impairment from using more than intended or problematic use in an attempt to alleviate negative mental states.

As with any health product, required regulations for labelling and packaging are needed to ensure product safety and to optimize patient outcomes. Countries in which cannabis is legal at a federal level, such as Canada, can be valuable resources to look to for examples on regulatory labelling practices. Generally, this pertains to providing concise, but detailed, information on the product that is easily viewable on the packaging. This may include product specifications such as the common name of the product, cannabinoid content (THC and CBD), packaging date, expiry date, net weight of cannabis, number of discrete units, and list of ingredients/food allergens. It is also useful to have an easily identifiable brand or producer with information on how to contact the producer if necessary. Additional labelling practices that may help both patients and providers include specifications on the intended use of the product and optimal storage conditions. It is also best practice to have a health warning message included, as there would be with any other health product. When assessing products, it is useful for healthcare providers and patients to be aware of the maximum amount of cannabinoids allowed per product within their jurisdiction. This can be helpful in spotting black market items, as they may often exceed legally allowed cannabinoid limits. The above specifications are potential indicators that can be used to assess product quality and safety, as well as assisting in safe dose titration.

Several principles outlined by Hammond [15] and Health Canada [19] may assist in the proper assessment of labelling (Table 31.1), including strategies to communicate "dose expression," so that consumers can appropri-

Table 31.1 Principles to guide cannabis labelling and packaging regulations

Principles to guide cannabis labelling and packaging regulations
Cannabinoid content (THC and CBD) clearly labelled For example: THC ## mg/g, Total THC ## per unit ## mg
Labelling provides guidance on THC amounts For example, communicating the number of tablets or capsules per dose, or the volume of product to be delivered
THC labelling reinforced by other packaging regulations, such as unit-dose packaging For example, if an edible product contained 10 mg of THC but was split into 5 servings, unit-dose or dose per serving would show 2 mg of THC
Labelling clearly identifies type of product and provides common basis for comparisons between products, to the extent possible While there is no standard THC dose or serving that can be used across all products, indications such as total THC content can be useful to give a broad comparison
Packaging has a security feature to indicate no opening prior to purchase
Labelling clearly indicates packaging and expiration date

ately titrate doses with as few impairments as possible.

It should be noted that specific labelling requirements differ based on geographical location. Each US state has different specifications and requirements. It is important for healthcare providers to know labelling requirements for each state they are practicing in. For labelling requirements by state, please visit "Cannabis Labelling Requirements by State" by Weber Packaging Solutions [20].

Concentrates and Potency

Changes in cannabis potency over the last two decades are well documented. Analysis of cannabis preparations seized by the US Drug Enforcement Administration between 1995 and 2014 showed that the potency of sinsemilla samples has increased. Overall, the potency of illicit cannabis plant material has consistently risen over time from approximately 4% THC in 1995 to 12% in 2014. On the other hand, the CBD content had fallen on average from 0.28% in 2001 to <0.15% in 2014 [21].

A more recent study showed that Δ9-THC concentration has increased dramatically over the last 10 years, from 8.9% in 2008 to 17.1% in 2017. The mean Δ9-THC/CBD ratio also rose substantially from 23 in 2008 to 104 in 2017. From 2008 to 2017, there was a marked increase in the proportion of hash oil samples (cannabis concentrates) from 0.5% to 4.7%, and their mean Δ9-THC concentration increased from 6.7% to 55.7%.

Generally, it is advised that for medical purposes, highly concentrated THC products are not used. Higher THC potency and increased dose are highly correlated with adverse events and side effects. Healthcare providers should be familiar with common extracts to assist in product evaluation and mitigation of risk to patients. Table 31.2 outlines common concentrates found

Table 31.2 Common cannabis concentrates

Cannabis concentrate	Description
Solvent-based extracts	
"Live" resin	Hydrocarbon extract. Extracted from fresh cannabis plant material. Preserves higher concentration of terpenes
Shatter	Hydrocarbon extract. A golden, translucent, brittle concentrate. Brittle due to crystallization of THCA in the extract Up to 90% potency
Wax	Hydrocarbon extract. Soft concentrate that varies in appearance, texture, and color depending on processing technique Common forms include: *Budder*: Whipped into a smooth consistency with a high terpene concentration. Also termed: *badder*, *frosting*, *icing*, and more *Crumble*: Purged wax (removal of any residual solvents) to create a drier texture concentrate. Have porous appearance like a honeycomb Both are generally 60–90% THC potency
CO2	Uses carbon dioxide under extreme temperature and pressure to extract cannabinoids and terpenes from plant. Commonly used to create cannabis oils and vape products Wide range of THC and CBD potency
Distillate	Viscous, translucent, flavorless oil. Concentrates made through an extensive refinement process in which crude extracts like CO2 and EtOH are distilled. Often used in edibles, topicals, and vape cartridges Generally, 70–90% THC potency
Isolate	Commonly uses a vacuum pump which pulls cannabis through fine sand filtration Cannabinoids can be isolated into concentrated crystalline structures or powder. Other cannabinoids and plant impurities removed. Can add cannabis terpenes to final product Nearly 100% THC or CBD potency

(continued)

Table 31.2 continued

Cannabis concentrate	Description
Solventless extracts	
Bubble hash/ice water hash	Created by agitating cannabis buds in ice water and filtering water through fine screen bags Water is then filtered and trichomes of the cannabis flower are collected leaving a paste known as "hash" Generally, 40–60% THC potency
Kief/dry sift	Kief: Flower is ground and sifted, leaving behind complete trichome glands Dry sift: Mechanically separated and collects resin glands from the cannabis flower using a series of different sized mesh screens. Only small trichome heads can pass through Generally, 50–80% THC potency
Rosin	Solventless concentrate extracted using high pressure and gentle heat to squeeze terpene-rich cannabinoid concentrate from cannabis flowers Generally, 40–75% THC potency

 Information gathered from Refs. [22, 23]

in both illicit and legal markets. Concentrates can be split into two categories, solvent-based extracts and solventless extracts. Hydrocarbon extracts (BHO) are a class of solvent-based extracts created using hydrocarbon solvents like butane and propane to extract cannabinoids and terpenes from cannabis with a closed-loop extraction system. Hydrocarbon extraction better preserves the cannabinoids and terpene profiles of a particular strain. Several common types of BHO extracts include shatter, wax, and "Live" resin. Other solvent-based extracts include CO2 oil, distillate, and isolate. Cannabis concentrates can also be made through solventless processes. Common solventless extracts include dry sift, hash, and rosin. Please see Table 31.2 for more details.

Product Safety and Clinical Applications: A Common Clinical Scenario

Patients commonly bring products to the clinic. For example, a bottle of oil or a syringe containing thick cannabis extract without a label. The instructions may be as vague as "I dose an amount of product the size of half a grain of rice." They may also indicate that they get the product "from a friend" who is an "organic" grower and it is "100% CBD" and "safe."

It is important for physicians and patients to understand that there is no way to have confidence when dosing an unknown product without a label, company name, or any of the other important details which are required to guarantee standardization and safety of the product for human consumption. Please see the below list of questions which can aid a healthcare provider in assessing a patient's cannabis product.

Cannabis laws vary by state and countries. In some jurisdictions, physicians can discuss cannabis and its use with patients, but may not be able to recommend specific products or help patients obtain them. Clinicians should review and encourage patients to implement the framework highlighted in Table 31.3 to help guide them in their decision-making regarding safe cannabis products. Additionally, see Fig. 31.1, an example of a cannabis dosing calculator, which may aid patients in determining their current dose of THC/CBD. Positioning of THC and CBD concentrations is not standard, ask your supplier if you are not sure (see Chap. 22 on Cannabinoid-Based Medicines: Dosing, Titration, and Monitoring for more information).

Table 31.3 Proposed framework for the safe selection of cannabis product

Proposed Framework for the safe selection of cannabis product
What are the product details (name of the product, grower/producer, distributor)? For dried flower or inhaled concentrates: What is the listed % of THC and CBD? For ingestible oils: How many mg of THC and CBD per ml of oil?
Does the patient have the product with them or a picture of the label? Confirm type of product (i.e., oil, flower, shatter, concentrate), labelling, date of packaging, expiry date
Does the company have a legitimate website? (is it only found on social media?)
Where was the product purchased? (online, dispensary, health food store, etc.)
Is it a legal, regulated product? (a) Know the cannabis regulations in your state (b) Research to assess if the patient has been using a regulated product or recommend one that is regulated.
What is the chemovar profile for the product? (i.e., what is the concentration of the other cannabinoids and terpenes?)
How long has the patient been taking the product? Has the response been consistent over time (i.e., batch to batch variability?)
What is the dose, route, frequency, and where possible total daily mgs of THC and CBD (for oils)? (please see Fig. 31.1 to aid in calculating dose if necessary)
What symptoms have improved with the product?
What adverse events have been experienced?

Summary

It is crucial to provide cannabis education in order to mitigate risks and promote patient safety, as many unwanted side effects can be avoided with proper education. Medical cannabis must be standardized to ensure consistent delivery of active components, namely, CBD and THC (among other cannabinoids and terpenes).

Quality control standards reduce exposure to harmful chemicals and contaminants such as pesticides, extractions, microorganisms, diluents, and fillers. These are important considerations when selecting cannabis products, and should not be overlooked by healthcare providers, medical patients, and cannabis consumers in general.

Regulated products from a legal source should always be recommended for use. This is particularly important for patients in at-risk populations such as immunocompromised or the elderly. Ensuring product safety and quality control should always be a top priority for healthcare providers looking to use cannabinoids in their practice.

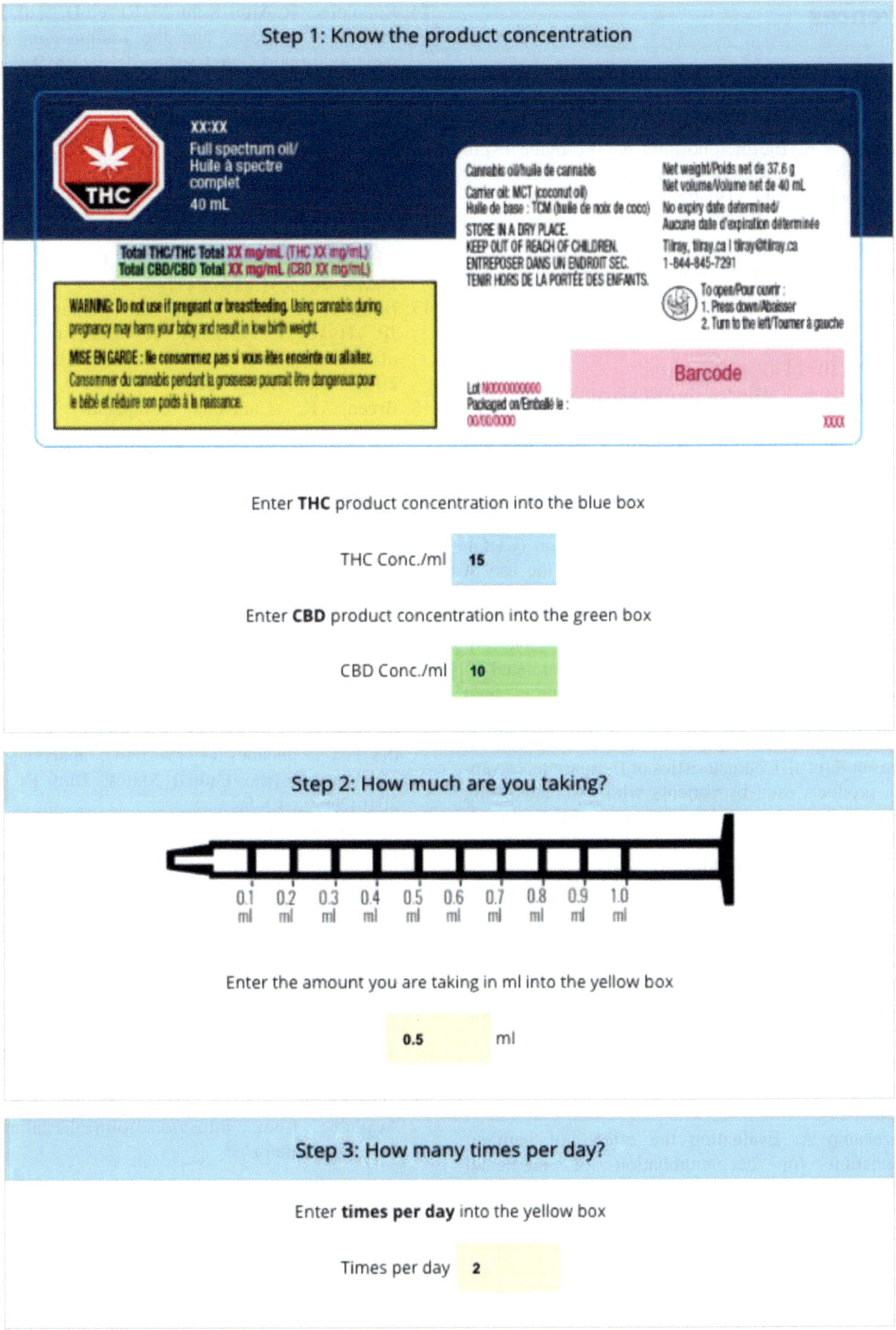

Fig. 31.1 Cannabis dosing calculator. (© Caroline MacCallum MD and Fonda Betts, used with permission) [24]
*Positioning of THC and CBD concentration on the label is not standardized. Ask your supplier if you are not sure

References

1. McLaren J, Swift W, Dillon O, Allsop S. Cannabis potency and contamination: a review of the literature. Addiction. 2008;103:1100–9.
2. Damalas CA, Eleftherohorinos IG. Pesticide exposure, safety issues, and risk assessment indicators. Int J Environ Res Public Health. 2011;8:1402–19.
3. Sarma ND, Waye A, ElSohly MA, Brown PN, Elzinga S, Johnson HE, et al. Cannabis inflorescence for medical purposes: USP considerations for quality attributes. J Nat Prod. 2020;83(4):1334–51.
4. Loflin M, Earleywine M. A new method of cannabis ingestion: the dangers of dabs? Addict Behav. 2014;39(10):1430–3.
5. Jensen RP, et al. Hidden formaldehyde in e-cigarette aerosols. NEJM. 2015;372(4):392–4.
6. Bertrand P, Bonnarme V, Piccirilli A, et al. Physical and chemical assessment of 1,3 Propanediol as a potential substitute of propylene glycol in refill liquid for electronic cigarettes. Sci Rep. 2018;8:10702.
7. Centers for Disease Control and Prevention (CDC). Outbreak of lung injury associated with the use of E-cigarette, or vaping, products. Centers for Disease Control and Prevention. 2020.
8. Layden J, Ghinai I, Pray I, Kimball A, Layer M, Tenforde MW, et al. Pulmonary illness related to E-cigarette use in Illinois and Wisconsin – final report. N Engl J Med. 2020;382:903–16.
9. Taylor J, Wiens T, Peterson J, Saravia S, Lunda M, Hanson K, et al. Characteristics of E-cigarette, or vaping, products used by patients with associated lung injury and products seized by law enforcement — Minnesota, 2018 and 2019. MMWR Morb Mortal Wkly Rep. 2019;68:1096–100.
10. Bloor RN, Wang TS, Španeˇl P, Smith D. Ammonia release from heated 'street' cannabis leaf and its potential toxic effects on cannabis uses. Addiction. 2008;103:1671–7.
11. Russo EB. Current therapeutic Cannabis controversies and clinical trial design issues. Front Pharmacol. 2016;7(309):1–19.
12. Health Canada. For health care professionals: Cannabis and cannabinoids. Government of Canada. 2018.
13. Hazekamp A. Evaluating the effects of gamma-irradiation for decontamination of medicinal Cannabis. Front Pharmacol. 2016;7:108.
14. Ruchlemer R, Amit-Kohn M, Raveh D, et al. Inhaled medicinal cannabis and the immunocompromised patient. Support Care Cancer. 2015;23:819–22.
15. Hammond D. Communicating THC levels and 'dose' to consumers: implications for product labelling and packaging of cannabis products in regulated markets. Int J Drug Policy. 2019; https://doi.org/10.1016/j.drugpo.2019.07.004.
16. Vandrey R, Raber JC, Raber ME, Douglass B, Miller C, Bonn-Miller MO. Cannabinoid dose and label accuracy in edible medical Cannabis products. JAMA. 2015;313(24):2491–3.
17. Bonn-Miller MO, Loflin M, Thomas BF, Marcu JP, Hyke T, Vandrey R. Labeling accuracy of Cannabidiol extracts sold online. JAMA. 2017;318(17):1708–9.
18. Breen, K. Cannabis companies facing proposed class-action lawsuit over alleged mislabelling. Global News. 2020, June 19. Retrieved from: https://globalnews.ca/news/7081677/cannabis-companies-proposed-lawsuit-potency/.
19. Health Canada. Packaging and labelling guide for cannabis products. Government of Canada. 2019.
20. Weber Packing Solutions. Cannabis Labeling Requirements By State. *Weber Packaging Solutions*. 2018. Retrieved From: http://www.weberpackaging.com/pdfs/Cannabis%20Laws%20by%20State.pdf.
21. ElSohly MA, Mehmedic Z, Foster S, Gon C, Chandra S, Church JC. Changes in Cannabis potency over the last 2 decades (1995–2014): analysis of current data in the United States. Biol Psychiatry. 2016;79(7):613–9.
22. Craft S, Winstock A, Ferris J, Mackie C, Lynskey MT, Freeman TP (2020). Characterising heterogeneity in the use of different cannabis products: latent class analysis with 55 000 people who use cannabis and associations with severity of cannabis dependence. Psychological Medicine 50, 2364–2373. https://doi.org/10.1017/S0033291719002460
23. Nickus L (2020). What are cannabis concentrates and how do you consume them? Weedmaps. https://weedmaps.com/learn/products-and-how-to-consume/cannabis-concentrates
24. MacCallum CA (2021). Dosing Calculator. Available from: https://drcarolinemaccallum.com/dosing-calculator/

Cannabinoids and Brain Development

32

Samer N. Narouze

There is evidence from human and animal studies that a vulnerable period for chronic cannabinoid administration exists during certain phases of development. Prenatal and early cannabis exposure result in measurable brain changes.

Since greater neuromaturation takes place during adolescence, there is evidence that the adolescent brain is at great deleterious risk, compared to the adult brain [42]. The deleterious effects of weekly cannabis use by teenagers are evident, which include lower IQ scores, decreased verbal memory, poorer executive function, decreased sustained attention, neurocognitive abnormalities, and abnormalities in brain morphometry [37].

The findings below signify the importance of identification of adolescent cannabis use and prenatal cannabis exposure to prevent and minimize damage to the developing brain.

Epidemiology of Youth Cannabis Use

The American population's perception of cannabis risk has significantly decreased. According to the Monitoring the Future Study, since 2016 there has been some leveling of inhalational cannabis trends among 10th and 12th graders, while some increase in use among 8th graders [33]. As cannabis usage increases and the public perception shifts, viewing cannabis as less harmful, likewise the age of first-time cannabis use declines [28]. Clinical criteria for cannabis use disorder may be met at any age; however, such criteria among users are met most often during adolescence or young adulthood [4, 15].

Risk and Prognostic Factors May Be Divided into Temperamental, Environmental, and Genetic Categories

Temperamental Risks

Certain personal temperamental risk factors increase the likelihood of adolescent cannabis use disorder. Internalizing or externalizing disorders, antisocial personality disorder, and conduct disorder in children and adolescents are associated with greater risk of future substance use disorders. Likewise, these factors also increase the likelihood of cannabis use disorder [3]. Behavioral disinhibition in young people is associated with early-onset substance abuse, including multiple substance involvement and conduct disorder [30].

Environmental Risks

Certain risks are categorized as environment risks, which increase the likelihood of cannabis and other substance abuse. Such risks include poor academic performance, unstable/abusive

S. N. Narouze (✉)
Western Reserve Hospital, Center For Pain Medicine, Cuyahoga Falls, OH, USA
e-mail: narouzs@hotmail.com
Twitter: @NarouzeMD

S. N. Narouze (ed.), *Cannabinoids and Pain*, https://doi.org/10.1007/978-3-030-69186-8_32

family situation, personal tobacco abuse, cannabis use by family members, family substance abuse, and low socioeconomic status. Since cannabis is readily available, this relative abundance within a community increases the risk of developing a cannabis use disorder [3]. Traditionally during early teens, adolescents start drinking alcohol and using illicit substances. Higher-risk communities have earlier onset of alcohol and substance use at elementary and early middle school periods [22]. Cannabis is frequently among the first drugs of adolescent experimentation in the United States, among all demographics [19].

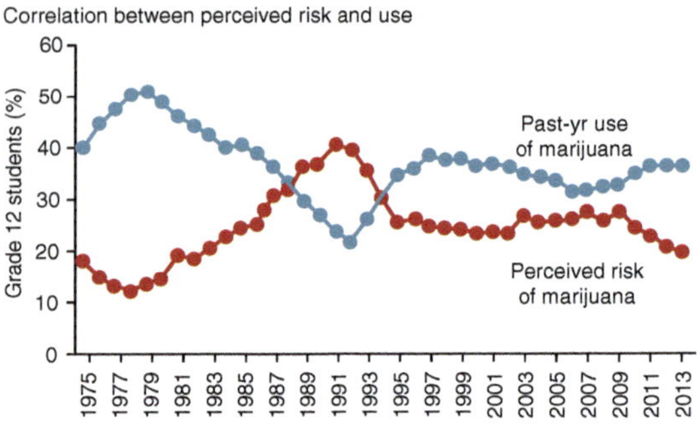

Fig. 32.1 Use of marijuana in relation to perceived risk among US students in grade 12, 1975–2013. There is inverse correlation between the perception of the risk associated with marijuana use and actual use [53]

Genetic and Physiological

Genetic factors are thought to influence the development of cannabis use disorders [1]. Heritable factors have been estimated to contribute between 30% and 80% of the total variance in risk, regarding cannabis disorders. Given the common environmental and genetic factors, shared between abusers of cannabis and other substances, there is likely a common genetic basis for conduct disorder and adolescent substance abuse.

Underage Cannabis Use in the Context of Other Substances

Lifetime use among American eighth graders (13–14-year-old cohort) includes alcohol (22.8%), electronic cigarettes (17.5%), cannabis (12.8%), tobacco cigarettes (9.8%), inhalants (7.7%), prescription amphetamines (5.7%), and prescription tranquilizers (3.0%) [34].

The Texas School Survey of Drug and Alcohol Use provides data for cohorts younger than age 12, grades 4–6. The Texas study reveals the lifetime use for the following drug categories within the fourth grader cohort: alcohol (12.7%), nicotine (2.8%), cannabis (0.8%), and inhalants (liquids, sprays, and gases that people sniff or inhale to get high) (11.1%). Among fourth graders, other drug categories were not evaluated. This survey also reveals that many fourth graders report that they never heard of cannabis (26.1%), inhalants (16%), nicotine (6%), and alcohol (3.6%). Given the lack of knowledge of many fourth graders and their lifetime use data, it can be hypothesized that many first initiate their use in late childhood (as young as 9), with increased incidence of usage into early adolescence [47].

According to the Monitoring the Future National Survey Results on Drug Use, 35.6% of 12th graders used cannabis within the past 12 months, ranking this drug as the second most commonly used [34]. There is an inverse correlation between the perception of the risk associated with marijuana use and actual use (Fig. 32.1) [53].

Animal Models of Early Cannabis Use

The dose-dependent toxicity of the main psychoactive component of cannabis, in brain regions rich in cannabinoid (CB1) receptors, is established in animal studies [28].

Healthy adult rats demonstrate enhanced binding of CB1 receptors within areas such as the prefrontal cortex (PFC) in comparison to juveniles. Researchers assessed ontogeny of CB1 receptor in adolescent and adult rats in vivo using positron emission tomography. These findings suggest that there is increased reliance on the cannabinoid system as an adolescent's brain develops [52]. Therefore regions undergoing maturation with CB1 receptors may be at increased risk for cannabis-induced alterations.

Using the rat model, cannabis use was associated with measurable brain changes. Cha et al. used male rats to illustrate that adolescent rats (postnatal age 30–32 days) were much more susceptible to cannabis exposure than adults (postnatal age 65–70 days), when exposed to delta9-tetrahydrocannabinol (THC). The effects of THC on male adolescent and adult rats in the Morris water maze were measured. Adolescent and adult rats were treated acutely with THC doses varying between 2.5 and 10 mg/kg or control vehicle while trained on the spatial version of the water. THC impaired both spatial and nonspatial learning more in adolescents more than in adults at all doses tested. The authors also mentioned that this chemically induced developmental sensitivity is analogous to the effects of ethanol [14].

In another study using the rats, Schneider and Koch concluded that chronic pubertal, but not adult chronic cannabinoid treatment impairs sensorimotor gating, recognition memory, and the performance in a progressive ratio task in adult rats. Adult and pubertal rats were exposed for 25 days to the synthetic cannabinoid agonist WIN 55,212-2 (1.2 mg/kg) or the control vehicle. The following endpoints were measured for each animal: object recognition memory, performance in a progressive ratio operant behavior task, locomotor activity, and prepulse inhibition of the acoustic startle response. Prepulse inhibition was significantly disrupted only by chronic peripubertal cannabinoid treatment. Interestingly, this long-lasting prepulse inhibition deficit was reversed by the medication haloperidol, a dopamine antagonist. Pubertal-treated rats also had lower break points in progressive ratio schedule. Adult rats exposed to the synthetic cannabinoids did not show any difference between controls. The study highlights the vulnerability of rats to cannabinoid agonists during puberty. The authors draw parallels to human disease. Since prepulse inhibition deficits, object recognition memory impairments, and anhedonia/avolition are among the endophenotypes of schizophrenia, they suggest that chronic cannabinoid administration during pubertal development may serve as an animal model for some aspects of schizophrenia [50].

Euphoria and reward processing involve amygdala and nucleus accumbens, observed in substance abuse models. Animal cannabis models have revealed that cannabinoid substances can alter the synaptic transmission of nucleus accumbens [38] and amygdala [5]. Rat model of THC exposure illustrates that structural abnormalities occur in the nucleus accumbens of THC-treated rats, similar to experiments which illustrated rat brain changes due to amphetamine exposure [35]. These findings suggest that cannabinoids promote dopamine activity in the mesolimbic dopamine system. Kolb et al. exposed rats to THC for 12 days, with either low dose (0.5 mg/kg) or escalating doses (0.5–4.0 mg/kg). Golgi-Cox staining was used to evaluate brain histology. All rats exposed to THC (regardless of dose) had increased length of the dendrites and increased number of dendritic branches in the shell of the nucleus accumbens in the medial prefrontal cortex, when compared with THC-naïve controls. Researchers did not appreciate the histological change in the hippocampus, striatum, orbital frontal cortex, parietal cortex, or occipital cortex, when comparing the two cohorts [35].

Human Evidence

Prenatal Cannabis Exposure

Cannabis consumption during pregnancy has been associated with gestational disorders such as preterm birth, intrauterine growth restriction, low birth weight, and increased risk of miscarriage [40]. However, the underlying biochemical mechanisms are not fully understood.

Garcia-Serra et al. revealed that only a small fraction of pregnant women using substances admitted their use. Of the 107 pregnant women evaluated, maternal hair analysis showed a 15.9% positivity for drugs of abuse (17 cases): 11 cannabis, 7 cocaine, 1 cannabis and ecstasy, and 1 cannabis and cocaine. Only one mother admitted to cannabis use and another one to cocaine use [25].

Cannabis and cigarettes are the most commonly used substances among pregnant women [43]. Early brain development is very susceptible to substances, even nicotine. The proposed mechanism for nicotine-related disruption of neurodevelopment is through the effects of acetylcholine. Jacobsen el at. evaluated white matter of adolescent smokers and nonsmokers with and without prenatal exposure to maternal smoking. Authors suggest that nicotine-induced disruption of the development of auditory corticofugal fibers may interfere with the ability of these fibers to modulate ascending auditory signals, leading to reduced efficiency of neurocircuitry that supports auditory processing [31].

Cannabis-induced neurobehavioral changes can be detected in newborns and persist into later stages of child development and adulthood. In utero cannabis exposure leads to impairments in specific functional domains including cognitive deficits, impairments in inhibitory control, impulsivity, hyperactivity, and increased risk of developing an addiction disorder later in life [16, 17, 43, 57] (Table 32.1).

THC concentrations in the fetus are lower than in mother [26]. Pregnant rhesus macaque monkeys were administered intravenous doses of 0.3 mg/kg THC, and fetal compartment distribution was measured. THC concentration peaked 15 minutes after maternal intravenous intake. Samples were analyzed for THC and a major metabolite, 11-nor-9-carboxy-THC, by radioimmunoassay. Fetal concentrations were 28% of the maternal measurements. THC half-life was greater in the fetal compartment, compared to the pregnant mother [6].

During early fetal development, the endocannabinoid system starts to develop, which is integrated with other neurotransmitter systems. Cannabis exposure during the prenatal period may cause changes in structures involved in the regulation of emotional systems and executive functions. Affected central nervous system regions, which have been implicated, include the mesolimbic system, prefrontal cortex, the hypothalamic-pituitary axis, and striatum [48].

Table 32.1 Summary of developmental effects associated with prenatal cannabis exposure in humans

Prenatal cannabis exposure	
Neonate	Tremors and exaggerated startle
9 months	Impaired mental development
3–4 years	Impaired short-term memory Impaired verbal, visual, abstract, and quantitative reasoning
6 years	Impaired sustained attention Increased impulsivity and hyperactivity
9–12 years	Impaired visual problem-solving and executive functioning Increased inattention, impulsivity, and hyperactivity
14–21 years	Increased risk for smoking and marijuana use

Used with permission from Samer Narouze, MD, PhD
Data compiled from Refs. [16, 17, 24, 43, 57]

The cannabinoid receptor one (CB1) is responsible for the effects of cannabis on motor and cognitive function in the CNS. Wang et al. used in situ hybridization to evaluate CB1 mRNA expression in normal human fetal (approximately 20 weeks of development) and adult brains. Fetal brains had distinct heterogeneous patterns of the CB1 mRNA expression in various regions. There was greater expression of the mRNA in the hippocampal cornu ammonis region and basal nuclear group of the amygdaloid complex. In the adult brain, the regions with positive gene expression were the same regions which were positive for CB1 mRNA in the fetal brain, such as the hippocampus. Additionally, the adult brain had greater gene expression in the cerebral cortex, caudate nucleus, putamen, and cerebellar cortex. The authors conclude that "the high CB1 mRNA expression in the fetal hippocampus and amygdala indicates that these limbic structures might be most vulnerable to prenatal cannabis exposure" [54].

In another study Wang et al. used in situ hybridization histochemistry to evaluate mRNA expression in mid-gestation (weeks 18–22) human fetal specimens. Pregnant women with evidence of cannabis use were compared to pregnant non-users (controls). Gene expressions for CB1 and dopamine receptor subtypes, D1 and D2, were evaluated. The targeted anatomic structures were striatum and mesocorticolimbic structures (amygdala and hippocampus). Fetuses of pregnant women who used cannabis had subsequent reduction of D2 mRNA expression in the amygdala basal nucleus. This effect was greater in male fetuses. The magnitude of this gene expression change was related to the amount of maternal cannabis intake during pregnancy. The authors state that "in utero cannabis exposure may impair distinct mesocorticolimbic neural systems that regulate emotional behavior" [55].

Maternal cannabis and alcohol exposure during pregnancy result in diminished opioid-related genes in the central nervous system. The mRNA expression for opioid peptide precursors preprodynorphin and preproenkephalin and opioid receptors (mu, kappa, and delta) were evaluated. Pregnant women who used cannabis had fetuses with increased mu receptor expression in the amygdala, reduced kappa receptor mRNA in mediodorsal thalamic nucleus, and reduced preproenkephalin expression in the caudal putamen. Alcohol use during pregnancy reduced kappa receptor mRNA in amygdala, claustrum, putamen, and insula cortex [56].

Prenatal cannabinoid exposure (PCE) can cause depression by decreasing serotonin levels while increasing dopamine levels. While cognitive impairment is mediated by an increase in norepinephrine and a decrease in glutamate level. On the other hand, locomotor impairment is mediated by changes in the GABA and glutamatergic systems (Fig. 32.2).

The relation of prenatal cannabis to brain morphology was evaluated by neuroimaging in children aged 6–8 years old. Prenatal cannabis exposure resulted in cortical thickness differences. Cannabis-exposed children in utero had thicker frontal cortexes, compared to controls. In utero maternal cannabis smoking resulted in cortical thinning of the superior frontal and superior parietal cortices [21].

The effects of prenatal marijuana exposure on delinquent behaviors are mediated by a decrease in neurocognitive functioning. A longitudinal study was performed by enrolling 580 pregnant women and monitoring the offspring for 14 years. Standardized methods (The Self Report Delinquency scale and Child Behavior checklist delinquency subscale) were used to measure outcomes, in addition to psychological, neurocognitive, social, environmental, and demographic characteristics. Women who used cannabis during pregnancy were significantly more likely to have children at age 10 with attention problems and clinical signs of depression. Consequently, child depressive symptoms and attention problems at age 10 significantly predicted delinquency at 14 years. At age 14, children of cannabis users during pregnancy (one or more joints per day) reported more delinquent behavior, odds ratio 1.76 (confidence interval 1.05–2.96) [17].

Three prospective longitudinal studies examining the effects of prenatal marijuana exposure and delinquent behaviors have been widely cited. The Ottawa Prenatal Prospective Study in the late 1970s enrolled 698 pregnant women.

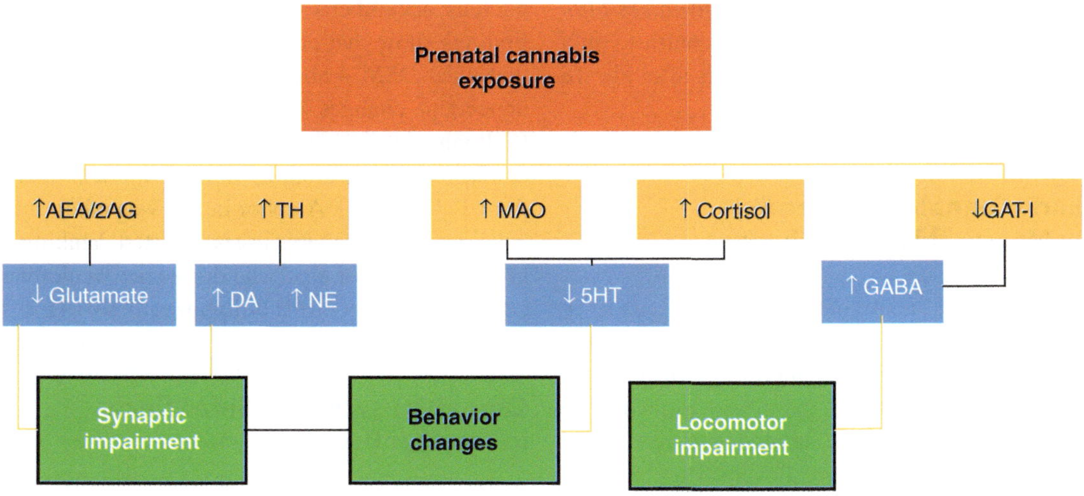

Fig. 32.2 Prenatal cannabinoid exposure (PCE) and possible neurotransmitter system changes. (Data compiled from Ref. [46]. 2-AG, arachidonyl glycerol; 5HT, serotonin; AEA, anandamide; DA, dopamine; NE, norepinephrine; GAT-1, GABA transporter type1; MAO, monoamine oxidase; TH, tyrosine hydroxylase. © Samer Narouze, MD, PhD, used with permission)

In 1982 Maternal Health Practices and Child Development Study in Pittsburgh enrolled 1360 women. The Generation R study in Rotterdam, the Netherlands, enrolled 9778 mothers, who delivered between 2002 and 2006. A summary of their findings is summarized in Table 32.1. Convergent findings link cannabis use during pregnancy to offspring behavioral issues [29].

Early-Onset Substance Use and Subsequent Substance Disorder

Adolescents are at great risk of substance use disorder (SUD) development with early substance exposure and use, making this age group particularly vulnerable and high risk [37].

Nicotine use disorder (NUD) is much more likely when children start using the substance regularly at age 10. Specifically, young female users are at greater risk of developing NUD, compared to other cohorts [36].

Adolescent alcohol use is associated with increased lifetime risk for developing an alcohol use disorder [41].

Likewise, early cannabis use is associated with an increased risk of developing cannabis use disorder (CUD): 11.5% of adults who used cannabis before age 14 developed the *Diagnostic and Statistical Manual of Mental Disorders Fifth Edition* (DSM-5) criteria for. In contrast, only 2.6% adults who first used cannabis after age 18 developed CUD [49].

Early Cannabis Use Results in Measurable Brain Changes

Since greater neuromaturation takes place at younger ages, the impact of cannabis on the brains of adolescents is more significant [28]. Zalesky et al. illustrated that heavy cannabis use resulted in impaired axonal connectivity in several regions of the corpus callosum. They revealed that the age of cannabis use onset impacted both radial and axial diffusivity. The severity of microstructural changes is correlated with earlier onset of cannabis use [58].

Cannabis use is quantitatively associated with nucleus accumbens and amygdala abnormalities in young adult recreational users (Gilman et al. 2014). There is great density of endogenous cannabinoid receptors (which bind to THC) located specifically in nucleus accumbens and amygdala [11]. The amygdala and nucleus accumbens are involved in reward processing. Euphoria associated with substance use involves these two structures. It has been established that the ventral tegmental area and the nucleus accumbens have critical roles in the processing of rewarding stimuli and consequently in drug addiction [38].

Gilman et al. evaluated right-handed young adult recreational cannabis users (versus controls) with high-resolution MRI. The authors specifically mentioned that "marijuana participants used marijuana at least once a week, but were not dependent, according a Structured Clinical Interview for the DSM-IV." Gray matter density, surface morphometry, and regional and total brain volumes were then measured. Young adult cannabis users had greater gray matter density in the left nucleus accumbens extending to subcallosal cortex, hypothalamus, sublenticular extended amygdala, and left amygdala. Dose-dependent volume changes were noted in left nucleus accumbens. Statistically significant shape differences were also detected in the left nucleus accumbens and right amygdala. These findings show that cannabis use, less than doses that meet DSM-4 abuse criteria, results in dose-dependent changes in neural reward structures (Gilman et al. 2014). This data is consistent with dendritic arborization in animal models mentioned above [35]. Alcohol intake was taken into consideration: cannabis users reported drinking a greater number of alcoholic drinks per week than cannabis-naïve controls (Gilman et al. 2014).

Cannabis Psychiatric Side Effects in Younger Users

Changes in energy levels affect stability, and eating habits are often observed with adolescent cannabis user. In this cohort dramatic decrease in academic performance, absenteeism, and decrease interest in school activities are often observed. These observations are likely due to acute intoxication and the subsequent coming-down effect. Actions taken by adolescents, in order to hide their cannabis usage, also result in behavior changes [39].

Cannabis usage before age 15 is a strong predictor for future cannabis abuse, risk of mental diseases, and abuse of other substances. These subsequent manifestations may be seen by early adulthood [23, 39].

Early cannabis use is associated with externalizing issues, such as conduct disorder. Adolescent use of marijuana is a predictor of internalizing problems, indicative that early use is an independent risk factor for the development of mental health disorders [18]. About a third of adolescents with cannabis use disorder have internalizing disorders (such as depression, anxiety, posttraumatic stress disorder), and about 60% have externalizing disorders (such as ADHD and conduct disorder) [3]. About 30% of bipolar patients also have current cannabis usage or dependence. Cannabis usage is related to earlier onset of first manic episode [7]. Cannabis usage during youth (adolescence) is correlated with greater prevalence of depression [13].

Marijuana smokers, ranging between 14 and 17 years old, are more impulsive. Dougherty et al. reported significantly higher Barratt Impulsiveness Scale scores in adolescent cannabis smokers relative to non-cannabis-smoking control subjects. 14–17-year-old subjects were evaluated on multiple cognitive and behavioral domains, including decision-making, attention, memory, and impulsivity. After controlling for performances across all measures, impaired short-term recall memory and consequence sensitivity impulsivity were associated with marijuana use. The authors conclude that their finding is consistent with previous observations that adolescent marijuana use is strongly associated with cognitive and behavioral impairments. They add that these specific performance deficits are potential therapeutic targets of intervention for vulnerable cohorts [20].

Cannabis is viewed as a "gateway" drug. Frequent cannabis users have a much higher lifetime probability of abusing other substances (such as cocaine and opioids), compared to non-users [19]. Cannabis use before age 17 is strongly correlated with substance use and the abuse of other illicit drugs use before age 18 [2]. Sixty-one percent of cannabis users below age 18 reported problematic use of other substances: alcohol (48%), cocaine (4%), methamphetamine (2%), and heroin/other opiates (2%) [3]. Adolescent medical cannabis users were approximately two times more likely to report the nonmedical use of prescription drugs and illicit substances, other than cannabis [10].

Adolescents and young adults who use multiple simultaneous substances have neurocognitive deficits above and beyond the impact of added single substances. Effects of multi-substance use are greater, when examining evidence of alcohol and nicotine, cannabis and nicotine, alcohol and cannabis, cannabis and methamphetamine, and alcohol and cocaine [37].

Early-Onset Cannabis Use Produces Greater Brain Morphologic Changes

Battistella et al. show gray matter changes, using voxel-based morphometry, in a group of regular cannabis smokers in comparison with a group of occasional smokers. The study shows that regular cannabis use is associated with gray matter volume reduction in the medial temporal cortex, temporal pole, parahippocampal gyrus, insula, and orbitofrontal cortex. These regions are associated with emotional, motivational, and affective processing, with ample cannabinoid CB1 receptors. Positive results correlated with the frequency of cannabis use. The magnitude of gray matter volume reductions correlated with either heavy use or adolescent onset use. In adolescent-onset cannabis subjects, significant gray matter volume reduction was observed, even if the current intake levels were classified as recreational (in distinction with heavy) use. The authors concluded that adolescent cannabis use affects developmental ontogenic processes, which are significant and long lasting [8].

Researchers have postulated that early cannabis use results in alterations in synaptic connections, leading to poorer cognitive functioning. Shollenbargera et al. examined the relationships between cannabis use and prefrontal cortex (PFC) and inferior parietal gyrification in subjects between 18 and 25 years old, divided into cannabis users and controls. (As previously mentioned, many in this cohort started during adolescence.) Those with comorbid psychiatric/neurologic disorders and other drug use were excluded. Cannabis use was correlated with decreased gyrification in ventral-medial prefrontal cortex, medial prefrontal cortex, and frontal poles. Significant differences were not found in hemispheric or inferior parietal local gyrification index, suggesting that aberrant gyrification may be localized to specific PFC regions in emerging adults. Cannabis use was associated with slightly decreased surface area in medial and ventral lateral prefrontal cortexes. The authors concluded that their findings have cognitive implications, since they found an association between cannabis use and reduced gyrification in regions associated with self-referential thought and social cognition [51].

Gruber et al. examined the relationship between age of onset of cannabis use, white matter microstructure, and reported impulsivity in chronic heavy cannabis smokers. Cannabis users had significantly greater self-reported impulsivity scores, compared to healthy controls. The Barratt Impulsiveness Scale (BIS) was used to quantify impulsivity tendencies. Each of the three BIS subscores and the total score reached statistical significance: attention ($t(41) = 1.89$, $p = 0.03$), motor ($t(41) = 1.91$, $p = 0.03$), non-planning ($t(41) = 1.92, p = 0.03$), and total impulsivity ($t(41) = 2.28, p = 0.01$) [28].

Early-onset cannabis users consume more cannabis, compared to later-onset users. Younger-onset cannabis smokers versus those who started older smoked more often (smokes/week; 18.76 vs. 15.51) and more than twice as much marijuana per week (grams/week; 14.65 vs. 6.66) [28].

There is a relationship between fractional anisotropy changes and behavioral impulsivity in cannabis smokers, especially in subjects who started before age 16. Cannabis users had significantly reduced fractional anisotropy in both left and right genu of the corpus callosum with statistically significantly higher Barratt Impulsiveness Scale scores, compared to non-user controls. This relationship was stronger among cannabis users who started before turning 16 years old, compared to those who started using cannabis after becoming 16 years old. A strong association was revealed between the cannabis onset age and fractional anisotropy in both the left and right genu, implicating cannabis as a cause for lower white matter fiber integrity in the anatomical areas. The authors postulate that the findings are due to alterations in cannabinoid receptors, disrupting normal adolescent white matter development [28]. This pre-16-year-old use cohort has demonstrated limited ability to inhibit inappropriate responses during cognitive assessments [27].

The pathophysiology of increased impulsivity may be alterations in the crossing of fibers through the genu [28]. These fibers connect the left and right dorsolateral prefrontal cortex, which have strong interconnections to the anterior cingulate cortex [44, 45]. Dorsolateral prefrontal cortex and anterior cingulate cortex are components of the cingulo-fronto-parietal cognitive attention network, which have roles in executive control, inhibition, attention, and feedback-based decision-making [12]. This study's limitation includes the concurrent use of tobacco by some subjects [28].

Human Study Limitations: Subjects Using Multiple Substances

Identification of early-onset cannabis side effects are challenging, due to study design limitations. Many studies are observational, not accounting for co-use of substances, which have unique impacts, potentially modifying outcomes. Lack of adequate control subjects also influences the strength of cannabis studies. Mostly cross-sectional studies do not allow for temporal conclusions, regarding cannabis exposure followed by neurocognitive findings. Many studies do not measure the potency of the cannabis products used by the subjects. Often unaccounted for is the strain of plant or type of cannabis products, tetrahydrocannabinol (THC) or cannabidiol (CBD) [37].

Many factors can impact findings, including total exposure (quantity/frequency), potency and content, route of administration, outcomes such as hangover symptoms, and co-use of substances. ABCD Substance Use module assesses the wide variety of available substances in society from OTC cough/cold medicines, caffeine, anabolic steroids, and tobacco products to various inhalants and various illicit substances. Regarding cannabis, researchers should account for the different variables associated with its usage: route of administration (smoked versus ingested versus inhaled), concentration, potency, synthetic cannabinoids, cannabis tinctures, cannabis-infused alcohol, and edible cannabis [37].

Brain changes noted in users of both cannabis and alcohol are complex. Altered white matter microstructure in adolescents was identified in alcohol and cannabis-using teenagers, compared with controls. Inferior frontal and temporal areas decrease in fractional anisotropy [9]. Jacous et al. compared adolescents who used cannabis and participated in binge-drinking and those who did not use cannabis and participated in binge-drinking. Binge-drinkers who used cannabis had higher fractional anisotropy values, which revealed some cannabis-related protection. This finding may have been due to cannabis functioning as a substitute for alcohol at times, further reducing the negative impact of alcohol-related oxidative stress [32].

References

1. Agrawal A, Lynskey MT. Candidate genes for cannabis use disorders: findings, challenges and directions. Addiction. 2009;104(4):518–32.
2. Agrawal A, Neale MC, Prescott CA, Kendler KS. A twin study of early cannabis use and subsequent use and abuse/dependence of other illicit drugs. Psychol Med. 2004;34:1227–37.
3. American Psychiatric Association. Diagnostic and statistical manual of mental disorders: DSM-5. 5th ed. Arlington: American Psychiatric Association; 2013.
4. Anthony JC. The epidemiology of cannabis dependence. In: Roffman RA, Stephens RS, editors. Cannnabis dependence: its nature, consequences and treatment. Cambridge: Cambridge University Press; 2006. p. 58–95.
5. Azad SC, Monory K, Marsicano G, Cravatt BF, Lutz B, Zieglgänsberger W, Rammes G. Circuitry for associative plasticity in the amygdala involves endocannabinoid signaling. J Neurosci. 2004;24:9953–61.
6. Bailey JR, Cunny HC, Paule MG, Slikker W. Fetal disposition of Δ9-tetrahydrocannabinol (THC) during late pregnancy in the rhesus monkey. Toxicol Appl Pharmacol. 1987;90(2):315–21.
7. Balley N, Zullino D, Aubry JM. Cannabis use and first manic episode. J Affect Disord. 2014;165:103–8.
8. Battistella G, Fornari E, Annoni JM, Chtioui H, Dao K, Fabritius M, Favrat B, Mall JF, Maeder P, Giroud C. Long-term effects of cannabis on brain structure. Neuropsychopharmacology. 2014;39:2041–8.
9. Bava S, Frank R, McQueeny T, Schweinsburg BC, Schweinsburg AD, Tapert SF. Altered white matter microstructure in adolescent substance abusers. Psychiatry Res. 2009;173:228–37.
10. Boyd CJ, Veliz PT, McCabe SE. Adolescents' use of medical marijuana: a secondary analysis of monitoring the future data. J Adolesc Health. 2015;57:241–4.
11. Burns HD, Van Laere K, Sanabria-Bohorquez S, Hamill TG, Bormans G, Eng WS, Gibson R, Ryan C, Connolly B, Patel S, Krause S, Vanko A, Van Hecken A, Dupont P, DeLepeleire I, Rothenberg P, Stoch SA, Cote J, Hagmann WK, Jewell JP, et al. [18F] MK-9470, a positron emission tomography (PET) tracer for in vivo human PET brain imaging of the cannabinoid-1 receptor. Proc Natl Acad Sci USA. 2007;104:9800–5.
12. Bush G, Spencer TJ, Holmes J, Shin LM, Valera EM, Seidman MN, Surman C, Aleardi M, Mick E, Biederman J. Functional magnetic resonance imaging of methylphenidate and placebo in attention-deficit/hyperactivity disorder during the multi source interference task. Arch Gen Psychiatry. 2008;65:102–14.
13. Cairns KE, Yap MBH, Pilkington PD, Jorn AF. Risk and protective factors for depression that adolescents can modify: a systematic review and meta-analysis of longitudinal studies. J Affect Disord. 2014;169:61–75.
14. Cha YM, White AM, Kuhn CM, Wilson WA, Swartzwelder HS. Differential effects of delta9-THC on learning in adolescent andadult rats. Pharmacol Biochem Behav. 2006;83:448–55.
15. Compton WM, Grant BF, Colliver JD, Glantz MD, Stinson FS. Prevalence of marijuana use disorders in the United States: 1991–1992 and 2001–2002. JAMA. 2004;291(17):2114–21.
16. Day NL, Goldschmidt L, Thomas CA. Prenatal marijuana exposure contributes to the prediction of marijuana use at age 14. Addiction. 2006;101(9):1313–22.
17. Day NL, Leech SL, Goldschmidt L. The effects of prenatal marijuana exposure on delinquent behaviors are mediated by measures of neurocognitive functioning. Neurotoxicol Teratol. 2011;33(1):129–36.
18. de Graaf R, Radovanovic M, van Laar M, Fairman B, Degenhardt L, Aguilar-Gaxiola S, Bruffaerts

R, de Girolamo G, Fayyad J, Gureje O, Haro JM, Huang Y, Kostychenko S, Lépine JP, Matschinger H, Mora ME, Neumark Y, Ormel J, Posada-Villa J, Stein DJ, Tachimori H, Wells JE, Anthony JC. Early cannabis use and estimated risk of later onset of depression spells: epidemiologic evidence from the population-based World Health Organization World Mental Health Survey Initiative. Am J Epidemiol. 2010;172(2):149–59.
19. Degenhardt L, Dierker L, Chiu WT, Medina-Mora ME, Neumark Y, Sampson N, Alonso J, Angermeyer M, Anthony JC, Bruffaerts R, de Girolamo G, de Graaf R, Gureje O, Karam AN, Kostyuchenko S, Lee S, Lépine JP, Levinson D, Nakamura Y, Posada-Villa J, Stein D, Wells JE, Kessler RC. Evaluating the drug use "gateway" theory using cross-national data: consistency and associations of the order of initiation of drug use among participants in the WHO World Mental Health Surveys. Drug Alcohol Depend. 2010;108(1–2):84–97.
20. Dougherty DM, Mathias CW, Dawes MA, Furr RM, Charles NE, Liguori A, Shannon EE, Acheson A. Impulsivity, attention, memory, and decision-making among adolescent marijuana users. Psychopharmacology. 2013;226:207–319.
21. El Marroun H, Tiemeier H, Franken IH, Jaddoe VW, van der Lugt A, Verhulst FC, et al. Prenatal cannabis and Tobacco exposure in relation to brain morphology: a prospective neuroimaging study in young children. Biol Psychiatry. 2016;79(12):971–9.
22. Feldstein-Ewing SW, Filbey FM, Loughran TA, Chassin L, Piquero AR. Which matters most? Demographic, neuropsychological, personality, and situational factors in long-term marijuana and alcohol trajectories for justice-involved male youth. Psychol Addict Behav. 2015;29:603–12.
23. Fergusson DM, Boden JM, Horwood LJ. Cannabis use and other illicit drug use: testing the cannabis gateway hypothesis. Addiction. 2006;101(4):556–69.
24. Fried P, Watkinson B, James D, Gray R. Current and former marijuana use: preliminary findings of a longitudinal study of effects on IQ in young adults. CMAJ. 2002;166(7):887–9.
25. Garcia-Serra J, Ramis J, Simo S, Joya X, Pichini S, Vall O, Garcia-Algar O. Matrices biológicas alternativas para detectar la exposición prenatal a drogas de abuso en el tercer trimestre de la gestación (Alternative biological materials to detect prenatal exposure to drugs of abuse in the third trimester of pregnancy). Anales de Pediatría. 2012;77(5):323–8.
26. Grant KS, Petroff R, Isoherranen N, Stella N, Burbacher TM. Cannabis use during pregnancy: pharmacokinetics and effects on child development. Pharmacol Ther. 2018;182:133–51.
27. Gruber SA, Dahlgren MK, Sagar KA, Gonenc A, Killgore WDS. Age of onset of marijuana use impacts inhibitory processing. Neurosci Lett. 2012;511:89–94.
28. Gruber SA, Dahlgren MK, Sagar KA, Gonenc A, Lukas SE. Worth the wait: effects of age of onset of marijuana use on white matter and impulsivity. Psychopharmacology. 2014;231:1455–65.
29. Huizink AC. Prenatal cannabis exposure and infant outcomes: overview of studies. Prog Neuropsychopharmacol Biol Psychiatry. 2014;52:45–52.
30. Iacono WG, Malone SM, McGue M. Behavioral disinhibition and the development of early-onset addiction: common and specific influences. Annu Rev Clin Psychol. 2008;4:325–48.
31. Jacobsen LK, Picciotto MR, Heath CJ, Frost SJ, Tsou KA, Dwan RA, Jackowski MP, Constable RT, Mencl WE. Prenatal and adolescent exposure to tobacco smoke modulates the development of white matter microstructure. J Neurosci. 2007;27:13491–8.
32. Jacobus J, McQueeny T, Bava S, Schweinsburg BC, Frank LR, Yang TT, Tapert SF. White matter integrity in adolescents with histories of marijuana use and binge drinking. Neurotoxicol Teratol. 2009;31:349–55.
33. Johnston LD, Miech RA, O'Malley PM, Bachman JG, Schulenberg JE, Patrick ME. Monitoring the Future National Survey Results on Drug Use, 1975-2020. 2020 Overview, Key Findings on Adolescent Drug Use. Institute for Social Research, The University of Michigan, Ann Arbor, MI. 2021.
34. Johnston LD, O'Malley PM, Miech RA, Bachman JG, Schulenberg JE. Monitoring the future national survey results on drug use, 1975–2016: overview, key findings on adolescent drug use. Ann Arbor: Institute for Social Research, The University of Michigan; 2017.
35. Kolb B, Gorny G, Limebeer CL, Parker LA. Chronic treatment with delta-9 tetrahydrocannabinol alters the structure of neurons in the nucleus accumbens shell and medial prefrontal cortex of rats. Synapse. 2006;60:429–36.
36. Lanza ST, Vasilenko SA. New methods shed light on age of onset as a risk factor for nicotine dependence. Addict Behav. 2015;50:161–4.
37. Lisdahl KM, Sher KJ, Conway KP, Gonzalez R, Feldstein Ewing SW, Nixon SJ, Tapert S, Bartsch H, Goldstein RZ, Heitzeg M. Adolescent brain cognitive development (ABCD) study: overview of substance use assessment methods. Dev Cogn Neurosci. 2018;32:80–96.
38. Lupica CR, Riegel AC, Hoffman AF. Marijuana and cannabinoid regulation of brain reward circuits. Br J Pharmacol. 2004;143:227–34.
39. Lynskey MT, Heath AC, Bucholz KK, Slutske WS, Madden PA, Nelson EC, Statham DJ, Martin NG. Escalation of drug use in early-onset cannabis users vs co-twin controls. JAMA. 2003;289(4):427–33.
40. Maia J, Midão L, Cunha SC, Almada M, Fonseca BM, Braga J, Gonçalves D, Teixeira N, Correia-da-Silva G. Effects of cannabis tetrahydrocannabinol on endo-

cannabinoid homeostasis in human placenta. Arch Toxicol. 2019;93:649–58.
41. Marshall EJ. Adolescent alcohol use: risks and consequences. Alcohol Alcohol. 2014;49(2):160–4.
42. Monti PM, Miranda R, Nixon K, Sher KJ, Swartzwelder HS, Tapert SF, White A, Crews FT. Adolescence: booze, brains and behavior. Alcohol Clin Exp Res. 2005;29:207–20.
43. Morris CV, DiNieri JA, Szutorisz H, Hurd YL. Molecular mechanisms of maternal cannabis and cigarette use on human neurodevelopment. Eur J Neurosci. 2011;34(10):1574–83.
44. Pandya DN, Seltzer B. Intrinsic connections and architectonics of posterior parietal cortex in the rhesus monkey. J Comp Neurol. 1982;204:196–210.
45. Park JH, Kim JJ, Lee SK, Seok JH, Chun J, Kim DI, Lee JD. Corpus callosal connection mapping using cortical gray matter parcellation and DT-MRI. Hum Brain Mapp. 2008;29:503–16.
46. Pinky PD, Bloemer J, Smith WD, Moore T, Hong H, Suppiramaniam V, Reed MN. Prenatal cannabinoid exposure and altered neurotransmission. Neuropharmacology. 2019;149:181–94.
47. Public Policy Research Institute. Texas school survey of drug and alcohol use: 2012. State: grades 4–6. College Station: Texas A&M University; 2012.
48. Roncero C, Valriberas-Herrero I, Mezzatesta-Gava M, Villegas JL, Aguilar L, Grau-López L. Cannabis use during pregnancy and its relationship with fetal developmental outcomes and psychiatric disorders. A systematic review. Reprod Health. 2020;17:25.
49. SAMHSA. National Survey on Drug Use and Health (NSDUH). Table 5.5A—Substance dependence or abuse in the past year among persons aged 12–17, by Demographic Characteristics: Numbers in Thousands, 2012 and 2013. 2013.
50. Schneider M, Koch M. Chronic pubertal, but not adult chronic cannabinoid treatment impairs sensorimotor gating, recognition memory, and the performance in a progressive ratio task in adult rats. Neuropsychopharmacology. 2003;28:1760–9.
51. Shollenbargera SG, Priceb J, Wiesera J, Lisdahl K. Reduced gyrification is correlated with poorer working memory. Dev Cogn Neurosci. 2015;16:46–53.
52. Verdurand M, Nguyen V, Stark D, Zahara D, Gregoire MC, Greguric I, Zavitsanou K. Comparison of cannabinoid CB1 receptor binding in adolescent and adult rats: a positron emission tomography study using [18F] MK-9470. Int J Mol Imaging. 2011;2011:548123. https://doi.org/10.1155/2011/548123.
53. Volkow ND, Baler RD, Compton WM, Weiss SRB. Adverse health effects of marijuana use. N Engl J Med. 2014;370:2219–27.
54. Wang X, Dow-Edwards D, Keller E, Hurd YL. Preferential limbic expression of the cannabinoid receptor mRNA in the human fetal brain. Neuroscience. 2003;118(3):681–94.
55. Wang X, Dow-Edwards D, Anderson V, Minkoff H, Hurd YL. In utero marijuana exposure associated with abnormal amygdala dopamine D2 gene expression in the human fetus. Biol Psychiatry. 2004;56(12):909–15.
56. Wang X, Dow-Edwards D, Anderson V, Minkoff H, Hurd YL. Discrete opioid gene expression impairment in the human fetal brain associated with maternal marijuana use. Pharm J. 2006;6(4):255–64.
57. Willford JA, Chandler LS, Goldschmidt L, Day NL. Effects of prenatal tobacco, alcohol and marijuana exposure on processing speed, visual-motor coordination, and interhemispheric transfer. Neurotoxicol Teratol. 2010;32:580–8.
58. Zalesky A, Solowij N, Yucel M, Lubman DI, Takagi M, Harding IH, Lorenzetti V, Wang R, Searle K, Pantelis C, Seal M. Effect of long-term cannabis use on axonal fibre connectivity. Brain. 2012;135:2245–55.

33 Cannabinoids and Mental Health Risks

Caroline A. MacCallum, Lauren de Freitas, and Shaohua Lu

Introduction

The relationship between cannabis and mental health is a highly debated and complex topic. While directionality between associations has yet to be determined, there does appear to be an association. Though there is evidence that in some individuals cannabis use may result in adverse mental health outcomes, there is also evidence to support the opposite, with cannabis being shown as beneficial for some conditions. An additional layer of complexity comes from differences between recreational and medical users. Intentions and patterns of use are inherently different between the two populations. As such, so are certain risks and considerations. To date, a large portion of the literature is from recreational studies. Translations to medical populations should be made with caution. Cannabis Recommending Clinicians (CRC) should be aware of both risks and potential benefits for cannabis and mental health.

Cannabis and Risk of Psychosis

One of the primary concerns resulting from the use of cannabis is risk of psychosis. The relationship between cannabis and psychosis is complex. Important considerations regarding cannabis use patterns, risk of precipitation or relapse of a psychotic illness, and the risk of exacerbation of residual psychosis are still not thoroughly understood, particularly for medical populations. These must be acknowledged when interpreting the evidence around psychosis risk and cannabis. Careful attention should be paid to how well evidence coming from recreational populations may transfer to medical populations.

In the stress-diathesis model of disease, psychiatric illness develops due to the intersection of one's genetic, biological, psychological, social vulnerabilities, and liabilities. The risk of developing or aggravating psychosis from cannabis use is dependent on the burden of biopsychosocial vulnerabilities and the presence of internal and external stressors.

The risk of initiation of a de novo psychotic episode or the development of a new psychotic

C. A. MacCallum (✉)
Department of Medicine, Faculty of Medicine, University of British Columbia, Vancouver, BC, Canada
e-mail: info@drcarolinemaccallum.com

L. de Freitas
Centre for Addiction and Mental Health, Toronto, ON, Canada

S. Lu
Department of Psychiatry, Faculty of Medicine, University of British Columbia, Vancouver, BC, Canada

S. N. Narouze (ed.), *Cannabinoids and Pain*, https://doi.org/10.1007/978-3-030-69186-8_33

illness in individuals without underlying risk factors or genetic predisposition appears to be low. Much of the literature pointing to increased psychosis comes from recreational cannabis users; who use higher THC doses, frequently used in adolescence, and have risk factors and/or a genetic predisposition to psychosis. The risk of cannabis and a psychosis relapse in those with previously stable psychosis, as well as the exacerbation of residual psychosis (in those with persistent psychotic illness), is less clear. Both of these groups may have other concurrent disorders or symptoms clusters including anxiety, depression, PTSD, insomnia, or pain, which may lead to self-medication with cannabis. Clinical observation and case reports show that for some patients, the use of cannabis may lead to reduced psychological distress from the burden of their psychotic illness. This reduction in psychological distress may be due to the alleviation of these secondary symptoms. It is therefore reasonable to balance the overall risks and benefits of cannabis use to patients with psychosis on a case-by-case basis. It is important to note that the risk of psychosis is related to THC dose. When weighing risks and benefits, the patterns of use must be taken into account.

It is important to distinguish cannabis intoxication-related perceptual disturbance from psychotic illness, which has functional implications. Psychotic illness in this context is defined in a broad sense, including schizophrenia and other psychotic-related illnesses. Brief psychosis and chronic psychotic illness may have different risk factors that are not well delineated. Bipolar affective disorders may have similar risk patterns, and therefore the above comments on psychosis may be applicable to bipolar affective conditions.

The National Academies of Sciences' comprehensive review in 2017 concluded that increased levels of cannabis use were associated with an increased risk of developing psychosis. This risk is further increased with genetic vulnerabilities, experiences of childhood trauma/maltreatment or early stressors in life, and early age of initiation and regular use, making some individuals more vulnerable to the effects of cannabis than others [1–3].

Genetic predisposition may account for 69–84% of the link between cannabis and psychosis [4]. A meta-analysis examining 30 studies of healthy controls compared to those at ultra-high risk (UHR) of psychosis revealed that not only did UHR individuals have increased rates of cannabis use and cannabis use disorder (CUD), but they also had increased positive symptomatology such as paranoia and unusual thought content compared to controls [5]. Twin studies also reveal heritability estimates for CUD ranging from 51% to 70%, with strong expression of a particular trait locus variant for cholinergic receptor nicotinic α2 subunit (CHRNA2) associated with increased risk of CUD, worsening cognitive performance, increased risk of schizophrenia, and attention deficit hyperactivity disorder (ADHD) [6]. Presence of a single nucleotide polymorphism in the AKT1 genotype or a catechol-O-methyl transferase (COMT) gene with a valine-to-methionine (Val/Met) polymorphism has been implicated in the development of psychosis and risk for cannabis-induced psychosis especially when use commences in adolescence [7, 8].

Among individuals with current psychosis and/or bipolar disorders, acute THC administration increases suspiciousness, perceptual disorganization, and paranoia compared to individuals without psychosis or bipolar disorder [9]. Ongoing recreational cannabis use in this population has been found to lead to an exacerbation of symptoms (including an increased number of episodes), decreased adherence to medications (including a reduced treatment response), and an overall poorer prognosis, especially with frequent, high-potent cannabis use [8]. Individuals with schizophrenia who were former frequent users of cannabis were significantly less likely to have a relapse in psychosis compared to those with schizophrenia currently using high-potent chemovars [10]. Moreover, benefits were observed among those using cannabis in smaller doses of less potency taken less often (less than monthly) [10]. High-potency chemovars may be preferred by patients with psychotic disorders in an attempt to control symptoms. In cannabis-using patients with schizophrenia, many reported the effects produced from high potency CBD and low potency THC chemovars were too short and weak.

Table 33.1 Risk factors for psychosis with recreational cannabis use

Genetic vulnerability/family history of psychosis; personal history of mental health illness [4–10]
Childhood traumas/maltreatment; early stressors in life [1–3]
Frequent (daily/near-daily), chronic, heavy use (amount used each time) [4, 8, 11–13]
High-potent use (high THC concentrations) [11, 14–17]
Use of cannabis in adolescence (see Chap. 34 on Cannabinoids and Adolescence) [18]
Continued use after experiencing a psychotic episode [1, 8]
Route of administration [19–21]
Intent of use
Combination of any of the above factors increases this risk further [1, 3, 8]

THC may precipitate psychosis in certain individuals with risk factors and high-risk patterns of use. However, the majority of medical cannabis users do not experience psychosis/schizophrenia. This is most likely, at least in part, due to intent of use and use patterns that favor less potent THC chemovars and lower overall quantities used. It remains important to understand the risk factors and prevalence of psychotic-like experiences and psychosis among the general population. Specifically, heavy and daily use of cannabis, combined with an early onset of use, personal/family history of psychosis, and continued use after experiencing a psychotic episode, can pose an increased risk for the onset of psychosis (Table 33.1).

In summary, it appears that the majority of new cases of psychosis involving cannabis use among those with psychosis risk factors including genetic predisposition. The risk of cannabis and its potential influence on the clinical course for either psychosis relapse or residual psychosis exacerbation is not clear from the literature, and likely varies on a case-by-case basis. CBD does not appear to pose the same inherent risk as THC and should be considered as a separate treatment option; it may be used as an adjuvant in the management of treatment-resistant psychosis. It is important for future research to clarify the distinction between association and causation between cannabis use and psychosis.

Cannabis Use Disorder (CUD)

Cannabis misuse can lead to clinically significant impairment or distress, known as cannabis use disorder (see Chap. 38 on Cannabis Use Disorder). Some clinical features of CUD include difficulty reducing use; expressions of concern from social networks; demanding prescriptions; poor work, school, and/or social functioning; mood, anxiety, or psychotic symptoms; other substance abuse; interference with completion of productive activities; and experiences of withdrawal symptoms (e.g., anxiety, fatigue). CUD is typically more prevalent among recreational users than medical users for a variety of reasons, including clinician monitoring, standardization of doses and products, etc.

It is important to screen for risk of CUD using validated questionnaires such as the Cannabis Use Disorder Identification Test-Revised (CUDIT-R) [22] or a modified Opioid Risk Tool (ORT) [23]. Only the CUDIT-R is specific to cannabis; however, the ORT highlights a number of important considerations for risk of opioid addiction which are relevant and similar to the risk for cannabis addiction. Each test has limitations that clinicians should be familiar with. For example, most medical cannabis patients use cannabis as medicine on a daily basis for their chronic condition(s). Good clinical judgment should be applied when scoring the CUDIT-R, in particular for medical patients, as they would receive an additional 4 points for using cannabis "4 or more times a week." Some risk factors for CUD include premorbid depression, current substance use (tobacco, alcohol, and/or illicit substances), childhood traumas, low socioeconomic status, and an early age of initiation of use. Interestingly, many of these same risk factors overlap with those for risk of psychosis with recreational cannabis.

Behavioral factors such as chronic use that is intensive (daily or near daily) are associated with worsening mental health trajectories. A more severe CUD diagnosis (out of mild, moderate, severe) is more strongly associated with mood and anxiety disorders compared to milder diagnoses [24]. Individuals with mood and anxiety disorders are more likely to engage in behaviors that contribute to this risk, such as using high-potency cannabis in an effort to mitigate their negative symptoms [25, 26]. However, high-potency cannabis use among this population can exacerbate symptoms of depression [27, 28] and anxiety [29–31], with doses as low as 5 mg of THC eliciting anxiogenic responses [32].

Like cannabis and psychosis, genetic predisposition may account for the association between cannabis and anxiety. Individuals with a short allele in the 5-HTLPR gene experience greater anxiety when using cannabis, particularly upon frequent, high-potency use [8]. Regular recreational cannabis users were found to experience a greater prevalence of current mental health distress compared to less frequent users (10.1% vs. 18.4%), and a greater incidence of a prior diagnosis of depression (18.4% vs. 29.9%) [31].

Cannabis Withdrawal Syndrome

Cannabis withdrawal syndrome (CWS) can lead to a variety of symptoms. CWS can develop between one and seven days post-cessation of use, and can last up to 28 days [33]. Cannabis withdrawal has been proposed to contribute to continued recreational cannabis use [34] and likely contribute to the development of addiction.

Cannabis withdrawal may produce irritability, nervousness/restlessness, low mood, reduced appetite, chills, and insomnia. CWS is not commonly seen in the medical population, especially in patients using chemovars with higher CBD content. Although there is some evidence for withdrawal among recreational populations, it is rarely serious enough to require medical intervention, [35] and typically is not observed frequently overall among individuals who use cannabis. Only one-third of recreational cannabis users in the general population experience withdrawal symptoms compared to 50–95% of heavy users in institutional or research settings [36]. Medical cannabis patients consume less than 2.5 g/day on average [37]. Clinically, CWS is not seen in patients staying within this appropriate medical cannabis dosing range, as symptoms are dose-dependently related to THC, and may not apply in the context of CBD. If withdrawal is responsible for symptomatology, physicians can alter dosing and cannabinoid composition to manage or treat these symptoms of anxiety [33]. For example, in patients consuming > 3–5 grams/day of dried flower, some clinicians may suggest a dose increase of CBD (usually in the form of oil) in order to facilitate THC dose reduction, or ultimately (where possible), a THC "washout" as a means of harm reduction. It has been observed in the author's clinical practice that a THC washout for at least five to seven days (ideally one to two weeks, but this is frequently not possible in these individuals) may be sufficient to serve as a "THC reset". After this intervention, these patients will commonly behave as if they were THC naive. If/when they restart THC (oil is preferred over inhaled for more consistent symptom control and to reduce the risk of euphoria), they have been observed to benefit from much lower doses of THC. These lower THC doses may be maintained over time without need for escalation (especially in combination with CBD oil). These patients are best cared for by physicians with the required cannabis expertise to manage the troubleshooting and complexities of these cases.

Other DSM-5 Cannabis-Induced Mental Health Disorders

Cannabis-Induced Psychotic Disorder [38, 39]

A. Presence of delusions or hallucinations.
B. Evidence from the history, physical examination, or laboratory findings of either one of the following:
   1. The symptoms in the first criterion developed during or soon after cannabis intoxication or withdrawal.
   2. The disturbance is not accounted for by a psychotic disorder that is not substance induced.
C. Evidence that the symptoms are accounted for by a psychotic disorder that is not substance induced might include the following:
   1. The symptoms precede the onset of substance use (or medication use).

2. The symptoms persist for a substantial period (e.g., about a month) after the cessation of acute withdrawal or severe intoxication, or are substantially more than what would be expected, given the type or amount of the substance used or the duration of use.
3. Other evidence suggests the existence of an independent non-substance-induced psychotic disorder (e.g., a history of recurrent non-substance-related episodes).
4. The disturbance does not occur exclusively during delirium.
5. The disturbance causes clinically significant distress or impairment in social, occupational, or other areas of functioning.

Cannabis-Induced Anxiety Disorder [38, 39]

A. Panic attacks or anxiety predominate in the clinical picture.
B. Evidence from the history, physical examination, or laboratory findings of either of the following:
   1. The symptoms in the first criterion developed during or soon after substance intoxication or withdrawal.
   2. The disturbance is not better accounted for by an anxiety disorder that is not substance induced. Evidence that the symptoms are better accounted for by an anxiety disorder that is not substance induced might include the following:
   3. The symptoms precede the onset of substance use.
   4. The symptoms persist for a substantial period (e.g., about a month) after cessation of acute withdrawal or severe intoxication or are substantially more than expected given the type or amount of the substance used or the duration of use.
   5. Other evidence suggests the existence of an independent non-substance-induced anxiety disorder (e.g., a history of recurrent non-substance-related episodes).
   6. The disturbance does not occur exclusively during delirium.
   7. The disturbance causes clinically significant distress or impairment in social, occupational, or other important areas of functioning.

Cannabis-Induced Sleep Disorder [38, 39]

A. A prominent and severe disturbance in sleep.
B. There is evidence from the history, physical examination, or laboratory findings of both of the following:
   1. The symptoms in the first criterion developed during or soon after cannabis intoxication or after withdrawal from or exposure to it.
   2. The disturbance is not better explained by a sleep disorder that is not substance/medication induced. Such evidence of an independent sleep disorder could include that:
   3. The symptoms precede the onset of cannabis use.
   4. The symptoms persist for a substantial period (i.e., about a month) after the cessation of acute withdrawal or severe intoxication.
   5. There is other evidence suggesting the existence of an independent non-substance-/medication-induced sleep disorder (i.e., a history of recurrent non-substance-/medication-related episodes).
   6. The disturbance does not occur exclusively during delirium.
   7. The disturbance causes clinically significant distress or impairment in social, occupational, or other important areas of functioning.

Efficacy of Cannabis for Mental Health

Anxiety and Depression

A recent systematic review and meta-analysis determined that pain symptoms (64%), anxiety (50%), and depression/mood (34%) were common reasons for medical cannabis use [40]. In a separate review, relaxation and anxiety relief were found to be the two most widely reported reasons for using cannabis both recreationally and for medical purposes, with a consistent anxiolytic effect of cannabis for therapeutic purposes observed [33]. Worsening of anxiety disorders among patients using cannabis may be attributed to baseline factors (clinical and sociodemographic parameters) rather than cannabis use itself or to patients obtaining and using alternative chemovars recreationally [33, 41]. Longitudinal evidence has shown either frequent recreational cannabis use preceding the onset of anxiety disorders, anxiety disorders preceding the use of cannabis for medical purposes, or evidence for no association between cannabis use and anxiety [33]. Therefore, it is crucial to assess patterns of use, level of consumption, and cannabinoids content when attributing the harms of use to cannabis.

THC should be used with caution among concurrent active mood, anxiety, and/or substance use disorders. THC is anxiolytic at low doses and anxiogenic at higher doses. Among a Canadian cohort taking medical cannabis for anxiety, depression, and/or agoraphobia/panic disorder ($n = 2032$ survey responses), 92% of the total participants stated that cannabis improved their symptoms, with 53.7% replacing non-psychiatric medication and 46.3% replacing psychiatric medication with cannabis for medical purposes [42].

CBD appears to be anxiolytic at all doses. There is evidence to suggest that CBD, with little or no THC, may be beneficial among some anxiety and depressive disorders [42]. A recent review examining six RCTs, one case series, and one case report concluded that CBD is well tolerated and has a promising role in alternative therapy for anxiety disorders with minimal adverse events other than sedation and fatigue [43]. The use of 300 mg of oral CBD among adolescents with social anxiety disorder (SAD) ($n = 37$) has been shown to be effective in reducing anxiety over a 4-week period [44] which has been observed in other SAD populations [45, 46]. Moreover, 600 mg of CBD may be beneficial in reducing social stress, even among a population that is considered clinically high-risk for developing psychosis [47]. In clinical practice, much lower doses of CBD, such as 50–100mg per day in two divided doses, have been noted to be helpful in reducing anxiety.

Post-Traumatic Stress Disorder

PTSD, although distinguished from anxiety disorders, is recognized as an anxious condition [33] in response to traumatic experience. Cannabis (THC) has been increasingly recognized to treat the symptoms associated with PTSD, which has been shown to be associated with improved sleep, negative affect management, and a reduction in nightmares and daytime flashbacks [33]. A recent systematic review and meta-analysis also points to some evidence for medical cannabis use among PTSD patients, particularly in reducing anxiety, altering memory-related processes, and improving sleep [48].

Another recent population-based cross-sectional study among Canadians, using data from the 2012 Canadian Community Health Survey-Mental Health, provided epidemiological evidence for a reduction in severe depressive and suicidal states among individuals with PTSD using cannabis compared to non-using patients [49]. Cannabis can be considered a harm-reduction strategy among individuals with PTSD, as it has been reported to reduce the use of other harmful drugs, such as opioids [50].

Similar to the evidence for anxiety, medicinal cannabis with CBD and little-to-no THC may reduce PTSD symptomatology including depressive symptoms and frequent nightmares [51]. Although a recent article published in *The Lancet* by Black et al. [52] suggests that cannabis is not effective in the treatment of mental disorders, it is not without methodological flaws [53]. While it is agreed that a large proportion of the evidence is still in its infancy, preliminary results are promising for the management of PTSD and anxiety-related disorders with cannabis.

Psychosis and Bipolar Disorder

As discussed in the section "Recreational Cannabis and Psychosis" above, THC may not be appropriate for those with psychosis and/or bipolar disorders. Evidence for the safety and efficacy of CBD in psychosis is still limited [54]. CBD has been investigated, up to 1500 mg, as an antipsychotic among individuals with psychosis with some promise [54, 55]. It was associated with increased anandamide concentrations [56, 57] and decreased side effects compared to other antipsychotics such as amisulpride [58]. Other clinical trials using CBD (1000 mg/day for 6 weeks) adjunctive to usual antipsychotic therapy among patients with chronic schizophrenia have observed reductions in positive, but not negative, symptoms among individuals taking CBD in comparison to placebo [59, 60]. A recent review of clinical trials concluded CBD (400–1000 mg/day) proved to have relatively good efficacy in managing positive symptoms, moderate efficacy in treating negative symptoms, and relatively low efficacy in managing the cognitive symptoms of schizophrenia [61], with sedation as the most common side effect reported [54]. Alternatively, CBD may produce cognitive benefits among patients with first-onset psychosis. CBD at a dose of 600 mg has been shown to decrease underlying learning and memory impairments among first-episode patients with schizophrenia [62] and among individuals at high risk of developing psychosis [63].

However, CBD monotherapy for patients with treatment-resistant schizophrenia (TRS) proved to be unsuccessful [64]; alternatively dronabinol may be useful clinically for TRS [65]. CBD monotherapy, at any dose, among bipolar disorders did not produce beneficial effects for managing manic episodes [54, 66]. More evidence is required in longitudinal trials with larger sample sizes to determine the role of CBD as adjunctive or monotherapy for those at risk or with treatment-resistant psychosis or bipolar disorder.

Summary

When treating individuals with mental health disorders, it is imperative to identify those with existing biopsychosocial vulnerabilities and mental health concerns prior to initiating cannabis treatment. The risks and benefits should be weighed by the physician on a case-by-case basis with the patient. As with any off-label prescription medication, and especially in high-risk patient populations, a shorter trial for cannabis initiation should be considered, with frequent monitoring and reassessment for efficacy, adverse events, drug interactions, etc. Chemovars high in CBD with little-to-no THC may be beneficial in some anxiety disorders (i.e., social anxiety disorder) as well as among cases of PTSD and insomnia. Additionally, CBD should be considered preferentially over THC in these populations. Observational studies show efficacy of cannabis in treating anxiety, PTSD, or insomnia; however, larger studies are needed.

Evidence has suggested that rates of mental health illness may be high in medical cannabis dispensary users, so the use of structured clinical assessments in conjunction with standardized symptom severity questionnaires may be beneficial in minimizing harms [67]. An assessment of one's ability to balance occupational, recreational, and personal responsibility is the best clinical indicator of risk versus harm.

References

1. National Academies of Sciences, Engineering, and Medicine. The health effects of cannabis and cannabinoids: the current state of evidence and recommendations for research. Washington, DC: National Academies Press; 2017.
2. Proal AC, Fleming J, Galvez-Buccollini JA, DeLisi LE. A controlled family study of cannabis users with and without psychosis. Schizophr Res. 2014;152(1):283–8.
3. Ragazzi TC, Shuhama R, Menezes PR, Del-Ben CM. Cannabis use as a risk factor for psychotic-like experiences: a systematic review of non-clinical populations evaluated with the Community Assessment of Psychic Experiences. Early Interv Psychiatry. 2018;12(6):1013–23.
4. Karcher NR, Barch DM, Demers CH, Baranger DA, Heath AC, Lynskey MT, Agrawal A. Genetic predisposition vs individual-specific processes in the association between psychotic-like experiences and cannabis use. JAMA Psychiat. 2019;76(1):87–94.
5. Carney R, Cotter J, Firth J, Bradshaw T, Yung AR. Cannabis use and symptom severity in individuals at ultra high risk for psychosis: a meta-analysis. Acta Psychiatr Scand. 2017;136(1):5–15.

6. Demontis D, Rajagopal VM, Thorgeirsson TE, Als TD, Grove J, Leppälä K, Gudbjartsson DF, Pallesen J, Hjorthøj C, Reginsson GW, Tyrfingsson T. Genome-wide association study implicates CHRNA2 in cannabis use disorder. Nat Neurosci. 2019;22(7):1066.
7. Williams HJ, Owen MJ, O'Donovan MC. Is COMT a susceptibility gene for schizophrenia? Schizophr Bull. 2007;33(3):635–41.
8. Halah MP, Zochniak MP, Barr MS, George TP. Cannabis use and psychiatric disorders: implications for mental health and addiction treatment. Curr Addict Rep. 2016;3(4):450–62.
9. Boggs DL, Nguyen JD, Morgenson D, Taffe MA, Ranganathan M. Clinical and preclinical evidence for functional interactions of cannabidiol and Δ9-tetrahydrocannabinol. Neuropsychopharmacology. 2018;43(1):142–54.
10. Schoeler T, Petros N, Di Forti M, Klamerus E, Foglia E, Ajnakina O, Gayer-Anderson C, Colizzi M, Quattrone D, Behlke I, Shetty S. Effects of continuation, frequency, and type of cannabis use on relapse in the first 2 years after onset of psychosis: an observational study. Lancet Psychiatry. 2016;3(10):947–53.
11. Colizzi M, Bhattacharyya S. Cannabis use and the development of tolerance: a systematic review of human evidence. Neurosci Biobehav Rev. 2018;93:1–25.
12. Scott JC, Slomiak ST, Jones JD, Rosen AF, Moore TM, Gur RC. Association of cannabis with cognitive functioning in adolescents and young adults: a systematic review and meta-analysis. JAMA Psychiat. 2018;75(6):585–95.
13. Ramaekers JG, Mason NL, Theunissen EL. Blunted highs: pharmacodynamic and behavioral models of cannabis tolerance. Eur Neuropsychopharmacol. 2020;36:191–205.
14. Levinsohn EA, Hill KP. Clinical uses of cannabis and cannabinoids in the United States. J Neurol Sci. 2020;411:116717.
15. Fischer B, Russell C, Sabioni P, Van Den Brink W, Le Foll B, Hall W, Rehm J, Room R. Lower-risk cannabis use guidelines: a comprehensive update of evidence and recommendations. Am J Public Health. 2017;107(8):e1–2.
16. World Health Organization. WHO Expert Committee on Drug Dependence: fortieth report. Geneva: World Health Organization; 2018.
17. Health Canada. Information for health care professionals: cannabis (marihuana, marijuana) and the cannabinoids. 2019. Available at: https://www.canada.ca/content/dam/hc-sc/documents/services/drugs-medication/cannabis/information-medical-practitioners/information-health-care-professionals-cannabis-cannabinoids-eng.pdf.
18. Bélanger RE, Grant CN. Counselling adolescents and parents about cannabis: a primer for health professionals. Paediatr Child Health. 2020;25(Supplement_1):S34–40.
19. Boisvert EE, Bae D, Pang RD, Davis JP, Kelley-Quon LI, Barrington-Trimis JL, Kirkpatrick MG, Chai SH, Leventhal AM. Subjective effects of combustible, vaporized, and edible cannabis: results from a survey of adolescent cannabis users. Drug Alcohol Depend. 2020;206:107716.
20. Newmeyer MN, Swortwood MJ, Abulseoud OA, Huestis MA. Subjective and physiological effects, and expired carbon monoxide concentrations in frequent and occasional cannabis smokers following smoked, vaporized, and oral cannabis administration. Drug Alcohol Depend. 2017;175:67–76.
21. Russell C, Rueda S, Room R, Tyndall M, Fischer B. Routes of administration for cannabis use–basic prevalence and related health outcomes: a scoping review and synthesis. Int J Drug Policy. 2018;52:87–96.
22. Marshall SE. The Cannabis use disorder identification test-revised (CUDIT-R): categorisation and interpretation. Doctoral dissertation, University of Tasmania. 2012.
23. Barclay JS, Owens JE, Blackhall LJ. Screening for substance abuse risk in cancer patients using the Opioid Risk Tool and urine drug screen. Support Care Cancer. 2014;22(7):1883–8.
24. Hasin DS, Kerridge BT, Saha TD, Huang B, Pickering R, Smith SM, Jung J, Zhang H, Grant BF. Prevalence and correlates of DSM-5 cannabis use disorder, 2012-2013: findings from the National Epidemiologic Survey on Alcohol and Related Conditions–III. Am J Psychiatr. 2016;173(6):588–99.
25. Borodovsky JT, Lee DC, Crosier BS, Gabrielli JL, Sargent JD, Budney AJ. US cannabis legalization and use of vaping and edible products among youth. Drug Alcohol Depend. 2017;177:299–306.
26. Hoch E, Bonnet U, Thomasius R, Ganzer F, Havemann-Reinecke U, Preuss UW. Risks associated with the non-medicinal use of cannabis. Dtsch Ärztebl Int. 2015;112(16):271–8.
27. Agrawal A, Nelson EC, Bucholz KK, Tillman R, Grucza RA, Statham DJ, Madden PA, Martin NG, Heath AC, Lynskey MT. Major depressive disorder, suicidal thoughts and behaviours, and cannabis involvement in discordant twins: a retrospective cohort study. Lancet Psychiatry. 2017;4(9):706–14.
28. Bahorik AL, Leibowitz A, Sterling SA, Travis A, Weisner C, Satre DD. Patterns of marijuana use among psychiatry patients with depression and its impact on recovery. J Affect Disord. 2017;213:168–71.
29. Mammen G, Rueda S, Roerecke M, Bonato S, Lev-Ran S, Rehm J. Association of cannabis with long-term clinical symptoms in anxiety and mood disorders: a systematic review of prospective studies. J Clin Psychiatry. 2018;79(4):17r11839.
30. Borodovsky JT, Budney AJ. Cannabis regulatory science: risk–benefit considerations for mental disorders. Int Rev Psychiatry. 2018;30(3):183–202.
31. Hall KE, Monte AA, Chang T, Fox J, Brevik C, Vigil DI, Van Dyke M, James KA. Mental health–related emergency department visits associated with cannabis in Colorado. Acad Emerg Med. 2018;25(5):526–37.

32. D'Souza DC, Abi-Saab WM, Madonick S, Forselius-Bielen K, Doersch A, Braley G, Gueorguieva R, Cooper TB, Krystal JH. Delta-9-tetrahydrocannabinol effects in schizophrenia: implications for cognition, psychosis, and addiction. Biol Psychiatry. 2005;57(6):594–608.
33. Walsh Z, Gonzalez R, Crosby K, Thiessen MS, Carroll C, Bonn-Miller MO. Medical cannabis and mental health: a guided systematic review. Clin Psychol Rev. 2017;51:15–29.
34. Hasin DS, Sarvet AL, Cerdá M, Keyes KM, Stohl M, Galea S, Wall MM. US adult illicit cannabis use, cannabis use disorder, and medical marijuana laws: 1991-1992 to 2012-2013. JAMA Psychiat. 2017;74(6):579–88.
35. Ronan PJ, Wongngamnit N, Beresford TP. Molecular mechanisms of cannabis signaling in the brain. In: Progress in molecular biology and translational science, vol. 137. Amsterdam: Academic Press; 2016. p. 123–47.
36. Hasin DS. US epidemiology of cannabis use and associated problems. Neuropsychopharmacology. 2018;43(1):195–212.
37. Ware MA, Wang T, Shapiro S, Collet JP, Boulanger A, Esdaile JM, Gordon A, Lynch M, Moulin DE, O'Connell C. Cannabis for the management of pain: assessment of safety study (COMPASS). J Pain. 2015;16(12):1233–42.
38. American Psychiatric Association. Diagnostic and statistical manual of mental disorders (DSM-5®). Arlington: American Psychiatric Publishing; 2013.
39. Patel J, Marwaha R. Cannabis use disorder. In: StatPearls [Internet]. Treasure Island: StatPearls Publishing; 2019.
40. Kosiba JD, Maisto SA, Ditre JW. Patient-reported use of medical cannabis for pain, anxiety, and depression symptoms: systematic review and meta-analysis. Soc Sci Med. 2019;233:181–92.
41. Feingold D, Rehm J, Factor H, Redler A, Lev-Ran S. Clinical and functional outcomes of cannabis use among individuals with anxiety disorders: a 3-year population-based longitudinal study. Depress Anxiety. 2018;35(6):490–501.
42. Turna J, Simpson W, Patterson B, Lucas P, Van Ameringen M. Cannabis use behaviors and prevalence of anxiety and depressive symptoms in a cohort of Canadian medicinal cannabis users. J Psychiatr Res. 2019;111:134–9.
43. Skelley JW, Deas CM, Curren Z, Ennis J. Use of cannabidiol in anxiety and anxiety-related disorders. J Am Pharm Assoc. 2020;60(1):253–61.
44. Masataka N. Anxiolytic effects of repeated cannabidiol treatment in teenagers with social anxiety disorders. Front Psychol. 2019;10:2466.
45. Bergamaschi MM, Queiroz RH, Chagas MH, De Oliveira DC, De Martinis BS, Kapczinski F, Quevedo J, Roesler R, Schröder N, Nardi AE, Martín-Santos R. Cannabidiol reduces the anxiety induced by simulated public speaking in treatment-naive social phobia patients. Neuropsychopharmacology. 2011;36(6):1219–26.
46. Crippa JA, Derenusson GN, Ferrari TB, Wichert-Ana L, Duran FL, Martin-Santos R, Simões MV, Bhattacharyya S, Fusar-Poli P, Atakan Z, Filho AS. Neural basis of anxiolytic effects of cannabidiol (CBD) in generalized social anxiety disorder: a preliminary report. J Psychopharmacol. 2011;25(1):121–30.
47. Appiah-Kusi E, Petros N, Wilson R, Colizzi M, Bossong MG, Valmaggia L, Mondelli V, McGuire P, Bhattacharyya S. Effects of short-term cannabidiol treatment on response to social stress in subjects at clinical high risk of developing psychosis. Psychopharmacology. 2020;237:1121–30.
48. Orsolini L, Chiappini S, Volpe U, De Berardis D, Latini R, Papanti GD, Corkery JM. Use of medicinal cannabis and synthetic cannabinoids in post-traumatic stress disorder (PTSD): a systematic review. Medicina. 2019;55(9):525.
49. Lake S, Kerr T, Buxton J, Walsh Z, Marshall BD, Wood E, Milloy MJ. Does cannabis use modify the effect of post-traumatic stress disorder on severe depression and suicidal ideation? Evidence from a population-based cross-sectional study of Canadians. J Psychopharmacol. 2020;34(2):181–8.
50. Cohen J, Wei Z, Phang J, Laprairie RB, Zhang Y. Cannabinoids as an emerging therapy for posttraumatic stress disorder and substance use disorders. J Clin Neurophysiol. 2020;37(1):28–34.
51. Elms L, Shannon S, Hughes S, Lewis N. Cannabidiol in the treatment of post-traumatic stress disorder: a case series. J Altern Complement Med. 2019;25(4):392–7.
52. Black N, Stockings E, Campbell G, Tran LT, Zagic D, Hall WD, Farrell M, Degenhardt L. Cannabinoids for the treatment of mental disorders and symptoms of mental disorders: a systematic review and meta-analysis. Lancet Psychiatry. 2019;6(12):995–1010.
53. Crippa JA, de Lima Osório F, Hallak J, Guimarães FS, Zuardi AW. Cannabinoids for the treatment of mental disorders. Lancet Psychiatry. 2020;7(2):125–6.
54. Bonaccorso S, Ricciardi A, Zangani C, Chiappini S, Schifano F. Cannabidiol (CBD) use in psychiatric disorders: a systematic review. Neurotoxicology. 2019;74:282–98.
55. Zuardi AW, Crippa JA, Hallak JE, Moreira FA, Guimaraes FS. Cannabidiol, a Cannabis sativa constituent, as an antipsychotic drug. Braz J Med Biol Res. 2006;39(4):421–9.
56. Rohleder C, Müller JK, Lange B, Leweke FM. Cannabidiol as a potential new type of an antipsychotic. A critical review of the evidence. Front Pharmacol. 2016;7:422.
57. Roser P, Vollenweider FX, Kawohl W. Potential antipsychotic properties of central cannabinoid (CB1) receptor antagonists. World J Biol Psychiatry. 2010;11(2–2):208–19.
58. Leweke FM, Piomelli D, Pahlisch F, Muhl D, Gerth CW, Hoyer C, Klosterkötter J, Hellmich M, Koethe D. Cannabidiol enhances anandamide signaling and

alleviates psychotic symptoms of schizophrenia. Transl Psychiatry. 2012;2(3):e94.
59. McGuire P, Robson P, Cubala WJ, Vasile D, Morrison PD, Barron R, Taylor A, Wright S. Cannabidiol (CBD) as an adjunctive therapy in schizophrenia: a multicenter randomized controlled trial. Am J Psychiatr. 2018;175(3):225–31.
60. McGuire P, Robson P, Cubała W, Vasile D, Morrison P, Barron R, Taylor A, Wright S. 17.1 A randomized controlled trial of cannabidiol in schizophrenia. Schizophr Bull. 2018;44(Suppl 1):S27.
61. Elsaid S, Kloiber S, Le Foll B. Effects of cannabidiol (CBD) in neuropsychiatric disorders: a review of pre-clinical and clinical findings. In: Progress in molecular biology and translational science, vol. 167. Amsterdam: Academic Press; 2019. p. 25–75.
62. O'Neill A, Wilson R, Blest-Hopley G, Annibale L, Colizzi M, Bhattacharyya S. S152. Cannabidiol induced modulation of mediotemporal activity during a verbal memory task in first-episode psychosis. Schizophr Bull. 2018;44(Suppl 1):S384.
63. Bhattacharyya S, Wilson R, Appiah-Kusi E, O'Neill A, Brammer M, Perez J, Murray R, Allen P, Bossong MG, McGuire P. Effect of cannabidiol on medial temporal, midbrain, and striatal dysfunction in people at clinical high risk of psychosis: a randomized clinical trial. JAMA Psychiat. 2018;75(11):1107–17.
64. Zuardi AW, Hallak JE, Dursun SM, Morais SL, Sanches RF, Musty RE, Crippa JA. Cannabidiol monotherapy for treatment-resistant schizophrenia. J Psychopharmacol. 2006;20(5):683–6.
65. Schwarcz G, Karajgi B, McCarthy R. Synthetic Δ-9-tetrahydrocannabinol (dronabinol) can improve the symptoms of schizophrenia. J Clin Psychopharmacol. 2009;29(3):255–8.
66. Zuardi AW, Crippa JA, Dursun SM, Morais SL, Vilela JA, Sanches RF, Hallak JE. Cannabidiol was ineffective for manic episode of bipolar affective disorder. J Psychopharmacol. 2010;24(1):135–7.
67. Yau JC, Yu SM, Panenka WJ, Pearce H, Gicas KM, Procyshyn RM, MacCallum C, Honer WG, Barr AM. Characterization of mental health in cannabis dispensary users, using structured clinical interviews and standardized assessment instruments. BMC Psychiatry. 2019;19(1):335.

Cannabinoids and Adolescence

34

Caroline A. MacCallum and Lauren de Freitas

Introduction

The impact of cannabis on the developing brain is an important consideration. The endocannabinoid system is involved in regulating neuronal development throughout different developmental stages from perinatal to young adulthood (Fig. 34.1). Depending on the stage of development, cannabis can potentially have varying influences on physiological and behavioral processes. A "critical period" theory emerged upon discovery of increased endocannabinoid system activity during the onset of puberty, when cognitive capacities are increasing throughout the brain (i.e., increased executive functioning due to prefrontal cortical maturation particularly in the frontal cortex and limbic system), making it potentially more vulnerable to cannabis' effects when used recreationally [1, 2]. Early, regular recreational cannabis use throughout crucial periods of neuronal development, such as adolescence, has been associated with cognitive impairments, including a lower IQ and school dropout, although this evidence is inconclusive [3–7]. The use of cannabis in adolescence is generally not recommended.

Medical Cannabis and Adolescence

In the vast majority of cases, the risk out weighs the benefit for the use of medical cannabis in adolescence. Although some adoelscence report using medical cannabis for mental health conditions, such as anxiety, evidence is not yet robust enough to support its efficacy or safety within this population. The use of CBD in epilepsy is one of the few excepts to this. It is strongly recommended that only experienced clinicians recommending cannabis (CRC) work with these patients.

Potential Risks of Cannabis Use in Adolescence

Even though medical cannabis use is not recommended in adolescence, many adolescents report using cannabis. As such, it is important for cli-

C. A. MacCallum (✉)
Department of Medicine, Faculty of Medicine, University of British Columbia, Vancouver, BC, Canada
e-mail: info@drcarolinemaccallum.com

L. de Freitas
Centre for Addiction and Mental Health, Toronto, ON, Canada

S. N. Narouze (ed.), *Cannabinoids and Pain*, https://doi.org/10.1007/978-3-030-69186-8_34

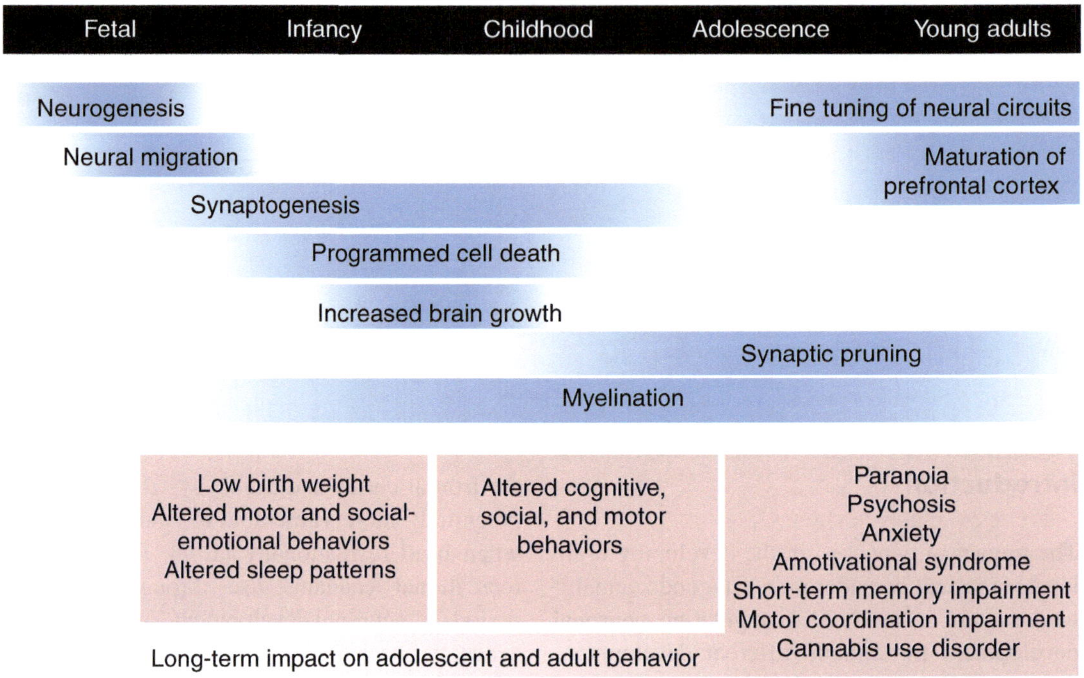

Fig. 34.1 Human brain development regulated by the endocannabinoid system. Exposure to cannabis at different growth stages from pregnancy to young adulthood affects the neurodevelopment processes (blue bars) impacting physiology and behavior. (Hurd [8])

nicians to be aware of associated risks. The use of cannabis in the early youth period (i.e., 10–15 years of age and using at least monthly) is strongly associated with adverse health impacts [9, 10]. Regular cannabis users under the age of 18 years old may be at increased risk for persistent cognitive effects, as well as increased social dysfunction, anxiety, and depression [11–15]. Heavy, frequent cannabis use among individuals 15 years old or younger is associated with both cognitive impairment and mental illness later in life [16]. Other evidence suggests that adolescent-onset cannabis users show slowed learning compared to controls when not acutely intoxicated, with associated deficits observed within the medial temporal and midbrain functioning [17]. Recent evidence suggests that these chronic cognitive deficits, such as learning or memory impairments, resulting from heavy cannabis use in adolescence may be overestimated in terms of magnitude and prevalence [18, 19]. Deficits have been shown to resolve following a period of abstinence [18, 19].

Finally, one of the greatest risks regarding adolescent cannabis use is the potential impact on mental health. Recent meta-analytic evidence suggests heavy cannabis use in adolescence may increase the risk of developing psychosis and/or substance use or abuse [20]. Among youth at risk, a younger age of first cannabis use may be associated with a younger age of onset of schizophrenia and/or bipolar disorder, in addition to other worsening psychological outcomes [11–15]. Regular recreational cannabis use under the age of 18 is also associated with an increased risk for developing major depression and increased suicidality early in adulthood (OR = 1.37 and 3.46, respectively) [21]. This association was not seen for developing anxiety or suicidal ideation later in life [21]. Potency of cannabis use, in addition to the frequency of use, is an important factor when considering the mental health risks of cannabis use in adolescence. A recent cohort study examining 1087 participants reporting past-year cannabis use determined that high-potency cannabis use is associated with increased frequency of use

(AOR = 4.38), cannabis problems (AOR = 4.08), and likelihood of an anxiety disorder (AOR = 1.92), compared to less-potent cannabis use [22]. More research is still greatly needed within the area. Currently, a large scale investigation, the Adolescent Brain Cognitive Development (ABCD) Study [23], is underway to conduct neurocognitive and neuroimaging assessments on children prior to cannabis use and following them longitudinally over time [24]. This will help clarify many of the risks discussed above.

Treatment-Resistant Epilepsy

There is conclusive evidence for the use of cannabidiol in treatment-resistant pediatric epilepsy, specifically regarding reduction in seizure frequency, spasticity (in severe complex motor disorder), sleep difficulties, pain, and quality of life improvement [25]. A recent systematic review examining four high-quality RCTs and 19 non-randomized studies concluded that there is moderate certainty that CBD reduced the frequency of seizures among drug-resistant pediatric epilepsy, but could not extend this conclusion to other cannabis-based medicines [26]. Accumulating evidence for the benefits of oral CBD in pediatric epilepsy has led to the development of Epidiolex®, a purified oral CBD solution approved for the treatment of Dravet syndrome and Lennox-Gastaut syndrome [27]. The use of CBD among pediatric patients may produce adverse events among this population compared to placebo including diarrhea, vomiting, fatigue, somnolence, decreased appetite, and much less commonly status epilepticus and abnormal liver function test results [28, 29].

In another recent study, Liver enzyme abnormalities were reported in a very small number of patients, which may have resulted from concomitant ingestion with three or more antiseizure medications known to be metabolized by the liver [30–34]. Specifically, among those who had increase in hepatic aminotransferase levels, it was found there was also concomitant administration of valproic acid [29]. This potential adverse event needs further investigation.

Discussing Cannabis use with Adolescents

In 2019, a Canadian survey revealed that 44% of youth aged 16–19 reported using cannabis within the past year [35]. As a result, it can be seen just how important it is to counsel patients on responsible cannabis use and provide resources they can utilize if they are concerned about their use. The Canadian Pediatric Society has outlined various ways that healthcare practitioners can counsel both young patients and their parents regarding responsible cannabis use, and may be a valuable resource for clinicians [10].

It is imperative to make the clinical setting a safe space for adolescents to discuss the use of psychoactive substances, such as cannabis, in order to converse about specific strategies for approaching cannabis use in both an effective and safe manner (Table 34.1). In order to do so, it is important to understand potential reasons adolescents may be turning to cannabis use. There is an association between youth who report self-medicating with cannabis and their perceptions of the inadequacies of the medical system and ineffective medical interventions. Many youths reported feeling invalidated by the medical system and dissatisfied by solutions and medications

Table 34.1 Recommendations for reducing cannabis-related harms

1. Start low and go slow
2. Consider appropriate time and place
3. Choose less risky cannabis products
4. Choose safer methods of cannabis consumption
5. Utilize safer smoking practices
6. Reduce the amount of cannabis used andt how frequently it is used
7. Avoid synthetic cannabis altogether
8. Avoid mixing cannabis with tobacco and alcohol
9. Don't drive high – have a plan for transportation before using cannabis
10. Consider your risk profile and avoid using cannabis if pregnant

Adapted from Valleriani et al. [36]

offered. Cannabis was framed by young people as the "better" and natural alternative to pharmaceuticals [37]. Youth report using cannabis for medical purposes as self-medication, including relief from depression, anxiety, insomnia, pain, and concentration difficulties [38]. Screening questionnaires such as the Cannabis Abuse Screening Test (CAST) [39], CRAFFT [40], and the Severity of Dependence Scale (SDS) [41] can be used to help identify at-risk patients who may require greater support or intervention.

The Canadian Students for Sensible Drug Policy (CSSDP) has also created a "Sensible Cannabis Education" toolkit for educating youth, which includes recommendations for reducing cannabis-related harms (Table 34.1) [36]. There is an opportunity to speak with youth about cannabis, but for this conversation to be effective, there are number of considerations and important questions to ask (Table 34.2).

Table 34.2 Considerations and Questions to address with youth regarding cannabis

Assure patient privacy and confidentiality
Decide on an approach (e.g., will it be conversation about "facts" or about their own experiences?)
Ask about cannabis use, after obtaining permission to do so. Six specific questions to ask include: 1. How long have you been using cannabis? 2. How often? 3. How do you consume cannabis? 4. What kind of product(s)? 5. When do you consume? 6. What about driving?
Listen to develop rapport. Ask open-ended questions and try not to interrupt
Answer all patient questions, and support healthy choices
Communicate your expectations clearly and set boundaries around use
Assess the impacts of cannabis use by applying a screening tool
Appraise patient willingness to change or reduce cannabis use
Focus on positive choices and future goals
Assist with specific goal-setting and a realistic timeframe
Arrange for a follow-up within weeks and regularly thereafter
Regularly engage about cannabis to encourage harm reduction and/or prevention
Acknowledge parental needs and concerns, when these arise

 Information gathered from [10, 36]

Summary

There are a number of significant risks associated with cannabis use in adolescence. Evidence on the efficacy and safety of medical cannabis in this population is limited, with the exception of treatment-resistant epilepsy. As such, the risks most often outweigh the benefits and medical cannabis use in adolescents is generally not recommended. Despite this, cannabis use is not uncommon in this population, with many reporting self-medication for mental health. It is imperative clinicians can provide a safe and supportive space to educate and discuss strategies to decrease risks. When possible, screening tools should be used to identify at-risk patients who may require greater support.

References

1. Schneider M. Puberty as a highly vulnerable developmental period for the consequences of cannabis exposure. Addict Biol. 2008;13(2):253–63.
2. Satterthwaite TD, Wolf DH, Erus G, Ruparel K, Elliott MA, Gennatas ED, et al. Functional maturation of the executive system during adolescence. J Neurosci. 2013;33(41):16249–61.
3. Meier MH, Caspi A, Ambler A, Harrington H, Houts R, Keefe RS, et al. Persistent cannabis users show neuropsychological decline from childhood to midlife. Proc Natl Acad Sci. 2012;109(40):E2657–64.
4. Mandelbaum DE, de la Monte SM. Adverse structural and functional effects of marijuana on the brain: evidence reviewed. Pediatr Neurol. 2017;66:12–20.
5. Hasin DS. US epidemiology of cannabis use and associated problems. Neuropsychopharmacology. 2018;43(1):195.
6. Fischer B, Russell C, Rehm J, Leece P. Assessing the public health impact of cannabis legalization in Canada: core outcome indicators towards an "index" for monitoring and evaluation. J Public Health. 2019;41(2):412–21.
7. Lorenzetti V, Hoch E, Hall W. Adolescent cannabis use, cognition, brain health and educational outcomes: a review of the evidence. Eur Neuropsychopharmacol. 2020;36:169–80.

8. Hurd YL. Cannabis and the developing brain challenge risk perception. J Clin Invest. 2020;130(8): 3947–9.
9. Hyshka E. Applying a social determinants of health perspective to early adolescent cannabis use–an overview. Drugs. 2013;20(2):110–9.
10. Bélanger RE, Grant CN. Counselling adolescents and parents about cannabis: a primer for health professionals. Paediatr Child Health. 2020;25(Supplement_1):S34–40.
11. Urbanoski KA, Strike CJ, Rush BR. Individuals seeking treatment for cannabis-related problems in Ontario: demographic and treatment profile. Eur Addict Res. 2005;11(3):115–23.
12. Nocon A, Wittchen HU, Pfister H, Zimmermann P, Lieb R. Dependence symptoms in young cannabis users? A prospective epidemiological study. J Psychiatr Res. 2006;40(5):394–403.
13. Dragt S, Nieman DH, Schultze-Lutter F, Van Der Meer F, Becker H, De Haan L, et al. Cannabis use and age at onset of symptoms in subjects at clinical high risk for psychosis. Acta Psychiatr Scand. 2012;125(1):45–53.
14. Crean RD, Crane NA, Mason BJ. An evidence based review of acute and long-term effects of cannabis use on executive cognitive functions. J Addict Med. 2011;5(1):1.
15. Fergusson DM, Horwood LJ, Swain-Campbell N. Cannabis use and psychosocial adjustment in adolescence and young adulthood. Addiction. 2002;97(9):1123–35.
16. Lubman DI, Cheetham A, Yücel M. Cannabis and adolescent brain development. Pharmacol Ther. 2015;148:1–16.
17. Blest-Hopley G, Giampietro V, Bhattacharyya S. Regular cannabis use is associated with altered activation of central executive and default mode networks even after prolonged abstinence in adolescent users: results from a complementary meta-analysis. Neurosci Biobehav Rev. 2019;96:45–55.
18. Scott JC, Slomiak ST, Jones JD, Rosen AF, Moore TM, Gur RC. Association of cannabis with cognitive functioning in adolescents and young adults: a systematic review and meta-analysis. JAMA Psychiat. 2018;75(6):585–95.
19. Kroon E, Kuhns L, Hoch E, Cousijn J. Heavy cannabis use, dependence and the brain: a clinical perspective. Addiction. 2019; 115(3);559-572.
20. Jacobson MR, Watts JJ, Boileau I, Tong J, Mizrahi R. A systematic review of phytocannabinoid exposure on the endocannabinoid system: implications for psychosis. Eur Neuropsychopharmacol. 2019;29(3):330–48.
21. Gobbi G, Atkin T, Zytynski T, Wang S, Askari S, Boruff J, et al. Association of cannabis use in adolescence and risk of depression, anxiety, and suicidality in young adulthood: a systematic review and meta-analysis. JAMA Psychiat. 2019;76(4):426–34.
22. Hines LA, Freeman TP, Gage SH, Zammit S, Hickman M, Cannon M, et al. Association of high-potency cannabis use with mental health and substance use in adolescence. JAMA Psychiatry. 2020;77(10):1044–51.
23. National Institute of Health. The Adolescent Brain Cognitive Development (ABCD) study. 2015. View at: https://www.addictionresearch.nih.gov/abcd-study.
24. Volkow ND, Koob GF, Croyle RT, Bianchi DW, Gordon JA, Koroshetz WJ, et al. The conception of the ABCD study: from substance use to a broad NIH collaboration. Dev Cogn Neurosci. 2018;32:4–7.
25. Chao YS, McCormack S. Medicinal and synthetic cannabinoids for pediatric patients: a review of clinical effectiveness and guidelines. Ottawa: Canadian Agency for Drugs and Technologies in Health; 2019.
26. Elliott J, DeJean D, Clifford T, Coyle D, Potter BK, Skidmore B, et al. Cannabis-based products for pediatric epilepsy: a systematic review. Epilepsia. 2019;60(1):6–19.
27. Burggren AC, Shirazi A, Ginder N, London ED. Cannabis effects on brain structure, function, and cognition: considerations for medical uses of cannabis and its derivatives. Am J Drug Alcohol Abuse. 2019;45(6):563–79.
28. Devinsky O, Marsh E, Friedman D, Thiele E, Laux L, Sullivan J, et al. Cannabidiol in patients with treatment-resistant epilepsy: an open-label interventional trial. Lancet Neurol. 2016;15(3):270–8.
29. Devinsky O, Cross JH, Laux L, Marsh E, Miller I, Nabbout R, et al. Trial of cannabidiol for drug-resistant seizures in the Dravet syndrome. N Engl J Med. 2017;376(21):2011–20.
30. Meier U, Dussy F, Scheurer E, Mercer-Chalmers-Bender K, Hangartner S. Cannabinoid concentrations in blood and urine after smoking cannabidiol joints. Forensic Sci Int. 2018;291:62–7.
31. Hundal H, Lister R, Evans N, Antley A, Englund A, Murray RM, et al. The effects of cannabidiol on persecutory ideation and anxiety in a high trait paranoid group. J Psychopharmacol. 2018;32(3):276–82.
32. Schoedel KA, Szeto I, Setnik B, Sellers EM, Levy-Cooperman N, Mills C, et al. Abuse potential assessment of cannabidiol (CBD) in recreational polydrug users: a randomized, double-blind, controlled trial. Epilepsy Behav. 2018;88:162–71.
33. Solowij N, Broyd S, Greenwood LM, van Hell H, Martelozzo D, Rueb K, et al. A randomised controlled trial of vaporised Δ^9-tetrahydrocannabinol and cannabidiol alone and in combination in frequent and infrequent cannabis users: acute intoxication effects. Eur Arch Psychiatry Clin Neurosci. 2019;269(1):17–35.
34. Chesney E, Oliver D, Green A, Sovi S, Wilson J, Englund A, et al. Adverse effects of cannabidiol: a systematic review and meta-analysis of randomized clinical trials. Neuropsychopharmacology. 2020;45(11):1799–806.
35. Health Canada. Canadian Cannabis Survey 2019 – summary. 2019. Retrieved from: https://www.canada.ca/en/health-canada/services/publications/drugs-health-products/canadian-cannabis-survey-2019-summary.html.

36. Valleriani J, Maghsoudi N, Nguyen-Dang M, Lake S, Thiessen M, Robinson J, Pavlova D. Sensible cannabis education: a toolkit for educating youth. Canadian students for sensible drug policy. 2018. Retrieved from: https://cssdp.org/uploads/2018/04/Sensible-Cannabis-Education-A-Toolkit-for-Educating-Youth.pdf.
37. Bottorff JL, Johnson JL, Moffat BM, Mulvogue T. Relief-oriented use of marijuana by teens. Subst Abuse Treat Prev Policy. 2009;4(1):1–10.
38. Nelemans SA, Hale WW, Raaijmakers QA, Branje SJ, van Lier PA, Meeus WH. Longitudinal associations between social anxiety symptoms and cannabis use throughout adolescence: the role of peer involvement. Eur Child Adolesc Psychiatry. 2016;25(5):483–92.
39. Legleye S, Piontek D, Kraus L, Morand E, Falissard B. A validation of the Cannabis Abuse Screening Test (CAST) using a latent class analysis of the DSM-IV among adolescents. Int J Methods Psychiatr Res. 2013;22(1):16–26.
40. Knight JR, Sherritt L, Shrier LA, Harris SK, Chang G. Validity of the CRAFFT substance abuse screening test among adolescent clinic patients. Arch Pediatr Adolesc Med. 2002;156(6):607–14.
41. Martin G, Copeland J, Gates P, Gilmour S. The Severity of Dependence Scale (SDS) in an adolescent population of cannabis users: reliability, validity and diagnostic cut-off. Drug Alcohol Depend. 2006;83(1):90–3.
42. Scott JC, Slomiak ST, Jones JD, et al. Association of Cannabis With Cognitive Functioning in Adolescents and Young Adults A Systematic Review and Meta-analysis. JAMA Psychiatry. 2018;75(6):6.

35 Cannabinoids and Child Development: During and After Pregnancy

Qian Cece Chen and Samer N. Narouze

Epidemiology

According to the most recent data from the National Surveys on Drug Use and Health (NSDUH), in 2018, it was estimated that 43.5 million of Americans reported using marijuana in the last 12 months, which corresponds to 15.9% of the total population in the United States [1]. When compared to data from 2002 to 2017, this estimate is thus far the highest. Among the illicit drugs used by pregnant women, marijuana use continues to be the highest. In 2017, for example, 7.1% of pregnant women reported marijuana use in the past month compared to 1.4% of opioid use and 0.4% of cocaine use (Fig. 35.1) [1, 2]. From 2015 to 2017, marijuana use has also increased more significantly from 3.4% to 7.1%, while opioid use increased from 0.8% to 1.4%, and cocaine use increased from 0.0% to 0.4% (Figs. 35.1 and 35.2) [1, 2].

Among the pregnant women who use marijuana, 16.2% reported almost daily use throughout their pregnancy [3]. In addition, overall an estimated 70% of women, including both pregnant and non-pregnant, believed there is a minimal or no risk for marijuana use [3]. Similarly, a study conducted on pregnant women in the United Kingdom showed that those who concurrently used both marijuana and other substances such as cocaine stopped cocaine use during pregnancy; however 48% of these women continued to use marijuana throughout their pregnancy, believing that it was safe to use and safer than the other illicit drugs and smoking cigarette [4].

Various studies show that there may be potential risk factors associated with increased marijuana use during pregnancy (Table 35.1). These risk factors include women who live in urban cities, are younger than 25 years of age, did not graduate from high school, are from a low socioeconomic background, have a history of cigarette use or other illicit drug use, and reported ongoing emotional stressors [5]. These emotional stressors may be due to trauma, financial burden, depression, and abuse. In addition to these risk factors, women who experienced significant nausea from motion sickness also reported higher rates of marijuana use [6].

Effect of Cannabis During Pregnancy

Research on the effect of marijuana on pregnant women, the fetus, and later child development is still limited and inconclusive. What is known is that when used in the inhalation form, the serum carbon monoxide level found in pregnant women

Q. C. Chen (✉)
Department of Anesthesiology, Perioperative Care, and Pain Medicine, NYU Langone Health, New York, NY, USA
e-mail: Qian.Chen2@nyulangone.org

S. N. Narouze
Western Reserve Hospital, Center For Pain Medicine, Cuyahoga Falls, OH, USA

S. N. Narouze (ed.), *Cannabinoids and Pain*, https://doi.org/10.1007/978-3-030-69186-8_35

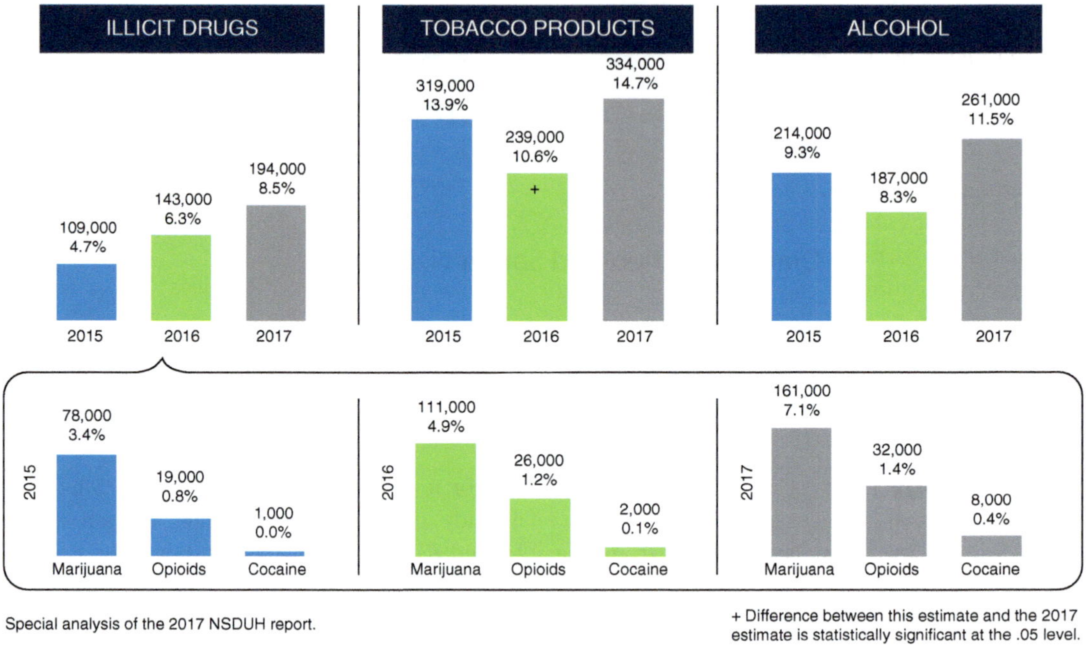

Fig. 35.1 Substance use among pregnant women. NSDUH National Findings Report 2017, SAMHSA [1, 2]

Fig. 35.2 Marijuana use among women. NSDUH National Findings Report 2017. SAMHSA [1, 2]

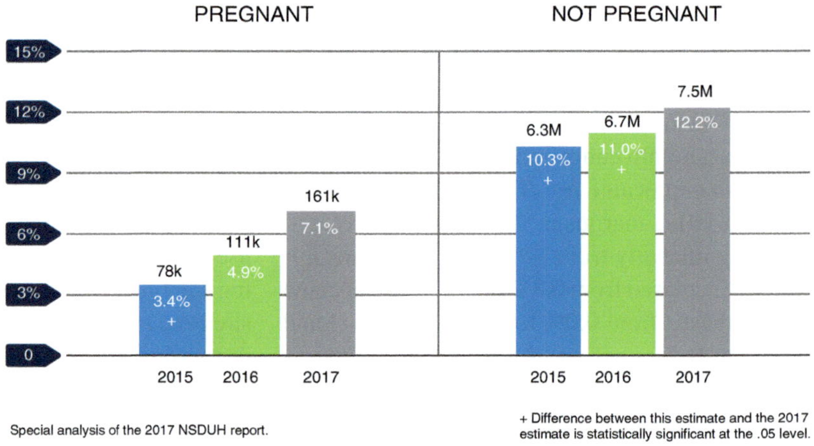

Table 35.1 Potential risk factors for increased cannabis use during pregnancy

Risk factors for increased cannabis use during pregnancy			
Demographic	Other substance use	Emotional stressors	Pregnancy-related symptoms
Urban cities No high school diploma Low socioeconomic background <25 years old	Also smokes cigarette Other illicit drugs including cocaine, heroin	Financial Trauma Depression Abuse	Nausea from motion sickness

is 5 times higher than the level found in those who smoked cigarettes [7]. Given that the fetal oxygenation depends solely on gas exchange with the mother, this can potentially lead to harmful effects on the fetus.

Marijuana can also affect the physiology of the placenta. It can increase the permeability of the placental barrier to pharmacologic agents and other recreational drugs used, consequently placing the fetus at higher risk from the effects of these agents used along with marijuana [8]. It is also believed to increase vascular resistance within the placenta, resulting in decreased circulation [9]. THC, the active compound that is found in marijuana and known for its psychoactive effects, has shown to readily cross the placental barrier. With maternal ingestion of marijuana, the concentration of THC found in fetal blood can be 1/3 to 1/10 of the level in the material circulation. THC is a highly lipophilic compound. When passed to the fetus, it can distribute and deposit into the brain and other fat-rich organs of the fetus [10].

Effect of Cannabis After Delivery

The studies that attempt to examine the effect of marijuana after delivery and during child development (Table 35.2) are often confounded by the concurrent maternal use of other illicit substances or cigarettes, which are known to affect fetal and child development. However marijuana is believed to hinder fetal growth rate, beginning in the second trimester of pregnancy, resulting in low birth weights in infants who were exposed in utero. These infants tend to be smaller in length and have smaller head circumferences compared to other infants. In addition, exposure to marijuana in utero may lead to stillbirth, low Apgar scores, and an overall increased risk of requiring NICU admission after delivery [11].

Table 35.2 Potential effects of cannabis at different developmental stages

Effects of cannabis at different developmental stages		
In utero	Infant	Childhood
Fetal growth restriction Stillbirth Preterm birth	Low birth weight Low Apgar scores Hyperactivity Abnormal arousal patterns Abnormal infant reflexes Poor habituation High-pitched cries Abnormal sleep patterns	Poor cognitive function Low verbal reasoning Poor language comprehension Memory deficits Visual impairment Poor impulse control Impaired attention

In later developmental stages, newborns with a history of marijuana exposure can exhibit abnormal arousal patterns, reflexes, excitability, poor habituation, abnormal high-pitched cries, and abnormal sleep patterns [12–14].

During the childhood stage, these children can be observed to have low verbal reasoning skills; deficits in language comprehension, memory, vision, and executive function; and poor impulse control and attention [15]. However due to potential confounding factors such as environmental influences on child development and demographic variables, which are often difficult to control in studies, a direct correlation between marijuana exposure and the above deficits cannot be concluded.

Cannabis and Breastfeeding

Cannabis is now the most commonly reported recreational drug used by pregnant and lactating women. Up to 36% of women report having used marijuana at some point in their pregnancy, and 18% report having used it while breastfeeding [16].

Bertrand et al. [17], using mass spectroscopy techniques, identified and quantified the concentration of several cannabinoids found in breast milk samples. They found measurable levels of THC in 63%, 11-hydroxy-Δ-9-tetrahydrocannabinol in 9%, and cannabidiol in 9% of the collected samples.

THC is highly lipophilic and can be expected to accumulate in fat-rich organs such as the brain.

Accordingly, cannabinoids may accumulate preferentially in brain tissue when brain growth and development are occurring rapidly and when breastfeeding most often occurs [18].

Summary

Although a direct correlation between marijuana use in pregnant women and fetal and child development cannot yet be defined, the potential risks already indicate a reason for concern. As a result, both the American College of Obstetricians and Gynecologists (ACOG) and the American Academy of Pediatrics (AAP) both advise against the use of marijuana during pregnancy and breastfeeding. State laws that legalize marijuana however do not currently list marijuana as a contraindication for pregnancy. In addition, advertisement and social media often promote various purported benefits of marijuana, including its use for motion sickness, that often are not supported by scientific evidence. As a result, prenatal education plays a vital role in reducing marijuana use during pregnancy. According to ACOG and AAP guidelines, all pregnant women are recommended to undergo routine screening for marijuana. Due to the still limited understanding of marijuana and its long-term effects, more research is needed to ensure safe use of this drug.

References

1. SAMHSA. NSDUH National Findings Report 2018. https://www.samhsa.gov/data/sites/default/files/cbhsq-reports/NSDUHNationalFindingsReport2018/NSDUHNationalFindingsReport2018.pdf.
2. SAMHSA. NSDUH National Findings Report 2017. https://www.samhsa.gov/data/sites/default/files/cbhsq-reports/NSDUHNationalFindingsReport2017/NSDUHNationalFindingsReport2017.pdf.
3. Ko JY, Farr SL, Tong VT, et al. Prevalence and patterns of marijuana use among pregnant and non-pregnant women of reproductive age. Am J Obstet Gynecol. 2015;213(2):201.e1–201.e10. https://doi.org/10.1016/j.ajog.2015.03.021.
4. Moore DG, Turner JD, Parrott AC, et al. During pregnancy, recreational drug-using women stop taking ecstasy (3,4-methylenedioxy-Nmethylamphetamine) and reduce alcohol consumption, but continue to smoke tobacco and cannabis: initial findings from the Development and Infancy Study. J Psychopharmacol. 2010;24(9):1403–10.
5. Ryan SA, et al. Marijuana use during pregnancy and breastfeeding: implications for neonatal and childhood outcomes. Pediatrics. 2018;142(3):e20181889. https://doi.org/10.1542/peds.2018-1889.
6. Roberson EK, Patrick WK, Hurwitz EL. Marijuana use and maternal experiences of severe nausea during pregnancy in Hawai'i. Hawaii J Med Public Health. 2014;73(9):283–7.
7. Wu TC, Tashkin DP, Djahed B, Rose JE. Pulmonary hazards of smoking marijuana as compared with tobacco. N Engl J Med. 1988;318(6):347–51.
8. Feinshtein V, Erez O, Ben-Zvi Z, et al. Cannabidiol enhances xenobiotic permeability through the human placental barrier by direct inhibition of breast cancer resistance protein: an ex vivo study. Am J Obstet Gynecol. 2013;209(6):573.e1–573.e15.
9. El Marroun H, Tiemeier H, Steegers EA, et al. A prospective study on intrauterine cannabis exposure and fetal blood flow. Early Hum Dev. 2010;86(4):231–6.
10. Grotenhermen F. Pharmacokinetics and pharmacodynamics of cannabinoids. Clin Pharmacokinet. 2003;42(4):327–60.
11. Gunn JK, Rosales CB, Center KE, et al. Prenatal exposure to cannabis and maternal and child health outcomes: a systematic review and meta-analysis. BMJ Open. 2016;6(4):e009986.
12. De Moraes Barros MC, Guinsburg R, de Araújo Peres C, Mitsuhiro S, Chalem E, Laranjeira RR. Exposure to marijuana during pregnancy alters neurobehavior in the early neonatal period. J Pediatr. 2006;149(6):781–7.
13. Fried PA, Watkinson B, Dillon RF, Dulberg CS. Neonatal neurological status in a low-risk population after prenatal exposure to cigarettes, marijuana, and alcohol. J Dev Behav Pediatr. 1987;8(6):318–26.
14. Lester BM, Dreher M. Effects of marijuana use during pregnancy on newborn cry. Child Dev. 1989;60(4):765–71. (49–52).
15. Fried PA, Watkinson B, Siegel LS. Reading and language in 9- to 12-year olds prenatally exposed to cigarettes and marijuana. Neurotoxicol Teratol. 1997;19(3):171–83.
16. Wang GS. Pediatric concerns due to expanded cannabis use: unintended consequences of legalization. J Med Toxicol. 2017;13(1):99–105. PMID: 2713970.
17. Bertrand KA, Hanan NJ, Honerkamp-Smith G, Best BM, Chambers CD. Marijuana use by breastfeeding mothers and cannabinoid concentrations in breast milk. Pediatrics. 2018;142(3):e20181076.
18. Ryan SA. A modern conundrum for the pediatrician: the safety of breast milk and the cannabis-using mother. Pediatrics. 2018;142(3):e20181921. https://doi.org/10.1542/peds.2018-1921.

Part VIII

Cannabis Impairment and Use Disorder

Cannabinoid-Related Adverse Events and Impairment

36

Caroline A. MacCallum, Lauren de Freitas, Lindsay A. Lo, Lauren Eadie, and Jeffrey R. Brubacher

Introduction

Cannabis can cause cognitive and psychomotor impairment in some individuals, as THC can produce acute psychoactive effects and intoxication upon use. Different clinical tests and batteries can be used to assess the degree of neurocognitive impairment, as there is no evidence of correlation between impairment and blood-THC or metabolite concentration. Cannabis impairment can impact daily life and/or cause harm when driving or performing safety sensitive tasks due to impaired psychomotor skills. Risk and extent of cannabis-induced impairment depends on both modifiable (eg. intent, administration route, tolerance, frequency, dose) and non-modifiable (genetics, metabolism, comorbidities) factors, making it an important discussion to have when trying to minimize patient impairment. Chronic adverse events of cannabis are due to heavy, repeated use over time, typically via smoking, which can lead to issues such as respiratory alterations, risk of worsening of mental health disorders in some individuals, and infrequently cannabinoid hyperemesis syndrome.

C. A. MacCallum (✉) · L. Eadie
Department of Medicine, Faculty of Medicine, University of British Columbia, Vancouver, BC, Canada
e-mail: info@drcarolinemaccallum.com

L. de Freitas
Centre for Addiction and Mental Health, Toronto, ON, Canada

L. A. Lo
Department of Psychology, Queen's University, Kingston, ON, Canada

J. R. Brubacher
Department of Emergency Medicine, Faculty of Medicine, UBC, Vancouver, BC, Canada

Acute Adverse Events

Cannabinoid-Related Adverse Events

Cannabinoids, such as CBD and THC, act on peripheral and central receptors, and are recognized for their anti-anxiety, antidepressant, analgesic, muscle relaxant, anti-inflammatory, antihistamine, and antiepileptic properties, among others. In addition to therapeutic benefits, some individuals also experience alterations in neuropsychological functioning following cannabis consumption. Acute adverse events are typically dose-dependent, reflect an individual's short-term response to consuming cannabis, and depend on the dose and route of administration among other factors, which are discussed in Table 36.1.

Cannabis Intoxication Syndromes

Cannabis (THC) use may lead to cannabis intoxication or cannabis intoxication delirium [1, 2].

Cannabis (THC) can produce acute psychoactive effects and feelings of intoxication upon use, such as altering an individual's level of consciousness, cognition, perceptions, and affect.

S. N. Narouze (ed.), *Cannabinoids and Pain*, https://doi.org/10.1007/978-3-030-69186-8_36

Table 36.1 Adverse events associated with cannabis use

Adverse events	Most common	Common	Rare
THC related			
Dizziness	✓		
Cognitive effects	✓		
Dry mouth	✓		
Anxiety	✓		
Drowsiness	✓		
Fatigue	✓		
THC and CBD related			
Nausea	✓		
THC related			
Euphoria		✓	
Blurred vision		✓	
THC and CBD related			
Headache		✓	
THC related			
Orthostatic hypotension			✓
Psychosis or paranoia			✓
Depression			✓
Ataxia or discoordination			✓
Tachycardia			✓
Cannabis hyperemesis syndrome			✓
Amotivational syndrome			✓
Route specific			
Diarrhea (due to carrier oil)			✓
Cough, phlegm, or bronchitis (due to smoking cannabis)			✓

© Caroline MacCallum, MD, used with permission. Information gathered from [9, 53, 92, 93]

These short-term effects can last anywhere from 1 to 5 hours, and vary in magnitude depending on the route of administration, dose consumed, current frequency of cannabis use and/or other drug use, as well as the "set and setting" (e.g., an individual's mood, expectations, and attitudes toward the effects of cannabis at time of use and the social setting cannabis is used in, respectively) [3].

Cannabis Intoxication Delirium

The diagnosis of cannabis intoxication delirium relies on the presence of delirium (an acute alteration in mental ability that is characterized by restlessness, incoherence of thought and speech, and illusions), and is appropriate when the following two symptoms predominate in someone who has taken cannabis [1, 2]:

1. Disturbance in attention (i.e., reduced ability to direct focus, sustain, and shift attention) and awareness (reduced orientation to the environment)
2. An additional disturbance in cognition (i.e., memory deficit, disorientation, language, visuospatial ability, or perception)

Similarly, the *International Statistical Classification of Diseases and Related Health Problems* [4] defines acute intoxication from cannabinoids as:

A. The general criteria for acute intoxication must be met.
B. There must be dysfunctional behavior or perceptual abnormalities, including at least one of the following:
   1. Euphoria and disinhibition
   2. Anxiety or agitation
   3. Suspiciousness or paranoid ideation
   4. Temporal showing (a sense that time is passing very slowly, and/or the person is experiencing a rapid flow of ideas)
   5. Impaired judgment
   6. Impaired attention
   7. Impaired reaction time
   8. Auditory, visual, or tactile illusions
   9. Hallucinations with preserved orientation

10. Depersonalization
11. Derealization
12. Interference with personal functioning

C. At least one of the following signs or symptoms must be present:
1. Increased appetite
2. Dry mouth
3. Conjunctival injection
4. Tachycardia

Acute Neurocognitive Impairment

Cannabis produces short-term alterations in neuropsychological functioning upon consumption among some individuals, known as acute impairment. Acute cannabis use, specifically THC and other cannabinoid receptor 1 (CB1) agonists, may impair learning, attention, concentration, memory, judgment, and decision-making in addition to producing acute alterations in psychomotor performance (i.e., reaction time, processing speed, coordination, motor control), drowsiness, and temporal slowing [5–7].

Clinical Tools and Metabolites to Measure Neurocognitive Impairment

Unlike alcohol, there is no clear evidence that cannabis impairment can be determined from "per se" levels of THC or other cannabinoid metabolites in bodily fluids. Verbal learning, memory, concentration, and psychomotor performance appear to be most impacted during cannabis impairment, particularly under informationally complex and time-pressured contexts [8]. Although this provides a general overview of typical symptoms, it does not accurately reflect the experiences of everyone who consumes cannabis. People who take cannabis regularly will develop tolerance, and as a result, medical cannabis patients may have elevated blood THC levels but still perform normally on cognitive and motor tests [9].

Assessing neurocognitive impairments and adjusting the associated doses of THC is imperative to improving patients' quality of life. Several general neurocognitive tests that can be administered to measure neurocognitive impairment [10–15] are shown in Table 36.2.

Table 36.2 Neurocognitive tests and cognitive domains

Neurocognitive test	Neurocognitive correlate assessed
Paced Auditory Serial Attention Test	Auditory information processing speed and working memory
Wechsler Adult Intelligence Scale Digit Symbol Test	Concentration, psychomotor speed, and graphomotor abilities
Trail Making Test A and B	Processing speed, visual attention, and task-switching
Grooved Pegboard Test (Dominant and Non-Dominant)	Fine motor coordination and speed
Hopkins Verbal Learning Test Revised with 20-minute delay	Learning/ability to retain, reproduce, and recognize information after a 20 minutes delay. Immediate and delayed recall of verbal information
Adult Memory and Information Processing Battery	*Spatial Recall Test*: Visuospatial memory *Symbol Digit Modalities Test*: Concentration, psychomotor speed, and graphomotor abilities *Paced Auditory Serial Addition Test*: Auditory information processing speed and working memory *Word Generation List*: Lexical fluency *Selective Reminding Test*: Verbal learning and memory
Brief Neurocognitive Battery	*Animal Fluency*: Semantic fluency and executive control *Boston Naming Test-15*: Expressive language *Coding*: Attention and visuomotor processing *Digit Span*: Auditory attention and working memory *Stroop Color Naming*: Attention and speed of information processing *Stroop Word Reading*: Attention and speed of word reading *Stroop Interference*: Inhibition and cognitive flexibility *Trails Making Test-A*: Simple attention, visual scanning and processing speed *Trails Making Test-B*: Visual scanning, divided attention and cognitive flexibility

Eadie et al. [20]

Driving and Safety-Sensitive Activities

An individual's ability to operate heavy machinery or drive safely may be negatively impacted by acute cannabis use, potentially leading to serious injury or death. This risk is especially high when cannabis is combined with alcohol [16, 17] or other impairing substances. General recommendations state that cannabis use should be separated from driving, and that drivers should never combine alcohol with cannabis. Individuals should not drive for at least four hours after inhaling cannabis, six hours after orally ingesting cannabis, and eight hours if euphoria is experienced after administration [17–19]. However, an important distinction that is often missed is separating THC from CBD. THC has known dose-dependent effects, and thus poses majority of the risk for impairment [20–22]. CBD, on the other hand, has shown no association with increase cognitive or psychomotor impairment for doses up to 100 mg of CBD [23, 24].

Cannabis impairs the psychomotor skills required for safe driving. Cannabis slows reaction time and impairs automated tasks such as reaction time, tracking ability (e.g., staying within a lane), or monitoring the speedometer and maintaining a constant speed [17, 25–32]. Expert panels compared experimental studies of cannabis vs. alcohol impairment, and concluded that a blood alcohol concentration (BAC) of 0.05% causes a similar degree of impairment as whole blood THC levels of 2–5 ng/mL, although the type of impairment differs [33–35]. Several recent meta-analyses all concluded that *cannabis increases the risk of crashing*, albeit to a relatively small extent (OR < 2) and to a lesser extent than with alcohol [17, 31, 36, 37]. However, previous research is limited by many technical difficulties involved with studying the collision risk associated with cannabis. Two recent high-quality studies found that low levels of THC (<5 ng/mL) were not associated with a statistically significant increased risk of collision [38, 39]. At higher THC levels (>5 ng/mL), the risk of collision was significantly increased in one study (OR = 3.2), [39] but not in the other (OR = 1.7, $p = 0.35$) [38].

Several caveats are required when applying the cannabis and collision risk data to the medical cannabis population. First, the vast majority of this evidence comes from people who take cannabis recreationally and not for medical reasons. The intent of recreational cannabis use is inherently different than when cannabis is taken for medical reasons. While medical cannabis patients take cannabis to alleviate their symptoms, the typical goal of those using cannabis recreationally is euphoria or relaxation – effects that are commonly achieved by using cannabis with high THC and minimal CBD content, and by inhalation instead of ingestion (see section "Factors Affecting Cognitive Impairment"). This difference makes for different cognitive and psychomotor outcomes in these two populations. In line with this is the mounting evidence that daily use of THC, as is seen in most medical cannabis patients, may increase tolerance to the impairing effects of THC [20, 21, 40]. However, many studies that are used as evidence for cannabis impairment are based upon naive or infrequent users. A study comparing infrequent to daily users found that at a 0.5 mg/kg dose of THC, there was significant impairment in all measures for infrequent users [21]. In contrast, daily users did not show acute impairment in almost all of the impairment tasks, with the one except being a decline in impulse control at high THC concentrations (>10 ng/ml) [21]. This highlights a major issue in translating findings from infrequent/non-medical users to medical populations. It is also important to recognize that medical cannabis patients may have some degree of psychomotor or cognitive impairment resulting from their underlying symptoms or illness. Many of the medical conditions treated with cannabis are associated with increased risk of motor vehicle collisions. For example, epilepsy, multiple sclerosis, schizophrenia, arthritis, insomnia, anxiety, and depression all have shown to increase risk of motor vehicle collisions [41–44]. Treating these conditions with cannabis may actually improve patients' neurocognitive and psychomotor functioning, especially as they develop tolerance to the impairing effects of THC (see section "Frequency of Use and Tolerance") [9]. Another consideration is that medications (such as benzodiazepines, antihistamines, antidepressants, and opioids), which may be used instead of cannabis in some patients, can also increase collision risk. In fact, the risk with many of these medications, although lower than with alcohol, appears to be as high as, or higher than, the risk associated with cannabis [38, 45–47]. There is a clear need for more research on collision risk in the medical cannabis population.

Chronic Adverse Events

Evidence remains varied on chronic adverse health effects associated with chronic cannabis use. It is important to note that much of the evidence comes from recreation users engaging in frequent, high THC potency cannabis use. As such, many of the risks identified may not be applicable to medical populations who have inherently different patterns of use. Among potential risks include worsening mental health, substance dependency, cognitive impairment, and respiratory harm (if cannabis is smoked) [48].

Long-term use of cannabis in some individuals has been associated with psychological impairments such as the worsening of mental health disorders, namely, psychosis or schizophrenia [49], and less clearly, depression, especially if use commenced in adolescence (see Chap. 34 on Cannabinoids and Adolescence) [50]. Dependency may also be a risk, and is estimated to have a lifetime risk of about 9% in cannabis users [51]. In some cases, this may lead to cannabis use disorder (CUD). For more information on the risk factors of CUD please see Chap. 38 on Cannabis Use Disorder.

The association between cannabis use and chronic cognitive deficits is highly debated. Though some evidence shows there may be neurocognitive deficits in long-term, frequent users, the directionality of the association remains unclear. Deficits in verbal learning, memory, and attention have been reported in long-term, heavy cannabis users, but these findings may be attributable to the acute not chronic impairing effects of THC [52, 48]. A recent systematic review and meta-analysis looking at cognivite function in cannabis-using adolescents and young adults found deficits resolved following a period of abstinence [52]. Similar findings in adults have shown full or partial recovery from cognitive deficits following abstinence as well [48]. As previously stated, much of the literature is from recreational populations, but medical cannabis users often have more conservative patterns of use, which are associated with less risk. In fact, one of the more comprehensive studies for medical cannabis, the Cannabis for Management of Pain: Assessment of Safety Study (COMPASS), reported improved cognitive function following year-long use of medical cannabis [53].

Finally, smoking cannabis is a known harm [50]. Chronic use of smoked cannabis has been associated with respiratory effects such as an irritation of the mucosa lining within the bronchi and lungs, as well as chronic bronchitis [50]. It is less clear whether chronic cannabis use is associated with lung cancer or chronic obstructive pulmonary disorder (COPD), as the evidence is typically confounded by tobacco use (see Chap. 23 on Patient Safety Considerations) [50].

Cannabinoid Hyperemesis Syndrome

Cannabis, THC in particular, can produce both antiemetic effects at low doses (i.e., reducing chemotherapy-induced nausea and vomiting) and hyperemetic effects within the gastrointestinal tract and central nervous system at high doses, known as cannabinoid hyperemesis syndrome (CHS) [54–56]. CHS is classified by persistent nausea and abdominal discomfort/pain, which can transition to frequent cyclical vomiting and subsequent weight loss [57] associated with chronic (one to >25 years of use), frequent (weekly to daily), high-dose THC use [56]. A review of CHS (N = 76 studies) in those over 18 years old (25% female) who used cannabis for an average of 12.9 years found that respondents began to notice symptoms of nausea and vomiting after having smoked cannabis for a mean of 9.4 years [54]. Cases of CHS resulting from synthetic cannabis use (i.e., K2, Kryptonite) have also

Table 36.3 Criteria for cannabinoid hyperemesis syndrome

Essential	Primary	Secondary
Chronic cannabis use		
	Severe cyclic nausea and vomiting	
	Cannabis cessation = resolution	
	Hot showers/baths = relief	
	Abdominal pain	
	Frequent (>weekly) cannabis use	
		<50 years old
		>5 kg weight loss
		Morning predominance of symptoms
		Normal bowel habits
		Laboratory, radiographic, endoscopic results = negative

Adapted from Lu and Agito [2]

been observed, which can cause adverse events at lower doses than THC [54, 56]. Although CHS is more common among recreational users with heavy cannabis use, heavy use is necessary but not sufficient to elicit CHS [58] (Table 36.3).

CHS has clinically been categorized into three phases: the prodromal phase (severe anxiety, agitation, and autonomic symptoms including sweating, flushing, thirst, and stomach pain); the hyperemetic/vomiting phase (debilitating abdominal pain, severe cyclical nausea, and vomiting that can happen without warning, taking hot showers or baths for symptom relief); and the recovery phase (resolution of compulsive bathing and other symptoms after prolonged cessation of cannabis use, which can be enhanced by intravenous fluid replacement) [55, 56].

The complex pathophysiology of CHS still remains unclear (Fig. 36.1). In addition to binding to cannabinoid receptors in the brain, THC also binds to cannabinoid receptors within the enteric nervous system. One theory suggests that chronic, heavy, use can cause cannabinoid receptor stimulation in the brain to be overridden by cannabinoid binding in the gut, leading to paradoxical hyperemesis [54]. Prolonged, high doses of THC can alter endocannabinoid functioning through the downregulation of cannabinoid receptor type 1 (CB1), dysregulating stress and anxiety responses, thermoregulation, the transient receptor potential vanilloid (TRPV) system, and certain neurotransmitter systems, thereby potentially mediating the pathophysiology of CHS [55, 56]. Excessive stimulation of enteric cannabinoid receptors may cause diffuse splanchnic vasodilation, potentially contributing to abdominal pain [55]. THC is also known to slow peristalsis and gastric emptying, which may be other contributing factors to the experience of CHS [54]. CHS may have a genetic component to it via hepatic drug-transforming enzymes that increase cannabinoid metabolite levels, promoting emesis [55]. Laboratory tests appear normal aside from mild leukocytosis, hypokalaemia, and ketonuria due to associated dehydration and acute renal failure [55, 59].

CHS prevalence is largely unknown due to symptomatic overlap with other disorders, most notably, cyclical vomiting syndrome (CVS), and therefore is often misdiagnosed [56]. Unlike CVS, CHS is associated with delayed gastric emptying, a relief of symptoms with hot showers and topical capsaicin, and a complete resolution of symptoms upon cessation of cannabis [56, 60].

No diagnostic tests have consistently shown efficacy in diagnosing CHS, including CT, MRI, X-ray, colonoscopies, gastric emptying, ultrasound, and barium swallow tests.

The only permanently effective treatment to date is cannabis abstinence, as confirmed by a recent review (low GRADE quality of evidence; [59]). Additionally, intravenous fluids can assist with rehydration [57]. Other treatments include capsaicin cream, applied topically to an individual's stomach, chest, back, or arms; sedative and anxiolytic medications;

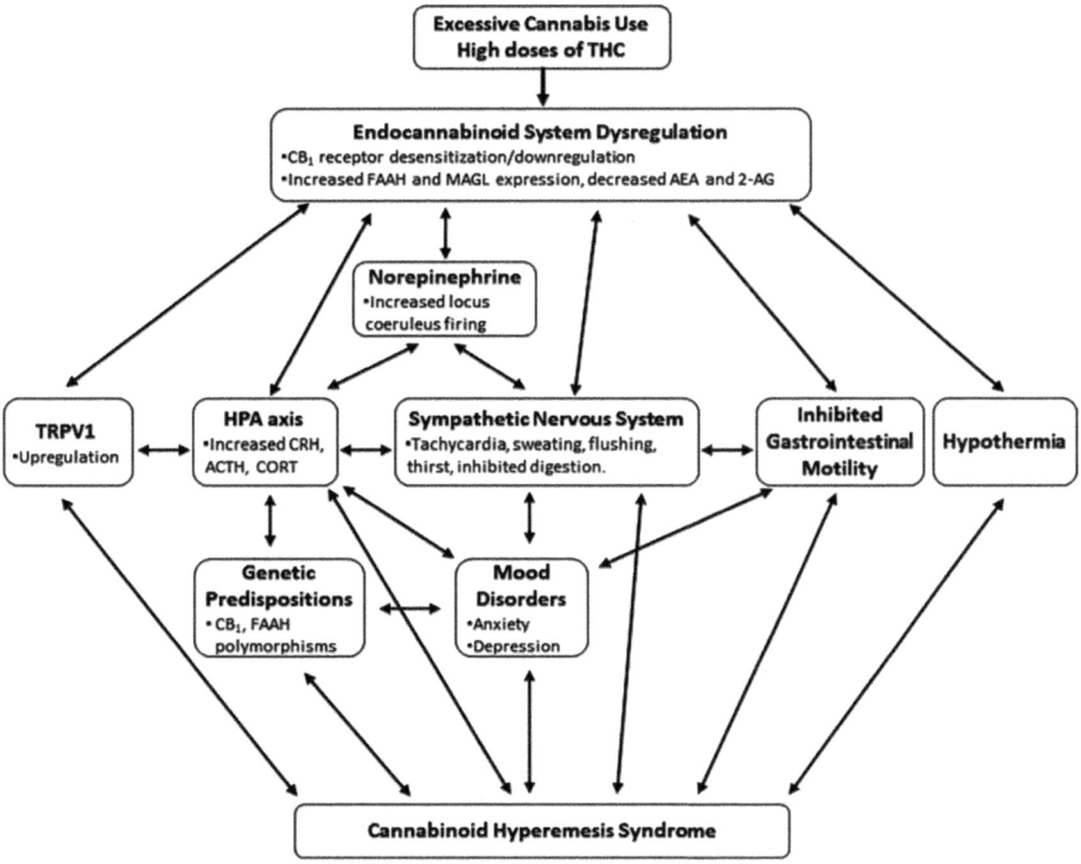

Fig. 36.1 Schematic representation of factors that may contribute to CHS [56]

and dopamine antagonists such as haloperidol, although they are not consistently as effective in reducing symptoms associated with CHS [57, 59, 60]. Conventional antiemetics (i.e., ondansetron, metoclopramide, prochlorperazine, and promethazine) have not been shown to be effective in treating CHS symptoms [55, 56]. Narcotic medications should be avoided when treating CHS, as opioid use can cause bowel dysfunction, potentially worsening CHS symptoms [59].

More research is needed to clarify risk factors associated with CHS, including the dose and duration of cannabis use prior to symptom onset and individuals who may be more sensitive to these effects, as the majority of cannabis users do not experience these effects.

Modifiable and Non-Modifiable Factors Influencing Impairment

It is important to differentiate impairment outcomes related to recreational and medicinal cannabis use. Among medical cannabis patients, symptom management is the primary goal of cannabis use, in comparison to the recreational intake of THC which is predominantly sought to produce euphoria or relaxation [61]. Some people also use recreational cannabis as a coping strategy for negative emotional states. There is evidence that using cannabis for this purpose could interfere with development of healthier coping mechanisms in adolescents and increase the risk of developing cannabis use disorder [62–65]. Supervised medical cannabis patients also typically follow a more consistent and standardized dosing procedure (i.e., "start low and go slow") and have different expectations and goals compared to recreational users [9]. The use of oral cannabis products, such as oils, allows for more precise dosing and is associated with less potential respiratory harm when compared to inhaled cannabis [66].

The way in which cannabis may produce impairment among certain individuals is dependent on several factors, which, when combined, may increase the risk for acute psychotomimetic and cognitive effects. Individualistic considerations encompass genetic and behavioral vulnerabilities that contribute to the increased risk for experiencing impairment upon cannabis consumption. Recent evidence suggests that genetics may account for 69.2–84.1% of correlated associations between cannabis use and psychotic-like experiences (PLEs), although it is largely influenced by frequency of use [49].

Factors influencing impairment include route of administration, chemovars, CBD content, dose, tolerance, alcohol use, and use of other substances, in addition to genetics and personal/family mental health history (Fig. 36.2), as discussed below.

Demographic and Genetic Variables

Genetics

An individual's "endocannabinoid tone," or the makeup and functioning of their endocannabinoid system, can largely influence how cannabis is experienced, particularly through CB1 receptor availability in regions such as the amygdala, hippocampus, and prefrontal cortex [67, 68]. CB1 receptor availability is positively correlated with modulation of amygdala function by THC, suggesting those with increased CB1 density, particularly within the limbic system of the brain, may experience more pronounced effects [68]. Similarly, genetic vulnerability to mental health disorders, including personal or family history of psychoses/mental health disorders, and/or those presenting with prodromal signs and symptoms may dictate ensuing experiences of cannabis use [69–75] as discussed in Chap. 32 on cannabinoids and brain development.

Age

The age at which an individual begins consuming cannabis is also important, as described in Chap. 34 on Cannabinoids and Adolescence. Impairment may be more pronounced among adolescents compared to adults due to brain development and cortical maturation. Differences in goals of use and risk perception between older and younger cannabis users may also influence the types of products, potencies, and routes of administration chosen. Older adults may be at risk for greater impairment due to decreased cognitive reserves and other potential medical complications (see Chap. 23 on Cannabinoid-Based Medicines: Patient Safety Considerations).

Other Sedating Substances

Common over-the-counter medications (e.g. dimenhydrinate, diphenhydramine), prescription medications (e.g. zopiclone, benzodiazepines, opioids, muscle relaxants), as well as other sedating substances, such as alcohol, can cause compounded impairment and sedation when used in combination with THC (see Chap. 23 on Cannabinoid-Based Medicines: Patient Safety Considerations).

Cannabis Potency and Dose

Adverse events are THC dose-dependent, with lower doses producing relatively mild neuropsychiatric and systemic impairment [7]. The use of high THC potency products may increase the risk for adverse events or impairment, due to the ability for a greater amount of THC to be consumed. To minimize cognitive impairment, doses should be based on the mg of THC, not the concentration or % (see Chap. 22 on Cannabinoid-Based Medicines: Dosing, Titration, and Monitoring). Health Canada warns of using products such as resin, hash oil wax, and distillates with high-potent THC [≥20% THC (200 mg/g)], as they can increase the risk of acute and chronic mental health problems [5]. In contrast to THC, CBD has been shown to have a much safer side effect profile, producing almost little to no impairment when administered as a pure isolate.

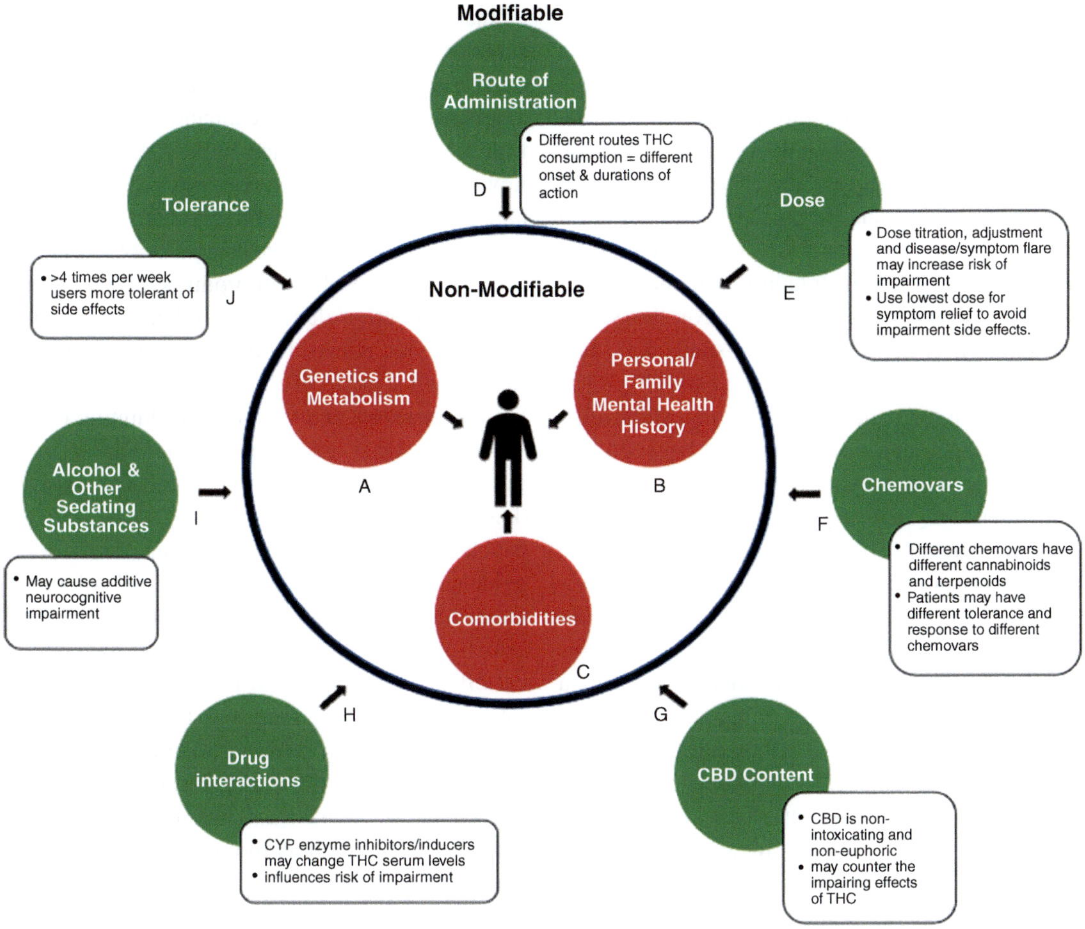

Fig. 36.2 Modifiable and non-modifiable factors influencing acute neurocognitive impairment in medical cannabis users. (**A**) Genetic and metabolic profiles can influence response to cannabinoids. (**B**) Predisposition to or history of mental health conditions may increase risk of impairment. (**C**) Comorbidities that produce symptoms like fatigue, dizziness, or cognitive slowing may compound impairment. (**D**) How cannabis is consumed influences the duration of impairments via differences in absorption and metabolism. (**E**) Severity of impairment is THC dose-dependent. (**F**) Chemical composition (level of various cannabinoids and metabolites) of a cannabis product influences degree of impairment (**G**) Amount of CBD contained in product may balance side effects of THC. (**H**) Drug interactions can alter serum THC levels. (**I**) Use of other sedating recreational or prescribed substances may cause additive impairment. (**J**) Pattern of regular consumption in medical cannabis users decreases drug response, and side effects, to cannabinoids [20]

CBD, when combined with THC, may reduce some of the psychological and cognitive impairments produced by the same dose of THC-only, while THC-induced cardiac effects (e.g., tachycardia) and subjective impairments (e.g., euphoria) remain relatively unchanged [76]. The Lower-Risk Cannabis Use Guidelines also recommend using high levels of CBD-to-THC to minimize impairment [77]. It should be noted that while CBD may decrease the degree of impairment for infrequent or low-dose THC users, there is some evidence that the co-use of high CBD products in individuals who regularly use high THC cannabis may actually cause greater acute impairment [78, 79]. As such, the proportions of CBD:THC play an important role regarding risk of impairment, and may differ depending on the individual.

Cannabis Products and Route of Administration

Each route of administration (e.g. inhalation, oral, oralmucosal) has unique pharmacokinetic properties that determine the onset and duration of action [9]. As such, the route of administration will determine how long an individual may be at risk for impairment. Inhalation methods, such as dried product vaporization, have the shortest duration of action which is usually less than 4 hours in medical cannabis patients [20]. Oral administration methods, such as ingestible oils, have a longer duration of action, between 6-8 hours [20]. This has important implications for individuals engaging in safety sensitive activities, as it dictates the amount of time needed to pass before it is safe to partake in such activities. Product type also impacts risk of impairment because it influences how accurate the cannabis can be dosed. Cannabis oils that come with a graduated syringe allow for patients to know the exact amount of THC mg's they are consuming, decreasing risk of accidental overconsumption. In contrast, smoked or vaporized dried cannabis flower is much harder to accurately dose, and thus may lead to a great risk of impairment (see Chap. 22 on Cannabinoid-Based Medicines: Dosing, Titration, and Monitoring).

Frequency of Use and Tolerance

Consistent, daily use of THC can increase tolerance to impairment [20]. As such, the effect of Cannabis will depend on an individuals pattern of use. Frequent users may be at a lower risk of impairment, especially at low or moderate doses of THC [20]. However, frequent use of high dose THC is associated with a host of adverse events and increased risk for imairment. Multiple definitions of "frequent cannabis use" exist in the literature. For instance, Newmeyer et al. [80] define "frequent" cannabis use as ≥5×/week plus a positive urine screen for metabolites. Whereas occasional use is described as consuming cannabis ≥2×/month and ≤3 times per week plus a positive urine test. In individuals who use cannabis less frequently, lack of tolerance may increase risk of impairment as well [69].

A recent systematic review concluded that the acute effects of a single cannabinoid administration are experienced by a greater degree among novice or occasional users compared to frequent and daily users [81]. Administration of THC in people who seldom used cannabis (<5 times of lifetime use) resulted in significantly increased anxiety, attention deficit, and other adverse psychotomimetic effects. Females in particular tended to experience physical effects such as tremors, pallor, hypotension, and symptoms of fainting [82].

With regular use, tolerance to the impairing effects of THC may be built. The greatest degree of tolerance to cannabis occurs in the psychomotor coordination domain, with some evidence that people can develop full tolerance. Other adverse events, such as acute intoxicating effects, psychological effects, and physiological effects, are blunted to a lesser extent (partial tolerance) [82]. For instance, frequent cannabis users (>4×/week) develop tolerance, showing no neurocognitive or motor impairment following cannabis intake [83–85]. Other important considerations, such as the intent of use, help to clarify the evidence. Cannabis Recommending Clinicians (CRC) can assist patients in building tolerance to the impairing or adverse events associated with THC by utilizing a low dose, slow titration cannabis initiation method (See Chap. 22 on Cannabinoid-Based Medicines: Dosing, Titration & Monitoring).

It may also be informative to compare side effects of medical cannabis with those of alternative therapies. Many of the first- or second-line therapies for chronic neuropathic pain (e.g., gabapentinoids, tricyclic antidepressants, or opioids) are frequently associated with morbidity, and even mortality, when taken in overdose, especially for opioids. This is in contrast to medical cannabis-related neurocognitive impairments, which appear to be minimal and are decreased overtime without reduced therapeutic benefit [52]. Evidence suggests that acute neurocognitive impairment related to medical cannabis use among chronic non-cancer pain or spasticity populations is dose-dependently related to THC and dissipates over time [12, 53, 86–90]. Unlike data pertaining to recreational populations, less than 0.5% of chronic, daily medical cannabis users experience euphoria or paranoia, [91] suggesting acute impairment dissipates as tolerance increases.

Summary

To minimize neurocognitive impairments, it is important to have a goal-setting discussion with patients in addition to completing a full history, including all risk factors mentioned above, including, but not limited to, age, sex, personal and family history of mental health illness (including substance use disorders), history of cannabis use (number of years used, frequency of use over those years), current frequency of use (number of days per month and/or number of times per day), dose used each time, chemovar composition (THC, CBD, other cannabinoids and terpenes), and, importantly, intent for use (including whether it is being used as a coping strategy for negative mental states).

References

1. American Psychiatric Association. Diagnostic and statistical manual of mental disorders. 5th ed. Arlington: American Psychiatric Association; 2013.
2. Patel J, Marwaha R. Cannabis use disorder. In: StatPearls [Internet]. Treasure Island: StatPearls Publishing; 2019.
3. World Health Organization. ICD-10, vol. 2. 5th ed. Geneva: World Health Organization; 2016.
4. Word Health Organization. The ICD-10 classification of mental and behavioural disorders: diagnostic criteria for research. Geneva: World Health Organization; 1993.
5. Health Canada. Information for health care professionals: cannabis (marihuana, marijuana) and the cannabinoids. 2019. Available at: https://www.canada.ca/content/dam/hc-sc/documents/services/drugs-medication/cannabis/information-medical-practitioners/information-health-care-professionals-cannabis-cannabinoids-eng.pdf.
6. Bloomfield MA, Hindocha C, Green SF, Wall MB, Lees R, Petrilli K, et al. The neuropsychopharmacology of cannabis: a review of human imaging studies. Pharmacol Ther. 2019;195:132–61.
7. Levinsohn EA, Hill KP. Clinical uses of cannabis and cannabinoids in the United States. J Neurol Sci. 2020;411:116717.
8. Broyd SJ, van Hell HH, Beale C, Yücel M, Solowij N. Acute and chronic effects of cannabinoids on human cognition—a systematic review. Biol Psychiatry. 2016;79(7):557–67.
9. MacCallum CA, Russo EB. Practical considerations in medical cannabis administration and dosing. Eur J Intern Med. 2018;49:12–9.
10. Brandt J. The Hopkins verbal learning test: development of a new memory test with six equivalent forms. Clin Neuropsychol. 1991;5:125–42.
11. Coughlan AK, Hollows SE. The adult memory and information processing battery (AMIPB). Leeds: St James University Hospital; 1985.
12. Olla P, Rykulski N, Hurtubise JL, Bartol S, Foote R, Cutler L, et al. Short-term effects of cannabis consumption on cognitive performance in medical cannabis patients. Appl Neuropsychol Adult. 2019:1–11.
13. Gronwall D. Paced auditory serial-addition task: a measure of recovery from concussion. Percept Mot Skills. 1977;44:367–73.
14. Wechsler D. Manual for the Wechsler adult intelligence scale. New York: Psychological Corporation; 1955.
15. Dominic A. Carone Ph.D. (2007) E. Strauss, E. M. S. Sherman, & O. Spreen, A Compendium of Neuropsychological Tests: Administration, Norms, and Commentary, Applied Neuropsychology. 2007;14(1): 62–63. https://doi.org/10.1080/09084280701280502.
16. Bondallaz P, Favrat B, Chtioui H, Fornari E, Maeder P, Giroud C. Cannabis and its effects on driving skills. Forensic Sci Int. 2016;268:92–102.
17. Rogeberg O, Elvik R. The effects of cannabis intoxication on motor vehicle collision revisited and revised. Addiction. 2016;111(8):1348–59.
18. College of Family Physicians of Canada. Authorizing dried cannabis for chronic pain or anxiety: preliminary guidance. 2014. Retrieved from: https://portal.cfpc.ca/resourcesdocs/uploadedFiles/Resources/_PDFs/Authorizing%20Dried%20Cannabis%20for%20Chronic%20Pain%20or%20Anxiety.pdf.
19. Health Canada. Canadian alcohol and drug use monitoring survey (CADUMS). Ottawa: Health Canada; 2013.
20. Eadie L, Lo LA, Christiansen A, Brubacher JR, Barr AM, Panenka WJ and MacCallum CA (2021) Duration of Neurocognitive Impairment With Medical Cannabis Use: A Scoping Review. Front. Psychiatry 12:638962. https://doi.org/10.3389/fpsyt.2021.638962.
21. Ramaekers JG, Kauert G, Theunissen EL, Toennes SW, Moeller MR. Neurocognitive performance during acute THC intoxication in heavy and occasional cannabis users. J Psychopharmacol. 2009;23(3):266-77. https://doi.org/10.1177/0269881108092393.
22. Curran HV, Brignell C, Fletcher S, Middleton P, Henry J. Cognitive and subjective dose-response effects

of acute oral Delta 9-tetrahydrocannabinol (THC) in infrequent cannabis users. Psychopharmacology (Berl). 2002;164(1):61-70. https://doi.org/10.1007/s00213-002-1169-0.
23. Arkell TR, Vinckenbosch F, Kevin RC, Theunissen EL, McGregor IS, Ramaekers JG. Effect of Cannabidiol and Δ9-Tetrahydrocannabinol on Driving Performance: A Randomized Clinical Trial. JAMA. 2020;324(21):2177-2186. https://doi.org/10.1001/jama.2020.21218.
24. Spindle TR, Cone EJ, Goffi E, Weerts EM, Mitchell JM, Winecker RE, Bigelow GE, Flegel RR, Vandrey R. Pharmacodynamic effects of vaporized and oral cannabidiol (CBD) and vaporized CBD-dominant cannabis in infrequent cannabis users. Drug Alcohol Depend. 2020;211:107937. https://doi.org/10.1016/j.drugalcdep.2020.107937.
25. Brands B, Mann RE, Wickens CM, Sproule B, Stoduto G, Sayer GS, et al. Acute and residual effects of smoked cannabis: impact on driving speed and lateral control, heart rate, and self-reported drug effects. Drug Alcohol Depend. 2019;205:107641.
26. Berghaus G, Scheer N, Schmidt P. Effects of cannabis on psychomotor skills and driving performance – a metaanalysis of experimental studies. Adelaide: International Council on Alcohol Drugs and Traffic Safety (ICADTS); 1995.
27. Ramaekers JG, Berghaus G, van Laar M, Drummer OH. Dose related risk of motor vehicle crashes after cannabis use. Drug Alcohol Depend. 2004;73(2):109–19.
28. Grotenhermen F, Leson G, Berghaus G, Drummer OH, Krüger HP, Longo M, Moskowitz H, Perrine B, Ramaekers J, Smiley A, Tunbridge R. Developing science-based per se limits for driving under the influence of cannabis (DUIC): findings and recommendations by an expert panel. Report. Washington, DC: International Association for Cannabis as Medicine; 2005.
29. Ronen A, Gershon P, Drobiner H, Rabinovich A, Bar-Hamburger R, Mechoulam R, Cassuto Y, Shinar D, Ronen A, Gershon P, Drobiner H, Rabinovich A, Bar-Hamburger R, Mechoulam R, Cassuto Y, Shinar D. Effects of THC on driving performance, physiological state and subjective feelings relative to alcohol. Accid Anal Prev. 2008;40(3):926–34.
30. Sewell RA, Poling J, Sofuoglu M, Sewell RA, Poling J, Sofuoglu M. The effect of cannabis compared with alcohol on driving. Am J Addict. 2009;18(3):185–93.
31. Hartman RL, Brown TL, Milavetz G, Spurgin A, Pierce RS, Gorelick DA, Gaffney G, Huestis MA. Cannabis effects on driving lateral control with and without alcohol. Drug Alcohol Depend. 2015;154:25–37.
32. Doroudgar S, Mae Chuang H, Bohnert K, Canedo J, Burrowes S, Perry PJ. Effects of chronic marijuana use on driving performance. Traffic Inj Prev. 2018;19(7):680–6.
33. Grotenhermen F, Leson G, Berghaus G, Drummer OH, Kruger HP, Longo M, Moskowitz H, Perrine B, Ramaekers JG, Smiley A, Tunbridge R. Developing limits for driving under cannabis. Addiction. 2007;102(12):1910–7.
34. Berghaus G, Sticht G, Grellner W, Lenz D, Naumann T, Wiesenmuller S. Meta-analysis of empirical studies concerning the effects of medicines and illegal drugs including pharmacokinetics on safe driving. 2010. Available from: http://www.druid-project.eu.
35. Vindenes V, Jordbru D, Knapskog A-B, Kvan E, Mathisrud G, Slordal L, Morland J. Impairment based legislative limits for driving under the influence of non-alcohol drugs in Norway. Forensic Sci Int. 2012;219(1–3):1–11.
36. Asbridge M, Hayden JA, Cartwright JL. Acute cannabis consumption and motor vehicle collision risk: systematic review of observational studies and meta-analysis. BMJ. 2012;344:e536.
37. Li MC, Brady JE, DiMaggio CJ, Lusardi AR, Tzong KY, Li G. Marijuana use and motor vehicle crashes. Epidemiol Rev. 2012;34:65–72.
38. Brubacher JR, Chan H, Erdelyi S, Macdonald S, Asbridge M, Mann RE, Eppler J, Lund A, MacPherson A, Martz W, Schreiber WE, Brant R, Purssell RA. Cannabis use as a risk factor for causing motor vehicle crashes: a prospective study. Addiction. 2019;114(9):1616–26.
39. Drummer OH, Gerostamoulos D, Di Rago M, Woodford NW, Morris C, Frederiksen T, Jachno K, Wolfe R. Odds of culpability associated with use of impairing drugs in injured drivers in Victoria, Australia. Accid Anal Prev. 2019;135:105389.
40. Ramaekers JG, Theunissen EL, de Brouwer M, Toennes SW, Moeller MR, Kauert G. Tolerance and cross-tolerance to neurocognitive effects of THC and alcohol in heavy cannabis users. Psychopharmacology (Berl). 2011;214(2):391-401. https://doi.org/10.1007/s00213-010-2042-1.
41. Freidel M, Tiel-Wilck K, Schreiber H, Prechtl A, Essner U, Lang M. Drug-resistant MS spasticity treatment with Sativex® add-on and driving ability. Acta Neurol Scand. 2015;131:9–16.
42. Charlton JL, Koppel S, O'Hare M, Andrea D, Smith G, Khodr B, et al. Influence of chronic illness on crash involvement of motor vehicle drivers. Monash University Accident Research Centre Reports, No. 213. 2004. p 482.
43. McGwin JG, Sims RV, Pulley L, Roseman JM. Relations among chronic medical conditions, medications, and automobile crashes in the elderly: a population-based case-control study. Am J Epidemiol. 2000;152:424–31.
44. Sagberg F. Driver health and crash involvement: a case-control study. Accid Anal Prev. 2006;38:28–34.
45. Compton RP, Berning A. Drug and alcohol crash risk. J Drug Addict Educ Erad. 2015;11(1):29.
46. Elvik R. Risk of road accident associated with the use of drugs: a systematic review and meta-analysis of evidence from epidemiological studies. Accid Anal Prev. 2013;60:254–67.
47. Hels T, Lyckegaard A, Simonsen KW, Steentoft A, Bernhoft IM. Risk of severe driver injury by driv-

ing with psychoactive substances. Accid Anal Prev. 2013;59:346–56.
48. Hall W, Degenhardt L. The adverse health effects of chronic cannabis use. Drug Test Anal. 2014;6(1-2):39-45
49. Karcher NR, Barch DM, Demers CH, Baranger DA, Heath AC, Lynskey MT, Agrawal A. Genetic predisposition vs individual-specific processes in the association between psychotic-like experiences and cannabis use. JAMA Psychiat. 2019;76(1):87–94.
50. National Academies of Sciences, Engineering, and Medicine. The health effects of cannabis and cannabinoids: the current state of evidence and recommendations for research. Washington, DC: National Academies Press; 2017.
51. Anthony J. Cannabis Dependence: Its Nature, Consequences and Treatment, (Eds: R.A. Roffman, R.S. Stephens). Cambridge University Press, Cambridge, 2006, pp. 58–105.
52. Scott JC, Slomiak ST, Jones JD, Rosen AF, Moore TM, Gur RC. Association of cannabis with cognitive functioning in adolescents and young adults: a systematic review and meta-analysis. JAMA Psychiat. 2018;75(6):585–95.
53. Ware MA, Wang T, Shapiro S, Collet JP, Boulanger A, Esdaile JM, et al. Cannabis for the management of pain: assessment of safety study (COMPASS). J Pain. 2015;16(12):1233–42.
54. Parekh JD, Wozniak SE, Khan K, Dutta SK. Cannabinoid hyperemesis syndrome. BMJ Case Rep. 2016;2016:bcr2015213620. 2016. https://doi.org/10.1136/bcr-2015-213620.
55. Lu ML, Agito MD. Cannabinoid hyperemesis syndrome: Marijuana is both antiemetic and proemetic. Cleve Clin J Med. 2015;82(7):429–34.
56. DeVuono MV, Parker LA. Cannabinoid Hyperemesis Syndrome: A Review of Potential Mechanisms. Cannabis and Cannabinoid Research. 2020;5(2):132–144.
57. Institute for Safe Medication Practices Canada. Medications Most Frequently Reported in Harm Incidents over the Past 5 Years (2015-2020). ISMP Canada. 2020:20(11).
58. Albert K, Sivilotti ML, Gareri J, Day A, Ruberto, AJ, Hookey LC. Hair cannabinoid concentrations in emergency patients with cannabis hyperemesis syndrome. Canad J Emerg Med. 2019:21(4);477–81.
59. Sorensen CJ, DeSanto K, Borgelt L, Phillips KT, Monte AA. Cannabinoid hyperemesis syndrome: diagnosis, pathophysiology, and treatment—a systematic review. J Med Toxicol. 2017;13(1):71–87.
60. Pergolizzi Jr JV, LeQuang JA, Bisney JF. Cannabinoid hyperemesis. Med Cannabis Cannabinoids. 2018;1(2):73–95.
61. Walsh Z, Callaway R, Belle-Isle L, et al. Cannabis for therapeutic purposes: patient characteristics, access, and reasons for use. Int J Drug Policy. 2013;24: 511–6.
62. Benschop A, Liebregts N, van der Pol P, Schaap R, Buisman R, van Laar M, van den Brink W, de Graaf R, Korf DJ. Reliability and validity of the Marijuana Motives Measure among young adult frequent cannabis users and associations with cannabis dependence. Addict Behav. 2015;40:91–5.
63. Colder CR, Lee YH, Frndak S, Read JP, Wieczorek WF. Internalizing symptoms and cannabis and alcohol use: between-and within-person risk pathways with coping motives. J Consult Clin Psychol. 2019;87:629–44.
64. Mitchell H, Zvolensky MJ, Marshall EC, Bonn-Miller MO, Vujanovic AA. Incremental validity of coping-oriented marijuana use motives in the prediction of affect based psychological vulnerability. J Psychopathol Behav Assess. 2007;29:277–88.
65. Moitra E, Christopher PP, Anderson BJ, Stein MD. Coping-motivated marijuana use correlates with DSM-5 cannabis use disorder and psychological distress among emerging adults. Psychol Addict Behav. 2015;29:627–32.
66. Halladay JE, Boyle MH, Munn C, Jack SM, Georgiades K. Sex differences in the association between cannabis use and suicidal ideation and attempts, depression, and psychological distress among Canadians. Can J Psychiatry. 2019;64(5):345–50.
67. Lorenzetti V, Solowij N, Yücel M. The role of cannabinoids in neuroanatomic alterations in cannabis users. Biol Psychiatry. 2016;79(7):e17–31.
68. Bhattacharyya S, Egerton A, Kim E, Rosso L, Barros DR, Hammers A, et al. Acute induction of anxiety in humans by delta-9-tetrahydrocannabinol related to amygdalar cannabinoid-1 (CB1) receptors. Sci Rep. 2017;7(1):15025.
69. Halah MP, Zochniak MP, Barr MS, George TP. Cannabis use and psychiatric disorders: implications for mental health and addiction treatment. Curr Addict Rep. 2016;3(4):450–62.
70. Borodovsky JT, Budney AJ. Cannabis regulatory science: risk–benefit considerations for mental disorders. Int Rev Psychiatry. 2018;30(3):183–202.
71. Bonner WA, Andkhoie M, Thompson C, Farag M, Szafron M. Patterns and factors of problematic marijuana use in the Canadian population: evidence from three cross-sectional surveys. Can J Public Health. 2017;108(2):e110–6.
72. Di Forti M, Sallis H, Allegri F, Trotta A, Ferraro L, Stilo SA, et al. Daily use, especially of high-potency cannabis, drives the earlier onset of psychosis in cannabis users. Schizophr Bull. 2013;40(6):1509–17.
73. Moore TH, Zammit S, Lingford-Hughes A, Barnes TR, Jones PB, Burke M, Lewis G. Cannabis use and risk of psychotic or affective mental health outcomes: a systematic review. Lancet. 2007;370(9584):319–28.
74. Schubart CD, Boks MPM, Breetvelt EJ, Van Gastel WA, Groenwold RHH, Ophoff RA, et al. Association between cannabis and psychiatric hospitalization. Acta Psychiatr Scand. 2011;123(5):368–75.
75. Hall KE, Monte AA, Chang T, Fox J, Brevik C, Vigil DI, et al. Mental health–related emergency department visits associated with cannabis in Colorado. Acad Emerg Med. 2018;25(5):526–37.

76. Freeman AM, Petrilli K, Lees R, Hindocha C, Mokrysz C, Curran HV, et al. How does cannabidiol (CBD) influence the acute effects of delta-9-tetrahydrocannabinol (THC) in humans? A systematic review. Neurosci Biobehav Rev. 2019;107:696–712.
77. Fischer B, Russell C, Sabioni P, van den Brink W, Le Foll B, Hall W, et al. Lower-risk cannabis use guidelines: a comprehensive update of evidence and recommendations. Am J Public Health. 2017;107(8):e1–e12.
78. Solowij N, Broyd S, Greenwood LM, van Hell H, Martelozzo D, Rueb K, et al. A randomised controlled trial of vaporised Δ9-tetrahydrocannabinol and cannabidiol alone and in combination in frequent and infrequent cannabis users: acute intoxication effects. Eur Arch Psychiatry Clin Neurosci. 2019;269(1):17–35.
79. Morgan CJ, Freeman TP, Hindocha C, Schafer G, Gardner C, Curran HV. Individual and combined effects of acute delta-9-tetrahydrocannabinol and cannabidiol on psychotomimetic symptoms and memory function. Transl Psychiatry. 2018;8(1):181.
80. Newmeyer MN, Swortwood MJ, Abulseoud OA, Huestis MA. Subjective and physiological effects, and expired carbon monoxide concentrations in frequent and occasional cannabis smokers following smoked, vaporized, and oral cannabis administration. Drug Alcohol Depend. 2017;175:67–76.
81. Colizzi M, Bhattacharyya S. Cannabis use and the development of tolerance: a systematic review of human evidence. Neurosci Biobehav Rev. 2018;93:1–25.
82. Colizzi M, Weltens N, McGuire P, Van Oudenhove L, Bhattacharyya S. Descriptive psychopathology of the acute effects of intravenous delta-9-tetrahydrocannabinol administration in humans. Brain Sci. 2019;9(4):93.
83. Ramaekers JG, Mason NL, Theunissen EL. Blunted highs: pharmacodynamic and behavioral models of cannabis tolerance. Eur Neuropsychopharmacol. 2020;36:191–205.
84. Desrosiers NA, Ramaekers JG, Chauchard E, Gorelick DA, Huestis MA. Smoked cannabis' psychomotor and neurocognitive effects in occasional and frequent smokers. J Anal Toxicol. 2015;39(4):251–61.
85. Nurmikko TJ, Serpell MG, Hoggart B, Toomey PJ, Morlion BJ, Haines D. Sativex successfully treats neuropathic pain characterised by allodynia: a randomised, double-blind, placebo-controlled clinical trial. Pain. 2007;133(1–3):210–20.
86. Wilsey B, Marcotte T, Tsodikov A, Millman J, Bentley H, Gouaux B, Fishman S. A randomized, placebo-controlled, crossover trial of cannabis cigarettes in neuropathic pain. J Pain. 2008;9(6):506–21.
87. Corey-Bloom J, Wolfson T, Gamst A, Jin S, Marcotte TD, Bentley H, Gouaux B. Smoked cannabis for spasticity in multiple sclerosis: a randomized, placebo-controlled trial. CMAJ. 2012;184(10):1143–50.
88. Notcutt W, Price M, Miller R, Newport S, Phillips C, Simmons S, Sansom C. Initial experiences with medicinal extracts of cannabis for chronic pain: results from 34 "N of 1" studies. Anaesthesia. 2004;59(5):440–52.
89. Wilsey B, Marcotte T, Deutsch R, Gouaux B, Sakai S, Donaghe H. Low-dose vaporized cannabis significantly improves neuropathic pain. J Pain. 2013;14(2):136–48.
90. Wilsey B, Marcotte TD, Deutsch R, Zhao H, Prasad H, Phan A. An exploratory human laboratory experiment evaluating vaporized cannabis in the treatment of neuropathic pain from spinal cord injury and disease. J Pain. 2016;17(9):982–1000.
91. Volkow ND, Swanson JM, Evins AE, DeLisi LE, Meier MH, Gonzalez R, et al. Effects of cannabis use on human behavior, including cognition, motivation, and psychosis: a review. JAMA Psychiat. 2016;73(3):292–7.
92. Wang T, Collet JP, Shapiro S, Ware MA. Adverse effects of medical cannabinoids: a systematic review. CMAJ 2008;178:1669–78.
93. Russo EB, Etges T, Stott C, Wright S, Mohammed A, Robson P. Sativex safety profile is improving over time. 21st Annual Symposium on the Cannabinoids. St. Charles, IL, USA: International Cannabinoid Research Society; 2011. p. GW1.

37 Cannabis Vaping Hazards

Qian Cece Chen and Samer N. Narouze

Introduction

Vaping is the practice of inhaling a vapor produced by a vaping device, often an electronic cigarette or e-cigarette. E-cigarettes are battery-powered devices that can turn substances into aerosol inhalants. These devices utilize cartridges purchased by the users that can contain liquid forms of nicotine or cannabis, in addition to flavoring and other chemicals. The device then heats the liquid in the cartridges, turning it into vapor that can be inhaled. Vaping marijuana involves inhaling heated THC and/or CBD oil [1].

E-cigarettes' popularity in the United States began in 2007, and since then e-cigarette has become the mostly commonly used product among the youth. It has been reported that from 2017 to 2018, usage among high school students increased from 11.7% to 20.8% [2]. These devices were originally created for inhaling nicotine, believed to be a safer alternative to traditional cigarette smoking. However according to the American Lung Association, inhalation of any type of substance can be injurious to the lungs [3]. People using e-cigarettes can be exposed to heavy metals, volatile organic compounds, and other ingredients that are currently being investigated for their potential harmful effect [2]. In 2019, an outbreak of multiple cases of severe lung injury associated with vaping prompted health authorities to begin a public health investigation [4].

Q. C. Chen (✉)
Department of Anesthesiology, Perioperative Care, and Pain Medicine, NYU Langone Health, New York, NY, USA
e-mail: Qian.Chen2@nyulangone.org

S. N. Narouze
Western Reserve Hospital, Center For Pain Medicine, Cuyahoga Falls, OH, USA

Effect of Vaping on Lungs

Though e-cigarettes have been popular for years, it was not until July of 2019 that health officials began to notice their health-damaging effects. Around that time both the Wisconsin Department of Health Services and Illinois Department of Public Health began to receive multiple reports of cases associated with vaping-related severe lung injury that was occurring in previously young health patients [2, 4]. A public health investigation was then begun, and since then, the Centers for Disease Control and Prevention (CDC) has recorded similar cases in at least 25 states in the United States [2].

By October 2019, 867 cases were reported. Of these, 86% of the patients used THC-containing e-cigarettes within 3 months of onset of symptoms. By December 2019, nearly 2561 cases of such lung injury have been reported, 55 of which resulted in deaths [2] (Fig. 37.1).

The culprits are believed to be harmful ingredients found in the vaping products, including vitamin E acetate, oils, and lipid components. Vitamin E acetate which is an additive used in vaping prod-

S. N. Narouze (ed.), *Cannabinoids and Pain*, https://doi.org/10.1007/978-3-030-69186-8_37

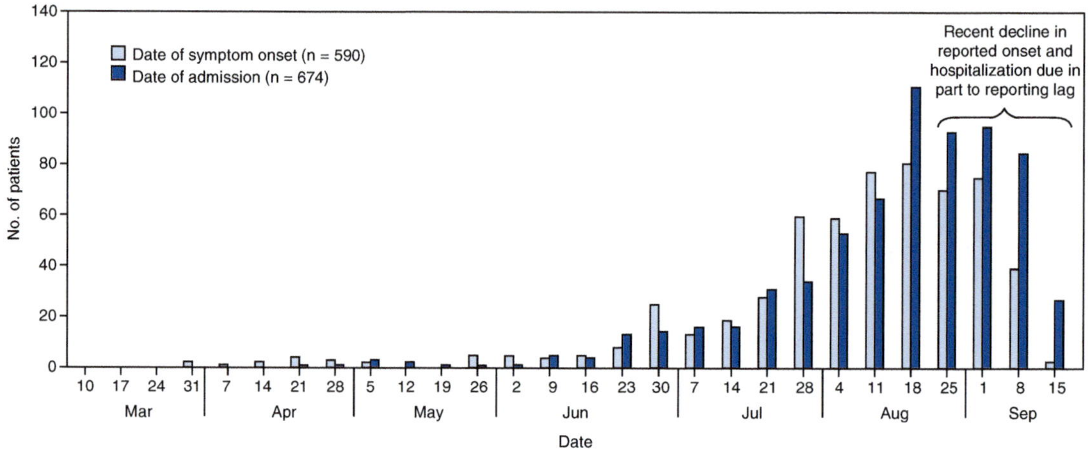

Fig. 37.1 CDC data on reported cases of vaping-associated lung injuries in the United States from March to Sept 2019 [1]

ucts is considered to be particularly harmful. The flavorings used also contain aldehydes and alcohols that when heated, mixed with other ingredients, and aerosolized can create compounds that may be harmful to the lungs. Whether there are additional ingredients that may also be toxic is still being investigated [5] (Fig. 37.2).

Patient Presentation

Patients who presented with EVALI (e-cigarette or *vaping* product use-associated *lung* injury) have presented with an array of symptoms that included dyspnea (87%), fever (81%), coughs (83%), chest pain (55%), nausea and vomiting (66%), and diarrhea (43%) [2, 7]. Of those who also presented with hypoxemia, 38% of the patients had oxygen saturation between 89% and 94% on room air, while 31% had oxygen saturation of less than 89% on room air. The above symptoms can develop and progress over a period of few days to 6 months [4].

Laboratory Findings

Lab findings in patients with EVALI can be variable and non-specific. According to one study, 87% of the patients presented with leukocytosis with >80% neutrophil count. Eosinophil count however tended to be <2% in these patients. There was also evidence of slightly elevated serum aminotransferase levels in 50% of the patients. About 30% of the patients had mild electrolyte changes including hyponatremia and hypokalemia [4].

Many of the EVALI patients also underwent bronchoscopy with bronchoalveolar lavage. The obtained samples commonly showed neutrophilia and lipid-laden macrophages [4].

Imaging Findings

On CT imaging, patients with EVALI commonly show bibasilar, ground-glass lung opacities. There tends to be also evidence of diffuse alveolar damage (Fig. 37.3). Some patients also had pneumomediastinum, pneumothorax, or pleural effusions. Finally in some cases, there was evidence of lipoid pneumonia, which is the result of an inflammatory response to the presence of lipids in the lungs that can occur from inhalation of oil-based products like CBD oil or other oil-based ingredients used in vaping products. Not all imaging findings occur acutely; some can develop over days to months [2, 4].

Fig. 37.2 Frequently reported brand names of tetrahydrocannabinol (THC) and nicotine-containing e-cigarette or vaping, products reported by patients with lung injury. (CDC data-Illinois and Wisconsin, 2019 [6])

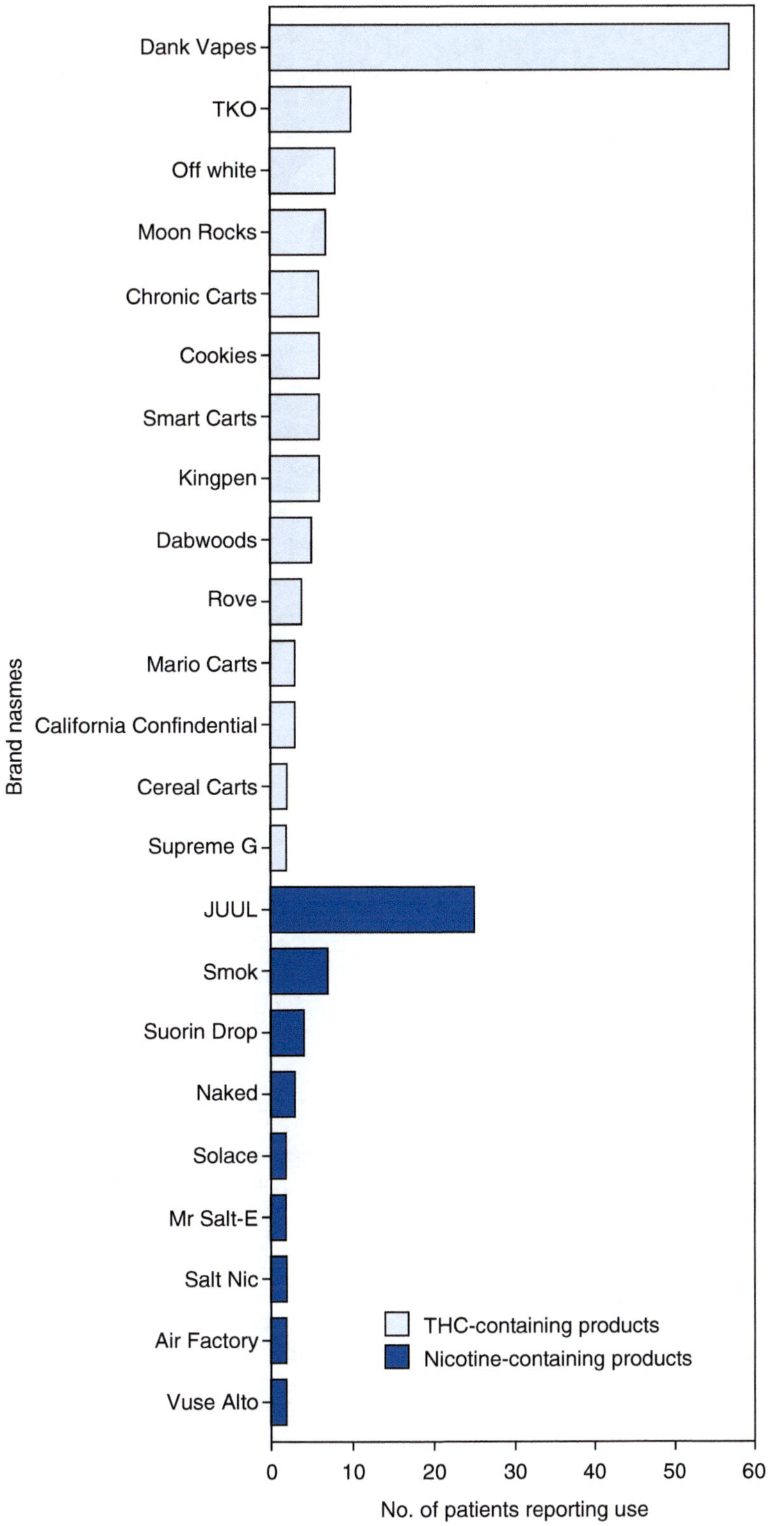

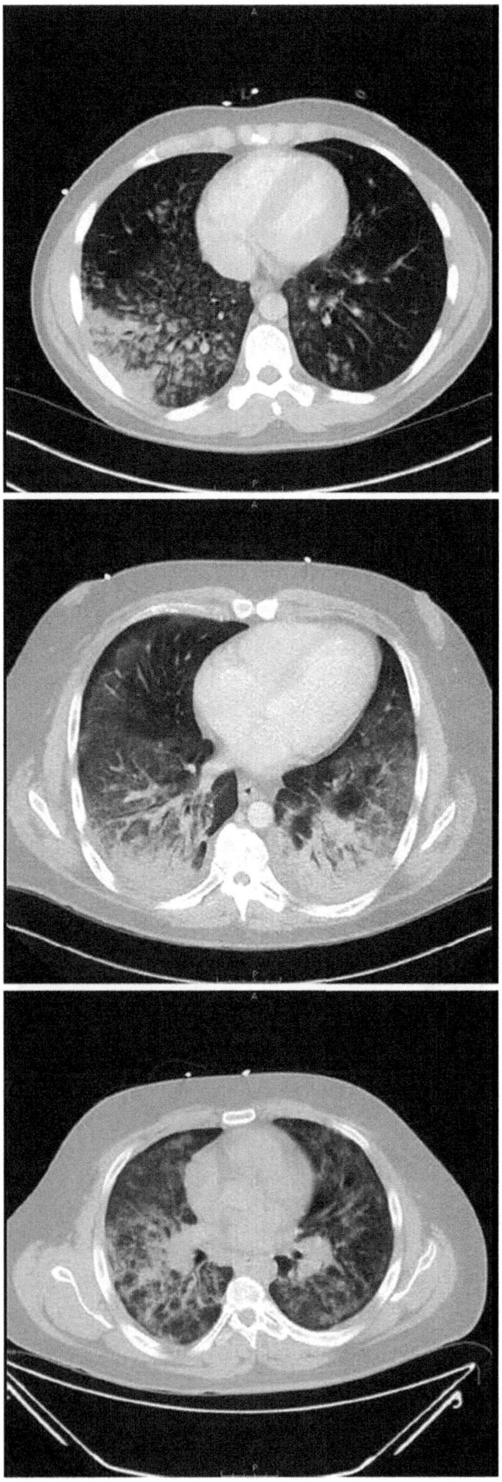

Fig. 37.3 Computerized tomography (CT) images showing diffuse lung infiltrates in three patients with e-cigarette-associated severe lung disease. (CDC data from North Carolina, July–August 2019 [8])

Pathological Findings

The pathological findings associated with EVALI are still poorly understood. A study that examined 17 cases showed histopathology findings consistent with acute fibrinous pneumonitis, diffuse alveolar damage, and organizing pneumonia. There was also evidence of foamy macrophages and pneumocyte vacuolization. Findings of prominent neutrophils with rare eosinophils are consistent with blood work results described in other studies. Unlike the findings from the imaging studies however, the pathological findings did not find any evidence of lipoid pneumonia. It is suspected that the lipids may be a sign of acute exposure but not evidence of developing disease [9] (Fig. 37.4).

Clinical Course

In a study that examined 53 patients who presented to the ER for vaping-related symptoms, 94% of the patients had to be hospitalized with a length of stay of about 1 week. 58% of the patients required ICU admission for respiratory failure, and 32% required intubation with ventilatory support. There were no patients that required conversion of an endotracheostomy tube to a tracheostomy. Out of the 53 patients, 15 had documented diagnosis of acute respiratory distress syndrome (ARDS). Two patients ultimately required conversion to extracorporeal membrane oxygenation (ECMO) with one eventual patient death [2].

Direct Effect of Marijuana on Lungs

In addition to the damaging effect of vaping, marijuana itself, when inhaled, has been found to also cause injurious effects on the lungs. When inhaled, marijuana can cause increased cough, sputum production, wheezing, acute bronchitis, and impaired ciliary and alveolar macrophage functions, potentially leading to higher risk for pulmonary infections [10]. Several cases have demonstrated that marijuana itself can cause spontaneous pneumothorax in otherwise healthy young patients [10, 11].

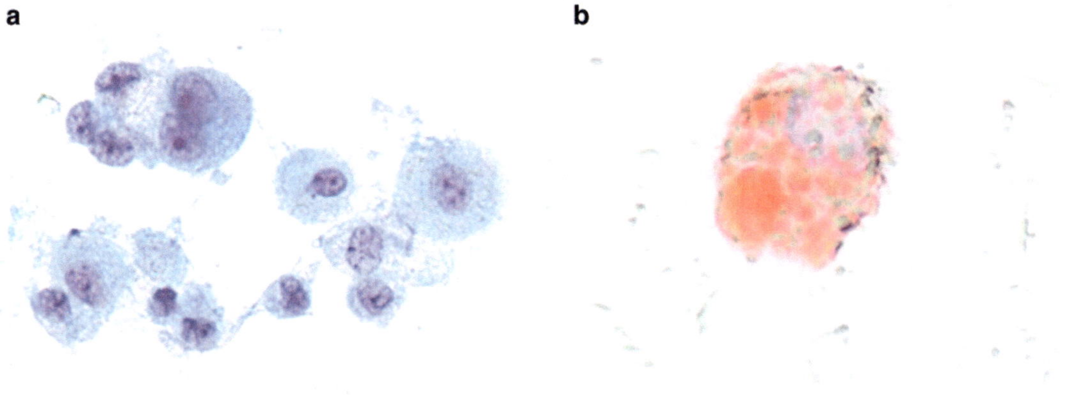

Fig. 37.4 Microscopic picture of a bronchoalveolar lavage sample (**a** Papanicolaou stain and **b** oil red O stain) from a patient with acute lung injury associated with vaping. (CDC data from North Carolina, during July–August 2019 [8])

Conclusion

All of the research and clinical findings thus far have strongly indicated the dangers of vaping THC and CBD. Though legalization of marijuana has increased over the years, some states are now warning the population of the health risks associated with using it in the vaping form. Because some users may be obtaining their vaping products through the black market, CDC has a particular warning against such products as the ingredients may be unknown or variable. Even with the products that are sold legally however, due to lack of regulation, there is still not a guarantee that the labels accurately reflect all of the ingredients [12]. One of the ingredients, vitamin E acetate, has been firmly established as one of the sources for vaping-associated lung injury. Until further research can investigate the other ingredients used in vaping products, CDC and other health organizations have delivered a general warning against all vaping products.

References

1. National Institute on Drug Abuse. "Vaping Devices (Electronic Cigarettes) DrugFacts." National Institute on Drug Abuse. Accessed on 16 June 2020.
2. Layden JE, Ghinai I, Pray I, Kimball A, Layer M, et al. Pulmonary illness related to E-cigarette use-final report. N Engl J Med. 2020;382(10):903–16.
3. "Marijuana and Lung Health." American Lung Association. www.lung.org/quit-smoking/smoking-facts/health-effects/marijuana-and-lung-health.
4. Henry TS, Kanne JP, Kligerman SJ. Imaging of vaping-associated lung disease. N Engl J Med. 2019;381(15):1486–7.
5. Blount BC, Karwowski MP, Morel-Espinosa M, Rees J, et al. Evaluation of bronchoalveolar lavage fluid from patients in an outbreak of E-cigarette, or vaping, product use–associated lung injury – 10 states, August–October 2019. MMWR Morb Mortal Wkly Rep. 2019;68(45):1040–1.
6. Ghinai I, Pray IW, Navon L, et al. E-cigarette product use, or vaping, among persons with associated lung injury — Illinois and Wisconsin, April–September 2019. MMWR Morb Mortal Wkly Rep. 2019;68:865–9. https://doi.org/10.15585/mmwr.mm6839e2.
7. Carlos WG, Crotty Alexander LE, Gross JE, Dela Cruz CS, et al. E-cigarette or vaping product use-associated lung injury (EVALI). Am J Respir Crit Care Med. 2019;200(7):P13–4.
8. Davidson K, Brancato A, Heetderks P, et al. Outbreak of electronic-cigarette-associated acute lipoid pneumonia – North Carolina, July–August 2019. MMWR Morb Mortal Wkly Rep. 2019;68(36):784–6. Published 2019 Sept 13. https://doi.org/10.15585/mmwr.mm6836e1.
9. Butt YM, Smith ML, Tazelaar HD, Vaszar LT, et al. Pathology of vaping-associated lung injury. N Engl J Med. 2019;381(18):1780–1.
10. Beshay M, Kaiser H, Niedhart D, Reymond MA, Schmid RA. Emphysema and secondary pneumothorax in young adults smoking cannabis. Eur J Cardiothorac Surg. 2007;32:834–8.
11. Tashkin DP. Effects of marijuana smoking on the lung. Ann Am Thorac Soc. 2013;10:239–47.
12. Stone W. Some states with legal weed embrace vaping bans, warn of black market risks. NPR. 26 Oct. 2019.

Cannabis Use Disorder

38

Samer N. Narouze, Caroline A. MacCallum, and Lauren de Freitas

Introduction

Adolescents and adults increasingly view cannabis as harmless. While the majority can use cannabis without harm, there are many potential problems including decline in educational or occupational functioning after early adolescent use, impaired driving, cannabis use disorders, cannabis withdrawal, and psychiatric comorbidity. There are limited evidence suggesting that medical marijuana laws have led to national increases in cannabis potency and prenatal and unintentional childhood exposure. Increased cannabis use in adults led to increase in cannabis-related emergency room visits, fatal vehicle crashes, and cannabis use disorder (CUD) [1].

S. N. Narouze (✉)
Western Reserve Hospital, Center For Pain Medicine, Cuyahoga Falls, OH, USA
e-mail: narouzs@hotmail.com
Twitter: @NarouzeMD

C. A. MacCallum
Department of Medicine, Faculty of Medicine, University of British Columbia, Vancouver, BC, Canada
e-mail: info@drcarolinemaccallum.com

L. de Freitas
Centre for Addiction and Mental Health, Toronto, ON, Canada

Epidemiology of Cannabis Use Disorder

Marijuana is the most commonly abused drug in the United States [2]. An estimated 26.0 million Americans aged 12 or older in 2017 were current users of marijuana. This corresponds to 9.6 percent of the population aged 12 or older. This is higher than the percentages from 2002 to 2016. This increase in marijuana use among people aged 12 or older reflects increases in marijuana use among both young adults aged 18 to 25 and adults aged 26 or older. In 2017, about 1 in 5 young adults aged 18 to 25 were current users of marijuana [2, 3]. Globally, approximately 4% of the population was using cannabis in 2015. Among teenagers, 8% in the United States and 16% in Europe report use cannabis [4].

As consumption increases among adults, so does the unintended consequence of childhood exposure [5]. Between 2005 and 2009, 985 unintentional exposures to children (median age of 1.7 years) were reported. States legalizing marijuana have had a 20-fold increase in calls to poison centers and admissions to critical care units for its exposure [6].

The prevalence of marijuana use more than doubled between 2001–2002 and 2012–2013, and this was accompanied by a large increase in marijuana use disorder. The past-year prevalence of marijuana use increased significantly from 4.1% in 2001–2002 to 9.5% in 2012–2013. Concomitantly, the past-year prevalence of DSM-IV marijuana

S. N. Narouze (ed.), *Cannabinoids and Pain*, https://doi.org/10.1007/978-3-030-69186-8_38

use disorder increased from 1.5% in 2001–2002 to 2.9% in 2012–2013. However, the prevalence of marijuana use disorder among marijuana users decreased from 35.6% in 2001–2002 to 30.6% in 2012–2013. Approximately, three out of ten marijuana users presented with marijuana use disorder in 2012–2013 [7].

Cannabis Use Disorder

Cannabis abuse is an outdated medical term that was used in the *Diagnostic and Statistical Manual of Mental Disorders* (DSM-IV) which divided substance use from substance dependence. The *Diagnostic and Statistical Manual of Mental Disorders* (DSM-5) uses the term "cannabis use disorder" defined by nine pathological patterns classified under impaired control, social impairment, risky behavior, or physiological dependence [8].

The DSM-5 cannabis use disorder (addictive disorder) provides 11 criteria to identify a problematic pattern of cannabis use leading to clinically significant impairment or distress as manifested by at least two of the 11 criteria occurring in a 12-month period. Criteria 1–9 represent the behavioral patterns for addictive use of marijuana. Criteria 10 and 11 represent the pharmacological phenomena of tolerance and dependence

Loss of control is represented by Criteria 1, 2, 3, and 4 and social impairment by criteria 5, 6, and 7. While high-risk use is presented by criteria 8 and 9 and pharmacological tolerance and dependence by criteria 10 and 11.

Cannabis abuse and dependence were combined in the DSM-5 into a single entity capturing the behavioral disorder that can occur with chronic cannabis use and named cannabis use disorder, it is defined as a problematic pattern of cannabis use leading to clinically significant impairment or distress, as manifested by at least two of the following 11 criteria, occurring within a 12-month period. The severity is graded as either mild (2–3 criteria), moderate (4–5 criteria), or severe (>6 criteria).

1. Cannabis is often taken in larger amounts or over a longer period than was intended.
2. There is a persistent desire or unsuccessful efforts to cut down or control cannabis use.
3. A great deal of time is spent in activities necessary to obtain cannabis, use cannabis, or recover from its effects.
4. Craving or a strong desire or urge to use cannabis.
5. Recurrent cannabis use results in failure to fulfill role obligations at work, school, or home.
6. Continued cannabis use despite having persistent or recurrent social or interpersonal problems caused or exacerbated by the effects of cannabis.
7. Important social, occupational, or recreational activities are given up or reduced because of cannabis use.
8. Recurrent cannabis use in situations in which it is physically hazardous.
9. Cannabis use continues despite knowledge of having a persistent or recurrent physical or psychological problem that is likely to have been caused or exacerbated by cannabis.
10. Tolerance manifested as markedly diminished effect with continued use of the same amount of cannabis or the need for markedly increased cannabis to achieve desired effects.
11. Characteristic withdrawal syndrome for cannabis, or cannabis is taken to relieve or avoid withdrawal symptoms.

Early Remission After full criteria for cannabis use disorder were previously met, none of the criteria for cannabis use disorder has been met for at least 3 months but less than 12 months (with an exception provided for craving).

Sustained Remission After full criteria for cannabis use disorder were previously met, none of the criteria for cannabis use disorder has been met at any time for 12 months or longer (with an exception provided for craving) [8, 9].

Clinical Presentation and Risk Factors for "Problematic Cannabis Use"

The clinical presentation for problematic cannabis use is summarized in Fig. 38.1, while the risk factors for problematic cannabis use and cannabis use disorder were summarized in Tables 38.1.

Cannabis Withdrawal

Cannabis withdrawal symptoms and signs may include irritability, anxiety, insomnia, nightmares, decreased appetite, depressed mood, tremors, sweating, or headaches (Table 38.2). Cannabis withdrawal is diagnosed if three or more of these signs and symptoms develop within 1 week after cessation of daily, heavy, prolonged cannabis use over a period of at least a few months [8–10].

Withdrawal occurs in only a subset of patients, and symptoms usually begin within the first 24 hours, peak by day 3, and can last for up to 2 weeks [11–13].

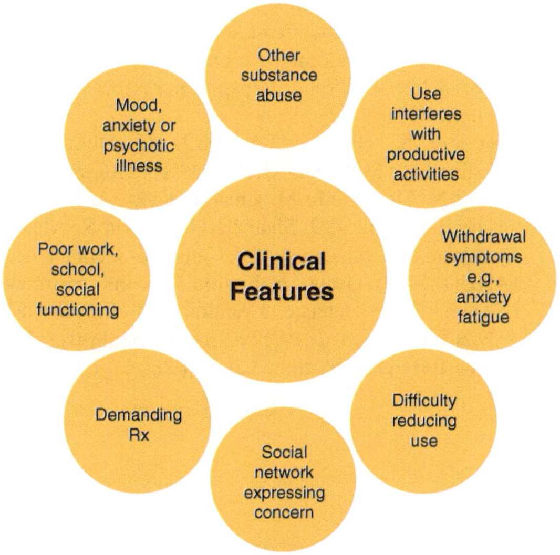

Fig. 38.1 Clinical features of problematic cannabis use. (© Dr. Caroline MacCallum used with permission)

Table 38.1 Risk factors for problematic cannabis use

Risk factors for "problematic cannabis use"
Regular chronic use in recreational cannabis users can increase the risk of cannabis dependence as well other illicit drugs and alcohol
The earlier the person starts recreational cannabis, the higher the risk of CUD
Current tobacco use and other illicit drugs
Male gender
Depression
Parental substance abuse
Childhood sexual abuse
Oppositional behaviors
Antisocial behaviors
Poor school performance

This is usually less of an issue with medical cannabis

Table 38.2 Cannabis withdrawal syndrome as defined by DSM-5 [8]

Cannabis withdrawal syndrome
The cessation of cannabis use that has been heavy and prolonged (i.e., usually daily or almost daily use over a period of at least a few months) with three or more of the following signs and symptoms developing within approximately 1 week after cessation: 1. Irritability, anger, or aggression 2. Nervousness or anxiety 3. Sleep difficulty (insomnia, disturbing dreams) 4. Decreased appetite or weight loss 5. Restlessness 6. Depressed mood At least one of the following physical symptoms causing significant discomfort: 1. Abdominal pain 2. Shakiness and tremors 3. Sweating 4. Fever 5. Chills 6. Headache The signs or symptoms cause clinically significant distress or impairment in social, occupational, or other important areas of functioning. The signs or symptoms are not attributable to another medical condition and are not better explained by another mental disorder, including intoxication or withdrawal from another substance.

Cannabinoid Agonists for Cannabis Use Disorder

Recently, it was shown that the cannabinoid (nabiximols), in combination with psychosocial interventions such as cognitive behavior therapy, is a safe approach for reducing cannabis use among individuals with cannabis dependence [14].

In a parallel double-blind randomized clinical trial of 128 participants, a 12-week course of nabiximols, a combination of tetrahydrocannabinol and cannabidiol, resulted in significantly fewer days of illicit cannabis use compared with placebo and was well tolerated by participants [15].

References

1. Hasin DS. US epidemiology of cannabis use and associated problems. Neuropsychopharmacology. 2018;43(1):195–212. https://doi.org/10.1038/npp.2017.198.
2. Key substance use and mental health indicators in the United States: results from the 2017 National Survey on Drug Use and Health. https://www.samhsa.gov/data/sites/default/files/cbhsq-reports/NSDUHFFR2017/NSDUHFFR2017.pdf. Accessed 28 May 2020.
3. The 2018 National Survey on Drug Use and Health (NSDUH). https://www.samhsa.gov/data/nsduh/reports-detailed-tables-2018-NSDUH. Accessed 7/8/2019.
4. Peacock A, Leung J, Larney S, Colledge S, Hickman M, Rehm J, Giovino GA, West R, Hall W, Griffiths P, Ali R, Gowing L, Marsden J, Ferrari AJ, Grebely J, Farrell M, Degenhardt L. Global statistics on alcohol, tobacco and illicit drug use: 2017 status report. Addiction. 2018;113(10):1905–26.
5. Volkow ND, Baler RD, Compton WM, Weiss SR. Adverse health effects of marijuana use. N Engl J Med. 2014;370(23):2219–27.
6. Wang GS, Roosevelt G, Le Lait MC, Martinez EM, Bucher-Bartelson B, Bronstein AC, Heard K. Association of unintentional pediatric exposures with decriminalization of marijuana in the United States. Ann Emerg Med. 2014;63(6):684–9.
7. Hasin DS, Saha TD, Kerridge BT, Goldstein RB, et al. Prevalence of marijuana use disorders in the United States between 2001–2002 and 2012–2013. JAMA Psychiat. 2015;72:1235–42.
8. American Psychiatric Association. Diagnostic and statistical manual of mental disorders: diagnostic and statistical manual of mental disorders. 5th ed. Arlington: American Psychiatric Association; 2013.
9. Patel J, Marwaha R. Cannabis use disorder. In: StatPearls. Treasure Island: StatPearls Publishing; 2020.
10. Bonnet U, Preuss UW. The cannabis withdrawal syndrome: current insights. Subst Abus Rehabil. 2017;8:9–37.
11. Preuss UW, Watzke AB, Zimmermann J, Wong JW, Schmidt CO. Cannabis withdrawal severity and short-term course among cannabis-dependent adolescent and young adult inpatients. Drug Alcohol Depend. 2010 Jan 15;106(2–3):133–41.
12. Budney AJ, Hughes JR, Moore BA, Vandrey R. Review of the validity and significance of cannabis withdrawal syndrome. Am J Psychiatry. 2004 Nov;161(11):1967–77.
13. Marshall K, Gowing L, Ali R, Le Foll B. Pharmacotherapies for cannabis dependence. Cochrane Database Syst Rev. 2014;(12):CD008940.
14. Trigo JM, Soliman A, Quilty LC, Fischer B, Rehm J, Selby P, Barnes AJ, Huestis MA, George TP, Streiner DL, Staios G, Le Foll B. Nabiximols combined with motivational enhancement/cognitive behavioral therapy for the treatment of cannabis dependence: a pilot randomized clinical trial. PLoS One. 2018;13(1):e0190768. https://doi.org/10.1371/journal.pone.0190768.
15. Lintzeris N, Bhardwaj A, Mills L, Dunlop A, Copeland J, McGregor I, Bruno R, Gugusheff J, Phung N, Montebello M, Chan T, Kirby A, Hall M, Jefferies M, Luksza J, Shanahan M, Kevin R, Allsop D, Agonist Replacement for Cannabis Dependence (ARCD) Study Group. Nabiximols for the treatment of cannabis dependence: a randomized clinical trial. JAMA Intern Med. 2019;179(9):1242–53. https://doi.org/10.1001/jamainternmed.2019.1993.

39 Cannabis Withdrawal

Yinan Chen and Christina Le-Short

Introduction

Cannabis is the most commonly used illicit substance worldwide. Although commonly considered to be a "soft drug," cannabis use is associated with mental and physical health problems. As use of cannabis increases over the past two decades, more research efforts have advanced our understanding of not only cannabis use disorder but also cannabis withdrawal [1]. Abrupt cessation of prolonged cannabis use can lead to a cannabis withdrawal syndrome (CWS), a new diagnosis included in the *Diagnostic and Statistical Manual of Mental Disorders – Fifth Edition* (DSM-5) [2] and as a criterion for cannabis use disorder. Symptoms of CWS occur reliably following a specific time course with cessation of cannabis use, are transient, can be ameliorated by readministration of cannabis, and are clinically significant.

Y. Chen
Department of Pain Medicine, Division of Anesthesiology and Critical Care, The University of Texas MD Anderson Cancer Center, Houston, TX, USA

C. Le-Short (✉)
Department of Pain Medicine, Division of Anesthesiology, Critical Care and Pain Medicine, The University of Texas MD Anderson Cancer Center, Houston, TX, USA
e-mail: cle2@mdanderson.org

Symptoms and Prevalence

Cannabis withdrawal syndrome (CWS) is diagnosed when within a week after cessation of heavy, prolonged use, ≥3 of 7 symptoms occur, including six behavioral or emotional symptoms and one or more of a list of physical symptoms (Table 39.1). It should be noted that if the symptoms are attributable to another medical condition or better explained by another mental disorder, including intoxication with or withdrawal from another substance, diagnosis of CWS is excluded. This makes the diagnosis of CWS even more challenging since the coexistence of mental disorder and other substance use disorder among cannabis users is not uncommon [3–5]. Onset of symptoms typically occurred between days 1 and 3, peak effects between days 2 and 6, and most effects lasted

Table 39.1 Cannabis withdrawal symptoms

Cannabis withdrawal symptoms
Nervousness or anxiety
Irritability or aggression
Insomnia or unpleasant dreams
Depressed mood
Decreased appetite or weight loss
Restlessness
Physical symptoms
Abdominal pain
Shakiness or tremors
Sweating
Fever
Chills
Headache

S. N. Narouze (ed.), *Cannabinoids and Pain*, https://doi.org/10.1007/978-3-030-69186-8_39

4–14 days, similar to tobacco and other withdrawal syndromes [6].

CWS was not included in DSM-IV-TR because its clinical significance was not recognized then. Budney et al. proposed the existence of CWS and reported that more than 50% of adults seeking treatment for marijuana dependence experienced withdrawal symptoms [7]. Allsop et al. demonstrated that CWS could be functionally impairing and patients with greater functional impairment were more likely to relapse [8, 9]. Another challenge to identify CWS is the lack of consensus on the best screening tool. Commonly used assessment instruments include the 22-item Marijuana Withdrawal Symptom checklist [7], the Cannabis Withdrawal Scale [8], the Marijuana Quitting Questionnaire [10, 11], the Customary Drinking and Drug Use Record [12], and clinical interviews involving the Time-Line-Flow-Back [13]. A recent metanalysis which included 23,158 participants in 47 studies showed no difference in prevalence estimation using different ascertainment methods [14]. However, this does not mean that all instruments to assess CWS are equal. The inclusion of diagnosis criteria in DSM-V will help to properly diagnose and treat CWS and prevent relapse.

The aforementioned metanalysis by Bahji and colleagues [14] identified a pooled prevalence of CWS of 47% with significant heterogeneity among studies when the data source was stratified. Population-based studies had the lowest prevalence of CWS of 17%, whereas outpatient and inpatient samples showed prevalence of 54% and 87%, respectively. Concurrent use of tobacco and other illicit drug was associated with significantly higher prevalence of CWS, as well as daily cannabis use. Like various individual studies, this metanalysis did not reveal association between CWS prevalence and gender, age, race/ethnicity, or geographic region. Unlike multiple individual studies, this metanalysis did not identify any association between CWS and psychiatric comorbidity. The authors, however, pointed out that cannabis use disorder (CUD) was more common among individuals with psychiatric comorbidity [15] including anxiety [16], mood [3], eating [17], and psychotic disorders [18, 19]. The association between CUD and psychiatric comorbidity is generally negative, especially in the settings of younger cannabis exposure age and heavier cannabis use [15]. The overlapping symptoms between CWS and psychiatric disorder make the differential diagnosis further challenging. For example, patients with anxiety may use cannabis for the acute anxiolytic effect, and the anxiety experienced during abstinence may be the manifestation of CWS, worsening of pre-existing anxiety, or the combination of both. Therefore, clinicians need to familiarize themselves with such association to provide patients with proper care and counseling.

Mechanism of Cannabis Withdrawal

Pharmacological studies identified delta-9-tetrahydrocannabinol (THC) as the primary psychoactive compound in cannabis that causes rewarding and addictive effect [20]. THC is a partial agonist of the cannabinoid receptor type 1 (CB1R) [21]. CB1 knockout mouse model and pharmacological blockade of CB1R demonstrated its role in modulating cannabis dependence and withdrawal [22, 23]. Regular use of cannabis has been shown to desensitize and downregulate CB1R. This effect starts to reverse within 2 days of cannabis cessation, and CB1R returns to baseline function within 4 weeks of abstinence [24, 25], which is consistent with the time course of CWS. Evidence supporting that THC plays critical role in CWS includes (1) a hysteresis effect between the decrease in plasma THC and onset of CWS [26], (2) withdrawal symptoms following oral THC [27, 28], and (3) alleviation of CWS by oral THC [29]. THC likely exerts its effect via a non-CB1R-dependent mechanism as well. For example, animal study showed that THC increased the potassium-evoked dopamine release in the rat caudate nucleus [30]. More research further demonstrated that cannabinoids and endocannabinoids could modulate both voltage-gated ion channels (calcium, sodium, and potassium) and ligand-gated ion channels (serotonin type 3, nicotinic acetylcholine, and glycine receptors) [31], as well as cell membrane proteins and neurotransmitter receptors [32]. The exact mechanism of such modulation is not clear, and more studies are warranted to provide potential treatment targets.

Although heavier cannabis users are more likely to develop CWS, some individuals develop CWS with short-term, less than daily exposure. This raised the question whether genetic background predisposes certain individuals to withdrawal. Earlier genetic epidemiology studies focused on CUD and concluded that it was highly heritable [33]. For example, the San Francisco family study found that not only cannabis use, abuse, and dependence but also age of first use was all heritable [34]. The same study also found that certain symptoms of CWS especially nervousness was heritable, too. More studies have been conducted since the inclusion of CWS in DSM-5. Twin study in Australia by Verweij and colleagues found that approximately 50% of variances in withdrawal were attributable to additive genetic factors (68% in abuse/dependence). The remaining variances were mainly due to unshared environmental influences [35]. The authors concluded that CWS is moderately heritable. More importantly, the genetic influences on cannabis withdrawal almost completely (99%) overlapped with those on abuse/dependence. This is reassuring for genetic informed studies that did not assess withdrawal.

Treatment of Cannabis Withdrawal

Cannabis withdrawal is considered a negative reinforcement for relapse, and patients have reported using other substances such as nicotine and alcohol as a reliever [6, 7, 10, 36]. Therefore, much effort has been made to identify treatment options for CWS.

Despite the growing interests and positive results from small-scale trials, there is no approved pharmacological treatment for CWS or CUD. Current candidates for CWS are through either the cannabinoid receptor or other neurotransmitters [37]. The most studied cannabinoids are THC and cannabidiol (CBD). While THC has psychoactive activity thus a narrow therapeutic window, CBD lacks psychotropic property and is considered a promising candidate for CUD and CWS treatment [20]. Animal study showed that CBD alleviated withdrawal symptoms and reversed gene expression changes induced by cannabis withdrawal including opioid μ receptor (Oprm1), cannabinoid CB1 receptor (Cnr1), and CB2 receptor (Cnr2) in the nucleus accumbens in mice [38]. Further study is necessary to determine whether CBD has similar therapeutic effect in human subjects. THC was able to decrease the intensity of withdrawal symptoms in several studies; however, it did not show efficacy in terms of abstinence maintenance in a recent metanalysis [39].

Among non-cannabinoid agents, bupropion caught early attention due to its approval for tobacco cessation. Although cannabis and nicotine withdrawal share notable overlapping symptoms, bupropion was reported to worsen CWS symptoms [40]. Serotonin reuptake inhibitors (SSRIs) and serotonin-norepinephrine reuptake inhibitors (SNRIs) produced mixed results based on both literature review and metanalysis [38, 39]. Some studies reported CWS symptom alleviation with SSRIs and SNRIs, while others showed no differenced as compared to placebos. Treatment with neither class resulted in increased likelihood of abstinence. Anticonvulsants such as gabapentin and topiramate showed promising results with decreased cannabis use and symptom intensity. However, studies so far are limited due to low power and poor completion rate [38]. Larger-scale, fully powered studies are necessary to provide more conclusive evidence for the role of anticonvulsants in treating CUD. N-Acetylcysteine (NAC) is another agent of interest given its role in regulating glutamate release and preliminary favorable results treating cocaine and cigarette craving. NAC yielded positive primary cessation outcome in cannabis-dependent adolescents and young adults (age 18–21) in both open-labeled pilot study [41] and double-blind, randomized control trial [42]. The same group replicated the study in adults (age 18–50) but could not reproduce the positive result, suggesting a possible age effect in treatment [43].

While the search for pharmacological agents for CWS treatment remains ongoing, psychotherapy studies have established several evidence-based models and promising techniques in CWS/CUD treatment. Cognitive behavioral therapy (CBT), motivational enhancement therapy (MET), and contingency management (CM) are studied the most and have all shown benefits in cannabis use outcome (decreased frequency and quantity of use during treatment). And the combination of the three modalities has the highest efficacy [44, 45]. However, abstinence rate remained modest and declined after treatment. Moreover, the increasing number of cannabis user, both recreational and medicinal, ensures that the volume of people developing CUD and/or experiencing CWS exceeds the capacity of substance abuse specialty services. Further investigation on brief intervention, computer/telephone-based intervention, and social media may improve the accessibility of psychotherapy. Psychotherapy should also be incorporated with pharmacological therapy to improve the efficacy of CWS treatment.

References

1. GBD 2016 Alcohol and Drug Use Collaborators. The global burden of disease attributable to alcohol and drug use in 195 countries and territories, 1990–2016: a systematic analysis for the Global Burden of Disease Study 2016 [published correction appears in Lancet Psychiatry. 2019 Jan;6(1):e2]. Lancet Psychiatry. 2018;5(12):987–1012. https://doi.org/10.1016/S2215-0366(18)30337-7.
2. American Psychiatric Association. Diagnostic and statistical manual of mental disorders. 5th ed. Arlington: American Psychiatric Association; 2013.
3. Arias F, Szerman N, Vega P, et al. Abuse or dependence on cannabis and other psychiatric disorders. Madrid study on dual pathology prevalence. Actas Esp Psiquiatr. 2013;41(2):122–9.
4. Banks DE, Rowe AT, Mpofu P, Zapolski TCB. Trends in typologies of concurrent alcohol, marijuana, and cigarette use among US adolescents: an ecological examination by sex and race/ethnicity. Drug Alcohol Depend. 2017;179:71–7. https://doi.org/10.1016/j.drugalcdep.2017.06.026.
5. Zuckermann AME, Williams G, Battista K, de Groh M, Jiang Y, Leatherdale ST. Trends of poly-substance use among Canadian youth. Addict Behav Rep. 2019;10:100189. Published 2019 May 10. https://doi.org/10.1016/j.abrep.2019.100189.
6. Budney AJ, Moore BA, Vandrey RG, Hughes JR. The time course and significance of cannabis withdrawal. J Abnorm Psychol. 2003;112(3):393–402. https://doi.org/10.1037/0021-843x.112.3.393.
7. Budney AJ, Novy PL, Hughes JR. Marijuana withdrawal among adults seeking treatment for marijuana dependence. Addiction. 1999;94(9):1311–22. https://doi.org/10.1046/j.1360-0443.1999.94913114.x.
8. Allsop DJ, Norberg MM, Copeland J, Fu S, Budney AJ. The Cannabis Withdrawal Scale development: patterns and predictors of cannabis withdrawal and distress. Drug Alcohol Depend. 2011;119(1–2):123–9. https://doi.org/10.1016/j.drugalcdep.2011.06.003.
9. Allsop DJ, Copeland J, Norberg MM, et al. Quantifying the clinical significance of cannabis withdrawal. PLoS One. 2012;7(9):e44864. https://doi.org/10.1371/journal.pone.0044864.
10. Levin KH, Copersino ML, Heishman SJ, et al. Cannabis withdrawal symptoms in non-treatment-seeking adult cannabis smokers. Drug Alcohol Depend. 2010;111(1–2):120–7. https://doi.org/10.1016/j.drugalcdep.2010.04.010.
11. Gorelick DA, Levin KH, Copersino ML, et al. Diagnostic criteria for cannabis withdrawal syndrome. Drug Alcohol Depend. 2012;123(1–3):141–7. https://doi.org/10.1016/j.drugalcdep.2011.11.007.
12. Greene MC, Kelly JF. The prevalence of cannabis withdrawal and its influence on adolescents' treatment response and outcomes: a 12-month prospective investigation. J Addict Med. 2014;8(5):359–67. https://doi.org/10.1097/ADM.0000000000000064.
13. Sherman BJ, McRae-Clark AL, Baker NL, et al. Gender differences among treatment-seeking adults with cannabis use disorder: clinical profiles of women and men enrolled in the achieving cannabis cessation-evaluating N-acetylcysteine treatment (ACCENT) study. Am J Addict. 2017;26(2):136–44. https://doi.org/10.1111/ajad.12503.
14. Bahji A, Stephenson C, Tyo R, Hawken ER, Seitz DP. Prevalence of cannabis withdrawal symptoms among people with regular or dependent use of cannabinoids: a systematic review and meta-analysis. JAMA Netw Open. 2020;3(4):e202370. Published 2020 Apr 1. https://doi.org/10.1001/jamanetworkopen.2020.2370.
15. Hanna RC, Perez JM, Ghose S. Cannabis and development of dual diagnoses: a literature review. Am J Drug Alcohol Abuse. 2017;43(4):442–55. https://doi.org/10.1080/00952990.2016.1213273.
16. Crippa JA, Zuardi AW, Martín-Santos R, et al. Cannabis and anxiety: a critical review of the evidence. Hum Psychopharmacol. 2009;24(7):515–23. https://doi.org/10.1002/hup.1048.
17. Bahji A, Mazhar MN, Hudson CC, Nadkarni P, MacNeil BA, Hawken E. Prevalence of substance use disorder comorbidity among individuals with eating disorders: a systematic review and meta-analysis. Psychiatry Res. 2019;273:58–66. https://doi.org/10.1016/j.psychres.2019.01.007.

18. Boggs DL, Kelly DL, Liu F, et al. Cannabis withdrawal in chronic cannabis users with schizophrenia. J Psychiatr Res. 2013;47(2):240–5. https://doi.org/10.1016/j.jpsychires.2012.10.010.
19. Koola MM, Kelly DL, McMahon RP, Boggs DL, Liu F, Gorelick DA. Psychoactive substance use by adults with schizophrenia before and during cannabis withdrawal. Prim Care Companion CNS Disord. 2016;18(5). Published 2016 Sep 1. https://doi.org/10.4088/PCC.16l01959.
20. Grotenhermen F. Pharmacokinetics and pharmacodynamics of cannabinoids. Clin Pharmacokinet. 2003;42(4):327–60. https://doi.org/10.2165/00003088-200342040-00003.
21. Cooper ZD, Haney M. Cannabis reinforcement and dependence: role of the cannabinoid CB1 receptor. Addict Biol. 2008;13(2):188–95. https://doi.org/10.1111/j.1369-1600.2007.00095.x.
22. Ledent C, Valverde O, Cossu G, et al. Unresponsiveness to cannabinoids and reduced addictive effects of opiates in CB1 receptor knockout mice. Science. 1999;283(5400):401–4. https://doi.org/10.1126/science.283.5400.401.
23. Lichtman AH, Martin BR. Marijuana withdrawal syndrome in the animal model. J Clin Pharmacol. 2002;42(S1):20S–7S. https://doi.org/10.1002/j.1552-4604.2002.tb05999.x.
24. Hirvonen J, Goodwin RS, Li CT, et al. Reversible and regionally selective downregulation of brain cannabinoid CB1 receptors in chronic daily cannabis smokers. Mol Psychiatry. 2012;17(6):642–9. https://doi.org/10.1038/mp.2011.82.
25. D'Souza DC, Cortes-Briones JA, Ranganathan M, et al. Rapid changes in CB1 receptor availability in cannabis dependent males after abstinence from cannabis. Biol Psychiatry Cogn Neurosci Neuroimaging. 2016;1(1):60–7. https://doi.org/10.1016/j.bpsc.2015.09.008.
26. Cone EJ, Huestis MA. Relating blood concentrations of tetrahydrocannabinol and metabolites to pharmacologic effects and time of marijuana usage. Ther Drug Monit. 1993;15(6):527–32. https://doi.org/10.1097/00007691-199312000-00013.
27. Jones RT, Benowitz NL, Herning RI. Clinical relevance of cannabis tolerance and dependence. J Clin Pharmacol. 1981;21(S1):143S–52S. https://doi.org/10.1002/j.1552-4604.1981.tb02589.x.
28. Budney AJ, Hughes JR, Moore BA, Vandrey R. Review of the validity and significance of cannabis withdrawal syndrome. Am J Psychiatry. 2004;161(11):1967–77. https://doi.org/10.1176/appi.ajp.161.11.1967.
29. Haney M, Hart CL, Vosburg SK, Comer SD, Reed SC, Foltin RW. Effects of THC and lofexidine in a human laboratory model of marijuana withdrawal and relapse. Psychopharmacology. 2008;197(1):157–68. https://doi.org/10.1007/s00213-007-1020-8.
30. Ng Cheong Ton JM, Gerhardt GA, Friedemann M, et al. The effects of delta 9-tetrahydrocannabinol on potassium-evoked release of dopamine in the rat caudate nucleus: an in vivo electrochemical and in vivo microdialysis study. Brain Res. 1988;451(1–2):59–68. https://doi.org/10.1016/0006-8993(88)90749-4.
31. Oz M. Receptor-independent effects of endocannabinoids on ion channels. Curr Pharm Des. 2006;12(2):227–39. https://doi.org/10.2174/138161206775193073.
32. Oz M. Receptor-independent actions of cannabinoids on cell membranes: focus on endocannabinoids. Pharmacol Ther. 2006;111(1):114–44. https://doi.org/10.1016/j.pharmthera.2005.09.009.
33. Agrawal A, Lynskey MT. The genetic epidemiology of cannabis use, abuse and dependence. Addiction. 2006;101(6):801–12. https://doi.org/10.1111/j.1360-0443.2006.01399.x.
34. Ehlers CL, Gizer IR, Vieten C, et al. Cannabis dependence in the San Francisco Family Study: age of onset of use, DSM-IV symptoms, withdrawal, and heritability. Addict Behav. 2010;35(2):102–10. https://doi.org/10.1016/j.addbeh.2009.09.009.
35. Verweij KJ, Agrawal A, Nat NO, et al. A genetic perspective on the proposed inclusion of cannabis withdrawal in DSM-5. Psychol Med. 2013;43(8):1713–22. https://doi.org/10.1017/S0033291712002735.
36. Cornelius JR, Chung T, Martin C, Wood DS, Clark DB. Cannabis withdrawal is common among treatment-seeking adolescents with cannabis dependence and major depression, and is associated with rapid relapse to dependence. Addict Behav. 2008;33(11):1500–5. https://doi.org/10.1016/j.addbeh.2008.02.001.
37. Brezing CA, Levin FR. The current state of pharmacological treatments for cannabis use disorder and withdrawal. Neuropsychopharmacology. 2018;43(1):173–94. https://doi.org/10.1038/npp.2017.212.
38. Navarrete F, Aracil-Fernández A, Manzanares J. Cannabidiol regulates behavioural alterations and gene expression changes induced by spontaneous cannabinoid withdrawal. Br J Pharmacol. 2018;175(13):2676–88. https://doi.org/10.1111/bph.14226Nielsen.
39. Nielsen S, Gowing L, Sabioni P, Le Foll B. Pharmacotherapies for cannabis dependence. Cochrane Database Syst Rev. 2019;1(1):CD008940. Published 2019 Jan 28. https://doi.org/10.1002/14651858.CD008940.pub3.
40. Haney M, Ward AS, Comer SD, Hart CL, Foltin RW, Fischman MW. Bupropion SR worsens mood during marijuana withdrawal in humans. Psychopharmacology. 2001;155(2):171–9. https://doi.org/10.1007/s002130000657.
41. Gray KM, Watson NL, Carpenter MJ, Larowe SD. N-acetylcysteine (NAC) in young marijuana users: an open-label pilot study. Am J Addict. 2010;19(2):187–9. https://doi.org/10.1111/j.1521-0391.2009.00027.x.
42. Gray KM, Carpenter MJ, Baker NL, et al. A double-blind randomized controlled trial of N-acetylcysteine in cannabis-dependent adolescents [published

correction appears in Am J Psychiatry. 2012 Aug 1;169(8):869]. Am J Psychiatry. 2012;169(8):805–12. https://doi.org/10.1176/appi.ajp.2012.12010055.

43. Gray KM, Sonne SC, McClure EA, et al. A randomized placebo-controlled trial of N-acetylcysteine for cannabis use disorder in adults. Drug Alcohol Depend. 2017;177:249–57. https://doi.org/10.1016/j.drugalcdep.2017.04.020.

44. Danovitch I, Gorelick DA. State of the art treatments for cannabis dependence. Psychiatr Clin North Am. 2012;35(2):309–26. https://doi.org/10.1016/j.psc.2012.03.003.

45. Sherman BJ, McRae-Clark AL. Treatment of cannabis use disorder: current science and future outlook. Pharmacotherapy. 2016;36(5):511–35. https://doi.org/10.1002/phar.1747.

Part IX

Cannabinoids Future Directions

Cannabinoids Future Research

40

Ignacio Badolia

Introduction

Written claims of cannabis as a medication for the treatment of pain date to around the fifteenth century BCE and can be found in the Chinese Pharmacopeia, the Rh-ya [1]. Spreading throughout the world over the next 2000 years, it made its way into western medicine around 1850 resulting in its inclusion in the US Pharmacopeia with a wide variety of indications for its use, most notably pain. These indications were not strictly evidenced based but based on anecdotal evidence. Despite this lack of evidence, cannabis was among the most highly prescribed drugs in the early twentieth century. However, by the early 1930s, opponents to cannabis use gained momentum resulting in the prohibition of cannabis by multiple states and ultimately the federal government outlawing its medical use. Despite its classification by the US government as having no medical use, cannabis-based medicine (CBM) has reentered mainstream medicine in the United States and many other countries especially over the last 25 years. This emerging interest by the public for cannabis products – specifically for medicinal use – has been stimulated by advocacy for its legalization for both medicinal and recreational use. One study reported that among adults, the prevalence of cannabis use increased from 10.4% to 13.3% with said increase due to growing social/legal acceptance, increased availability, and a decrease in the perception of risk [2]. As of March 2020, 11 states and the District of Columbia have legalized both medicinal and recreational forms of cannabis, while over 30 states have legalized medicinal use of cannabis [3]. Ironically as more individuals gain access to cannabis for medicinal use, researchers in the United States continue to face regulatory hurdles when attempting to study cannabis partly due to its classification as a schedule 1 drug under the controlled substances act. Limitations in available products to study (most of which are not synchronous to what consumers are using medicinally) and extensive regulations on storage and dispensing of research cannabis add to the difficulty.

While many other states have active legislative bills to legalize/decriminalize cannabis, indications for medical use are based on low-grade evidence. These indications are not congruent between states highlighting the lack of a good evidence base. For example, cannabis can be used to treat glaucoma in New Jersey but not New York. However, pain is almost a universal indication. Unlike the traditional pathway to drug approval, cannabis has bypassed the normal due diligence required for drug approval and entered the therapeutic arena mostly via advocacy [4]. Politics and advocacy have surpassed solid clinical evidence; however clinical

I. Badolia (✉)
Anesthesiology and Critical Care, University of Pennsylvania, Philadelphia, PA, USA
e-mail: Ignacio.Badiola@pennmedicine.upenn.edu

S. N. Narouze (ed.), *Cannabinoids and Pain*, https://doi.org/10.1007/978-3-030-69186-8_40

providers must provide guidance on science not on hype. Thus, there is an urgent need for quality research.

Difficulties in Cannabis Research

Despite the changes in policy at the state level and the increasing use and decreasing stigma associated with cannabis in general and CBM specifically, the federal government classifies cannabis as a schedule I drug under the controlled substances act [5]. Agents listed under class 1 substances have no currently accepted medical use in the United States, a lack of accepted safety under medical supervision and a high potential for abuse. Therein lies the conundrum. In order to study the purported effects of cannabis based on thousands of years of use, the US government has already determined that cannabis has no medical use and classified it as such.

Scientific truth is not affected by political circumstance, but science is shaped by the political climate in which it takes place. These restrictive policies at the federal level make research into the benefits or harm of the cannabis products that most Americans have available to them difficult leaving clinicians and patients without the evidence they need to make sound clinical decisions. This includes best indications, best product, cannabinoid and non-cannabinoid ratios, dosing, routes of administration, and subtypes of pain. Federal money into the research of cannabis is only approved under very specific circumstances by multiple agencies, and until recently all marijuana used in federally funded research was produced from a single approved facility which produced marijuana dissimilar to what patients were taking and state approved dispensaries were dispensing. Easement of these barriers will help make research into what the public mostly uses medical cannabis for, pain, more fruitful so that providers and patients can make more informed decisions as to whether cannabis will help, or harm, in their particular case. Cannabis is best thought as not a medicine like a traditional prescription drug, but as a broad category of various agents that vary in what they target, how the host responds, and the side effects they produce.

State laws vary widely for which conditions medicinal cannabis is approved for. For most of these conditions, approval has relied on lower-quality evidence, anecdotal reports, individual testimonials, and public opinion, with differences in states reflecting inconsistencies in evaluating and applying the current evidence toward decision-making about qualifying indications for medical cannabis use [4]. Pain is one of the most common indications for the use of medical cannabis. Estimates of mean prevalence indicate that almost 70% of individuals report using medical cannabis for pain, while mean prevalence of the highly associated anxiety and depression is around 50% and about 35%, respectively [6].

Regarding current data, it is important to realize that the lack of evidence of benefit does not always equate with evidence of a lack of benefit. In clinical practice, patients using cannabis frequently attest to analgesic benefit, and many case reports/case series purport analgesic benefit as well. However, much research remains to be done. Unanswered questions remain in almost all aspects of cannabis use in pain management. This includes cannabis use in acute pain states – for example, postoperative pain and the perioperative setting. Although chronic pain remains one of its most common uses, not all chronic pain is the same, and further research into what specific types of chronic pain cannabis works well for is desperately needed.

All of this needs to be done using current cannabis formulations that are available for and currently in use by patients. In general, current research into cannabis for pain is significantly flawed and requires longer study periods with larger sample sizes and with better methodology. Some population studies have shown reduction in opioid use in states with legal cannabis, although like all cannabis-based research, this is far from conclusive [7–9]. If this is the case, further clinical research into whether this can be extrapolated into individual patients must be performed. Although western medicine and pharmaceuticals have over abundantly evaluated medications using isolated molecules, the cannabis plant has over 100 cannabinoids and hundreds of other compounds. Are any other molecules, or even the whole plant, needed to obtain maximal analgesic benefit? Exploration of this "entourage effect" from a clinical perspective requires further study. Tolerance, an effect well-known in reducing analgesic effects of opioids, has also been described in cannabis users for pain as has a cannabis-induced hyperalgesia [10]. Preclinical and experimental studies have also uncovered a possible worsening of pain depending on dose. Clinical dose-response information is desperately needed. Cannabis use is known to produce downregulation and desensitization of cannabinoid receptors. As all humans have this endocannabinoid system, are some pain states due to dysregulation of this system? Can novel molecules that inhibit breakdown of endocannabinoids help regulate this important system? We will touch on some of these topics in this chapter.

Cannabis in Acute Pain/Perioperative Pain Medicine

Acute postoperative pain is ubiquitous following almost all surgical procedures, and it is particularly recalcitrant to current therapy. Some estimate a prevalence of over 80% of poorly managed postoperative pain [11]. Opioids have served as the cornerstone of postoperative pain management until recently as multimodal therapy using various modalities/medications has become more commonplace, in part due to the opioid epidemic. There is evidence that opioid exposure following surgery increases risk of continued and prolonged opioid use [12]. Although opioids can play a part in postoperative pain management, better non-opioid options are needed, and multimodal therapy has dramatically changed the way postoperative pain is managed. Cannabinoids impact the endocannabinoid system, a system known to be involved in pain modulation, and current therapies used in multimodal perioperative pain management do not take advantage of this system. This begs the question as to whether exogenous cannabinoids can play a part. As current pain therapies remain far from optimal, molecules that work on alternative mechanisms of action are desperately needed. Given effects of cannabis on some forms of chronic pain, the question remains whether we can extrapolate that and add it to the multimodal armamentarium for patients and clinicians dealing with acute postoperative pain. Unfortunately, the literature needed to answer this broad question is sparse at best. Experimental pain studies on acute pain provide some evidence of a therapeutic window of modest pain relief, especially in some acute neuropathic pain models [13]. However, a systematic review of 7 studies with 611 patients undergoing various surgical procedures failed to demonstrate an overall benefit in using cannabinoids for acute postoperative pain. Of the seven studies, five demonstrated equivalent analgesia to that of placebo with only one of the seven suggesting benefit [14]. A more recent systematic review and meta-analysis, which included studies not in the previously discussed review, included six trials using oral formulation (five trials) and an intramuscular formulation (1 trial). Results noted a small but significant reduction in acute pain especially with the intramuscular formulation [15]. Furthermore, a SR/MA of 8 randomized controlled trials with over 900 patients and 4000 patients in observational studies noted a very limited role in perioperative cannabinoids [16]. However, the studies used in these SR/MA evaluated cannabis preparations which vary significantly from those that are available from cannabis dispensaries. Thus, much like other areas of pain, much more research is needed to see if currently available cannabinoids provide any benefit in acute pain conditions.

Interestingly, and in contradistinction, there is preliminary evidence that prior cannabis use may in fact worsen postoperative pain outcomes and complicate postoperative pain management. A retrospective cohort of propensity-matched preoperative cannabis users noted higher pain scores and poorer quality of sleep following major orthopedic surgery [17]. Two more retrospective studies on patients following traumatic injury and following elective inflammatory bowel surgery noted higher opioid use in those using chronic cannabis [18, 19]. As previously noted, cannabis may have a therapeutic window with higher doses of THC worsening pain. These studies were mostly retrospective and suffer typical limitations of retrospective studies including quantification of cannabis use. Prospective studies evaluating current cannabis products are needed when used alone and as part of a multimodal postoperative pain approach as well as whether those using cannabis prior to surgery experience worse postoperative pain outcomes. Dose-response relationships of cannabis used need to be assessed as well. Furthermore, does cannabis withdrawal contribute to worsening pain acute pain outcomes in the perioperative period? Most hospitals do not allow inpatients to use cannabis. Do those chronic cannabis users admitted to the hospital suffer cannabis withdrawal and experience worse pain? Symptoms of withdrawal can include insomnia, mood changes (anxiety, depression), and physical discomfort [20]. All of this can lead to a worsening pain perception in this patient population.

Cannabis and Opioid Reduction

The thought of using cannabis to mitigate the opioid epidemic seems counterintuitive to many. Are we replacing one addictive substance with another? One epidemic for another? However, at face value if cannabis helps treat chronic pain, then shouldn't patients rely less on opioids? Would this reduction in opioid prescriptions reduce opioid overdoses and opioid-related deaths? Like everything discussed in this chapter, the answer is not definitive, and more research is needed. This is also complicated because chronic pain is multidimensional, and it is well-known that patients use opioids to treat other dimensions aside from pain (i.e., mood disorders). A systematic review and metanalysis of 19 preclinical studies suggested a median effective dose of morphine administered in combination with cannabinoids was 3.6 times lower than the median effective dose of morphine alone [21]. This makes sense, at least theoretically, as CB1 receptors are much more abundant (around ten times) compared to mu opioid receptors in the brain [22, 23]. There is co localization of these endocannabinoid receptors in various regions of the central nervous system associated with pain transmission and modulation suggesting augmentation of the analgesia produced by opioids. On an ecological and population perspective, a 2014 time series analysis of medical cannabis state laws and state level death certificates between 1999 and 2010 noted an almost 25% lower mean annual opioid overdose mortality rate when compared to states without medical cannabis laws [8]. Up until 2010, 13 states had medical cannabis laws. A more recent study replicated the 2014 study extending the analysis to 2017. Interestingly, the association between state medical cannabis laws and opioid overdose mortality reversed direction [9]. It must be kept in mind that these were population-based/ecological studies and are prone to the ecological fallacy. From an individual level perspective, there is some evidence that cannabis may reduce opioid use especially noted in case series and preclinical/experimental studies. However, the evidence for clinical based research is less robust [21]. Nevertheless, there is some clinical evidence suggesting an opioid sparring effect of cannabis; however most are flawed by small sample size and study design [24, 25]. In contrast other clinical evidence points toward the opposite with evidence suggesting that cannabis users experienced no reduction in pain nor a reduction in opioid use [26]. In summary it is too early to make definitive conclusions, and it is unknown if medical cannabis has an opioid sparring effect and if it does whether this translates to a reduction in opioid prescriptions and overdose deaths. Further observational studies, or ideally clinical trials, would help answer this question rather than relying on ecological data.

Herbal Synergy/Entourage Effect

Cannabis-based medicine differs from the traditional single molecule pharmaceuticals common in western medicine. Although the general public typically thinks of cannabis in terms of its THC or CBD content, the cannabis plant has hundreds of molecules usually divided into cannabinoids (binds to cannabinoid receptors) and non-cannabinoids (those that do not bind to cannabinoid receptors). Can a cannabis preparation of a single molecule (i.e., THC) be too pure to confer analgesic and medical benefit? As noted, the cannabis plant contains over 100 cannabinoid molecules including cannabigerols and cannabichromes. It also contains hundreds of non-cannabinoids including terpenes, nitrogenous compounds, alcohols, ketones, steroids, and hundreds of other compounds [27]. Most of the existing research has focused on THC and CBD, largely ignoring these hundreds of other molecules. Some proponents suggest that so as to achieve the maximal medicinal benefit from cannabis, isolated molecules will not do. Instead a combination of these molecules – and for some the entire plant – is needed to obtain maximal benefit. This contrasts with the traditional western medical model of isolating individual molecules from plants and developing them into branded pharmaceuticals. THC analogues nabilone and dronabinol are currently FDA-approved exemplars of this traditional path.

This dynamic interaction of various phytocannabinoids and non-cannabinoids has come to be known as herbal synergy, akin to the entourage effect where active and inactive metabolites effect each other pharmacologically. This effect was originally described in 1998 as an explanation for some biological observations that endocannabinoid ligand activity was affected by other lipids concurrently released by cells [28, 29]. Early examples from the 1970s by Carlini et al. demonstrated how CBD may interfere with THC both in humans and how cannabis extracts produced greater effect than that of pure THC at the same doses contained in the extracts [30, 31]. Preclinical studies are not all concordant with this concept with some suggesting no effect of common terpenes on cannabinoid receptors or on modulating THC on these receptors, while others do suggest a synergistic effect [29, 32, 33]. Clinical studies specifically looking at analgesic outcomes when comparing whole plant cannabinoid use to single molecules are lagging. Thus, despite strong support by some, there are many limitations at this point to definitively state whether or not the entire cannabis plant is required to produce maximal analgesic benefit compared to some of the plant's constituent molecules. If the entourage effect does indeed exist, it is still unknown which specific compounds drive this effect. Currently there are no specific trials in humans looking at the entourage effect on analgesia. However, many studies evaluating pain outcomes have used nabiximols – a formulation that contains a mixture of 1:1 THC:CBD – and whole plant *Cannabis sativa* showing modest analgesic relief with no analgesic relief following nabilone alone [34, 35].

However, other clinical studies focusing on other medical conditions have found minimal to no differences when comparing synthetic cannabinoids to herbal preparations, suggesting no entourage effect. Nevertheless, using these findings to dismiss the potential for an entourage effect is premature and arguing from the null hypothesis [27, 36–38].

In defense of the single molecule approach, single molecule cannabinoid chemistry/pharmacology also holds promise as pharmacologists and chemists can modify cannabinoid molecules to make very specific and selective mechanisms of action and improve efficacy and reduce possible adverse effects relative to nonselective phytocannabinoids.

Other Mechanisms of Action

Most articles and textbooks discuss how cannabinoids interact/modulate the endocannabinoid receptors found throughout the body. However, it is well-known that cannabinoids also interact with various other receptors known to be involved in pain transmission and modulation [39]. For example, THC is purported to reduce NMDA response, a well-known mechanism involved in difficult to treat hyperalgesic pain syndromes including fibromyalgia [40]. CBD also interacts with various receptors and ion channels including TRPV1 (agonist), modulation of glycine receptors and opioid receptors, serotonin agonism, and antagonism of human enzymes which break down endocannabinoids (i.e., fatty acid amide hydrolase) [41–44]. The more common "minor" cannabinoids include cannabichromene (CBC), cannabinol (CBN), cannabigerol (CBG), and tetrahydrocannabivarin/cannabidvarin (THCV/CBDV) and may be involved in pain modulation. There are preclinical studies suggesting evidence of anti-inflammatory and analgesic properties of some of these compounds. For example, CBG may stimulate various receptors important for pain, inflammation, and heat sensitization, while CBC can induce nociception when used by itself while potentiating the analgesic/antinociceptive effects when used with THC [39]. No well-powered clinical studies are available to evaluate the potential of these "minor" cannabinoids in providing analgesia in various pain states. The NIH recognizing the potential of these molecules with the National Center for Complementary and Integrative Health awarding various research grants into investigating their potential [45].

Methodology/Design of Research

Although the acceptance of cannabis in the medical community and public continues to grow, most of the research driving clinical decisions is plagued by methodological flaws. The gold standard of clinical research has classically been the double-blind randomized controlled clinical trial. Like other psychoactive substances, cannabis presents a challenge in blinding of subjects due to its inherent psychoactivity. The placebo arm of trials evaluating smoked, oral, or vaporized cannabis typically consists of inactive cannabis. Although this may look and taste like cannabis, many participants can distinguish between the intervention and placebo – presumably because the psychoactive properties of the cannabis do not present in the placebo. For example, in a randomized crossover trial, participants enrolled in the treatment arm were given cannabis cigarettes. More than 90% were able to guess their treatment assignment compared to 38% of those who received placebo first. But at crossover more than 90% of those initially in the placebo arm guessed correctly when given the cannabis intervention [47]. Lack of effective blinding has the possibility to produce results overestimating the effectiveness of cannabis [48]. Various ways to reduce this bias have been proposed including use of a psychoactive control that is known to not be an analgesic, recruitment of cannabis-naïve users (less likely to be familiar with the psychoactive effect of cannabis), assessment of blinding during each trial to help with post hoc evaluation of bias, and performance of trials evaluating the non-psychoactive cannabis strains (i.e., high CBD and low THC) [48].

Other imitations to current studies include small sample sizes. A systematic review and met-analysis of 104 studies noted that only about 20% of the included studies had at least 100 subjects per arm and that in some estimates effect sizes were larger for studies having less than 30 participants per treatment arm. Also noted is the short duration of those studies with a median duration of only 8 weeks. Interestingly reductions in pain intensity were highest for 1 day studies and were smaller and non-significant in studies of 13 weeks or longer suggesting the possibility of diminishing analgesia with time [34]. Other limitations in methodology that could be improved include poor recording of cannabinoid dosing (most studies record only a maximum recommended dose as opposed to what the subject actually consumes) as well as studies that evaluate the long-term risks and public health outcomes of currently available cannabis preparations.

Conclusions

The science of cannabis is rapidly evolving with further research anticipated to improve its use in various medical conditions including pain. This will require academic, industry, and governmental support. Research from the ground up is needed including studies on mechanisms of action, evaluation in various pain states (i.e., acute, chronic somatic, chronic neuropathic), dose-response evaluations, cannabinoid combination studies, and long-term health outcomes of chronic medical cannabis use.

With increasing cannabis use for medical reasons throughout the United States, we should take advantage of this massive natural history of experiment with millions enrolled to evaluate effects on pain as well as public health outcomes. Although randomized clinical trials are considered, the gold standard in helping prove causation other studies including observational studies and pragmatic studies can be executed using patients being managed in customary clinical care environments. This would help generate real-world data and information.

Bibliography

1. Lipman AG. Medical cannabis for pain: anecdote or evidence. J Pain Palliat Care Pharmacother. 2017;31(2):96–7.
2. Compton WM, Han B, Jones CM, Blanco C, Hughes A. Marijuana use and use disorders in adults in the USA, 2002-14: analysis of annual cross-sectional surveys. Lancet Psychiatry. 2016;3(10):954–64.
3. Map of Marijuana Legality by State [Internet]. [cited 2020 Jul 5]. Available from: https://disa.com/map-of-marijuana-legality-by-state.
4. D'Souza DC, Ranganathan M. Medical marijuana: is the cart before the horse? JAMA. 2015;313(24):2431–2.
5. Kenny BJ, Zito PM. Controlled substance schedules. In: StatPearls. Treasure Island: StatPearls Publishing; 2020.
6. Kosiba JD, Maisto SA, Ditre JW. Patient-reported use of medical cannabis for pain, anxiety, and depression symptoms: systematic review and meta-analysis. Soc Sci Med. 2019;233:181–92.
7. Khan SP, Pickens TA, Berlau DJ. Perspectives on cannabis as a substitute for opioid analgesics. Pain Manag. 2019;9(2):191–203.
8. Bachhuber MA, Saloner B, Cunningham CO, Barry CL. Medical cannabis laws and opioid analgesic overdose mortality in the United States, 1999–2010. JAMA Intern Med. 2014;174(10):1668–73.
9. Shover CL, Davis CS, Gordon SC, Humphreys K. Association between medical cannabis laws and opioid overdose mortality has reversed over time. Proc Natl Acad Sci U S A. 2019;116(26):12624–6.
10. Touil N, Lavand'homme P. Cannabis hyperalgesia: a phenomenon underestimated in the peri-operative period? Eur J Anaesthesiol. 2019;36(9):623–4.
11. Gan TJ. Poorly controlled postoperative pain: prevalence, consequences, and prevention. J Pain Res. 2017;10:2287–98.
12. Hah JM, Bateman BT, Ratliff J, Curtin C, Sun E. Chronic opioid use after surgery: implications for perioperative management in the face of the opioid epidemic. Anesth Analg. 2017;125(5):1733–40.
13. Wallace M, Schulteis G, Atkinson JH, Wolfson T, Lazzaretto D, Bentley H, et al. Dose-dependent effects of smoked cannabis on capsaicin-induced pain and hyperalgesia in healthy volunteers. Anesthesiology. 2007;107(5):785–96.
14. Stevens AJ, Higgins MD. A systematic review of the analgesic efficacy of cannabinoid medications in the management of acute pain. Acta Anaesthesiol Scand. 2017;61(3):268–80.
15. Gazendam A, Nucci N, Gouveia K, Abdel Khalik H, Rubinger L, Johal H. Cannabinoids in the management of acute Pain: a systematic review and meta-analysis. Cannabis Cannabinoid Res. 2020;5:290–7.
16. Abdallah FW, Hussain N, Weaver T, Brull R. Analgesic efficacy of cannabinoids for acute pain management after surgery: a systematic review and meta-analysis. Reg Anesth Pain Med. 2020;45:509–19.
17. Liu CW, Bhatia A, Buzon-Tan A, Walker S, Ilangomaran D, Kara J, et al. Weeding out the problem: the impact of preoperative cannabinoid use on pain in the perioperative period. Anesth Analg. 2019;129(3):874–81.
18. Salottolo K, Peck L, Tanner Ii A, Carrick MM, Madayag R, McGuire E, et al. The grass is not always greener: a multi-institutional pilot study of marijuana use and acute pain management following traumatic injury. Patient Saf Surg. 2018;12:16.
19. Jamal N, Korman J, Musing M, Malavade A, Coleman BL, Siddiqui N, et al. Effects of pre-operative recreational smoked cannabis use on opioid consumption following inflammatory bowel disease surgery: a historical cohort study. Eur J Anaesthesiol. 2019;36(9):705–6.
20. Echeverria-Villalobos M, Todeschini AB, Stoicea N, Fiorda-Diaz J, Weaver T, Bergese SD. Perioperative care of cannabis users: a comprehensive review of pharmacological and anesthetic considerations. J Clin Anesth. 2019;57:41–9.
21. Nielsen S, Sabioni P, Trigo JM, Ware MA, Betz-Stablein BD, Murnion B, et al. Opioid-sparing effect of cannabinoids: a systematic review and meta-analysis. Neuropsychopharmacology. 2017;42(9):1752–65.
22. Marijuana and Medicine: Assessing the Science Base. Institute of Medicine. 1999. Washington, DC: The National Academies Press. https://doi.org/10.17226/6376.
23. Sim LJ, Selley DE, Xiao R, Childers SR. Differences in G-protein activation by μ- and δ-opioid, and cannabinoid, receptors in rat striatum. Eur J Pharmacol. 1996;307(1):97–105.
24. Boehnke KF, Litinas E, Clauw DJ. Medical cannabis use is associated with decreased opiate medication use in a retrospective cross-sectional survey of patients with chronic pain. J Pain. 2016;17(6):739–44.
25. Lynch ME, Clark AJ. Cannabis reduces opioid dose in the treatment of chronic non-cancer pain. J Pain Symptom Manag. 2003;25(6):496–8.
26. Campbell G, Hall WD, Peacock A, Lintzeris N, Bruno R, Larance B, et al. Effect of cannabis use in people with chronic non-cancer pain prescribed opioids: findings from a 4-year prospective cohort study. Lancet Public Health. 2018;3(7):e341–50.
27. Bonn-Miller MO, ElSohly MA, Loflin MJE, Chandra S, Vandrey R. Cannabis and cannabinoid drug development: evaluating botanical versus single molecule approaches. Int Rev Psychiatry. 2018;30(3):277–84.

28. Cogan PS. The "entourage effect" or "Hodge-Podge Hashish": the questionable rebranding, marketing, and expectations of cannabis polypharmacy. Expert Rev Clin Pharmacol. 2020:1–11.
29. Finlay DB, Sircombe KJ, Nimick M, Jones C, Glass M. Terpenoids from cannabis do not mediate an entourage effect by acting at cannabinoid receptors. Front Pharmacol. 2020;11:359.
30. Carlini EA, Karniol IG, Renault PF, Schuster CR. Effects of marihuana in laboratory animals and in man. Br J Pharmacol. 1974;50(2):299–309.
31. Karniol IG, Shirakawa I, Kasinski N, Pfeferman A, Carlini EA. Cannabidiol interferes with the effects of Δ9-tetrahydrocannabinol in man. Eur J Pharmacol. 1974;28(1):172–7.
32. Santiago M, Sachdev S, Arnold JC, McGregor IS, Connor M. Absence of entourage: terpenoids commonly found in Cannabis sativa do not modulate the functional activity of Δ9-THC at human CB1 and CB2 receptors. Cannabis Cannabinoid Res. 2019;4(3):165–76.
33. Blasco-Benito S, Seijo-Vila M, Caro-Villalobos M, Tundidor I, Andradas C, García-Taboada E, et al. Appraising the "entourage effect": antitumor action of a pure cannabinoid versus a botanical drug preparation in preclinical models of breast cancer. Biochem Pharmacol. 2018;157:285–93.
34. Stockings E, Campbell G, Hall WD, Nielsen S, Zagic D, Rahman R, et al. Cannabis and cannabinoids for the treatment of people with chronic noncancer pain conditions: a systematic review and meta-analysis of controlled and observational studies. Pain. 2018;159(10):1932–54.
35. Meng H, Johnston B, Englesakis M, Moulin DE, Bhatia A. Selective cannabinoids for chronic neuropathic pain: a systematic review and meta-analysis. Anesth Analg. 2017;125(5):1638–52.
36. Cannabis-In-Cachexia-Study-Group, Strasser F, Luftner D, Possinger K, Ernst G, Ruhstaller T, et al. Comparison of orally administered cannabis extract and delta-9-tetrahydrocannabinol in treating patients with cancer-related anorexia-cachexia syndrome: a multicenter, phase III, randomized, double-blind, placebo-controlled clinical trial from the Cannabis-In-Cachexia-Study-Group. J Clin Oncol. 2006;24(21):3394–400.
37. O'Neil ME, Nugent SM, Morasco BJ, Freeman M, Low A, Kondo K, et al. Benefits and harms of plant-based cannabis for posttraumatic stress disorder: a systematic review. Ann Intern Med. 2017;167(5):332–40.
38. Haney M, Gunderson EW, Rabkin J, Hart CL, Vosburg SK, Comer SD, et al. Dronabinol and marijuana in HIV-positive marijuana smokers. Caloric intake, mood, and sleep. J Acquir Immune Defic Syndr. 2007;45(5):545–54.
39. Marcu JP. An overview of major and minor phytocannabinoids. In: Neuropathology of drug addictions and substance misuse: Elsevier; 2016. p. 672–8.
40. Hampson AJ, Bornheim LM, Scanziani M, Yost CS, Gray AT, Hansen BM, et al. Dual effects of anandamide on NMDA receptor-mediated responses and neurotransmission. J Neurochem. 1998;70(2): 671–6.
41. Russo EB, Burnett A, Hall B, Parker KK. Agonistic properties of cannabidiol at 5-HT1a receptors. Neurochem Res. 2005;30(8):1037–43.
42. Ahrens J, Demir R, Leuwer M, de la Roche J, Krampfl K, Foadi N, et al. The nonpsychotropic cannabinoid cannabidiol modulates and directly activates alpha-1 and alpha-1-Beta glycine receptor function. Pharmacology. 2009;83(4):217–22.
43. De Petrocellis L, Ligresti A, Moriello AS, Allarà M, Bisogno T, Petrosino S, et al. Effects of cannabinoids and cannabinoid-enriched Cannabis extracts on TRP channels and endocannabinoid metabolic enzymes. Br J Pharmacol. 2011;163(7):1479–94.
44. Baron EP. Medicinal properties of cannabinoids, terpenes, and flavonoids in cannabis, and benefits in migraine, headache, and pain: an update on current evidence and cannabis science. Headache. 2018;58(7):1139–86.
45. NIH to investigate minor cannabinoids and terpenes for potential pain-relieving properties | National Institutes of Health (NIH) [Internet]. [cited 2020 May 21]. Available from: https://www.nih.gov/news-events/news-releases/nih-investigate-minor-cannabinoids-terpenes-potential-pain-relieving-properties
46. Russo EB. Current therapeutic cannabis controversies and clinical trial design issues. Front Pharmacol. 2016;7:309.
47. Ellis RJ, Toperoff W, Vaida F, van den Brande G, Gonzales J, Gouaux B, et al. Smoked medicinal cannabis for neuropathic pain in HIV: a randomized, crossover clinical trial. Neuropsychopharmacology. 2009;34(3):672–80.
48. Casarett D. The achilles heel of medical cannabis research-inadequate blinding of placebo-controlled trials. JAMA Intern Med. 2018;178(1):9–10.

Index

A
Absorption
  oral, 74
  oro-mucosal and intranasal, 74
  rectal, 75
  smoking, 74
  transcutaneous, 75
Accepted medical use, 10
Acute neurocognitive impairment, 294
  clinical tools and metabolites, 295
Acute nociceptive pain, 208
Acute pain, 327, 328
Adolescence
  medical use of, 282, 283
    anxiety, 283
    treatment resistant epilepsy, 283
  recreational cannabis use and developing brain, 281, 282
  resources for, 283, 284
Alcohol exposure, 263
α-Amino-3-hydroxy-5-methyl-isoxazole propionic acid receptor (AMPAR), 50–51
Amendment 64, 244
Amygdala, 261
Anandamide, 63, 191, 192
  biosynthesis and breakdown pathways, 63, 64
  chemical structure, 63
  endocannabinoid signaling, plasticity of, 66, 67
  endocannabinoids mechanism of action, 66
  pain, endocannabinoids in
    peripheral mechanisms, 67
    spinal mechanisms, 67
    supraspinal mechanisms, 68
Antiepileptic drugs (AEDs), 97
Antiepileptics, cannabis drug interactions, 97
Anxiety
  adolescence, 283
  mental health risks, 275, 276
Anxiety disorder, 182
2-Arachidonoylglycerol (2-AG), 192, 193
  chemical structure, 63
  biosynthesis and breakdown pathways, 65
  endocannabinoid signaling, plasticity of, 66, 67
  endocannabinoids mechanism of action, 66
  pain, endocannabinoids in
    peripheral mechanisms, 67
    spinal mechanisms, 67
    supraspinal mechanisms, 68

B
Barratt Impulsiveness Scale, 265
Biologics, 180
Bipolar disorders, 277
  patient safety, 185
Bonferroni method, 21
Brain development, 259
  context of substances, underage cannabis use in, 260
  early cannabis use, animal models of, 260, 261
  early onset cannabis use, 265, 266
  early onset substance use and subsequent substance disorder, 264
  environment risks, 259, 260
  genetic and physiological, 260
  human evidence
    prenatal cannabis exposure, 261–263
  human study limitations, 266, 267
  measurable brain changes, early cannabis use, 264
  temperamental risks, 259
  younger users, cannabis psychiatric side effects in, 264, 265
  youth cannabis use, epidemiology of, 259
Brain stem rostral ventromedial medulla, 51
Breastfeeding, 289
  patient safety, 185, 186
Buprenorphine, 96
Bupropion, 319

C
Calcineurin inhibitors, 180
Calcitonin gene-related peptide (CGRP), 213
Canadian Students for Sensible Drug Policy (CSSDP), 284
Cancer pain, 208, 211
  cannabinoids, future of, 216
  clinical considerations, 215, 216
  clinical studies, 213–215
  clinical trial, 217–218
  relevant mechanisms of, 212, 213
  survivorship population, cancer survivors, 212

S. N. Narouze (ed.), *Cannabinoids and Pain*, https://doi.org/10.1007/978-3-030-69186-8

Cancer-related pain, nabiximols, 121, 122
Cannabichromene (CBC), 90
Cannabidiol (CBD), 5, 34, 73, 79, 115, 198–200
applied pharmacology and pharmacokinetics, 80, 81
cannabidiol interaction with tetrahydrocannabinol, 83
chemical structure, 80
elimination, 82
and mental health, 276
metabolism, 82
natural cannabis, 157–158
oral, 81
pharmacodynamics of, 80
safety profile and side effects, 82, 83
smoking, 81
transcutaneous, 81, 82
and various clinical effects, 79, 80
volume of distribution, 82
Cannabidiol (Epidiolex), 113
abuse potential, 116
adverse effects, 116
chemical structure of, 114
clinical trials of, 114
dosage and administration, 115
initiation, titration, and monitoring, 115
monitoring, 116
pharmacology and pharmacokinetics, 114, 115
Cannabigerol (CBG), 34, 88, 89
Cannabinoid-based medicines, 33, 154
cannabinoid prescription, barriers for, 146
cannabis use, social stigma for, 145, 146
clinical use of, 145
lack of knowledge, 148, 149
limited medical cannabis education, 149
medical cannabis education programs, development of, 149, 150
myths *vs.*realities, 146–148
natural cannabis, 156
inhalation, 156, 157
oral administration, 157
therapeutic properties of cannabinoids, 157, 158
prescription/pharmaceutical cannabinoids, 154–156
research gaps and limitations, 147, 148
Cannabinoid receptor 1 (CB1), 47–49, 262
distribution, 50
hippocampus, 50
hypothalamic, 51
midbrain periaqueductal gray, brain stem rostral ventromedial medulla, 51
neocortex, 50
ligands, 52
physiology, pathology and pharmacology, 47, 48
signaling, 48, 49
signaling and biased agonism, 50
tolerance, 51, 52
Cannabinoid receptors, 35
Cannabinoid-2 receptor (CB2), 55
chronic pain models, 57, 58
distribution, 56, 57
ligands, 58, 59
modulation of neuronal functions, 55
physiology and pharmacology, 55, 56
signaling, 57
tolerance, 58
Cannabinoid-related adverse effects and impairment, 293, 294
Cannabinoids (CB), 5, 87, 191, 212
algorithm, use of, 232–234
anti-inflammatory action of, 191
endocannabinoids and pain modulation, 192
anandamide and 2-AG synergistic effect, 194, 195
peripheral mechanisms, 192
spinal mechanisms, 192, 194
supraspinal mechanisms, 194
endocannabinoids mechanism of action
2-arachidonoylglycerol, 192, 193
anandamide, 191, 192
endocannabinoids receptors
CB1 receptors, 195, 196
central CB2 receptors, 197
peripheral CB2 receptors, 195, 197
and endocannabinoid system, 88
GPR55, 196–198
minor cannabinoids
cannabichromene, 90
cannabigerol, 88, 89
cannabinol, 88
tetrahydrocannabivarin, 90
TRPV1, 197, 198
Cannabinol (CBN), 34, 88
Cannabis, 3, 31, 33, 212
acceptance and availability of, 7, 231
in acute pain/perioperative pain medicine, 327
cannabinoid-based medicines or treatments, 33
cannabinoids, 130
CBD, 6
chemovars, practical guidance, 133
classification, 132
chemovar, 132
strain, 132
compounds, 131
cultivars, 34
cultivation and trichomes, 129
importance of, 130
education, 179
entourage effect of, 131
guidelines and algorithms, 231
vs. Hemp, 32, 33
mechanisms of action, 327, 328
medical cannabis, 34
medicinal use of, 5
methodology/design of research, 328
National Organization for the Reform of Marijuana Laws, 5
North American cultivation and use, 4
and opioid reduction, 328
origins, 3, 4
pharmaceutical or prescription cannabinoids, 33
preclinical studies, 5
preparations, tinctures, and anointments, 4
prevalence of, 4

products and accessories
concentrates, 35
extracts, 35
historical slang, 35
pipe or bong, 35
vaporizer, 35
prohibition, 4
research, difficulties in, 324, 325
science of, 328
selection for clinicians, 132
state cannabis policies, map of, 6
terpenoids, 130, 131
Cannabis-based medicine (CBM), 325
Cannabis drug interactions
anticoagulants and antiplatelets blood thinners, 98
clopidogrel, 98
direct oral anticoagulants, 98
heparin and fondaparinux, 99
warfarin, 98
antiepileptics, 97
cannabinoids drug interactions, 94
medication, 99
neuropathic agents, 95, 96
opiates, 96, 97
over-the-counter analgesics, 94, 95
psychotropics, 97, 98
routes of administration, 93, 94
Cannabis impairment, clinical application, potential contributors for, 303
Cannabis indica, 32, 129
Cannabis-induced anxiety disorder, 275
Cannabis-induced psychotic disorder, 274
Cannabis-induced sleep disorder, 275
Cannabis intoxication, short-term effects of, 244
Cannabis intoxication syndromes, 293
delirium, 293, 294
intoxication, 293
Cannabis oil dosing, 172–174
Cannabis plant, aspects of, 31, 32
Cannabis ruderalis, 129
Cannabis sativa, 32, 71, 113, 129
Cannabis use disorder (CUD), 272, 273, 318
abuse and dependence, 314
cannabinoids agonists for, 314
cannabis withdrawal, 315
clinical presentation and risk factors, 315
diagnostic and statistical manual of mental disorders, 314
early remission, 314
epidemiology of, 313
loss of control, 314
patient safety, 184
sustained remission, 314
Cannabis withdrawal syndrome (CWS), 274
mechanism of, 318, 319
symptoms and prevalence, 317
treatment of, 319
Cardiovascular disease (CVD), 183
patient safety, 184
Cardiovascular effects, 237, 238
Catechol-O-methyl transferase (COMT) gene, 272
CB1 agonists, 232
CBD-A, 34
Central CB1 receptors, 41, 195–197
Central CB2 receptors, 41, 48, 197
yin-yang relationship of, 60
Centralized pain disorders, 205
Certification of analysis (COA), 250
Cesamet, 111
Chemotherapy, 109
Chemotherapy-induced nausea and vomiting (CINV), 109
Chemovar, 132
Chemovars, practical guidance, 133
Child development
breastfeeding, 289
delivery, cannabis after, 289
epidemiology, 287, 288
pregnancy, cannabis effect during, 287, 289
Chronic adverse effects of cannabis, 296
Chronic induced neuropathic pain (CIPN), 214
Chronic kidney disease, patient safety, 180, 181
Chronic neuropathic pain, 207
Chronic non-cancer pain (CNCP), 205–207, 223
Chronic pain, 326–328
nabiximols, 123, 124
Chronic pain models, CB2, 57, 58
Chronic pain syndromes, 211
Clinical evidence
acute nociceptive pain, 208
cancer pain, 208
chronic neuropathic pain, 207
chronic non-cancer pain, 205–207
fibromyalgia, 207
rheumatoid arthritis, 207, 208
Clobazam, 115
Clopidogrel, 98
Cognitive behavioral therapy (CBT), 320
Cognitive impairment, factors affecting, 296, 297
age, 298
cannabis potency and dose, 301
cannabis products and route of administration, 299
consumption of food, medications/substances, 298
frequency of use and tolerance, 302
genetics, 297
intent, 300
sex, 300
Colorado Department of Public Health and Environment (CDPHE), 243
Colorado experience, 243–245
annual and average monthly sales, 245
health and safety effects, 244
legislative, social, and economic reform, 246
long-term psychological and physiological effects, 246
prohibition, 247
recreational, 244
total taxes, licenses and fees, 246
Colorado Medical Marijuana Enforcement Division (CMED), 243–244
Complete Freund's adjuvant (CFA) model, 57
Comprehensive medical marijuana program, 19

Contract research organization, 137
Controlled Substances Act (CSA), 6, 9
Correlation matrix, 24

D
Delirium, cannabis intoxication syndromes, 293, 294
Delivery, cannabis after, 289
Delta-9-tetrahydrocannabinol (THC), 34, 72, 198
  mechanism of action of, 72, 73
Dependence, 314
Depression, mental health risks, 275, 276
Desensitization, 48, 198
Direct oral anticoagulants, 98
Distribution, phytocannabinoids, 75
Dravet syndrome (DS), 113, 283
Driving, 295, 296
Dronabinol (Marinol®), 105, 156
  drug-drug interactions, 106
  empirical and structural formulas, 105
  mechanism of action, 105
  pharmacokinetics, 106
  safety, toxicity and adverse effects, 106
  therapeutic use, 106
Drug Enforcement Agency (DEA) Schedule, 16, 247
Drug interactions, 238, 239
DSM-5 cannabis-induced mental health disorders
  cannabis-induced anxiety disorder, 275
  cannabis-induced psychotic disorder, 274
  cannabis-induced sleep disorder, 275

E
E-cigarettes, 183, 307
E-cigarette/vaping product use-associated lung injury (EVALI), 308
Elimination
  cannabidiol, 82
  phytocannabinoids, 75
Endocannabinoid system (ECS), 33, 34, 39
  cannabinoids and, 88
  cannabis and hemp, history of, 39, 40
  CB1 and CB2 receptor, 41
  complexity of, 41
  components of, 40
  eCBs and signal transduction pathways, 40, 41
  enzymes, 43
  functions of, 44
  physiological actions of, 43, 44
  signaling and metabolism, 43
  transporters, 43
Endocannabinoids, 35
  and pain modulation, 192
    anandamide and 2-AG synergistic effect, 194, 195
    peripheral mechanisms, 192
    spinal mechanisms, 192, 194
    supraspinal mechanisms, 194
Endocannabinoids receptors
  central CB1 receptors, 195, 196
  central CB2 receptors, 197
  peripheral CB1 receptors, 196
  peripheral CB2 receptors, 195, 197
Endogenous cannabinoids(eCBs), 40–41
Entourage effect, 32, 34, 131, 328, 329
Epidiolex®, 80, 83, 97, 156, 283
Epilepsy, adolescence, 283
Euphoria, 261
E-cigarette or vaping product use-associated lung injury (EVALI), 308
Evil weed, 4

F
Fatty acid amide hydrolase (FAAH), 43
Federal regulations, 9–11
Fibromyalgia, 207
Fondaparinux, 99
Functional selectivity, 57

G
G protein-coupled receptor (CX5), 41
Gabapentin, 95
Gabapentinoids, 96
Gamma radiation, product safety and quality control, 252
  and clinical applications, 255–257
  concentrates and potency, 254, 255
  labelling, 252–254
Genetic predisposition, 272
Good manufacturing processes (GMP), 250
GPR55, 41, 196–198

H
Hemostatic effects, 238
Hemp, 32, 33, 39, 40
Heparin, 99
Himmunocompromised patientsct, 328
Hippocampus, 50
Human brain development, 282
Hypothalamic pro-opiomelanocortin, 51

L
Lennox-Gastaut syndrome (LGS), 113, 283
Ligands
  CB1, 52
  CB2, 58, 59

M
Marijuana, 4
Maternal cannabis, 263
Medical cannabis, 34
  dosing
    cannabis flower dosing, 171, 172
    cannabis oil dosing, 172–174
    cannabis reduction, 174, 175
    concentration and potency, 170, 171
    optimal therapeutic dose and cannabis rotation, 174
  methods of administration, 167, 168
    oral, 169
    oromucosal preparations, 169, 170
    smoking and vaporizing, 167, 169

monitoring, 175, 176
practical recommendations for, 153
topical, 170
treatment algorithm, 177
Medical cannabis clinic, 135
cannabis regulations, 136
comprehensive and multidisciplinary team, 136
continuing medical education, 141
contract research organization and, 137
direct access/self-referral, 137, 138
follow-up and monitoring, 139
initial visit, 138, 139
ongoing development and expansion, 135
patient-centered interventions and prescription, 136
patient education and physician communication, 139, 140
protocols and procedure guidelines, 140, 141
referral, 137
research development, 141, 142
Medical cannabis education, 15
duty and responsibility, 16
knowledge gap, 16
knowledge, risks and effectiveness, 16
lack of preparedness and training, 15
stigma, 16
Medical marijuana, 15
Medical marijuana laws (MCLs), 225
Mental health risks
cannabis withdrawal syndrome, 274
DSM-5 cannabis-induced mental health disorders
cannabis-induced anxiety disorder, 275
cannabis-induced psychotic disorder, 274
cannabis-induced sleep disorder, 275
medical uses of
anxiety and depression, 275, 276
CBD and, 276
post-traumatic stress disorder, 276, 277
psychosis and bipolar disorder, 277
THC and, 276
recreational cannabis and cannabis use disorder, 273
recreational cannabis and psychosis, 271–273
Mesopotamian, 4
Metabolism
cannabidiol, 82
phytocannabinoids, 75
Microglia, 56, 58
Midbrain periaqueductal gray, 51
Monoacylglycerol lipase (MAGL), 43
Morphine, 96, 326
Motivational enhancement therapy (MET), 320
Motor vehicle accidents (MVA), 244
MS-related neuropathic pain, nabiximols, 120, 121
MS-related spasticity, nabiximols, 120, 121
Multidisciplinary team, 136, 142

N

Nabilone (Cesamet®), 109, 154, 233
abuse potential, 111
adverse effects, 111
chemical structures, 109
clinical trials, 110
dosage and administration, 111
drug interactions, 111
pharmacology and pharmacokinetics, 110, 111
Nabiximol, 80, 227, 233
Nabiximols (Sativex®), 74, 119, 156
administration, 124
approval and indications, 120
cancer-related pain, 121, 122
contraindication, 120
dosage form, 125
dosing, 124
for chronic pain, 123–124
for MS-related neuropathic pain, 120, 121
for MS-related spasticity, 120, 121
production, 119
storage and stability, 125
tolerability, 123, 124
N-arachidonoyl-phosphatidylethanolamine (NAPE), 64
National Academies of Sciences, Engineering and Medicine (NASEM), 28
National Organization for the Reform of Marijuana Laws (NORML), 5
Neocortex, 50
Neurokinin 1 (NK-1) antagonists, 110
Neuromaturation, 259
Neuropathic agents, cannabis drug interactions, 95, 96
Neuropathic pain, 57
algorithm, pharmacological management of, 226
Nicotine use disorder (NUD), 264
Nociception, 212
Nonsteroidal anti-inflammatory drugs (NSAID), 95
Nucleus accumbens, 261

O

Opiates, cannabis drug interactions, 96, 97
Opioids, 213, 223, 327
clinical and meta-analytic evidence, 225–227
observational and epidemiological evidence, 224, 225
preclinical evidence, 224
proposed cannabis adjunct initiation trial, 228
reduction, cannabis and, 326
taper, 228
Oral CBD, 81
Oro-mucosal, 74–75
Oromucosal preparations, medical cannabis, 169, 170
Orphan G protein-coupled receptor, 41
Over-the-counter (OTC) analgesics, cannabis drug interactions, 94, 95
Oxycodone, 96

P

Pain physicians and medical cannabis
applied questionnaire, development and description of, 20, 21
attitudes, knowledge and beliefs, 23
correlation matrix, 24, 26
domains of the questionnaire and overall scores, 24
limitations, study, 28
medical cannabis program, participants, 23

Pain physicians and medical cannabis (cont.)
National Academies of Sciences, Engineering and Medicine, 28
participants, demographic and professional characteristics of, 22, 24, 25
participants, scores of, 22
positive association, 24
principal questionnaire domains, 22
recommendation, 26
registration of participants, 25
statistical analysis, 21
survey, 27, 28
Pain, endocannabinoids in
peripheral mechanisms, 67
spinal mechanisms, 67
supraspinal mechanisms, 68
Patient education, medical cannabis clinic, 139, 140
Patient safety, 179
calcineurin inhibitors, protein disulfide isomerase inhibitors, and biologics, 180
cannabis use disorder, 184
cannabis use, practical considerations for, 179
cardiovascular disease, 185
chronic kidney disease, 180, 181
immunocompromised patients, 180
individuals under age of 25, 184
older adults and patients, 181
polypharmacy and drug interactions, 181, 182
potential cannabinoid drug interactions, 182
precautions
cardiovascular disease, 183
concurrent active mood or anxiety disorder, 182, 183
E cigarette use, 183
sedation or cognitive impairment, 183
tobacco use, 183
pregnancy and breastfeeding, 186
psychosis and bipolar disorders, 185
respiratory disease, 184, 185
substance use disorder and consideration for harm reduction, 184
Pepcan-12, 61
Perioperative management
cardiovascular effects, 237, 238
drug interactions, 238, 239
evaluation, 239
hemostatic effects, 238
pulmonary effects, 237
temperature regulation, 238
Peripheral CB1 receptors, 196–197
Peripheral CB2 receptors, 197
Peroxisome proliferator-activated receptors (PPARs), 41
Pertussis toxin, 55
Pest control products act (PCPA), 252
Pesticides, 250–252
product safety and quality control, 251, 252
Pharmaceutical cannabinoids, 154
Pharmaceutical/prescription cannabinoids, 33
Phytocannabinoids, 34, 71
absorption
oral, 74
oro-mucosal and intranasal, 74
rectal, 75
smoking, 74
transcutaneous, 75
active and inactive forms of, 71
applied pharmacology and pharmacokinetics, 73
biosynthesis of, 87
cannabidiol, 198, 199
Δ9-tetrahydrocannabinol, 198
distribution, 75
metabolism and elimination, 74, 75
pain modulation, mechanisms of action in
CBD, 199, 200
THC, 199, 200
THC, 72
mechanism of action of, 72, 73
Polypharmacy, 181, 182
Post-traumatic stress disorder (PTSD), 276, 277
Practical recommendations, medical cannabis
cannabinoid-based medicines, 154
clinical evidence, 159
natural cannabis, 156–158
prescription of, 158, 159
prescription/pharmaceutical cannabinoids, 154–156
systematic approach, 159–160
history of previous cannabis use, 160
medical document or prescription, 161
medical history, 160
pharmacological and non-pharmacological treatments, 160
precautions and/or contraindications, 160, 161
side effects and follow-up visits, 162
treatment objectives and manage expectations, 161
treatment plan, 161
Preclinical evidence, opioids, 224
Pregabalin, 95
Pregnancy
cannabis effect during, 287, 289
patient safety, 185, 186
Prenatal cannabis exposure, 261–263
Prescription/pharmaceutical cannabinoids, 154–156
Product safety and quality control
and clinical applications, 255–257
concentrates and potency, 254, 255
contaminant, 250, 251
gamma radiation, 252
labelling, 252–254
microorganisms, 251
"natural" medicine, cannabis as, 249
pesticides, 251, 252
standardization and, 249, 250
Pro-opiomelanocortin (POMC), 51
Protein disulfide isomerase (PD1) inhibitors, 180

Psychosis, 271–273, 277
  patient safety, 185
Psychotropics
  cannabis drug interactions, 97, 98
Pulmonary effects, 237

R
Radiation, 212
Recreational cannabis, 271–273
  adolescence
    and developing brain, 281, 282
  and cannabis use disorder, 273
Regulations, cannabis, 9
  federal regulations, 9–11
  research expansion, 12, 13
  state cannabis laws, 11, 12
Respiratory disease, patient safety, 184, 185
Rheumatoid arthritis, 207, 208

S
Safety sensitive activities, 295, 296
Sativex, 207
Sedation/cognitive impairment, patient safety, 183
Serotonin-norepinephrine reuptake inhibitors (SNRIs), 319
Serotonin reuptake inhibitors (SSRIs), 319
Signal transduction pathways, 40–41
Smoking, 74
  cannabidiol, 81
Social anxiety disorder (SAD), 276
State cannabis laws, 11, 12
Statistical analysis, medical cannabis, 21
Strain, 132
Substance P, 110
Substance use disorder (SUD), 264
  patient safety, 184

T
Temperature regulation, 238
Terpenes, 34
Terpenoids, 130, 131
Tetrahydrocannabinol, 75
  cannabidiol interaction with, 83
Tetrahydrocannabinol (THC), 5, 199, 200, 237
  and mental health, 276
  natural cannabis, 157–158
Tetrahydrocannabivarin (THCV)
  cannabinoids, 90
Tolerance, CB2, 58
Transcutaneous CBD, 81, 82
Trichomes, 129–130
  importance of, 130
TRPV1, 197, 198

U
Ultra-high risk (UHR) of psychosis, 272
Upper limit of normal (ULN), 116

V
Vaping, 307
  lungs, effect of, 305–307
    clinical course, 310
    laboratory findings, 308
    marijuana, 310
    pathological findings, 310
    patient presentation, 308
Vaporization, 74, 81, 185

W
Warfarin, 98
Women, marijuana use among, 288